Practical Management of Thyroid Cancer

Ujjal K. Mallick · Clive Harmer
Ernest L. Mazzaferri · Pat Kendall-Taylor
Editors

Practical Management of Thyroid Cancer

A Multidisciplinary Approach

Second Edition

Springer

Editors
Ujjal K. Mallick
Consultant (Hon)
Northern Centre for Cancer Care
Freeman Hospital
Newcastle upon Tyne
United Kingdom

Ernest L. Mazzaferri†

Clive Harmer
London
United Kingdom

Pat Kendall-Taylor
Newcastle upon Tyne
United Kingdom

ISBN 978-3-030-06285-9 ISBN 978-3-319-91725-2 (eBook)
https://doi.org/10.1007/978-3-319-91725-2

1st edition: Springer-Verlag London Limited 2006

Softcover re-print of the Hardcover 2nd edition 2018

This Springer imprint is published by the registered company Springer Nature Switzerland AG
The registered company address is: Gewerbestrasse 11, 6330 Cham, Switzerland

This edition is dedicated to all who happened to have had Thyroid Cancer, hoping it might provide some incremental benefit and support.

Preface

"Think globally, act locally" is a contemporary maxim with wide implications for many fields including medicine. In our increasingly connected world, knowledge is constantly flowing across national boundaries. This book is a collective endeavour to facilitate access to cutting-edge internationally approved thyroid cancer treatment recommendations and its evidential basis. Written by world authorities from many countries, this edition, like the previous one, is also directed at a global readership.

The foundation of contemporary thyroid cancer management, and especially its areas of controversy, rests upon sound clinical judgement. Well-informed clinician/patient shared decision-making is mandatory. We hope the practical management information detailed in this book, adapted to local needs and resources, will help optimisation of this process.

First published in 2006, this book was conceived at a thyroid cancer conference in Newcastle. Significant and dramatic advances since then have demanded the need for publication of this second edition.

Newcastle upon Tyne, UK — Ujjal K. Mallick
London, UK — Clive Harmer

Contents

Contributors

Nicola Jane Armstrong The Newcastle upon Tyne Hospitals, NHS Foundation Trust, Freeman Hospital, Newcastle upon Tyne, UK

Thomas C. Beadnell Endocrinology, Metabolism and Diabetes, University of Colorado, Aurora, CO, USA

A. Berdelou Gustave Roussy, Villejuif, France

R. D. Bliss The Newcastle upon Tyne Hospitals, NHS Foundation Trust, Newcastle upon Tyne, UK

James D. Brierley Department of Radiation Oncology, Princess Margaret Cancer Centre, University of Toronto, Toronto, ON, Canada

Maria E. Cabanillas Department of Endocrine Neoplasia and Hormonal Disorders, University of Texas MD Anderson Cancer Center, Houston, TX, USA

Nadine R. Caron Department of Surgery, University of British Columbia, Prince George, BC, Canada

John D. Casler Department of Otorhinolaryngology—Head and Neck Surgery, Mayo Clinic, Jacksonville, FL, USA

Maria Grazia Castagna Department of Medical, Surgical and Neurological Sciences, University of Siena, Siena, Italy

Orlo H. Clark Department of Surgery, University of California, San Francisco, San Francisco, CA, USA

Mary Comiskey Palliative Medicine, The Newcastle upon Tyne Hospitals NHS Foundation Trust, Newcastle-upon-Tyne, UK

Gilbert Cote Department of Endocrine Neoplasia and Hormonal Disorders, University of Texas MD Anderson Cancer Center, Houston, TX, USA

Ramona Dadu Department of Endocrine Neoplasia and Hormonal Disorders, University of Texas MD Anderson Cancer Center, Houston, TX, USA

Rossella Elisei Endocrine Unit, Department of Clinical and Experimental Medicine, University Hospital of Pisa, Pisa, Italy

K. A. Farnell Butterfly Thyroid Cancer Trust, Tyne and Wear, UK

Shireen Fatemi Kaiser Permanente, Panorama City, CA, USA

Sudheer Kumar Gara Endocrine Oncology Branch, National Cancer Institute, National Institutes of Health, Bethesda, MD, USA

Sana A. Ghaznavi Department of Medicine, Memorial Sloan Kettering Cancer Center, New York, NY, USA

Meredith E. Giuliani Department of Radiation Oncology, Princess Margaret Cancer Centre, University of Toronto, Toronto, ON, Canada

Heribert Hänscheid Department of Nuclear Medicine, University Hospital Würzburg, Würzburg, Germany

Eun Ju Ha Department of Radiology, Ajou University School of Medicine, Suwon, South Korea

Allan Hackshaw Cancer Research UK and UCL Cancer Trials Centre, University College London, London, UK

Clive Harmer Previously Head of Thyroid Unit, Department of Radiotherapy, Royal Marsden Hospital, London, UK

Bryan R. Haugen Division of Endocrinology, Metabolism, and Diabetes, Department of Medicine, University of Colorado Cancer Center, University of Colorado Health Sciences Center, Denver, CO, USA

Marie Claude Hofmann Department of Endocrine Neoplasia and Hormonal Disorders, University of Texas MD Anderson Cancer Center, Houston, TX, USA

Hiro Ishii Department of Head and Neck, ENT Surgery, St. George's Hospital, London, UK

Yasuhiro Ito Department of Surgery, Kuma Hospital, Kobe, Japan

Sarah J. Johnson Department of Pathology, Royal Victoria Infirmary, Newcastle upon Tyne Hospitals, NHS Foundation Trust, Newcastle upon Tyne, UK

A.I. Kaleva Ipswich Hospital NHS Trust, Ipswich, UK

Dipti Kamani Division of Thyroid and Parathyroid Endocrine Surgery, Department of Otolaryngology – Head and Neck Surgery, Massachusetts Eye and Ear Infirmary, Harvard Medical School, Boston, MA, USA

Electron Kebebew Endocrine Oncology Branch, National Cancer Institute, National Institutes of Health, Bethesda, MD, USA

Department of Surgery, The George Washington University School of Medicine and Health Sciences, Washington, DC, USA

Katherine Kendell The Newcastle upon Tyne Hospitals, NHS Foundation Trust, Freeman Hospital, Newcastle upon Tyne, UK

Ji-hoon Kim Department of Radiology, Seoul National University Hospital, Seoul National University College of Medicine, Seoul, South Korea

Dae S. Kim Department of Head and Neck, ENT Surgery, St. George's Hospital, London, UK

Joanna Klubo-Gwiezdzinska Metabolic Disease Branch, National Institute of Diabetes and Digestive and Kidney Diseases, National Institutes of Health, Bethesda, MD, USA

Yevgenia Kushchayeva Diabetes, Obesity and Endocrinology Branch, National Institute of Diabetes and Digestive and Kidney Diseases, National Institutes of Health, Bethesda, MD, USA

Michael Lassmann Department of Nuclear Medicine, University Hospital Würzburg, Würzburg, Germany

S. Leboulleux Gustave Roussy, Villejuif, France

Markus Luster Department of Nuclear Medicine, University Hospital Marburg, Marburg, Germany

Ujjal K. Mallick Chief Investigator UK National "IoN" and HiLo Trials, Past clinical oncologist and Chair Regional Thyroid MDT, Northern Centre for Cancer Care, Freeman Hospital, Newcastle upon Tyne, United Kingdom

Claudio Marcocci Department of Clinical and Experimental Medicine, University of Pisa, Endocrine Unit 2, University Hospital of Pisa, Pisa, Italy

Antonio Matrone Endocrine Unit, Department of Clinical and Experimental Medicine, University Hospital of Pisa, Pisa, Italy

Michael E. Menefee Department of Internal Medicine, Division of Hematology and Oncology, Mayo Clinic, Jacksonville, FL, USA

Akira Miyauchi Department of Surgery, Kuma Hospital, Kobe, Japan

Dong Gyu Na Department of Radiology, GangNeung Asan Hospital, Gangneung-si, Gangwon-do, South Korea

I.J. Nixon NHS Lothian, Edinburgh, UK

Furio Pacini Department of Medical, Surgical and Neurological Sciences, University of Siena, Siena, Italy

Maria G. Pavlatou Department of Endocrinology, Royal Victoria Infirmary, Newcastle upon Tyne Hospitals, NHS Foundation Trust, Newcastle upon Tyne, UK

Petros Perros Department of Endocrinology, Royal Victoria Infirmary, Newcastle upon Tyne Hospitals, NHS Foundation Trust, Newcastle upon Tyne, UK

Fabián Pitoia Division of Endocrinology, Hospital de Clínicas, University of Buenos Aires, Buenos Aires, Argentina

David N. Poller Department of Pathology, University of Portsmouth, Portsmouth, UK

Queen Alexandra Hospital, Portsmouth, UK

Gregory W. Randolph Division of Thyroid and Parathyroid Endocrine Surgery, Department of Otolaryngology – Head and Neck Surgery, Massachusetts Eye and Ear Infirmary, Harvard Medical School, Boston, MA, USA

Thyroid Surgery Oncology, Harvard Medical School, Boston, MA, USA

Department of Surgery, Endocrine Surgery Service, Massachusetts General Hospital, Boston, MA, USA

Sara L. Richer Northeast Medical Group, Yale New Haven Health, New Haven, CT, USA

M. Schlumberger Gustave Roussy, Villejuif, France

Rebecca E. Schweppe Endocrinology, Metabolism and Diabetes, University of Colorado, Aurora, CO, USA

A.R. Shaha Memorial Sloan Kettering Cancer Center, New York, NY, USA

Robert C. Smallridge Department of Internal Medicine, Division of Endocrinology and Metabolism, Mayo Clinic, Jacksonville, FL, USA

Carole Spencer University of Southern California, USC Endocrine Laboratory, Pasadena, CA, USA

Cord Sturgeon Department of Surgery, Section of Endocrine Surgery, Northwestern University, Chicago, IL, USA

R. Michael Tuttle Department of Medicine, Memorial Sloan Kettering Cancer Center, New York, NY, USA

Steven G. Waguespack Department of Endocrine Neoplasia and Hormonal Disorders, University of Texas MD Anderson Cancer Center, Houston, TX, USA

Tracy S. Wang Department of Surgery, Section of Endocrine Surgery, Medical College of Wisconsin, Milwaukee, WI, USA

Jonathan D. Wasserman Division of Endocrinology, Hospital for Sick Children, University of Toronto, Toronto, ON, Canada

John C. Watkinson Department of Ear, Nose and Throat (ENT) Surgery, University Hospitals Birmingham NHS Foundation Trust, Queen Elizabeth Hospital Birmingham, Birmingham, UK

1 Pragmatism, Personalised Oncology, International Partnership for Research and Quality: The New Paradigm for Thyroid Cancer

Ujjal K. Mallick and Clive Harmer

"Nothing truly valuable can be achieved except by the unselfish co-operation of many individuals. … The best way to serve the cause of internationalism is by co-operating in some life -giving work"—Einstein.

Curing cancer and particularly thyroid cancer may not have to be a Panglossian dream anymore [1]. The advances in clinical, basic and translational research, faster transfer of discoveries from the bench to the bedside, better orgnanisation of patient centered national cancer services, and multicenter international trials are making incremental transformational changes in the cancer landscape [2–10].

Mandatory specialist multidisciplinary team approach to diagnosis and therapy, initial and dynamic risk assessment, pragmatic guideline based risk adapted treatment involving surveillance, surgery, radioiodine, patient -doctor shared individualised treatment plan, new tissue and blood biomarkers, next generation sequencing and detailed genetic analysis of individual tumours, precision oncology, and immune checkpoint inhibition specially for resistant tumours, multicenter national and international concerted effort for clinical trials addressing the unresolved issues in management, translational research and guideline implementation, patient doctor partnership, quality survivorship programmes, cost-effective risk based long term follow up, and specialist palliative care are all central to the contemporary management of thyroid cancer. Against this background the book has been designed with each of the chapters being written by leading international authorities on the subject hoping to help improve the outcome of thyroid cancer patients.

The vision of effective cancer management in all countries has a common theme of improving quality and consequently the outcome. The NHS UK Cancer management strategy document specifies that all high quality treatments should be effective, safe, efficient, offered early in a timely fashion, have patient focus and equity of access and delivered by the right workforce with the right competences in right numbers in place; this is similar in essence to the aim of the Institute of Medicine's (IOM) quality initiative, the statement - "the right patient should have the right treatment at the right time, every time" and the vision of the American Society of Clinical Oncologists (ASCO, https://www.asco.org/) [11–13].

U. K. Mallick (✉)
Chief Investigator UK National "IoN" and HiLo Trials, Past clinical oncologist and Chair Regional Thyroid MDT, Northern Centre for Cancer Care, Freeman Hospital, Newcastle upon Tyne, United Kingdom
e-mail: Ujjal.mallick@nuth.nhs.uk

C. Harmer
Previously Head of Thyroid Unit, Department of Radiotherapy, Royal Marsden Hospital, London, UK

U. K. Mallick et al. (eds.), *Practical Management of Thyroid Cancer*,
https://doi.org/10.1007/978-3-319-91725-2_1

This book written by internationally recognised thyroid cancer experts, is one small collaborative effort to follow precisely that common goal across geographic boundaries. It is a compilation of their collective wisdom detailing the state of the art practical management of thyroid cancer focusing on the many areas of existing controversy surrounding key aspects of management. Its aim, like the first edition, is to provide valuable and updated information for the "core" and "extended" members of the thyroid cancer multi disciplinary team (MDT) as well as to non specialist clinicians and trainees wherever they might be practising.

In these days of rapidly expanding sphere of scientific discovery it is hard for practising professionals to keep up to date in their field of expertise as well as to keep abreast with the recent developments and wider horizons of knowledge in that field. It is our fervent hope that it will be of some assistance to them, adapted to the local needs and priorities, regardless of geographic boundaries. This might help serving their patients on a day to day basis, with optimal and high quality care embedded in the principles of up to date evidence based guideline recommendations to improve their outcome in a small way.

We also hope that it will be of interest to patients or families with thyroid cancer by acting as a reliable resource book written by international experts enabling them to take part in a more informed shared decision making process. A special feature of the book is a chapter authored by a patient about her remarkable personal cancer journey providing valuable information for patients and her outstanding contributions to thyroid cancer patient support.

Unfortunately our friend and respected colleague Late Professor Ernie Mazzaferri, a giant in the field of thyroid cancer, whose pioneering work lit the way to the achievements of modern thyroid cancer management to the fabric of which his clinical research contributed so much, is sadly no longer with us. It was our great honour and pleasure to have had the opportunity to collaborate for the first edition of this book with Ernie focusing on the "Practical Patient- Centered Multi-Disciplinary" approach. It is also a big privilege and a great delight to collaborate with so many colleagues from different countries and to be able to put together the second edition of the book, trying to maintain the same approach at its core.

As in the first edition this project is the product of a phenomenal amount of self-less, hard work and kindness of colleagues who despite their busy professional schedules have taken precious time to take part and make contributions of the highest quality. Also without the keen interest, enthusiasm, tremendous support, hard work and high level of professionalism by Evgenia Koutsouki, Rekha Udaiyar, Saranya Sargunan and colleagues on behalf of Springer this book would not have seen the light of day. If the book is successful in its aim of helping our patients and colleagues in a small way it is because of their efforts.

The editors take this opportunity to extend their most grateful thanks to all who have contributed towards this collaborative attempt aiming to improve the outcome of our thyroid cancer patients wherever they might be.

Our grateful thanks go to our wives and family as well for their support and understanding during the preparation of this book.

References

1. Voltaire A, Cameron N. Candide (penguin popular classics) (translator - Norman Cameron). London: Penguin Books; 2007.
2. Burstein HJ, Krilov L, Aragon-Ching JB, Baxter NN, Gabriela Chiorean E, et al. Clinical cancer advances 2017: annual report on progress against cancer from the American Society of Clinical Oncology. J Clin Oncol. 2017;35(12):1341–67.
3. Lowy DR, Collins FS. Aiming high — changing the trajectory for cancer. N Engl J Med. 2016;374:1901–4.
4. Lancet. Launching a plan for the cancer moonshot. Lancet. 2016;388(10050):1130.
5. Perros P, Boelaert K, Colley S, Evans C, Evans RM, Gerrard Ba G, Gilbert J, Harrison B, Johnson SJ, Giles TE, Moss L, Lewington V, Newbold K, Taylor J, Thakker RV, Watkinson J, Williams GR, British Thyroid Association. Guidelines for the management of thyroid cancer. Clin Endocrinol. 2014;81(Suppl 1):1–122.
6. Haugen BR, Alexander EK, Bible KC, Doherty GM, Mandel SJ, Nikiforov YE, Pacini F, Randolph GW, Sawka AM, Schlumberger M, Schuff KG, Sherman SI, Sosa JA, Steward DL, Tuttle RM, Wartofsky L. American Thyroid Association management

guidelines for adult patients with thyroid nodules and differentiated thyroid cancer: the American Thyroid Association guidelines task force on thyroid nodules and differentiated thyroid cancer. Thyroid. 2016;26(1):1–133.
7. Cabanillas ME, McFadden DG, Durante C. Thyroid cancer. Lancet. 2016;388(10061):2783–95.
8. Fagin JA, Wells SA Jr. Biologic and clinical perspectives on thyroid cancer. N Engl J Med. 2016;375:1054–67.
9. Cancer Genome Atlas Research Network. Integrated genomic characterization of papillary thyroid carcinoma. Cell. 2014;159(3):676–90.
10. Bertagnolli MM, Sartor O, Chabner BA, Rothenberg ML, Khozin S, Hugh-Jones C, Reese DM, Murphy MJ. Advantages of a truly open-access data-sharing model. N Engl J Med. 2017;376:1178–81.
11. Achieving world-class cancer outcomes: taking the strategy forward. May 2016. https://www.england.nhs.uk/wp-content/uploads/2016/05/cancer-strategy.pdf.
12. Institute of Medicine (US) Committee on Quality of Health Care in America. Crossing the quality chasm: a new health system for the 21st century. Washington (DC): National Academies Press (US); 2001.
13. Clancy C. Healthcare quality and who decides? March 2009. www.hhs.gov/asl/testify/2009/03/3716.html.

Part I

Multidisciplinary Approach to Management of Thyroid Cancer

2 The UK Evidence-Based Guidelines for the Management of Thyroid Cancer: Key Recommendations

Maria G. Pavlatou, Sarah J. Johnson, and Petros Perros

Introduction

Towards the end of the last millennium a group of thyroid cancer experts, motivated by an obvious and random variance in clinical practice and poor published survival figures [1], drafted the first UK based guidance for managing patients with thyroid cancer [2]. It was followed by a formal national guideline embraced by professional bodies, first published in 2002 [3]. Updates were produced in 2007 [4] and 2014 [5]. Although the guidelines became more voluminous, and the number of recommendations expanded, the shift in the strength of evidence was modest, most still remaining expert opinions. As scientific evidence accumulated, the guidelines moved to an evidence-based consensus. A notable trend in the UK guidelines has been increasing focus towards a more individualized approach and less aggressive treatments for indolent tumors, which reflects the evolution of evidence over the past 15 years. One further characteristic of the UK guidelines is an appreciation of the existence of many areas of uncertainty and the use of shared decision making as an appropriate tool for tackling this common and difficult area [6]. Here, we review the most important key recommendations of the latest edition of the UK British Thyroid Association (BTA) guidelines, focusing on differentiated thyroid cancer (DTC), which compromises the vast majority of all thyroid cancers.

Multidisciplinary Management and Personalized Decision Making

The 2014 BTA guidelines emphasize and define the role of multidisciplinary teams (MDT). Multidisciplinary management of thyroid cancer has been practiced by many major centers for years and is generally accepted by clinicians to be a valuable model for reaching consensus. The MDTs should consist of an endocrinologist, a surgeon, and an oncologist or a nuclear medicine physician with support from a pathologist, a radiologist, and a specialist nurse, all with expertise and interest in thyroid cancer management. The teams should meet regularly and discuss all patients who have newly diagnosed or recurrent or persistent thyroid cancer. This approach ensures accurate and immediate care of patients, minimizing anxiety and misdiagnoses. The evidence, however, that this approach leads to better patient outcomes is lacking (reflected in the low grade of recommendation in the BTA guidelines), and it is demanding on clinicians' time and therefore costly. In the UK, MDTs are mandatory

M. G. Pavlatou (✉) · P. Perros
Department of Endocrinology, Royal Victoria Infirmary, Newcastle upon Tyne Hospitals, NHS Foundation Trust, Newcastle upon Tyne, UK

S. J. Johnson
Department of Pathology, Royal Victoria Infirmary, Newcastle upon Tyne Hospitals, NHS Foundation Trust, Newcastle upon Tyne, UK

U. K. Mallick et al. (eds.), *Practical Management of Thyroid Cancer*,
https://doi.org/10.1007/978-3-319-91725-2_2

in managing cancers and have become an integral part of the National Health Service. A key component of the multidisciplinary management of thyroid cancer is personalized decision making which involves individualization of management based on consideration of individual risk factors, comorbidities, clinical and cyto-or histo-pathological parameters as well as personal circumstances.

Ultrasound for Initial Assessment of Thyroid Nodules

High-resolution ultrasound (US) is an extremely sensitive tool for detection and characterization of thyroid nodules [7]. The current guidelines emphasize the use of US for initial assessment and risk stratification of thyroid nodules. As soon as a nodule is discovered or suspected, a thyroid US should be employed to determine the nature of the nodule and to decide whether or not a fine needle aspiration (FNA) should be performed. With the use of US increasing over the years, it has contributed to an epidemic of over-diagnosis of low risk incidental thyroid cancer [8, 9]. On the other hand, if the thyroid US is performed by an expert, it can, most of the time, accurately define the risk of thyroid cancer and determine the need for proceeding to FNA, minimizing the number of unnecessary and costly investigations and procedures that can follow overdiagnosis, increasing patient's anxiety and waiting times [10]. The BTA guidelines recommend a scoring system based on TIRADS [11], which divides US findings into five (U1–U5) categories with increasing risk of malignancy. As Tables 2.1 and 2.2 describe, nodules with benign features can be regarded as reassuring and not normally requiring FNA [12–14]. Nodules categorized as U3, U4 and U5 should undergo FNA for cytology diagnosis. A raised U score can also direct to repeating cytology after an initial benign FNA. Moreover, the BTA guidelines suggest that when reported by an expert sonographer and following the above classification system, size of nodule alone is not a criterion that mandates FNA. This recommendation is based on a body of literature pointing towards nodule size by itself being a poor predictor of malignancy [15–18].

Table 2.1 Ultrasound features indicative of benign and malignant nodule

US features indicative of benign nodule
Spongiform or honeycomb appearance (micro-cystic spaces with thin walls, comprising >50% of the nodule)
Purely cystic nodule and nodules with a cystic component containing colloid (hyper-echoic foci with a 'ring-down' sign)
Egg shell type calcification around the periphery of a nodule
Iso-echoic or (mildly) hyper-echoic in relation to the surrounding normal thyroid tissue and typically with a surrounding hypo-echoic halo
Peripheral vascularity on colour flow or power Doppler

US features indicative of malignant nodule
Papillary and medullary cancers:
A solid hypo-echoic (i.e. hypo-echoic relative to the normal thyroid tissue) nodule, which may contain hyper-echoic foci (i.e. micro-calcification)
An irregular margin, intra nodular vascularity and absence of an associated halo
A 'taller than wide' shape referring to anterior/posterior (AP) > transverse (TR) diameter when imaged in the axial plane. AP diameter > TR diameter increasing the likelihood of malignancy
An irregular or spiculated margin and a 'taller than wide' shape have both been shown to have good positive predictive value for malignant nodules
Egg shell type calcification around the periphery of a nodule with a broken calcified rim where there is extension beyond the calcified rim of a hypo-echoic mass
Follicular lesions:
Typically hyper-echoic and homogenous in echo texture with a well-defined halo
Hypo-echogenicity and loss of the associated halo-associated with carcinoma

US ultrasound, *AP* anterior/posterior diameter

Table 2.2 Thyroid nodules-ultrasound (U) classification

U1. Normal:	
U2. Benign:	(a) Halo, iso-echoic/mildly hyper-echoic (b) Cystic change ± ring down sign (colloid) (c) Micro-cystic/spongiform (d & e) peripheral egg shell calcification (f) Peripheral vascularity
U3. Indeterminate/ equivocal:	(a) Homogenous, hyper-echoic (markedly), solid, halo (follicular lesion) (b) Hypo-echoic, equivocal echogenic foci, cystic change (c) Mixed/central vascularity
U4. Suspicious:	(a) Solid, hypo-echoic (cf thyroid) (b) Solid, very hypo-echoic (cf strap muscle) (c) Disrupted peripheral calcification, hypo-echoic (d) Lobulated outline
U5. Malignant:	(a) Solid, hypo-echoic, lobulated/irregular outline, micro-calcification (papillary carcinoma) (b) Solid, hypo-echoic, lobulated/irregular outline, globular calcification (medullary carcinoma) (c) Intra-nodular vascularity (d) Shape (taller > wide) (AP > TR) (e) Characteristic associated lymphadenopathy

AP anterior/posterior diameter, *TR* transverse diameter

Cytology of Thyroid FNAs and Histology of Thyroid Cancer

The cytology of thyroid FNA samples should be reported by cytopathologists with experience in these samples and with access to colleagues with additional experience for second opinions. Reporting should follow the Royal College of Pathologists Guidance, updated in 2016 [19], and should contain a descriptive prose section and a Thy numerical category. The Thy categories align well with the categories in The Bethesda System and other international reporting systems [19, 20]. Interpretation of thyroid cytology can be difficult and subjective, especially in the atypical categories, and central review increases accuracy [21, 22]. Local audit of correlation with subsequent histology is important [23]. It is anticipated that at least the suspicious and diagnostically malignant cases are discussed in an MDT meeting. The role of molecular testing to refine cytological diagnosis is an important development and is further discussed elsewhere in this book (Chap. 5). Similarly, histo-pathologists reporting thyroid cancer should have a special interest in this field and also access to further expertise for second opinion. Reporting should follow the current dataset from The Royal College of Pathologists [24], and reports should clearly state the tumour type; the features required to allocate risk such as extra-thyroidal extension, vascular invasion and margin status; and give the pathological TNM staging. New thyroid cancer entities are being defined [25] and it is important that these are understood and recognized, including the recent reclassification of a subset of non-invasive encapsulated follicular variant of papillary thyroid carcinoma as non-invasive follicular thyroid neoplasm with papillary-like nuclei (NIFTP) [26]. New changes include the publication in December 2016 of the eighth edition of TNM staging, which does include changes for thyroid cancer [27]; in the UK, the Royal College of Pathologists has advised that reports clearly state which edition of UICC TNM is being used and that TNM8 is addressed in revisions to cancer datasets, for use from 2018. Eagerly anticipated is the publication later in 2017 of the revised WHO Classification of Tumours of the Thyroid Gland, following which the Royal College of Pathologists will revise the thyroid cancer histology reporting dataset.

Less Aggressive Surgery for Less Aggressive Tumors

Recommendations for the extent of surgery for biopsy proven DTC are significantly different from previous editions. A total thyroidectomy was previously recommended for nearly all DTCs >1 cm, independent of the presence or not of loco-regional or distant metastases or additional risk factors. The current guidelines recommend a less aggressive initial therapeutic surgery for thyroid cancers smaller than 4 cm and no other risk factors. For carefully selected patients with unifocal DTC >1 cm and <4 cm without extra-thyroidal extension (T1b-T2) and no clinical evidence of lymph node metastases (cN0), the initial procedure may be either a bilateral procedure (near total or total thyroidectomy) or a unilateral procedure (lobectomy). This is based on retrospective studies showing that when patients are properly selected, survival, recurrence rates and overall prognosis are similar between lobectomy and total thyroidectomy ([28–32]). Individual patient characteristics that include age over 45 years old, thyroid nodules in the contralateral lobe, history of radiation exposure to the head or neck, a family history of DTC, and patient choice, tip the balance in favor of total thyroidectomy. A new chapter discusses papillary thyroid micro-carcinomas and thyroid lobectomy is also recommended for papillary micro-carcinoma (<1 cm), which is unifocal, intrathyroidal, has no clinically detectable cervical nodal metastases (cN0) or extra-thyroidal extension and no other risk factors.

Post-operative Risk Stratification, Use of Radioiodine Remnant Ablation or Therapy and Degree of Initial TSH Suppression

After surgery, it is important to assess the risk of death, and of recurrence, and the overall prognosis, using scoring and prognostic systems to tailor treatment to the individual so as to minimize the risk of death and recurrence, but also to avoid unnecessary therapies, which may impact quality of life. The TNM staging (from histological examination of the excised tumour) predicts the risk of death, not the risk of recurrence, and does not take into account the response to treatment, which may affect prognosis. The post-operative risk stratification system for risk of recurrence of DTC proposed by the current BTA guidelines is based on the 2009 American Thyroid Association guidelines stratification system [33] which divides patients as having low, intermediate, or high risk of recurrence/persistence (Table 2.3). This system can identify those patients who should and should not undergo radioiodine remnant ablation (RRA). Current evidence suggests

Table 2.3 Post-operative risk stratification for risk of recurrence of DTC (adapted from ATA)

Low-risk patients have the following characteristics:
No local or distant metastases
All macroscopic tumour has been resected i.e. R0 or R1 resection (pathological definition)
No tumour invasion of loco-regional tissues or structures
The tumour does not have aggressive histology (tall cell, or columnar cell PTC, diffuse sclerosing PTC, poorly differentiated elements), or angioinvasion
Intermediate-risk patients have any of the following characteristics:
Microscopic invasion of tumour into the perithyroidal soft tissues (T3) at initial surgery
Cervical lymph node metastases (N1a or N1b)
Tumour with aggressive histology (tall cell, or columnar cell PTC, diffuse sclerosing PTC, poorly differentiated elements) or angioinvasion
High-risk patients have any of the following characteristics:
Extra-thyroidal invasion
Incomplete macroscopic tumour resection (R2)
Distant metastases (M1)

DTC differentiated thyroid cancer, *ATA* american thyroid association, *PTC* papillary thyroid cancer, *R0* no residual primary tumour, *R1* microscopic residual primary tumour, *R2* macroscopic residual primary tumour, *N1a* Metastases to Level VI (pretracheal, paratracheal, and prelaryngeal/Delphian lymph nodes), *N1b* metastases to unilateral, bilateral, or contralateral cervical (Levels I–IV, or V) or retropharyngeal or superior mediastinal lymph nodes (Level VII), *M1* distant metastasis

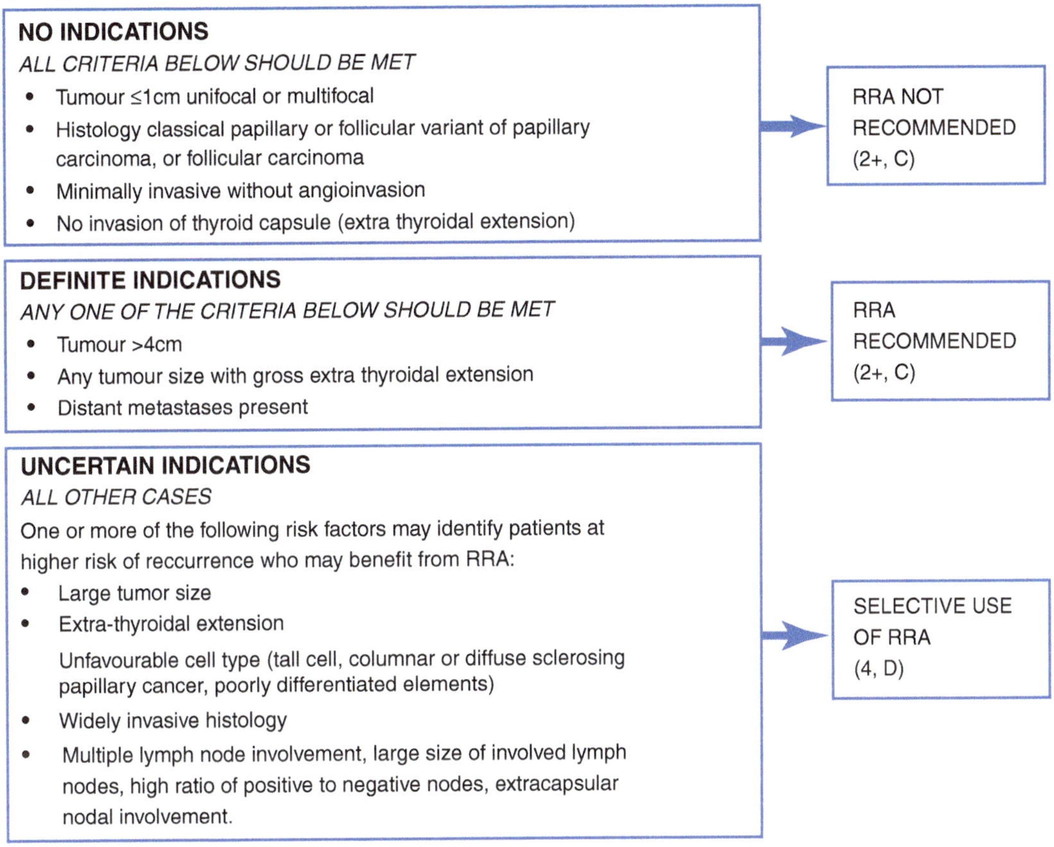

Fig. 2.1 Indications for radioactive iodine ablation (RRA)

that some patients with DTC will benefit from RRA, while others will not. A significant proportion of patients fall in the intermediate risk group, where the evidence for or against RRA is unclear and individualized decision-making is recommended. Figure 2.1 summarizes the indications for RRA. Recombinant thyrotropin is recommended as the standard means of preparation for RRA, thus avoiding iatrogenic hypothyroidism. In addition to the more restricted rather than universal use of RRA, the current guidelines suggest that lower RRA activities are equally effective to the higher activities used in the past, whereas the use of I^{131} to treat persistent, recurrent or metastatic disease requires higher activities, as described in Table 2.4. Following initial treat-

Table 2.4 Recommended I^{131} activity

I^{131} Ablation/ adjuvant activity	*Recommended I^{131} activity*	
For pT1-2, N0, R0	1.1 GBq	30 mCi
For pT3 and/or N1	On an individual case	>30 ≤150 mCi
^{131}I therapy activity	*Recommended I^{131} activity*	
Mainly empiric: 3.7–5.5 GBq		

I^{131} radioactive iodine 131, *GBq* becquerel, *mCi* millicurie, *pT1* tumour ≤2 cm in greatest dimension limited to the thyroid, *pT2* tumour >2 cm but ≤4 cm in greatest dimension, limited to the thyroid, *pT3* tumour >4 cm in greatest dimension limited to the thyroid or any tumour with minimal extra-thyroidal extension (e.g. extension to sternothyroid muscle or perithyroid soft tissues), *N0* no regional lymph node metastasis, *N1* regional lymph node metastasis, *R0* no residual primary tumour

ment with total thyroidectomy and RRA, and before evaluation of the patient's response to treatment after 9–12 months, TSH should be suppressed to below 0.1 mU/l in all patients. However, patients who have not received RRA because they fall in the 'no indication for RRA' group do not require TSH suppression and the serum TSH should be maintained in the low-normal range between 0.3 and 2.0 mU/l.

Dynamic Risk Stratification

Although the initial risk stratification of patients into three categories helps tremendously with initial management decisions, it only gives a static, single-point estimation of patients' status, based on the data available at the time of their initial therapy. However, it doesn't assess the risk of recurrence after RRA, based on re-evaluation of serum thyroglobulin (Tg) and US examination. Therefore, the concept of Dynamic Risk Stratification [34] has been incorporated in the BTA guidelines. This also stratifies patients into three groups: excellent (low risk), indeterminate (intermediate risk) and incomplete (high risk) response to initial therapy (Table 2.5). According to this reclassification, patients who achieve an excellent response to therapy can be reassured of their improved prognosis and have an adjustment in the intensity and frequency of follow up and the degree of TSH suppression, while those in the other groups require more intensive monitoring and reassessment.

Post Treatment Follow-Up

The recommended method for surveillance for tumor recurrence is clinical examination, serum thyroglobulin monitoring and US of the neck. The frequency of such follow-up depends on the dynamic risk stratification. The BTA guidelines take a holistic approach that includes guidance on management of post-operative hypoparathyroidism (frequently neglected), and managing the risk of osteoporosis and atrial fibrillation in patients receiving long-term TSH suppressive therapy. In patients with post-thyroidectomy hypocalcaemia, an attempt should be made to wean them off supplements in an outpatient setting. Patients on long-term alfacalcidol/calcitriol treatments should be monitored for adverse effects, which include hypercalcaemia, hypercalciuria, renal impairment, nephrocalcinosis and kidney stones. In specific at risk patient groups such as post-menopausal women, assessment of the 10-year probability of osteoporotic fragility fracture should also be performed using the WHO Fracture Risk Assessment Tool (FRAX). The degree of long-term TSH suppression depends on the individual patient's risk for recurrence. Figure 2.2 describes the proposed long-term management of DTC patients, based on their dynamic risk stratification. Patients with a higher risk of recurrence are monitored more intensively because it is believed that early detection of recurrent disease offers the best opportunity for effective treatment. On the other hand, patients unlikely to experience disease recurrence are followed with a less intensive plan that is more cost effective, safe

Table 2.5 BTA reclassification of patients with DTC based on their response to initial treatment with total thyroidectomy, R0 excision and RRA

Excellent response	Indeterminate response	Incomplete response
All the following • Suppressed and stimulated Tg < 1 lg/l* • Neck US without evidence of disease • Cross-sectional and/or nuclear medicine imaging negative (if performed)	Any of the following • Suppressed Tg < 1 lg/l* and stimulated Tg ≥1 and <10 lg/l* • Neck US with nonspecific changes or stable sub centimetre lymph nodes • Cross-sectional and/or nuclear medicine imaging with nonspecific changes, although not completely normal	Any of the following • Suppressed Tg ≥ 1 lg/l* or stimulated Tg ≥ 10 lg/l* • Rising Tg values • Persistent or newly identified disease on cross-sectional and/or nuclear medicine imaging
Low risk	Intermediate risk	High risk

*Assumes absence of interference in the Tg assay

BTA British thyroid association, *DTC* differentiated thyroid cancer, *RRA* radioactive iodine ablation, *US* ultrasound, *Tg* thyroglobulin, *R0* no residual primary tumour, *RRA* radioactive iodine ablation

- In patients with an *incomplete response,* the serum TSH should be suppressed below 0.1 mU/l indefinitely in the absence of specific contra-indications
- In patients with an *indeterminate response,* the serum TSH should be maintained between 0.1 and 0.5 mU/l for 5–10 years at which point re-evaluation is needed
- In patients with an *excellent response,* the serum TSH should be maintained □in the low-normal range between 0.3–2 mU/l.
- For historical patients who *have not undergone* Dynamic Risk Stratification, serum TSH should be suppressed below 0.1 mU/l for 5–10 years. This suppression can then be relaxed as appropriate, based on clinical, radiological or bio- chemical assessment of response.□
- Patients who have undergone *hemithyroidectomy only because of tumour ≤ 1* cm and low risk of recurrence do not require TSH suppression or long-term follow-up other that annual thyroid function testing
- Patients with low risk tumours *>1 to <4 cm treated with hemithyroidectomy,* may have a slightly higher risk of local recurrence than patients treated with total thyroidectomy, usually detectable within 3–5 years and mostly by 8–10 years. Low risk cases with tumour >1 to <4 cm treated with hemoithyroidectomy do not require TSH suppression, but Personalised Decision Making

BTA British thyroid association, *TSH* Thyroid-stimulating hormone

Fig. 2.2 BTA Long-term management based on dynamic risk stratification

and associated with a better quality of life. Thus, patients who are at low risk of recurrence and have reached 5 years following initial treatment with no evidence of disease, may be followed up in primary care provided there are clear protocols and re-referral pathways in place.

Recurrent and Persistent DTC

The choice of imaging should be guided in the first instance by the symptoms and clinical assessment of the patient, which may point to a particular anatomical area, bearing in mind that the commonest sites of recurrent disease are cervical/mediastinal lymph nodes, lungs and bones. Surgery with curative intent is the treatment of choice for recurrent disease confined to the neck. Metastases involving lungs and soft tissues are usually not amenable to surgery and should be treated with ^{131}I therapy. On the other hand, extensive bone metastases are generally not curable by ^{131}I therapy alone. External beam radiation therapy with/without resection and/or embolization/thermal ablation or cement injection may be beneficial in selected cases. External beam radiation therapy also has an important role in the management of spinal cord compression due to vertebral metastases in addition to surgery. Bisphosphonates are mainly used in the palliative setting. Cerebral metastases, which have a very poor prognosis, are managed with surgical resection or radiosurgery.

In suitable cases of unresectable iodine refractory metastatic DTC and unresectable metastatic MTC, especially if they are progressive and symptomatic, NICE approved Kinase Inhibitors should be considered by the MDT and if recommended they must be used under the supervision of a clinician experienced in using these drugs. New targeted agents should only be used in the context of clinical trials and studies.

In summary, the 2014 BTA guidelines have incorporated new developments in the field and translated them into recommendations that facilitate the management of patients with thyroid cancer. Notable trends are the central role of US in investigating thyroid nodules, use of therapies to match the aggressiveness of the cancer and individualised overall management. Patients' engagement is encouraged and shared decision-making promoted, thus reflecting a pragmatic response to the many uncertainties in the field. Ultimately the intention is to improve survival, reduce recurrence rates and maintain patient quality of life.

References

1. Teppo L, Hakulinen E, Eurocare Working Group. Variation in survival of adult patients with thyroid cancer in Europe. Eur J Cancer. 1998;34:2238–52.
2. Mallick UK, Ball S, Fenwick JD, James RA, Johnson SJ, Lennard TWJ, Lucraft HH, Proud G, Perros P, Weightman DR. Northern cancer network guide-

lines for management of thyroid cancer. Clin Oncol. 2000;12:373–91.
3. Kendall-Taylor P, Beckett GJ, Clark, Clarke EM, Collins R, Farndon J, Franklyn J, Owen Hafiz C, Harmer C, GAW H, Kabala J, Lawrence J, AM MN, Mallick UK, Ponder B, Prentice M, Proud G, Sturgeon C, Watkinson J, Weetman AP, Williams J, Vini L. Guidelines for the management of thyroid cancer in adults. London: RCP; 2002.
4. Perros P, Clarke SEM, Franklyn J, Gerrard G, Harrison B, Hickey J, Kendall-Taylor P, McNicol AM, Mallick UK, Prentice M, Thakker RV, Watkinson J, Weetman AP. Guidelines for the management of thyroid cancer. 2nd ed. London: RCP; 2007.
5. Perros P, Boelaert K, Colley S, Evans C, Evans R, Gerrard B, Gilbert J, Harrison B, Johnson S, Giles T, Moss L, Lewington V, Newbold K, Taylor J, Thakker R, Watkinson J, Williams G, Thyroid B. Guidelines for the management of thyroid cancer. Clin Endocrinol (Oxf). 2014;81:1–122.
6. Politi MC, Dizon DS, Frosch DL, Kuzemchak MD, Stiggelbout AM. Importance of clarifying patients' desired role in shared decision making to match their level of engagement with their preferences. BMJ. 2013;347:f7066.
7. Guth S, Theune U, Aberle J, Galach A, Bamberger C. Very high prevalence of thyroid nodules detected by high frequency (13 MHz) ultrasound examination. Eur J Clin Investig. 2009;39:699–706.
8. Aschebrook-Kilfoy B, Schechter RB, Shih YC, Kaplan EL, Chiu BC, Angelos P, Grogan RH. The clinical and economic burden of a sustained increase in thyroid cancer incidence. Cancer Epidemiol Biomark Prev. 2013;22:1252–9.
9. Vaccarella S, Franceschi S, Bray F, Wild C, Plummer M, Dal Maso L. Worldwide thyroid-Cancer epidemic? The increasing impact of overdiagnosis. N Engl J Med. 2016;375:614–7.
10. Smith-Bindman R, Lebda P, Feldstein V, Sellami D, Goldstein R, Brasic N, Jin C, Kornak J. Risk of thyroid cancer based on thyroid ultrasound imaging characteristics: results of a population-based study. JAMA Intern Med. 2013;173:1788–96.
11. Horvath E, Majilis S, Rossi R, Franco C, Nied- mann J, Castro A, Dominguez M. An ultrasonogram reporting system for thyroid nodules stratifying cancer risk for clinical management. J Clin Endocrinol Metab. 2009;90:1748–51.
12. Hambly N, Gonen M, Gerst S, Li D, Jia X, Mironov S, Sarasohn D, Fleming S, Hann L. Implementation of evidence-based guidelines for thyroid nodule biopsy: a model for establishment of practice standards. AJR Am J Roentgenol. 2011;196:655–60.
13. Lee Y, Kim D, In H, Park J, Kim S, Eom J, Kim B, Lee E, Rho M. Differentiation between benign and malignant solid thyroid nodules using an US classification system. Korean J Radiol. 2011;12:559–67.
14. Moon W, Jung S, Lee J, Na D, Baek J, Lee Y, Kim J, Kim H, Byun J, Lee D, Study T. Benign and malignant thyroid nodules: US differentiation--multicenter retrospective study. Radiology. 2008;247:762–70.
15. Albuja-Cruz MB, Goldfarb M, Gondek SS, Allan BJ, Lew JI. Reliability of fine-needle aspiration for thyroid nodules greater than or equal to 4 cm. J Surg Res. 2013;181:6–10.
16. Mehanna R, Murphy M, McCarthy J, O'Leary G, Tuthill A, Murphy MS, Sheahan P. False negatives in thyroid cytology: impact of large nodule size and follicular variant of papillary carcinoma. Laryngoscope. 2013;123:1305–9.
17. Shi H, Bobanga I, McHenry CR. Are large thyroid nodules classified as benign on fine needle aspiration more likely to harbor cancer? Am J Surg. 2017;213:464–6.
18. Shrestha M, Crothers BA, Burch HB. The impact of thyroid nodule size on the risk of malignancy and accuracy of fine-needle aspiration: a 10-year study from a single institution. Thyroid. 2012;22:1251–6.
19. The Royal College of Pathologists. Guidance on the reporting of thyroid cytology specimens. London: The Royal College of Pathologists; 2016.
20. Poller DN, Baloch ZW, Fadda G, Johnson SJ, Bongiovanni M, Pontecorvi A, Cochand-Priollet B. Thyroid FNA: new classifications and new interpretations. Cancer Cytopathol. 2016;124:457–66. https://doi.org/10.1002/cncy.21703.
21. Gerhard R, Boerner SL. The value of second opinion in thyroid cytology: a review. Cancer Cytopathol. 2014;122:611–9.
22. Kocjan G, Chandra A, Cross PA, et al. The interobserver reproducibility of thyroid fine-needle aspiration using the UK Roal College of Pathologists classification system. Am J Clin Pathol. 2011;135: 852–9.
23. Parkinson D, Aziz S, Bentley R, Johnson SJ. Thyroid cytology-histology correlation using the RCPath terminology for thyroid cytology reporting. J Clin Pathol. 2017;70(8):648–55. https://doi.org/10.1136/jclinpath-2016-204022.
24. The Royal College of Pathologists. Dataset for thyroid cancer histopathology reports. London: The Royal College of Pathologists; 2014.
25. Poller D, Johnson SJ. Recent developments in the pathology of thyroid cancer. Clin Oncol (R Coll Radiol). 2017;29(5):278–82. https://doi.org/10.1016/j.clon.2017.01.006.
26. Nikiforov YE, Seethala RR, Tallini G, Baloch ZW, Basolo F, Thompson LDR, Barletta JA, Wenig BM, Al Ghuzlan A, Kakudo K, Giordano TJ, Alves VA, Khanafshar E, Asa SL, El-Naggar AK, Gooding WE, Hodak SP, Lloyd RV, Maytal G, Mete O, Nikiforova MN, Nosé V, Papotti M, Poller DN, Sadow PM, Tischler AS, Tuttle RM, Wall KB, VA LV, Randolph GW, Ghossein RA. Nomenclature revision for encapsulated follicular variant of papillary thyroid carcinoma: a paradigm shift to reduce overtreatment of indolent tumors. JAMA Oncol. 2016;2(8):1023–9. https://doi.org/10.1001/jamaoncol.2016.0386.

27. Brierley JD, Gospodarowicz MK, Wittekind C, for UICC, editors. The TNM classification of malignant tumours. 8th ed. Chichester: Wiley-Blackwell; 2016.
28. Hay ID, McConahey WM, Goellner JR. Managing patients with papillary thyroid carcinoma: insights gained from the Mayo Clinic's experience of treating 2,512 consecutive patients during 1940 through 2000. Trans Am Clin Climatol Assoc. 2002;113: 241–60.
29. Matsuzu K, Sugino K, Masudo K, Nagahama M, Kitagawa W, Shibuya H, Ohkuwa K, Uruno T, Suzuki A, Magoshi S, Akaishi J, Masaki C, Kawano M, Suganuma N, Rino Y, Masuda M, Kameyama K, Takami H, Ito K. Thyroid lobectomy for papillary thyroid cancer: long-term follow-up study of 1,088 cases. World J Surg. 2013;38:68–79.
30. Nixon I, Ganly I, Patel S, Palmer F, Whitcher M, Tuttle R, Shaha A, Shah J. Thyroid lobectomy for treatment of well differentiated intrathyroid malignancy. Surgery. 2011;151:571–9.
31. Hassanain M, Wexler M. Conservative management of well-differentiated thyroid cancer. Can J Surg. 2010;53:109–18.
32. Mendelsohn AH, Elashoff DA, Abemayor E, St John MA. Surgery for papillary thyroid carcinoma: is lobectomy enough? Arch Otolaryngol Head Neck Surg. 2010;136:1055–61.
33. Cooper D, Doherty G, Haugen B, Kloos R, Lee S, Mandel S, Mazzaferri E, McIver B, Pacini F, Schlumberger M, Sherman S, Steward D, Tuttle R. Revised American thyroid association management guidelines for patients with thyroid nodules and differentiated thyroid cancer. Thyroid. 2009;19:1167–214.
34. Tuttle R, Tala H, Shah J, Leboeuf R, Ghossein R, Gonen M, Brokhin M, Omry G, Fagin J, Shaha A. Estimating risk of recurrence in differentiated thyroid cancer after total thyroidectomy and radioactive iodine remnant ablation: using response to therapy variables to modify the initial risk estimates predicted by the new American Thyroid Association staging system. Thyroid. 2010;20:1341–9.

3 The 2015 American Thyroid Association Evidence-Based Guidelines for Management of Patients with Thyroid Nodules and Differentiated Thyroid Cancer: Key Recommendations

Bryan R. Haugen

The 2015 American Thyroid Association (ATA) Evidence-Based Guidelines for Management of Patients with Thyroid Nodules and Differentiated Thyroid Cancer (DTC) have significant changes from the 2006 and 2009 ATA guidelines [1–3]. The recommendations are rated as *Strong* or *Weak* based on an adapted grading system from the American College of Physicians [4], citing high-quality, moderate-quality or low-quality evidence. These guidelines generated eight new questions, 21 new recommendations and 21 significantly changed recommendations. That said, 59 of the recommendations from the 2009 guidelines were not substantively changed based on no new evidence or continued evidence supporting the existing recommendation.

Thyroid Nodules

There are many new or changed recommendations that could be reviewed, but I would like to highlight a few that are the most controversial or may make the greatest impact on our care for our patients with thyroid nodules and DTC. *Recommendation 8* outlines five sonographic risk patterns and provides recommendations for size cutoff for considerations of FNA: high risk (>1 cm), intermediate risk (>1 cm), low risk (>1.5 cm), very-low risk (>2 cm), benign (no need for diagnostic FNA). This recommendation is accompanied by Fig. 3.1, which was generated to help clinicians find the appropriate sonographic risk category for each patient. This recommended approach should reduce the unnecessary FNA generated by previous recommendations from different group suggesting all thyroid nodule >1 cm undergo FNA. It should also be noted that the very-low risk patients, including those with the spongiform pattern, do not require diagnostic FNA for any size nodule, but if one is considering FNA, it should be in nodules >2 cm. *Recommendation 12* which states "If a cytology result is diagnostic for primary thyroid malignancy, surgery is *generally* recommended." This is often overlooked, but the word 'generally' was very purposefully added to the 2009 version of the recommendation, to begin to 'open the door' for consideration of active monitoring of a carefully selected subset patients with micropapillary carcinoma based on emerging evidence that many of these patients have no disease progression.

B. R. Haugen
Division of Endocrinology, Metabolism, and Diabetes, Department of Medicine, University of Colorado Cancer Center, University of Colorado School of Medicine, Aurora, Colorado, USA
e-mail: Bryan.Haugen@ucdenver.edu

U. K. Mallick et al. (eds.), *Practical Management of Thyroid Cancer*,
https://doi.org/10.1007/978-3-319-91725-2_3

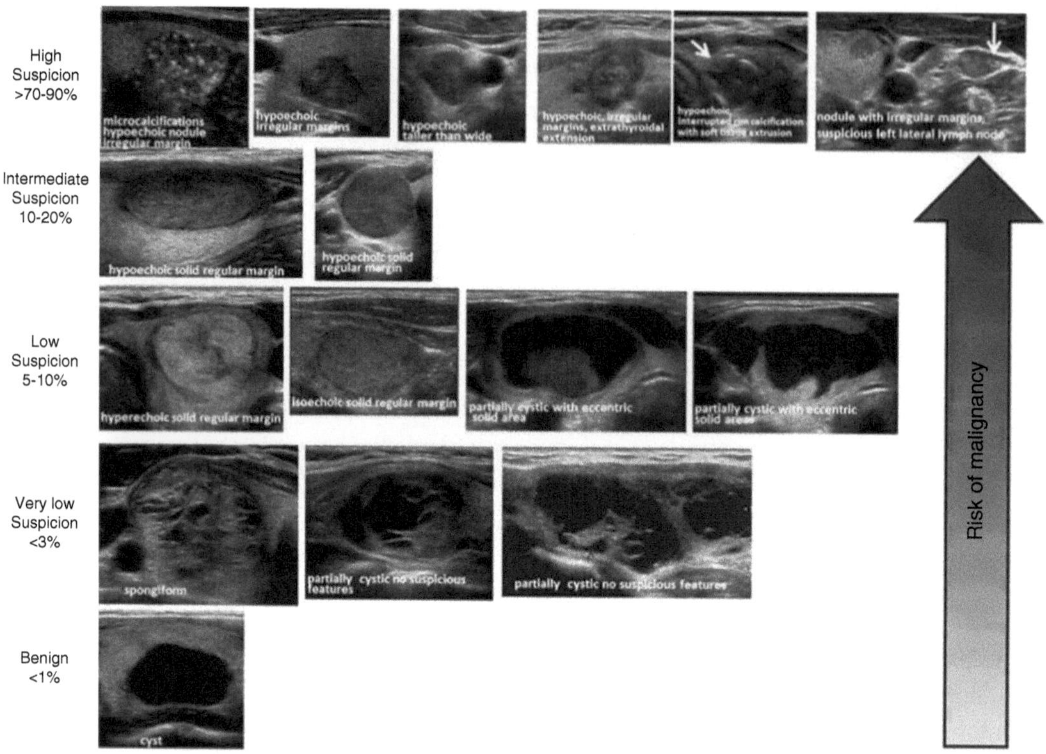

Fig. 3.1 ATA nodule sonographic patterns and risk of malignancy

Thyroid Cancer

Recommendation 33 should be noted as a shift in preoperative imaging from previous iterations of these guidelines. This recommendation endorses use of preoperative cross-sectional imaging (CT or MRI *with intravenous contrast* for patients with clinical suspicion for advanced disease. The factors raising this clinical suspicion are outlined and this recommendation pointedly notes that CT neck with contrast is both appropriate and needed in these patients and the contrast 'wash-out' of 4–8 weeks should not interfere with subsequent radioiodine therapy. *Recommendation 35B* may be the most controversial recommendation in the guidelines. This recommendation allows the consideration of a lobectomy or thyroidectomy for patients with 1–4 cm thyroid cancer without clinical or radiographic evidence of extrathyroidal extension or involved lymph nodes. This recommendation is based on five recent database studies [1], which we felt were of moderate-quality evidence demonstrating similar clinical outcomes between the two procedures in 'properly selected patients.' Many readers interpreted this as a mandate for lobectomy in these patients, but we merely allowed consideration of either procedure based on moderate-quality evidence. We also noted in the text that high-volume surgeons have better surgical outcomes than low-volume surgeons. For practical reasons, we did not elevate this to a specific recommendation about surgeon referral. We do note, however, that one should 'consider sending patients with more extensive disease … to a high-volume surgeon ….

Recommendations 48 and 49 are noteworthy in that they add an initial risk stratification for recurrence (high, intermediate, low) and a response to therapy (excellent, indeterminate, biochemical incomplete, structural incomplete) that complement the classic AJCC/TNM staging system to help guide treatment and monitoring of patients

Table 3.1 TSH targets for patients with DTC based on response to therapy and risk of TSH suppression

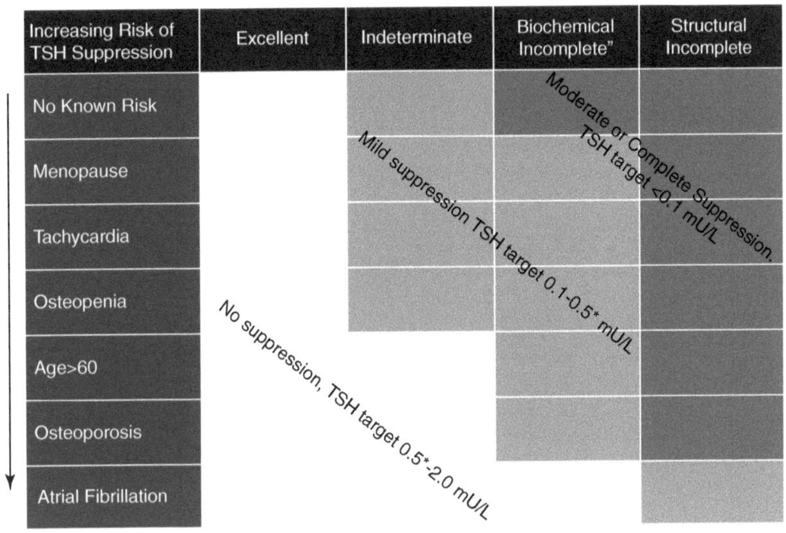

*0.5 mU/L represents the lower limit of the reference range for the TSH assay which can be 0.3-0.5 mU/L depending on the specific assay

** TSH target for patients with a biochemical incomplete response can be quite different based on original ATA risk, Tg level, Tg trend over time and risk of TSH suppression

No suppression. TSH target 0.5*-2.0 mU/L

Mild suppression, TSH target 0.1-0.5* mU/L

Moderate or Complete suppression. TSH target <0.1 mU/L

with DTC. We strongly recommend that these approaches should be incorporated into clinical management algorithms for these patients.

Recommendations 51 and 55 focus on the use of radioiodine in DTC. They are set on the foundation of determining the reason for the use of radioiodine: remnant ablation, adjuvant therapy or therapy. Based on these oncologic principles, RAI remnant ablation therapy is not routinely recommended for ATA low-risk DTC patients, and if used as remnant ablation in low- and intermediate-risk patients, a low administered activity of approximately 30 mCi (1.1 GBq) is recommended. This is a departure from previous guidelines where a more liberal use and higher administered activities of RAI were recommended. TSH goals have been somewhat changed in Recommendation 70, which are based on response to therapy and risk of TSH suppression (Table 3.1). For example, a patient with an indeterminate response to therapy (low level Tg, Tg antibodies, indeterminate LN on US) who is >60 years old, may be best served with a TSH of 0.5–2 mU/L and not aggressive suppression.

Finally, there is a new section at the end of the guidelines (*Recommendations 91–101*) addressing the definition and management of patients with RAI-refractory DTC. This section is meant to help guide the monitoring of these patients, as well as choices of directed therapy, systemic therapy and entry into clinical trials.

References

1. Haugen BR, Alexander EK, Bible KC, Doherty GM, Mandel SJ, Nikiforov YE, Pacini F, Randolph GW, Sawka AM, Schlumberger M, Schuff K, Sherman SI, Sosa JA, Steward DL, Tuttle RM, Wartofsky LM. 2015 American Thyroid Association management guidelines for adult patients with thyroid nodules and differentiated thyroid cancer. Thyroid. 2016;26:1–133. PMID 26462967.
2. Cooper DS, Doherty GM, Haugen BR, Kloos RT, Lee SL, Mandel SJ, Mazzaferri EL, McIver B, Sherman

SI, Tuttle RM. Management guidelines for patients with thyroid nodules and differentiated thyroid cancer. Thyroid. 2006;16:109–42.
3. Cooper DS, Doherty GM, Haugen BR, Kloos RT, Lee SL, Mandel SJ, Mazzaferri EL, McIver B, Pacini F, Schlumberger M, Sherman SI, Steward DL, Tuttle RM. Revised American Thyroid Association guidelines for patients with thyroid nodules and differentiated thyroid cancer. Thyroid. 2009;19:1167–214.
4. Qaseem A, Snow V, Owens DK, Shekelle P. The development of clinical practice guidelines and guidance statements of the American College of Physicians: summary of methods. Ann Intern Med. 2010;153:194–9.

4 Thyroid Cancer: One Doctor-Patient Partnership—The Newcastle Butterfly Model

Kathleen A. Farnell, Richard D. Bliss, and Ujjal K. Mallick

Introduction

The doctor-patient partnership is a huge, rapidly expanding area within medicine and the benefits of close working relationships between physician and patient are now being widely recognized. Shared decision making between the parties (as opposed to paternalistic and informed) should now be an integral part of medicine as patient satisfaction and behavior including compliance and clinical outcomes are all improved with closer working relationships [1]. It is also a requirement for the UK's medical regulatory body, the GMC, that "for a relationship between doctor and a patient to be effective, it should be a partnership based on openness, trust and good communication…" [2, 3]. The object of this chapter, therefore, is to review how a good doctor-patient partnership can produce outstanding results to the benefit of both parties by reviewing one such example in thyroid cancer rather than rehearse the arguments for different types of doctor-patient relationships.

At the time of writing, it is almost 17 years since I (KAF) was diagnosed with thyroid cancer. Looking back, so much has happened since then, much of which has been very positive, but my family and I were devastated by my diagnosis at the time. It was a very busy time in my life. I was working with my husband in his very busy dental practice, our son was 12 years old and would soon be preparing for important examinations at school, and my father was chronically ill.

Any patient will confirm that waiting to have the final diagnosis of a thyroid nodule which could be cancer, albeit in a very small (about 5%) proportion of patients, is a very stressful time. My diagnosis from fine needle aspiration was inconclusive (THY3); this led to hemithyroidectomy, which confirmed a diagnosis of minimally invasive follicular carcinoma of the thyroid. Completion thyroidectomy followed 1 week later. A 2.5-cm tumour in an awkward position led to difficult surgery with rupture of the tumour and I sustained a laryngeal nerve injury which produced a left-sided vocal cord palsy; the resulting laryngeal spasms and stridor attacks are exceptionally unpleasant. I also developed protracted hypocalcaemia (but was successfully weaned off calcium supplementation after 6 years!). Then came radioiodine ablation with hypo-thyroidism (Thyrogen was not available at that time), and treatment in isolation leading to depression and anxiety.

K. A. Farnell (✉)
Butterfly Thyroid Cancer Trust, Tyne and Wear, UK

R. D. Bliss
The Newcastle upon Tyne Hospitals, NHS Foundation Trust, Newcastle upon Tyne, UK

U. K. Mallick
Chief Investigator UK National "IoN" and HiLo Trials, Past clinical oncologist and Chair Regional Thyroid MDT, Northern Centre for Cancer Care, Freeman Hospital, Newcastle upon Tyne, United Kingdom
e-mail: Ujjal.mallick@nuth.nhs.uk

U. K. Mallick et al. (eds.), *Practical Management of Thyroid Cancer*,
https://doi.org/10.1007/978-3-319-91725-2_4

Although I was told repeatedly that this was a highly curable cancer (5-year survival 95–100%), it was very difficult to accept this as I had not had contact with anyone who had had this rare cancer, and 5 years seemed a long way off.

I was very lucky to have the support of a wonderful family and excellent doctors. I plagued my surgeon and oncologist with endless questions about the disease and my prognosis, and they were exceptionally patient and did their utmost to support me. I was very anxious and depressed during the initial 6 months; the only way I could cope was to find out everything I could about my disease, and I learned fairly quickly that this information needed to be sourced from my professional medical team and not the internet!

I was troubled by this issue, and realised through my own experiences that if patients were well informed with reliable information from the start and given the opportunity to have contact with other patients, it would be beneficial to their well-being. I started to meet with hospital managers and my medical team to talk about improving the situation for patients with thyroid cancer. They could not have been more open or supportive.

Development of Butterfly Thyroid Cancer Trust

My surgeon telephoned me about 12 months post diagnosis, and asked if I would talk with a young, newly diagnosed patient who was struggling. That was the beginning of the first patient support organisation in the UK for patients with thyroid cancer, the Butterfly Thyroid Cancer Trust. This young woman was in her 20s and understandably devastated by her diagnosis. We talked together, I shared my experiences about the treatment and what was involved, visited her in hospital and went to scan appointments with her. As well as helping her, this also helped me. She was the first person I knew who was going through what I had gone through. That was 16 years ago and much has happened since then, all of which has been good!

My doctors started to 'refer' newly diagnosed patients, and I gave up work at the dental practice to concentrate on setting up Butterfly on a full-time basis. It has taken a lot of hard work and determination to succeed, but the reward in seeing what good support can do for other patients is wonderful. Butterfly is the first registered charity in the UK solely dedicated to the support of people affected by thyroid cancer, and is recognised by and has the full support of the healthcare professionals treating patients in the region.

The Butterfly website (www.butterfly.org.uk) details what the charity can offer, but to a newly diagnosed patient, the opportunity to meet someone who has had the same disease as them and who is well/cured so many years later is priceless.

No one diagnosed with this rare cancer in the UK needs to go through their cancer journey feeling alone or isolated. Butterfly can offer support, information and encouragement whenever needed.

Honorary Thyroid Cancer Patient Advisor in Weekly Thyroid Cancer Clinic

Butterfly is a patient support charity, but perhaps the most important aspect of my work is to offer a unique service as a team member in my local hospital oncology clinic, offering on-site clinical support from a fellow patient. This is a unique partnership between a patient (myself) and the thyroid cancer care team in Newcastle referred to as 'The Butterfly Model'. I was given an honorary contract by The Newcastle upon Tyne Hospitals NHS Foundation Trust as a Thyroid Cancer Patient Advisor and work in clinic alongside the clinical team to support patients. Patient audit of this service returned outstanding results and our work has been recognised with many national awards including:

- Pfizer Excellence in Oncology Peoples Award 2006
- NHS Innovations Award—first prize 2006
- Best Oncology Team of the Year Award (Hospital Doctor) 2007
- Highly commended by the National Peer Review Team 2007 and invited to present at National Sharing Good Practice Event 2008

- Pfizer Excellence in Oncology Award (Commended) 2009
- Advancing Healthcare Awards (Runner-up) 2015
- National Royal Television Society Awards (runner-up) 2015
- BMA Patient Information Awards (highly commended) 2016
- As is evident by the chronology, the work never stops and future projects are both equally exciting and innovative.

Current Roles of BTCT

Butterfly Thyroid Cancer Trust works to support all patients diagnosed with thyroid cancer of any type. To this end, the Trust provides patient support in many forms, as well as supporting the medical professionals by helping deliver information and advice. On a larger scale however, BTCT appreciates the rapidly increasing number of patients being diagnosed with differentiated thyroid carcinoma and so works towards increasing the awareness of this in the general public and earlier detection to reduce the risk of significant complications and so improve the cancer patient's journey and outcome.

Membership of the Thyroid Oncology Team

I continue to attend the regional Thyroid Oncology Clinic held weekly at the local cancer centre. The clinic offers an opportunity to meet old friends and patients helping them with any ongoing problems as well as meeting newly diagnosed and recent referrals to the clinic.

I work closely with the Clinical Nurse Specialist in assessing the holistic needs of the patients supporting them with practical and personal help from the patients' perspective. A significant contribution of BTCT to the medical staff is that I am able to have more informal and social in-depth relationships and discussions with the patients and so help assist the medical and nursing staff to identify those patients struggling to come to terms with their diagnosis or potential complications of their treatment and would benefit from additional psychological support. I also support the patients at the time of their RAI treatment and introduce them to the facilities and medical physics team.

The oncology team include me as a patient representative in business meetings and continuing professional and educational programmes so that I am able to relay the most up-to-date information and consensus recommendations of the team to my patients and members.

My presence in the weekly clinic and in business meetings has most certainly facilitated improved communication with patients. It has also helped to deliver regular patient feedback and suggestions for service improvements, service developments, and may have played a part in reducing patient disatisfaction and potential complaints.

The special aspects of this doctor patient collaboration are:

- I was provided with an initial period of education/evidence based information in allowing me to attend local meetings and permitting supervised attendance as an observer (after obtaining patient consent) to gain experience directly from the consultants communicating with patients in the clinics and on the wards.
- This was followed up by continuous in–service training and CME by allowing and supporting me to attend and speak in national and international conferences.

This ensured that the service I was providing was with consultant supervision in the initial phase and that the information I was providing to patients was up to date guideline based information approved by the MDT. So I was more or less working within a kind of "regulatory framework" of the Hospital Trust where the clinical responsibility lay with the clinicians and the clinician was available next door if there were any issues; This form of "regulation and supervision" and arrangement at least in the initial phase gave me a lot of confidence and helped maintaining a high quality service trusted by patients.

Activities of BTCT

A dedicated telephone help line is organized by BTCT. This is manned as much as possible between volunteers but if no-one is able to give immediate 1-to-1 support, then the call will always be returned to allow direct support and advice whenever possible. If this is not immediately possible (for example, a clinical question) then BTCT will contact medical advisors who can usually suggest a local expert or give direct advice based on the information available.

The BTCT website has a lot of useful information and contacts for patients and medical staff as well as directing readers to an appropriate source.

Patient Support contacts across the UK with the development of a "Buddy System" to give more personalized support and ensure that patients going through treatment for thyroid cancer are not alone.

We believe strongly that BTCT should act as an advocate for patients and therefore support and contribute directly to the medicine regulatory bodies in the UK providing evidence for new treatments for thyroid cancer.

We have built strong professional relationships with pharmaceutical companies and receive news on new medicines at the earliest opportunity.

Excellent working relationships have been formed with other support organisations here in the UK and in other countries, especially the USA.

This enables us to share best practices and information.

Patient Information Pack including the patient information DVDs for newly diagnosed patients and those with advanced disease. The DVDs are comprehensive, covering the modern management of differentiated thyroid cancer and approved by professional associations such as the British Association of Endocrine and Thyroid Surgeons, the British Thyroid Association, British Medical Association and Cancer Research UK. To date, more than 8000 copies have been provided free of charge to newly diagnosed thyroid cancer patients across the UK.

Other innovations supporting clinicians in delivering first-class care to their patients include the development of TSH-suppression cards which have now been nationally adopted by thyroid cancer clinics across the UK. These alert cards are carried at all times by the patients so their primary care physicians or emergency physicians are aware of any ongoing requirements for TSH-suppression.

BTCT also supports patients once they have completed their treatment with ongoing counselling and support including the funding of holidays for those unable to fund themselves and allow a break in their circumstances and recharge their batteries.

We facilitate those patients who would like the added reassurance of a second medical opinion in complex cases.

BTCT is active in supporting the desire of Public Health England and Commissioning Groups to improve the awareness of cancers and increase the proportion of patients with early Stage I and II disease. BTCT has raised the awareness of thyroid cancer among the population of the UK by running television advertisements advising patients with undiagnosed neck lumps to seek a medical opinion and investigate as appropriate. More locally, a "Neck Check" event was organized in the largest shopping mall in the UK where passers-by could have a medical professional examine their neck. Thirteen physicians supported this event and over 1000 patients were seen resulting in 38 patients having undiagnosed thyroid nodules and requiring further investigation, with two new malignancies detected.

In a more general role supporting the future improvement of the patients' pathway, we support patient-centred research with grants for well-regarded medical and surgical studies.

As a patient representative, I am an extended member of the multidisciplinary team and also of the Regional Cancer Alliance Patient Advisory Panel. I am also invited to attend selected meetings of the National Cancer Research Institute's Thyroid Cancer Subgroup, and provide patients' perspectives on national thyroid cancer trial proposals for Cancer Research (UK).

We continue to undertake surveys of the patients' experience across the UK each year and present the results to professional medical staff at their Association's annual meeting (BAETS) to ensure that the patients voice continues to be heard.

First Global Workshop on the Role of TKI's

In 2014, I led on the first global workshop on the role of TKI's which was held in Paris and attended by world leaders but perhaps more importantly two terminally ill patients who were able to share their cancer journeys with the doctors.

First Patient Doctor Thyroid Cancer Conference in the UK in 2016

BTCT organized the first Patient Doctor Thyroid Cancer Conference in the UK in 2016. The audience was made up patients and doctors who enjoyed a programme delivered by expert patients and national professionals in all disciplines of the management of thyroid cancer. This allowed formal and informal meetings of physicians and surgeons with patients and ensured that patients were able to ask any questions worrying them as well as delivering the patients perspective to them. Social support and meeting other patients was also very beneficial to those who were able to attend. An integral part of the meeting included the presentation of the most recent BTCT patient survey highlighting significant inequalities in treatment and information offered to patients across the UK. The proceedings of the meeting are available to anyone via the Butterfly website.

BTCT in conjunction with the Newcastle team have arranged regular survivorship meetings with patients to examine to issues that Thyroid Cancer survivors face.

Wider Recognition of BTCT Work

Patient Involvement in Research and Trials

I am also invited to attend selected meetings of the National Cancer Research Institute's Thyroid Cancer Subgroup, and provide patients' perspectives on national thyroid cancer trial proposals and patient information leaflets for National Cancer Research Network (NCRN) trials funded by Cancer Research (UK). My contribution to the first successful randomised Thyroid Cancer Trial in the UK during its design and conduct was acknowledged by my inclusion in the authorship of the publication in the New England Journal of Medicine highlighting the increasing recognition of the positive impact of Patient involvement in trials [4, 5].

Invited Guest Speaker National and International Conferences

I have been invited to deliver teaching seminars to medical professional and pharmaceutical staff across Europe describing the work and activities of BTCT centred primarily on highlighting the patient journey. This ensures that the patient's perspective is delivered to a wide audience and so the patient's experience is always included when planning treatment and in particular when changes are being made to the patient pathway.

BTCT is regularly invited to present at international meetings in Europe and North America including the World Thyroid Cancer Congress, 2013. I was delighted to be invited to open the Congress with Dr. Mike Tuttle, from Memorial-Sloane Kettering Medical Center, New York, a world-recognised medical authority in the management of thyroid cancer.

I have been invited to present at numerous national and international thyroid cancer conferences, including the first global TKI patient doctor meeting in Paris 2014, the World Thyroid Cancer Congress in Toronto in August 2009. This resulted in meeting people who run patient organisations in a number of countries worldwide.

Conducting the First International Survey of Thyroid Cancer Patients

This led to the first ever International Survey of Thyroid Cancer Patients. The results initially were presented with Prof Marcus Luster in Paris to an audience of >900 clinicians in 2010, later published in *Hormones* [6].

Honour for Services

In 2014, I was honoured by Her Majesty the Queen and received an MBE for services to Thyroid Cancer.

My thanks to my care team for their expertise, their compassion and their will to continue to strive to improve the care of patients with this disease. I regularly witness their dedication and willingness to go above and beyond the call of duty in the care of our patients. I look forward to our continuing partnership!

I hope that my input enthusiasm and dedication to the cause of thyroid cancer patients has led in some way to improving the standard of care across the UK and the understanding of the thyroid cancer patients' pathway. Since BTCT was founded, we have supported thousands of patients, many of whom have been a source of inspiration and admiration in the manner in which they have borne the disease, complications of its treatment and occasionally with a very sad albeit unavoidable outcome.

Conclusions

The opportunity that I have been given to support patients with this disease is humbling and space is too limited to thank everybody individually.

I could not do this without the tremendous support of my fellow patients of BTCT locally, nationally and beyond; my doctors, in particular my oncologist, my family (particularly my husband and son), my surgeon, members of the Newcastle Hospital MDT and Trust Management; many national and international experts, individuals and organisations continue to be outstanding with their support, donations, advice, active participation, donations and fund raising.

Editorial Comment

This particular model has most definitely stood the test of time for the Newcastle regional thyroid cancer team. Initially started as an experimental model, it has been successful beyond any expectations and has hugely benefited the community of thyroid cancer patients and professionals at the regional, national and also at the international level.

Kate's personal experience with thyroid cancer, her continuing educational activities, previous nursing background, sheer enthusiasm, dedication and hard work were obviously key to its success as were the continuing active participation and contribution of hundreds of patients. There was also a commitment from the thyroid cancer MDT and hospital management to work together in a Doctor-Patient Partnership to improve the management of this relatively rare but highly curable disease with a long natural history.

References

1. Charles C, Whelan T, Gafni A. What do we mean by partnership in making decisions about treatment. BMJ. 1999;310:780–2.
2. General Medical Council. Good medical practice. London: GMC; 2013.
3. General Medical Council. Consent: doctors and patients making decisions together. London: GMC; 2008.
4. Mallick U, Harmer C, Yap B, Wadsley J, Clarke S, Moss L, Nicol A, Clark PM, Farnell K, McCready R, Smellie J, Franklyn JA, John R, Nutting CM, Newbold K, Lemon C, Gerrard G, Abdel-Hamid A, Hardman J, Macias E, Roques T, Whitaker S, Vijayan R, Alvarez P, Beare S, Forsyth S, Kadalayil L, Hackshaw A. Ablation with low-dose radioiodine and thyrotropin alfa in thyroid cancer. N Engl J Med. 2012;366(18):1674–85.
5. Department of Health. Research governance framework for health and social care. 2nd ed. London: Department of Health; 2005.
6. Banoch R, Bartes B, Farnell K, et al. Results of the thyroid cancer alliance international patient/survivor survey: psychosocial/informational support needs, treatment side effects and international differences in care. Hormones. 2013;12:428–38.

Part II

The Diagnosis of Thyroid Cancer

Molecular Diagnosis of Thyroid Nodules

5

David N. Poller

Introduction

Our understanding of the molecular pathology of the thyroid gland has advanced significantly in recent years, with the publication in 2014 of the Thyroid Cancer Genome Atlas [1], and the widespread introduction of molecular techniques, including next-generation DNA and RNA sequencing [2]. The availability of newer DNA and RNA techniques makes it feasible to undertake targeted mutational analysis of any given thyroid nodule via a thyroid fine needle aspirate and to predict with a high degree of certainty whether any given nodule is benign or malignant Other approaches include a proprietary micro-RNA panel which can be used as 'rule-out' test for carcinoma in indeterminate thyroid nodules. The application of preoperative molecular diagnostic testing for thyroid nodules is discussed.

Background

The thyroid gland lies at the base of the neck. Thyroid nodules are extremely common and most thyroid nodules are benign. Approximately 10% of thyroid nodules are malignant although the risk of thyroid malignancy in any given thyroid nodule depends on the patient age, genetics, and previous history including radiation exposure. The most common primary thyroid cancers are papillary thyroid carcinoma, differentiated follicular carcinoma, poorly differentiated carcinoma, anaplastic carcinoma, and parafollicular C-cell derived medullary carcinoma. In contrast other benign and malignant tumours of the thyroid are all relatively rare; e.g. hyalinising trabecular tumour, solitary fibrous tumour, teratoma, benign or malignant paraganglioma, leiomyoma or leiomyosarcoma, schwannoma or malignant peripheral nerve sheath tumour, spindle cell tumour with thymus-like differentiation, carcinoma showing thymus-like differentiation, salivary type tumours of the thyroid, squamous cell carcinoma or primary thyroid lymphoma. Metastatic tumours to the thyroid gland are an important differential diagnosis as these are identified in 1.4–3.0% of suspected thyroid cancer patients [3]. Parathyroid carcinoma and other head and neck tumours may also involve the thyroid.

The molecular pathology of thyroid cancer and its clinical applications are reviewed in much greater detail elsewhere [4, 5]. Thyroid tumours are thought to arise as a result of multiple mutational events. Diagnostic molecular methods for thyroid nodules ideally should take account of the wide differential diagnosis of thyroid nodules; follicular and papillary carcinoma, poorly differentiated and anaplastic carcinoma, medullary carcinoma, and other tumours which may involve

D. N. Poller
Department of Pathology, University of Portsmouth, Portsmouth, UK

Queen Alexandra Hospital, Portsmouth, UK
e-mail: david.poller@porthosp.nhs.uk

U. K. Mallick et al. (eds.), *Practical Management of Thyroid Cancer*,
https://doi.org/10.1007/978-3-319-91725-2_5

the thyroid region such as parathyroid carcinoma. Other approaches include assessment of TSHR mRNA as a molecular test for thyroid cancer particularly for recurrent thyroid cancer [6] and proteomic profiling [7].

Papillary Thyroid Carcinoma

Papillary thyroid carcinoma is the commonest type of thyroid carcinoma occurring in 85% or so of cases in modern series. Papillary thyroid carcinoma morphologically is divided into classical type papillary carcinoma and variants of classical type papillary carcinoma (tall cell, columnar cell, diffuse sclerosing, Warthin-like) and follicular variant of papillary thyroid carcinoma. Classical type papillary carcinoma shows somatic mutations in the mitogen activated protein kinase (*MAPK*) pathway with activations occurring due to *RAS* or *BRAF* mutations, or re-arrangements of *RET* or *NTRK1*. Papillary carcinomas usually show single mutations, with either *BRAF* mutations in 40–45%, *RET/PTC* rearrangements in 10–20% and *RAS* point mutations in 10–20% (Table 5.1) [8]. The prognosis of papillary thyroid carcinoma if the tumour is small and localised to the thyroid gland is typically excellent although larger tumours or tumours showing extrathyroidal extension or lymphatic or vascular invasion have adverse prognosis. Tumours with multiple gene mutations, e.g. *BRAF* V600E and *TERT* promoter, *PIK3CA*, *AKT1*, *TP53* mutations in addition to *BRAF* V600E mutation alone have been shown to predict adverse prognosis (Fig. 5.1) [9–14].

Follicular Variant of Papillary Thyroid Carcinoma (FVPTC)

FVPTC typically shows a genotype more similar to that of follicular carcinoma and follicular adenoma [8, 15] with *RAS* mutations, *BRAF* K601E mutations, and *PAX8/PPARG* rearrangements which are common in follicular carcinomas and rare in classical papillary thyroid carcinoma (Table 5.1 and Fig. 5.2).

Table 5.1 Mutational profiles seen in thyroid tumours

Mutation(s)	Follicular adenoma	NIFTP	eFVPTC	Follicular carcinoma	Classical papillary carcinoma	Anaplastic carcinoma
BRAF V600E					+++	++
BRAF K601E		+	+++	+		
NRAS	++	++	+++	++		+
HRAS	++	++	++	+		
KRAS	++	+	++	+	+	
PTEN	++			+		+
TSHR	++			+		
GNAS	++					
Gene fusions						
RET/PTC					++	
PAX8/PPARG		++	++	++		
ALK fusions					+	++
BRAF fusions					+	
ETV6/NTRK3					++	
NTRK1/3 fusion					+	

Note that the profiles of follicular adenoma and NIFTP overlap considerably with encapsulated follicular variant of papillary carcinoma and follicular carcinoma (follicular mutational group) with classical type papillary carcinoma showing a different mutational profile with *BRAF* V600E mutation among other mutations

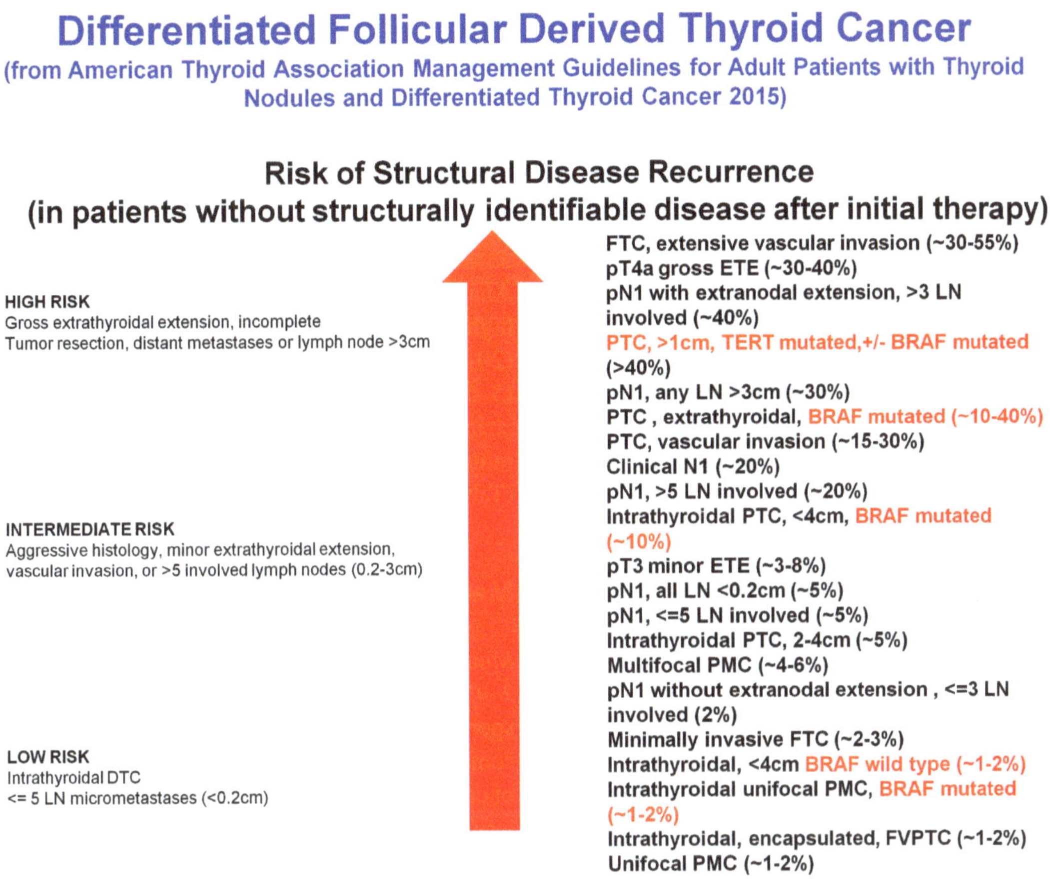

Fig. 5.1 Illustration based on the 2015 American Thyroid Association management guidelines for adult patients with thyroid nodules and differentiated thyroid carcinoma; risk of structural disease recurrence in patients without structural identifiable disease after initial therapy. Note that molecular profiling; *BRAF* V600E mutation and TERT promoter mutation can be used to prognostically profile thyroid nodules

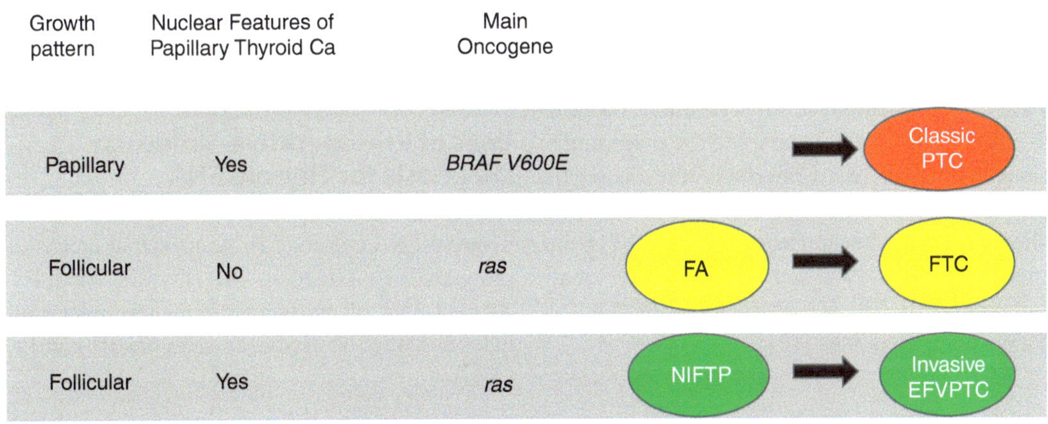

Fig. 5.2 Putative molecular pathogenic pathway for thyroid tumours, note that classical type papillary carcinoma is typically *BRAF* V600E driven, whereas follicular adenoma, follicular thyroid carcinoma and NIFTP are *ras* driven lesions

NIFTP Tumours

Recently a subset of follicular papillary thyroid carcinomas comprising approximately 20% of all newly diagnosed thyroid cancers in North America previously diagnosed as non-invasive or circumscribed encapsulated follicular variant of papillary carcinoma has now been re-designated as a much lower risk tumour entity, *'the non-invasive follicular thyroid neoplasm with papillary like nuclei—NIFTP'*. These tumours based on the data available appear to have very low risk of recurrence and are therefore no longer recognised or designated as carcinomas. NIFTP tumours show a phenotype similar to that of follicular carcinomas with absence of *BRAF* V600E mutations and presence of *RAS* mutations, *PAX8/PPARG* translocations and *THADA* fusions (Table 5.1 and Fig. 5.2) [16].

Follicular Thyroid Carcinoma

Follicular carcinomas of the thyroid are the second most common type of thyroid cancer, accounting for around 10% or less of thyroid carcinomas diagnosed in modern series [17]. *BRAF* V600E mutations are very unusual in follicular carcinoma although *BRAF* K601E mutations may occur. Follicular thyroid carcinoma shows a molecular phenotype similar to that of follicular adenoma with mutations seen in *NRAS*, *HRAS*, and *KRAS* genes in approximately 40–50% of cases (Table 5.1). *PAX8/PPARG* rearrangement is also common occurring in 30–35% of cases, *PTEN* point mutations or small deletions occur in 5–10% or so of cases, and *PIK3CA* point mutations in 5–10% [8]. Conversely the oncocytic (Hurthle cell) subtype of follicular carcinoma shows a much lower frequency of *RAS* point mutations (10–15%) and *PAX8/PPARG* rearrangements (0–5%) and absence of *PIK3CA* and PTEN point mutations [18].

Poorly Differentiated Carcinoma and Anaplastic Carcinoma

Poorly differentiated carcinoma is a rare subtype of tumour accounting for 1% or less of thyroid tumours characterised by mutations of *RAS* in around 30%, *BRAF* in 15% with mutations of TP 53 and β-catenin in around 25–30% of cases. Anaplastic carcinoma typically tends to show high frequencies of *RAS* (20–40%), *BRAF* V600E (20–40%), *TP53* (50–80%) and beta-catenin (5–60%) mutations. Anaplastic carcinoma is also characterised by *PIK3CA*, *PTEN*, *AKT1* and *APC* mutations, and fusions of *ALK* and other genes (Table 5.1) [8, 19].

Medullary Thyroid Carcinoma

Medullary carcinoma accounts approximately 2–4% of thyroid malignancies, most cases are sporadic, familial cases are inherited in an autosomal dominant pattern and accounts for 15–30% of cases, MEN 2A, MEN 2B, and familial medullary thyroid carcinoma. Medullary carcinoma is characterised by *RET/PTC* translocations in over 95% of cases [8]. Familial medullary carcinomas are associated with gain of function mutations in the *RET* gene. Somatic *RET* mutations may occur in 30–60% of sporadic medullary carcinomas. *RAS* mutations also occur in sporadic medullary carcinomas and evidence suggests that these are non-overlapping mutations with *RET* and *RAS* gene mutations [20].

Uses of Pre-operative Molecular Diagnosis for Thyroid FNA

Thyroid FNA cytology is the principal means of preoperative diagnosis of thyroid nodules. Around 25% of thyroid aspirates are indeterminate; classified as Bethesda category III and IV, (in the United Kingdom broadly equivalent to Thy3a and Thy3F) with a published risk of malignancy ranging from 5% to 30%. A diagnostic test may function as either a 'rule-in' or a 'rule-out' test for malignancy. The performance of the test depends on the positive predictive value (PPV) and the negative predictive value (NPV). PPV and NPV depend on the pre-test probability of malignancy in any given sample and therefore individual institutional rates of malignancy for the relevant FNA category.

Afirma

The *Afirma Gene Expression Classifer* (Veracyte, South San Francisco, USA) uses microarray technology to assess mRNA profiles of cytologically indeterminate nodules [21]. It requires two dedicated passes to be collected into vial of RNA preservative in addition to FNA passes for routine cytology. The GEC test is most useful for patients with indeterminate FNA's with no other reason to operate, e.g. larger nodule size, patient preference, or symptomatic goitre. Except for a few academic centres the manufacturer requires the cytology specimen to be interpreted in a centralised cytology laboratory. An initial panel of six 'cassettes' comprising 25 genes screens for expression profiles of less common entities in the thyroid such as metastatic lesions, parathyroid tissue, medullary thyroid carcinoma and oncocytic lesions. The main gene expression classifer comprises a 142 gene mRNA panel, and both parts compose 167 gene *Afirma* test. If one of the six preliminary screening cassettes is triggered the sample is automatically reported as a 'suspicious' gene expression profile without further analysis by the main gene expression classifer—for example medullary thyroid carcinoma would be flagged in the report as having a positive *Afirma* test. This test was validated in a blinded prospective multicentre trial of 265 nodules with indeterminate cytology and histological follow-up [21]. The current practice in centres using *Afirma* is to use it as a 'rule-out' test for indeterminate thyroid nodules, Bethesda class III and IV, and if the GEC result is benign the risk of malignancy based on published series is around 5–6%. A meta-analysis of seven studies confirms the value of GEC as a rule-out test showing a pooled sensitivity of 95.7% and pooled specificity of 30.5% [22]. For aspirates suspicious for malignancy the negative predictive value is around 85%, with the validation study showing a low positive predictive value for malignancy among the cytologically indeterminate nodules, 38% for Bethesda category III and 37% for Bethesda category IV. For nodules with a pre-test probability of malignancy below 25% the high NPV of a benign GEC result reduces the risk of malignancy to range of 5–6% which is comparable to that of a benign aspirate. Given this level of risk a patient can be managed by watchful waiting with ultrasound monitoring. For a category IV FNA a benign GEC test result removes the need for surgery, although for category III FNA as the management of these lesions does not necessarily require surgery there may be no benefit in performing the GEC test. Subsequent studies of the GEC show very few carcinomas in a few cases that have undergone excision after a benign GEC diagnosis. In 2015 Nishino [23] reported that 31 of 363 (8.5%) benign GEC cases in the literature had undergone surgery with only three benign GEC cases found to be histologically malignant; a 6 mm papillary carcinoma, a 32 mm follicular carcinoma and a 28 mm cystic papillary carcinoma. The risk of malignancy for a suspicious GEC result is lower for aspirates with oncocytic cytology [23]. In 2014 Veracyte added the malignancy classifiers—Afirma MTC and Afirma BRAF, both of these are mRNA classifiers, the identification of the gene expression signature of medullary thyroid carcinoma [24] and BRAF adds to this test. The Afirma BRAF test sensitivity and specificity is comparable to PCR reaction based tests for *BRAF* V600E mutations [25].

Mutational Tests

The molecular pathology of thyroid cancer is now comparatively well documented so it is feasible to use a variety of approaches for molecular testing ranging from simple single gene *BRAF* V600E testing to a comprehensive mutational panel test as both a rule-out and a rule-in test for cancer in thyroid nodules. *BRAF* V600E is >99% specific for diagnosis of thyroid cancer. The author implemented reflex testing for *BRAF* V600E for higher-risk fine-needle aspirates 4 years ago in Portsmouth, UK. *BRAF* V600E testing is comparatively easy to implement, but is only useful for higher risk FNA's where nuclear features of papillary carcinoma are suspected but the cytological diagnosis remains uncertain with a diagnosis of Thy3F or Thy4 (equivalent to Bethesda category IV or V) when a confident diagnosis of malignancy cannot be made. In these cases companion testing for *BRAF* V600E using a PCR technique will identify *BRAF* V600E mutations in 40–50% of Thy4 FNA's (equivalent to Bethesda Category V). The results achieved in Portsmouth, UK, are comparable to those of a meta-analysis of 47 studies of *BRAF* V600E testing of FNA cytology specimens showing a pooled sensitivity for *BRAF* V600E testing in thyroid FNA of 52% (95% CI 39–64%) [26]. Sensitivity when reported in individual studies was 100% but pooled sensitivity for indeterminate FNA (category III–V) in the six studies where this could be calculated was 31% (95% CI, 6–56%) [26]. *BRAF* V600E testing is also useful because NIFTP tumours, which are follicular derived *RAS* driven thyroid lesions never show *BRAF* V600E mutations and so confirmation of the presence of a *BRAF* V600E mutation can be used to exclude a NIFTP tumour in a higher risk thyroid FNA. The *American Thyroid Association Statement on Application of Molecular Profiling for Thyroid Nodules: Current Impact on Perioperative Decision Making* has recently reviewed the role of perioperative molecular profiling [27]. This document discusses some of the advantages and problems of molecular testing in the thyroid, including a discussion of the Seven Gene Test, The Afirma Gene Classifier and ThyroSeq2 [27]. Mutational testing is evolving from a simple system using a single mutational marker (*BRAF* V600E) via seven gene panels (*BRAF* V600E, *HRAS*, *KRAS*, *NRAS*, *RET/PTC* and *PAX8/PPARG* translocations) to next generation sequencing panels such as ThyroSeq [11, 28, 29]. The ThyroSeq v2 panel uses NGS for the simultaneous analysis of multiple genes in a cost-effective and high-throughput manner. The panel includes mutations and gene fusions from the seven-gene panel as well as additional genes that have been implicated in thyroid cancer. Overall, ThyroSeq v2 tests for point mutations and small insertions/deletions in 14 genes, 42 types of gene fusions, and expression levels of 16 genes. The ThyroSeq v2 panel can additionally detect mutations in *RET* which are seen in medullary thyroid carcinoma. *TERT* promoter mutation is an important alteration also present in the ThyroSeq v2 panel. These mutations, while occuring in well-differentiated papillary thyroid and follicular carcinomas, are also present at increased frequency in aggressive tumours such as poorly differentiated carcinoma, anaplastic thyroid carcinoma, and widely invasive oncocytic carcinoma [6–9]. Furthermore, studies have found an association of *TERT* promoter mutation with increased risk for distant metastases, persistent disease, and cancer-specific mortality (Fig. 5.1) [9]. This marker offers not only diagnostic, but also prognostic information. In addition, the ThyroSeq v2 panel also includes *TP53*, *PIK3CA*, and *AKT1* genes, which are also associated with aggressive behaviour and tumour progression, particularly when found in combination with early driver events like *BRAF* or *RAS* [10–17]. The list of gene fusions is also extended beyond the most common *RET/PTC1*, *RET/PTC3*, and *PAX8-PPARG* fusions to include additional fusions involving *RET*, *BRAF*, *NTRK1* and *3*, *ALK*, and other genes. In addition to the primary diagnostic markers, gene expression markers are used to assess the quality of samples, and specifically the

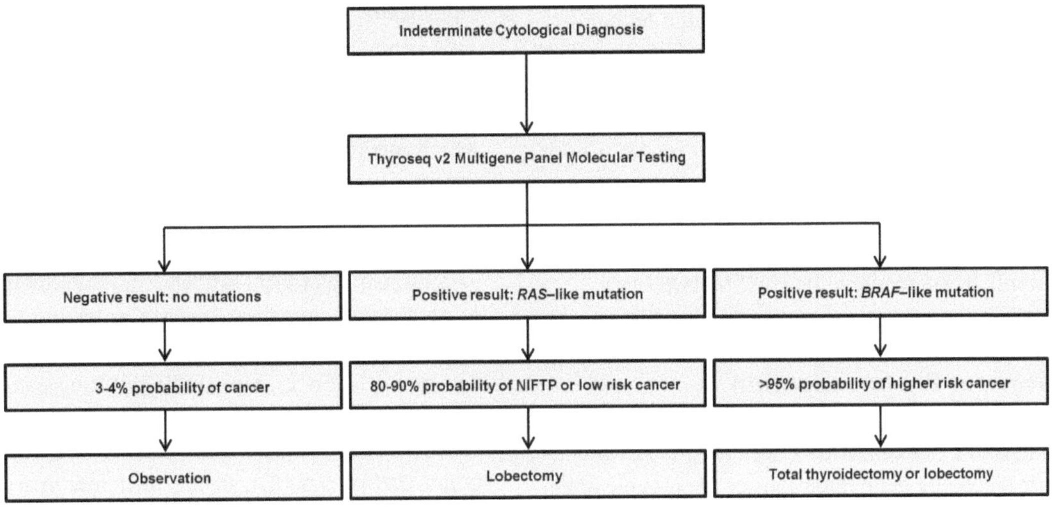

Fig. 5.3 Example of a decision tree algorithm for management of indeterminate thyroid FNA using a next-generation multigene panel ThyroSeq2 based on Nikiforov YE, JAMA Oncol. 2016 Aug 1;2(8):1098–9. doi: 10.1001/jamaoncol.2016.2205

proportion of thyroid follicular cells, and also the expression of the calcitonin and parathyroid hormone genes, which helps to diagnose medullary thyroid carcinoma and parathyroid lesions.

ThyroSeq v2 assesses cancer probability in a given thyroid nodule based on a specific mutated or fused gene, mutation hotspot, and proportion of cells carrying the mutation or multiple mutations. The performance of ThyroSeq v2 was initially validated in a single institution, combined retrospective and prospective study of 143 FN/SFN cytology thyroid nodules [28]. Results from this study showed overall very good performance with a specificity of 93%, sensitivity of 90%, PPV of 83% and NPV of 96% [28]. In a follow-up, single institution, prospective study of 465 AUS/FLUS thyroid nodules, similar good performance of the assay was seen, with sensitivity of 90.9%, specificity of 92.1%, PPV of 76.9%, and NPV of 97.2% [29].

The type(s) and combination(s) of mutations detected by ThyroSeq not only predict the probability of cancer, but also estimate the cancer aggressiveness, offering additional information to inform the surgical approach and other aspects of patient management. The finding of a *RAS* or *RAS*-like mutation predicts a high probability (~80%) of either low-risk cancer or NIFTP (Fig. 5.3). In many situations, the surgical approach for these patients may be limited to a lobectomy. The test positivity for isolated *BRAF* V600E or other *BRAF* V600E-like mutations confers a very high (>99%) probability of cancer, which is expected to be of intermediate risk for disease recurrence. These patients may undergo total thyroidectomy or lobectomy, depending on specific clinical situation (Fig. 5.3). ThyroSeq positivity for multiple mutations or high-risk mutations such as TERT is virtually diagnostic of cancer and an increased risk of disease recurrence and possibly cancer-related mortality. Therefore, these patients would benefit from total thyroidectomy.

As the number of genes in the panel increases so does the cost, the complexity of interpretation and the informatics required. A recently published *Template for Reporting Results of Biomarker Testing for Patients with Suspected Thyroid Carcinoma* produced by the College of American Pathologists gives a series of practical explanatory notes on the clinical significance of identified mutations of *BRAF* V600E, *RAS, PIK3 A, AKT1, TP53, CTNNB1, RET, ALK, NTRK1, NTRK3 and PPARG* [30]. Five to ten percent of thyroid cancers do not appear to have a specifically identifiable driver gene mutations that can be identified using existing molecular techniques and there is an overlap in the mutational profiles of benign and malignant thyroid lesions. The overlap of mutational profiles of benign and malignant lesions is particularly a problem with follicular lesions as follicular adenoma and follicular carcinoma as both may show identical point *RAS* gene mutations and much less commonly translocations for *PAX8/PPARG.*

Tumour Prognostication

Thyroid FNA can be used as a prognostic indicator if specific gene mutations or phenotypic alterations can be identified. While *BRAF* V600E mutation alone may confer slightly adverse prognosis in any given case, the adverse effect of this mutation alone is small [31] although recent evidence indicates that a combination(s) of *BRAF* V600E mutation with other gene mutations e.g. *BRAF* V600E and TERT promoter mutation, or coexistent mutations of *BRAF* V600E and *TP53, PIK3CA, AKT1 or ALK* fusions conveys significant adverse prognosis (Fig. 5.1) [9, 10, 14] all of which can be identified using multigene next-generation sequencing panels [29].

Tumour Therapy

Although there is much literature now on the use of *RAF* kinase inhibitors in iodine refractory thyroid cancer the published studies as far appear to show no particular benefit in preoperative testing for *BRAF* V600E in patients prior to therapy. The reason for this is not totally clear but is most likely related to the fact that the kinase inhibitor efficacy pathways are multifactorial and not solely depending on *BRAF* V600E mutation alone. *ALK* fusions are documented as single driver mutations in a small proportion of thyroid cancers and anecdotal evidence suggests that iodine refractory tumours that show *ALK* fusions may respond to drugs such as crizotinib. This effect has been shown in both in anaplastic thyroid cancer [32] and also in medullary thyroid carcinoma [20].

Conclusion

This chapter briefly summarises some of the existing molecular techniques for diagnosis, prognosis, and therapy of thyroid cancer which are relevant to pathologists. The field continues to evolve. The difficult issues appear to be the complexity and cost of the technology and the validation of the datasets required to demonstrate clinical efficacy. In other areas of pathology companion molecular testing to guide targeted therapy is now commonplace e.g. breast (*HER* 2), non-small cell lung cancer (*EGFR, ALK & KRAS*), colorectal cancer (*TP53, KRAS, NRAS, PIK3CA*), and melanoma (*BRAF* V600E). In the next few years molecular testing of thyroid FNA will also become much more widespread, specifically for diagnosis of indeterminate thyroid nodules, and as a tool for guiding targeted drug therapies.

Acknowledgement The author is grateful to Prof Y. Nikiforov for critical advice in the preparation of this article and for the section discussing *ThyroSeq2*.

References

1. Cancer Genome Atlas Research Network. Integrated genomic characterization of papillary thyroid carcinoma. Cell. 2014;159(3):676–90.
2. Goodwin S, McPherson JD, McCombie WR. Coming of age: ten years of next-generation sequencing technologies. Nat Rev Genet. 2016;17(6):333–51.
3. Chung AY, Tran TB, Brumund KT, Weisman RA, Bouvet M. Metastases to the thyroid: a review of the literature from the last decade. Thyroid. 2012;22(3):258–68.
4. Nikiforov YE, Biddinger PW, Thompson LDR. Diagnostic pathology and molecular genetics of the thyroid. 2nd ed. Philadelphia: Lippincott Williams and Wilkins; 2012.
5. Fagin JA, Wells SA Jr. Biologic and clinical perspectives on thyroid cancer. N Engl J Med. 2016;375(11):1054–67.
6. Milas M, Shin J, Gupta M, Novosel T, Nasr C, Brainard J, et al. Circulating thyrotropin receptor mRNA as a novel marker of thyroid cancer: clinical applications learned from 1758 samples. Ann Surg. 2010;252(4):643–51.
7. Krause K, Jessnitzer B, Fuhrer D. Proteomics in thyroid tumor research. J Clin Endocrinol Metab. 2009;94(8):2717–24.

8. Nikiforov YE, Nikiforova MN. Molecular genetics and diagnosis of thyroid cancer. Nat Rev Endocrinol. 2011;7(10):569–80.
9. Liu X, Qu S, Liu R, Sheng C, Shi X, Zhu G, et al. *TERT* promoter mutations and their association with *BRAF* V600E mutation and aggressive clinicopathological characteristics of thyroid cancer. J Clin Endocrinol Metab. 2014;99(6):E1130–6.
10. Melo M, da Rocha AG, Vinagre J, Batista R, Peixoto J, Tavares C, et al. *TERT* promoter mutations are a major indicator of poor outcome in differentiated thyroid carcinomas. J Clin Endocrinol Metab. 2014;99(5):E754–65.
11. Nikiforova MN, Wald AI, Roy S, Durso MB, Nikiforov YE. Targeted next-generation sequencing panel (ThyroSeq) for detection of mutations in thyroid cancer. J Clin Endocrinol Metab. 2013;98(11):E1852–60.
12. Ricarte-Filho JC, Ryder M, Chitale DA, Rivera M, Heguy A, Ladanyi M, et al. Mutational profile of advanced primary and metastatic radioactive iodine-refractory thyroid cancers reveals distinct pathogenetic roles for *BRAF*, *PIK3CA*, and *AKT1*. Cancer Res. 2009;69(11):4885–93.
13. Xing M, Clark D, Guan H, Ji M, Dackiw A, Carson KA, et al. *BRAF* mutation testing of thyroid fine-needle aspiration biopsy specimens for preoperative risk stratification in papillary thyroid cancer. J Clin Oncol. 2009;27(18):2977–82.
14. Xing M, Liu R, Liu X, Murugan AK, Zhu G, Zeiger MA, et al. *BRAF* V600E and *TERT* promoter mutations cooperatively identify the most aggressive papillary thyroid cancer with highest recurrence. J Clin Oncol. 2014;32(25):2718–26.
15. Xu B, Ghossein R. Encapsulated thyroid carcinoma of follicular cell origin. Endocr Pathol. 2015;26(3):191–9.
16. Nikiforov YE, Seethala RR, Tallini G, Baloch ZW, Basolo F, Thompson LD, et al. Nomenclature revision for encapsulated follicular variant of papillary thyroid carcinoma: a paradigm shift to reduce overtreatment of indolent tumors. JAMA Oncol. 2016;2(8):1023–9.
17. Sobrinho-Simoes M, Eloy C, Magalhaes J, Lobo C, Amaro T. Follicular thyroid carcinoma. Mod Pathol. 2011;24(Suppl 2):S10–8.
18. Nikiforov YE, Ohori NP. Follicular carcinoma. In: Nikiforov YE, Biddinger PW, Thompson LDR, editors. Diagnostic molecular pathology and molecular genetics of the thyroid. 2nd ed. Philadelphia: Wolters Kluwer; 2012.
19. Xu B, Ghossein R. Genomic landscape of poorly differentiated and anaplastic thyroid carcinoma. Endocr Pathol. 2016;27(3):205–12.
20. Ji JH, Oh YL, Hong M, Yun JW, Lee HW, Kim D, et al. Identification of driving ALK fusion genes and genomic landscape of medullary thyroid Cancer. PLoS Genet. 2015;11(8):e1005467.
21. Alexander EK, Kennedy GC, Baloch ZW, Cibas ES, Chudova D, Diggans J, et al. Preoperative diagnosis of benign thyroid nodules with indeterminate cytology. N Engl J Med. 2012;367(8):705–15.
22. Santhanam P, Khthir R, Gress T, Elkadry A, Olajide O, Yaqub A, et al. Gene expression classifier for the diagnosis of indeterminate thyroid nodules: a meta-analysis. Med Oncol. 2016;33(2):14.
23. Nishino M. Molecular cytopathology for thyroid nodules: a review of methodology and test performance. Cancer Cytopathol. 2016;124(1):14–27.
24. Kloos RT, Monroe RJ, Traweek ST, Lanman RB, Kennedy GC. A genomic alternative to identify medullary thyroid cancer preoperatively in thyroid nodules with indeterminate cytology. Thyroid. 2016;26(6):785–93.
25. Diggans J, Kim SY, Hu Z, Pankratz D, Wong M, Reynolds J, et al. Machine learning from concept to clinic: reliable detection of *BRAF* V600E DNA mutations in thyroid nodules using high-dimensional RNA expression data. Pac Symp Biocomput. 2015;2015:371–82.
26. Fnais N, Soobiah C, Al-Qahtani K, Hamid JS, Perrier L, Straus SE, et al. Diagnostic value of fine needle aspiration *BRAF* (V600E) mutation analysis in papillary thyroid cancer: a systematic review and meta-analysis. Hum Pathol. 2015;46(10):1443–54.
27. Ferris RL, Baloch Z, Bernet V, Chen A, Fahey TJ 3rd, Ganly I, et al. American Thyroid Association statement on surgical application of molecular profiling for thyroid nodules: current impact on perioperative decision making. Thyroid. 2015;25(7):760–8.
28. Nikiforov YE, Carty SE, Chiosea SI, Coyne C, Duvvuri U, Ferris RL, et al. Highly accurate diagnosis of cancer in thyroid nodules with follicular neoplasm/suspicious for a follicular neoplasm cytology by ThyroSeq v2 next-generation sequencing assay. Cancer. 2014;120(23):3627–34.
29. Nikiforov YE, Carty SE, Chiosea SI, Coyne C, Duvvuri U, Ferris RL, et al. Impact of the multigene ThyroSeq next-generation sequencing assay on cancer diagnosis in thyroid nodules with atypia of undetermined significance/follicular lesion of undetermined significance cytology. Thyroid. 2015;25(11):1217–23.
30. Chiosea S, Asa SL, Berman MA, Carty SE, Currence L, Hodak S, et al. Template for reporting results of biomarker testing of specimens from patients with thyroid carcinoma. Arch Pathol Lab Med. 2016;141(4):559–63.
31. Xing M, Alzahrani AS, Carson KA, Shong YK, Kim TY, Viola D, et al. Association between *BRAF* V600E mutation and recurrence of papillary thyroid cancer. J Clin Oncol. 2015;33(1):42–50.
32. Godbert Y, Henriques de Figueiredo B, Bonichon F, Chibon F, Hostein I, Perot G, et al. Remarkable response to crizotinib in woman with anaplastic lymphoma kinase-rearranged anaplastic thyroid carcinoma. J Clin Oncol. 2015;33(20):e84–7.

6 Ultrasonography in Diagnosis and Management of Thyroid Cancer: Current International Recommendations

Dong Gyu Na, Ji-hoon Kim, and Eun Ju Ha

The management of thyroid nodules has become a matter of debate worldwide with the increasing incidence of thyroid carcinomas. The rate of detection of thyroid carcinoma has increased with the widespread use of ultrasonography (US) for its diagnosis [1]. With the technological advance of US machines, high resolution US has been used for the neck and thyroid gland using a high frequency (>10-MHz) linear probe, which increases the detection of small lesions and provides detailed characterization of thyroid nodules and cervical lymph nodes. The role of US has become increasingly important for assessing malignancy risk, fine-needle aspiration (FNA) decision, and management decision after FNA in patients with thyroid nodules. US also has an essential role for preoperative staging of primary tumor and cervical lymph nodes and for postoperative surveillance in patients with thyroid cancer.

Recently, the role of US has been further emphasized for the personalized management of patients with thyroid nodules. Many international society guidelines have been recently updated for a more personalized management strategy. This chapter documents the evidence-based consensus and debatable issues of recently updated international society guidelines regarding the role of US in the diagnosis and management of thyroid cancer, which include current guidelines of the American Thyroid Association (ATA), American Association of Clinical Endocrinologist/American College of Endocrinology/Associazione Medici Endocrinologi (AACE/ACE/AME), British Thyroid Association (BTA), National Comprehensive Cancer Network (NCCN), Korean Thyroid Association/Korean Society of Thyroid Radiology (KTA/KSThR), American College of Radiology (ACR), and European Thyroid Association (ETA) [2–10].

US-based Risk Stratification of Thyroid Nodules

Various international societies have developed risk stratification systems for thyroid nodules to provide practitioners with evidence-based recommendations [2–10]. Many studies, including meta-analyses and multicenter studies, have consistently reported that several US features are strongly associated with thyroid cancer [11–17]. Recent international society guidelines have proposed US-based risk stratification systems for the management of thyroid nodules.

D. G. Na (✉)
Department of Radiology, GangNeung Asan Hospital, Gangneung-si, Gangwon-do, South Korea

J.-h. Kim
Department of Radiology, Seoul National University Hospital, Seoul National University College of Medicine, Seoul, South Korea

E. J. Ha
Department of Radiology, Ajou University School of Medicine, Suwon, South Korea

U. K. Mallick et al. (eds.), *Practical Management of Thyroid Cancer*,
https://doi.org/10.1007/978-3-319-91725-2_6

US Lexicon and US Features Predictive of Malignancy

The US lexicon for nodule characterization has been described in many literatures; several international groups/societies have proposed consensus statements of US lexicon for a standardized reporting [8, 18–20]. However, although the major US lexicons have found wide acceptance, the US terminology for thyroid nodules has not yet been standardized.

The major US lexicons for thyroid nodules include composition (or internal content), echogenicity, shape (shape and orientation), margin, calcifications (or echogenic foci), spongiform, and size. Both vascularity and elastography may also be useful in the differential diagnosis of thyroid nodules; however, the contributions of such data remain controversial. Nodular composition, defined as the ratio of the cystic to the solid portion, is categorized as solid (pure solid or nearly entirely solid with <10% of the cystic portion), predominantly solid (≤50% of the cystic portion), predominantly cystic (>50% of the cystic portion) and cystic (pure cyst or nearly entirly cystic with >90% of the cystic portion) [2, 8–10]. Thyroid cancers are mostly solid (84.8–95.1%); the malignancy risk of solid nodules is higher (16.6–35.4%) than that of partially cystic nodules (4–7.3%) [15–17].

Nodule echogenicity is that of the solid component and is categorized relative to that of reference structures (the thyroid parenchyma and strap muscles) as markedly hypoechoic (relative to the strap muscle); mildly hypoechoic (relative to the thyroid parenchyma); isoechoic (same echogenicity as the thyroid parenchyma); and hyperechoic (relative to the thyroid parenchyma). The reported echogenicity is generally the predominant echogenicity when the solid component is heterogeneous. However, the presence of any hypoechoic tissue classifies the nodule as a hypoechoic nodule and intermediate risk at ETA guideline [10]. Thyroid cancers are generally mildly or markedly hypoechoic (76.9–94.0%), and the risk of malignancy of hypoechoic nodules is higher (16.7–60.7%) than that of isohyperechoic nodules (3.7–8.5%) [15–17]. The malignancy risk increases as nodule echogenicity decreases [15–17].

A nodule is defined as taller than wide shape or nonparallel orientation, when the anteroposterior diameter of a nodule is longer than its transverse on a transverse plane [2, 6, 9] or when the anteroposterior diameter of a nodule is longer than its transverse or longitudinal diameter on a transverse or longitudinal plane [8, 21]. This US feature is highly suggestive of malignancy, associated with a specificity of 88.2–98.7% and a positive predictive value of 65.3–77.5% [14–16]. Nodule margins are categorized as smooth, spiculated (irregular or infiltrative), microlobulated (lobulated), or ill-defined. A smooth or ill-defined margin is not specific for either benign or malignant nodules. The spiculated (irregular) or microlobulated (lobulated) margin is highly specific and predictive of malignancy, with a specificity of 91.8–98.4% and a positive predictive value of 32.1–86.7% [14–17].

Calcifications are categorized as microcalcifications (punctuate echogenic foci ≤1 mm in diameter); macrocalcifications (echogenic foci >1 mm in diameter with posterior acoustic shadowing); and rim calcifications (peripheral curvilinear or eggshell calcifications). Microcalcification evident on US (punctate hyperechoic foci) has been reported to be both specific and predictive of malignancy, with a specificity of 84.4–92.4% and a positive predictive value of 26.5–77.9% [14–17]. Although microcalcification has been widely used to describe punctate echogenic foci within the solid portion of a nodule, such foci can be manifested by colloid materials within a benign nodule and by psammomatous microcalcifications of thyroid cancer. Punctate echogenic foci in the wall of the cystic space are frequently found in benign nodules, and nonshadowing linear echogenic foci are generally present in benign nodules [22]. Intracystic echogenic foci with comet tail artifacts are found exclusively in benign nodules [22, 23]. Macrocalcification slightly increases the risk of malignancy [14–16], but seems not an independent predictor for malignancy [15, 16]. The malignancy risk of isolated macrocalcification may be low to intermediate [24, 25], but lacking sufficient data, and peripheral or rim calcifications are not significantly associated with malignancy [14–16].

A spongiform (honeycomb) appearance is a typical US feature of benign nodules [26], it is generally defined as an aggregation of multiple microcystic components in >50% of the nodule [3, 8, 14, 20]. A nodule exhibiting multiple microcystic spaces separated by thin septa or isoechoic parenchyma can be regarded as benign; the specificity is 99.7–100% [14–16]. Therefore, isoechoic spongiform nodule was proposed for the lexicon of spongiform appearance to enhance the specificity for benignity [3, 8]. As the extent of intranodular vascularity is variable in both benign and malignant tumors [27–29], the ATA, KTA/KSThR, ACR, and ETA guidelines do not include the vascularity pattern in their risk stratifications of thyroid nodules. Also, the added value of US elastography is still controversial.

Nodules should be measured in three dimensions. Although a recent systematic review suggested that larger nodules were associated with a greater pretest risk of malignancy [30], the questions of whether larger nodules are associated with a greater malignancy risk, and whether nodule size predicts malignancy, remain controversial [31, 32]. Nodule growth is not a reliable predictor of malignancy; many benign nodules grow over time [33]. Nodule growth is generally defined when a 20% increase in nodular diameter accompanied by a minimum increase in two or more dimensions of at least 2 mm, or an increase >50% of nodule volume, is apparent [2].

In summary, solid composition and hypoechogenicity are highly sensitive predictors of malignancy (>80%), associated with low-to-intermediate specificities (27–46% and 52–72%, respectively) [14–17]. The microcalcification, spiculated/microlobulated (irregular) margin, and a taller-than-wide shape (nonparallel orientation) are strongly predictive of malignancy, with a high specificity (>80%) and a low-to-intermediate sensitivity (15–50%) [14–17]. The predictive values of such suspicious US features are dependent on composition and echogenicity of nodules [15–17]. Although all suspicious US features were independent predictors of malignancy with a high malignancy risk (>70%) in solid hypoechoic nodules, the malignancy risks of microcalcification and taller-than-wide shape (nonparallel orientation) were only low-to-intermediate (10–30%) in partially cystic or isohyperechoic nodules [15, 16]. Partially cystic or isohyperechoic nodules rarely have spiculated/microlobulated (irregular) margins [15, 16].

US-based Risk Stratification System

Although several US features are strongly predictive of malignancy, no single feature affords both high sensitivity and specificity. As the malignancy risk of a thyroid nodule cannot be determined by a single US feature, most international guidelines utilize US-based risk stratification systems devised using a pattern-based approach, thus employing combinations of US features [2–8, 10] (Table 6.1).

The risk stratification systems of the ATA, BTA, and KTA/KSThR guidelines focus on US patterns created principally by combinations of composition, echogenicity, and US features predictive of malignant or benign status [2, 4, 8]. The ATA and KTA/KSThR guidelines propose the use of five- and four-tier risk stratification systems yielding malignancy risk values for each category of thyroid nodules. These suggested malignancy risks were well-correlated in large population-based studies; however, some nodules did not meet the criteria for any specific pattern of the ATA guidelines (for example, an isohyperechoic nodule with any suspicious US feature). Such an unclassified US pattern may be associated with an intermediate (18.2–19%) malignancy risk based on the data of previous studies [34, 35]. In the KTA/KSThR risk stratification system, the malignancy risks are stratified by the Thyroid Imaging Reporting and Data System (TIRADS) by solidity, echogenicity, and three suspicious US features. Although the BTA guidelines propose the use of a similar four-tier risk stratification system, termed the U-score, these guidelines do not yield malignancy risks for each category of nodules. The AACE/ACE/AME guidelines were developed using a simplified three-tier approach in which a high-risk nodule is identified by the presence of any suspicious US feature, regardless of the composition or echogenicity. The ETA guideline proposes a simplified TIRADS mainly based on specific US features for thyroid malignancy and nodule echogenicity. However, the ACR guidelines propose the use of a points-based, five-tier risk, stratification system; a point score (ranging from 0–3) is assigned to each US feature and the values are summed. The

Table 6.1 Risk stratification systems and FNA criteria for thyroid nodules in international society guidelines

Guidelines	Recommendations	Estimated risk of malignancy (%)	FNA size cutoff (nodules ≥1.0 cm)
ATA			
High suspicion	– Solid hypoechoic nodule or solid hypoechoic component of a partially cystic nodule with one or more of the following features: irregular margins (infiltrative, microlobulated), microcalcifications, taller than wide shape, rim calcifications with small extrusive soft tissue component, evidence of extrathyroidal extension	>70–90	≥1.0 cm
Intermediate suspicion	– Hypoechoic solid nodule with smooth margins without microcalcifications, extrathyroidal extension or taller than wide shape	10–20	≥1.0 cm
Low suspicion	– Isoechoic or hyperechoic solid nodule, or partially cystic nodule with eccentric solid areas, without microcalcification, irregular margin or extrathyroidal extension, or taller than wide shape.	5–10	≥1.5 cm
Very low suspicion	– Spongiform or partially cystic nodules without any of the sonographic features described in low, intermediate, or high suspicion patterns	<3	Consider FNA at ≥2.0 cm or observation without FNA
Benign	– Purely cystic nodules (no solid component)	<1	Not indicated
AACE/ACE/AME			
High-risk	– Nodules with at least 1 of the following suspicious features: marked hypoechogenicity, spiculated or microlobulated margins, microcalcifications, taller than wide shape, evidence of extrathyroidal growth or pathologic adenopathy	50–90	≥1.0 cm
Intermediate-risk	– Slightly hypoechoic nodules (cf. surrounding thyroid tissue) and isoechoic nodules with ovoid-to-round shape and smooth or ill-defined margins – Intranodular vascularization, elevated stiffness at elastography, macro- or continuous rim calcifications, or hyperechoic spots of uncertain significance may be present	5–15	>2.0 cm
Low-risk	– Mostly cystic (>50%) nodules with reverberating artifacts that are not associated with suspicious US signs – Isoechoic spongiform nodules confluent or with regular halo	1	>2.0 cm (selective)[a]
BTA[b]			
Malignant (U5)	(a) Solid, hypoechoic, lobulated/irregular outline, microcalcification (b) Solid, hypoechoic, lobulated/irregular outline, globular calcification (c) Intranodular vascularity (d) Shape (tall > wide) (AP > TR) (e) Characteristic associated lymphadenopathy	–	≥1.0 cm
Suspicious (U4)	(a) Solid, hypoechoic (cf thyroid) (b) Solid, very hypoechoic (cf strap muscle) (c) Disrupted peripheral calcification, hypoechoic (d) Lobulated outline	–	≥1.0 cm
Indeterminate/ equivocal (U3)	(a) Homogeneous, hyperechoic (markedly), solid, halo (b) Hypoechoic (?), equivocal echogenic foci, cystic change (c) Mixed/central vascularity	–	≥1.0 cm
Benign (U2)	(a) Halo, isoechoic, mildly hyperechoic (b) Cystic change ± ring-down sign (c) Microcystic/spongiform (d, e) Peripheral eggshell calcification (f) Peripheral vascularity	–	Not indicated
NCCN 2014			
	Solid with suspicious US features[c]	–	≥1.0 cm
	Solid without suspicious US features[c]	–	≥1.5 cm
	Mixed cystic and solid with suspicious US features[c]	–	≥1.5–2.0 cm
	Mixed cystic and solid without suspicious US features[c]	–	≥2.0 cm
	Spongiform nodule	–	≥2.0 cm
	Simple cyst	–	Not indicated

Table 6.1 (continued)

Guidelines	Recommendations	Estimated risk of malignancy (%)	FNA size cutoff (nodules ≥1.0 cm)
KTA/KSThR			
High suspicion (K-TIRADS 5)	– Solid hypoechoic nodule with any of 3 suspicious US features[d]	>60	≥1.0 cm
Intermediate suspicion (K-TIRADS 4)	– Solid hypoechoic nodule without any of 3 suspicious US features[d] – Partially cystic or isohyperechoic nodule with any of 3 suspicious US features[d]	15–50	≥1.0 cm
Low suspicion (K-TIRADS 3)	– Partially cystic or isohyperechoic nodule without any of 3 suspicious US features[d]	3–15	≥1.5 cm
Benign (K-TIRADS 2)	– Spongiform, partially cystic nodule with comet tail artifact, pure cyst	<3	≥2.0 cm (selective)[e]
ACR[f]			
Highly suspicious (TR 5)	7 points or more	>20	≥1.0 cm
Moderately suspicious (TR 4)	4 to 6 points	5–20	≥1.5 cm
Mildly suspicious (TR 3)	3 points	5	≥2.5 cm
Not suspicious (TR 2)	2 points	<2	Not indicated
Benign (TR 1)	0 points	<2	Not indicated
ETA			
High risk (EU-TIRADS 5)	– At least 1 of the following features of high suspicion: irregular shape, irregular margins, microcalcifications, marked hypoechogenicity (and solid)	26–87	>1.0 cm
Intermediate risk[g] (EU-TIRADS 4)	– Ovoid, smooth, mildly hypoechoic, no features of high suspicion	6–17	>1.5 cm
Low risk (EU-TIRADS 3)	– Ovoid, smooth, entirely isoechoic/hyperechoic, no features of high suspicion	2–4	>2.0
Benign (EU-TIRADS 2)	– Pure cyst, entirely spongiform	≅0	Not indicated

Note. *ATA* American Thyroid Association, *AACE/ACE/AME* American Association of Clinical Endocrinologist/American College of Endocrinology/Associazione Medici Endocrinologi, *BTA* British Thyroid Association, *NCCN* National Comprehensive Cancer Network, *KTA/KSThR* Korean Thyroid Association/Korean Society of Thyroid Radiology, *K-TIRADS* Korean Thyroid Imaging Reporting and Data System, *ACR* American College of Radiology, *ETA* European Thyroid Association, *EU-TIRADS* European Union Thyroid Imaging Reporting and Data System, *TR* Thyroid Imaging Reporting and Data System

[a]Not routinely indicated, only when >20 mm and increasing in size or associated with a risk history and before thyroid surgery or minimally invasive ablation therapy

[b]Described US features of each category indicate corresponding US patterns which are described as graphics in the published guideline [4]

[c]Hypoechoic, microcalcifications, increased central vascularity, infiltrative margins, taller than wide in transverse plane

[d]Microcalcification, nonparallel orientation (taller than wide), spiculated/microlobulated margin

[e]Not routinely indicated, FNA may be selectively considered only for a spongiform nodule when the nodule size ≥2 cm, and before ablation therapy

[f]Sum of points assigned for each US feature including composition, echogenicity, shape, margin, and echogenic foci in a nodule

[g]In case of heterogeneous echogenicity of the solid component, the presence of any hypoechoic tissue classifies the nodule as intermediate risk

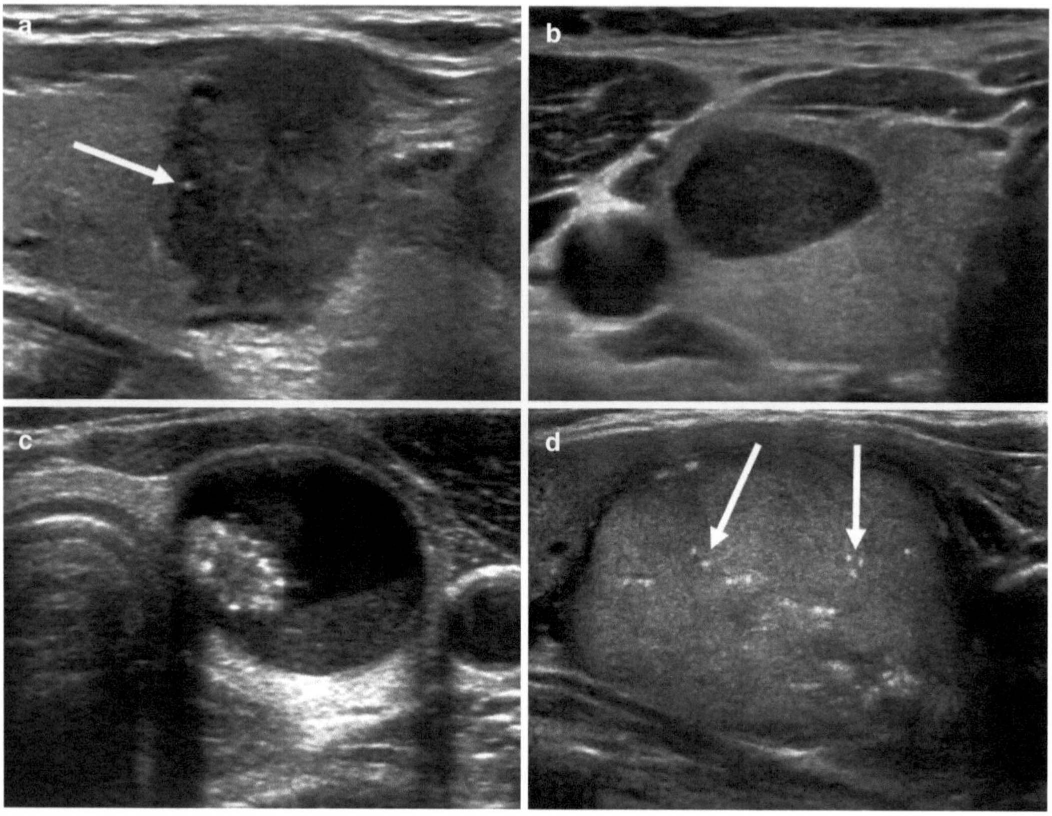

Fig. 6.1 US-based risk stratifications of thyroid nodules according to international society guidelines. (**a**) Solid hypoechoic nodule with a microcalcification (arrow), non-parallel orientation (taller than wide shape), and spiculated (irregular) margin, which is classified as high suspicion by ATA and KTA/KSThR, high-risk by AACE/ACE/AME, malignant by BTA, highly suspicious by ACR, and high risk by ETA guidelines. Diagnosis: papillary carcinoma. (**b**) Solid hypoechoic nodule without suspicious US feature, which is classified as intermediate suspicion by ATA and KTA/KSThR, intermediate-risk by AACE/ACE/AME, suspicious by BTA, moderately suspicious by ACR, and intermediate risk by ETA guidelines. Diagnosis: papillary carcinoma. (**c**) Partially cystic isoechoic nodule with multiple microcalcifications, which is classified as intermediate suspicion by KTA/KSThR, high-risk by AACE/ACE/AME, indeterminate/equivocal by BTA, moderately suspicious by ACR, high risk by ETA, and unclassified by ATA guidelines. Diagnosis: benign follicular nodule. (**d**) Solid isoechoic nodule with microcalcifications (arrows), which is classified as intermediate suspicion by KTA/KSThR, high-risk by AACE/ACE/AME, indeterminate/equivocal by BTA, moderately suspicious by ACR, high risk by ETA, and unclassified by ATA guidelines. Diagnosis: follicular carcinoma

ACR risk stratification system has been internally validated in a multi-institutional study on 3422 nodules; 85% of all nodules were within 1% of the specified TI-RADS risk thresholds [17] (Figs. 6.1 and 6.2).

Pattern-based systems categorize thyroid nodules using various combinations of individual US features. These systems vary in complexity, depending on the combinations of US features chosen, and may have the advantage that clinical application is both intuitive and easy if the risk stratification system is simplified. However, such simplified systems may compromise accuracy when malignancy risks of individual nodules are assessed. The point-based system sums the points awarded to the individual US features of a nodule, with the advantage that the system may more accurately estimate the malignancy risks of individual nodules. However, the system is less intuitive than the pattern-based systems, and requires rather complex calculations. Indeed, clinical applications of complex point-based systems will be aided by the application of computer-based algorithms [36].

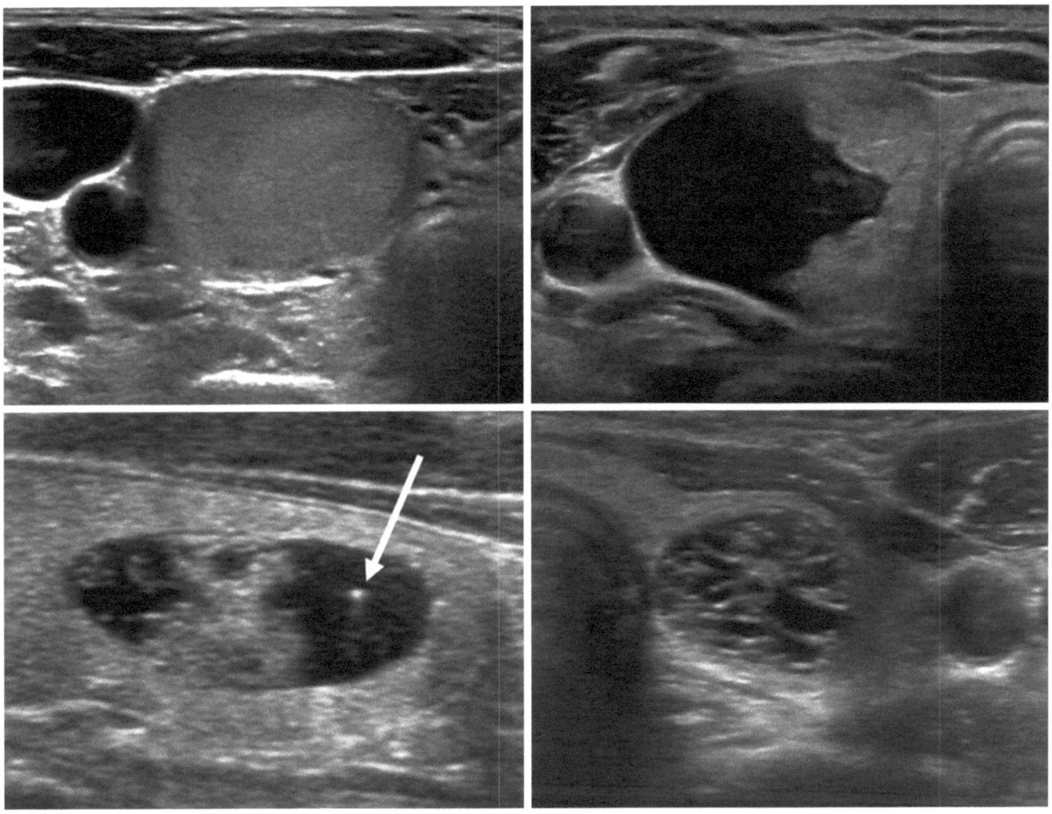

Fig. 6.2 US-based risk stratifications of thyroid nodules according to international society guidelines. (**a**) Solid isoechoic nodule without suspicious US feature, which is classified as low suspicion by ATA and KTA/KSThR, intermediate-risk by AACE/ACE/AME, benign by BTA, mildly suspicious by ACR, and low risk by ETA guidelines. Diagnosis: benign follicular nodule. (**b**) Partially cystic isoechoic nodule with eccentric solid areas and no suspicious US features, which is classified as low suspicion by ATA and KTA/KSThR, intermediate-risk by AACE/ACE/AME, benign by BTA, not suspicious by ACR, and low risk by ETA guidelines. Diagnosis: benign follicular nodule. (**c**) Partially cystic isoechoic nodule with intracystic comet tail artifact, which is classified as very low suspicion by ATA, benign by KTA/KSThR, low-risk by AACE/ACE/AME, benign by BTA, not suspicious by ACR, and low risk by ETA guidelines. Diagnosis: benign follicular nodule. (**d**) Partially cystic isoechoic nodule with spongiform appearance, which is classified as very low suspicion by ATA, benign by KTA/KSThR, low-risk by AACE/ACE/AME, benign by BTA, not suspicious by ACR, and benign by ETA guidelines. Diagnosis: benign follicular nodule

Recommendations for FNA of Thyroid Nodules

The US-based risk stratification systems have essential roles for FNA decision in thyroid nodules. The indications for FNA of thyroid nodules should be determined to screen clinically significant thyroid cancer with minimizing unnecessary FNAs. Although FNA is a safe, reliable, and effective method for diagnosis of thyroid malignancies, unnecessary FNA may impose significant burdens on healthcare systems and anxiety on patients. Therefore, the indications for FNA should be determined after careful consideration of the malignant and prognostic risk of a nodule, allowing sensitive detection of clinically significant thyroid malignancies while minimizing unnecessary evaluation. As thyroid cancers are slow-growing, and less aggressive than other malignancies, most guidelines suggest that FNA is not routinely indicated for thyroid nodules <1 cm. However, most current guidelines [2–8] recommend FNA of subcentimeter nodules in the presence of poor prognostic factors which includes suspected cervical lymph node metastasis or gross extrathyroidal tumor, and possibly in the patient with proven distant metastasis of a thyroid cancer.

The current guidelines recommend that different FNA decision-making criteria should be applied primarily based on the US risk categories and nodule size in thyroid nodules ≥1 cm (Table 6.1). The ATA guideline [2] recommends that FNA should be performed for high or intermediate suspicion nodules when the nodule size is ≥1 cm, for low suspicion nodules when the nodule size is ≥1.5 cm, and FNA may be considered for very low suspicion nodules when the nodule size is ≥2 cm. The BTA guideline recommends FNA for nodules ≥1 cm if the US appearances are equivocal/indeterminate, suspicious of malignancy, and malignant (U3–U5). The KTA/KSThR guideline [7, 8] recommends FNA for high or intermediate suspicion nodules when the nodule size is ≥1 cm, for low suspicion nodules when the nodule size is ≥1.5 cm. However, the ACE/ACE/AME and ACR guidelines [3, 9] have taken more conservative positions on FNA. The ACE/ACE/AME guideline recommends that FNA be performed for high-risk nodules when the nodule size ≥1.0 cm, for intermediate-risk nodules when the nodule size is >2 cm, and does not routinely recommend FNA for low-risk nodules. The ACR guideline [9] suggests that nodule sizes of 2.5 and 1.5 cm should be the treatment cutoffs for mildly and moderately suspicious nodules, respectively; these values are higher than those advocated by the ATA, BTA, and KTA/KSThR. The ETA guideline [10] recommends FNA for high risk nodules when the nodule size is >1 cm, for intermediate risk nodules when the nodule size is >1.5 cm, and for low risk nodules when the nodule size is >2.0 cm.

Although international guidelines are useful when making FNA decisions, it is important to further validate the diagnostic performances of the various stratification systems, and their applicabilities, in real-world clinical settings. A recent study showed that the diagnostic performance of the FNA criteria was 70.9–94.5% for sensitivity and 26.4–62.4% for specificity, depending on the guidelines used [35]. The ATA and KTA/KSThR guidelines afforded higher diagnostic sensitivities (up to 94.0%) than did the AACE/ACE/AME (80.4%) and ACR (74.7%) guidelines; however, the latter guidelines afforded higher specificity and lower rate of unnecessary FNA (25.3–32.5%) than the former ones (51.7–56.9%). As the diagnostic utilities of US-based FNA criteria vary among the international guidelines, physicians need a deep understanding of the benefits and risks of the US-based FNA criteria in different guidelines to select the best management plan for each case.

Recently, management paradigms for thyroid nodules have tended to become more conservative. The ATA guideline recommends that active surveillance can be considered as an alternative to immediate surgery in patients with very low-risk thyroid cancer (e.g., papillary microcarcinomas without clinically evident metastases or local invasion, and no convincing cytological evidence of aggressive disease); those at high surgical risk due to comorbidities; those with short remaining lifespans; and those with concurrent medical or surgical issues [2]. The AACE/ACE/AME guideline recommends that FNA sampling or watchful waiting can be considered on the basis of the clinical setting and patient preference for small (5–10 mm) nodules with suspicious US signs (high US risk thyroid lesions), and specifically, FNA is recommended for nodules if there is subcapsular or paratracheal location, suspicious lymph nodes or extrathyroid spread, positive personal or family history of thyroid cancer, and coexistent suspicious clinical findings [3]. Observational trials have suggested that active surveillance rather than immediate surgery is appropriate for adult patients with low-risk papillary thyroid microcarcinomas [37, 38]. The ATA guideline discourages FNA of asymptomatic subcentimeter thyroid nodules even when the nodules are highly suspicious for malignancy on the US images [2]. This avoids immediate admittance for surgical treatment due to a definite diagnosis of thyroid cancer [39]. However, the question of whether FNA could be used to evaluate highly suspicious subcentimeter nodules prior to initiation of active surveillance remains controversial. FNA may avoid unnecessary long-term active surveillance of some patients with benign nodules exhibiting US features mimicking malignancy. Also, the FNA result of high grade malignancy may change the decision of active surveillance to surgery, although such cases are rare.

Role of US in the Management of Thyroid Nodules After FNA

The management strategies after FNA should be determined based on the US results, clinical factors, results of molecular study (if performed), and the FNA result for the optimal personalized management of patients with thyroid nodules. The malignancy risk of thyroid nodules depends on US features and may differ among nodules with non-diagnostic [40], benign [41–43], and indeterminate [44–48] FNA results. US plays a supplementary role and malignancy risk needs to be evaluated by combination of cytology results and US features when deciding on the management of thyroid nodules [49]. Therefore, current guidelines recommend considering US features for the management of thyroid nodules after FNA. Table 6.2 summarized the recommendations of the major international thyroid societies according to FNA cytology results [2–4, 50–52].

Table 6.2 Comparison of ATA, AACE/ACE/AME, and BTA recommendations for nodules after FNA

	Management		
FNA cytology result	ATA	AACE/ACE/AME	BTA
Nondiagnostic (BSRTC I, TIR 1, Thy 1)			
– Initial nondiagnostic	– Repeat FNA	– Repeat FNA with US guidance if solid nodule	– When there is clinical suspicion of malignancy and/or indeterminate or suspicious US features, repeat FNA is mandatory
– Repeatedly nondiagnostic	– Close observation or surgery if not high suspicion US pattern – Consider surgery if high suspicion US pattern or nodule growth detected during US surveillance or presence of clinical risk factors for malignancy	– Core needle biopsy if solid nodule – Consider surgery for persistently nondiagnostic solid nodules – Clinical and US follow-up if cystic or predominantly cystic nodules with no suspicious clinical or US features	
Benign, nonmalignant, nonneoplastic, (BSRTC II, TIR2, Thy 2)			
– Not suspicious US feature	– Very low suspicion US pattern: US surveillance is not mandatory. – Low to intermediate suspicion US pattern: (1) Repeat US at 12–24 month (2) continued US follow up or repeat FNA if nodule growth or development of new suspicious US feature (3) repeated FNA if continued nodule growth	– Clinical follow-up unless symptomatic – Repeat clinical and US follow-up with TSH measurement at 12 month in accordance with clinical setting – Repeat FNA if nodule growth >50% of volume or symptomatic during follow-up – In asymptomatic nodules with a repeated benign cytology and no suspicious clinical or US features routine follow-up may be avoided	– Correlate with clinical and US features – No follow-up if no suspicious US features and no clinical suspicion of thyroid cancer

(continued)

Table 6.2 (continued)

	Management		
FNA cytology result	ATA	AACE/ACE/AME	BTA
– Suspicious US feature	– High suspicion US pattern: repeat FNA within 12 month	– Repeat FNA in nodules with suspicious clinical or US features	– Repeat FNA if there is any clinical suspicion of malignancy and/or when the US is indeterminate or suspicious
AUS/FLUS, low-risk indeterminate lesion, neoplasm possible (BSRTC III, TIR 3A, Thy 3a-atypia)	– Repeat FNA or molecular testing – Surveillance or diagnostic surgery depending on clinical factors, US pattern, and patient preference if repeat FNA or molecular testing is not performed or inconclusive	– Consider conservative management in the case of favorable clinical criteria, such as personal or family history, lesion size, and low-risk US and elastography features – Repeat FNA – Core needle biopsy may be considered (routine use is currently not recommended) – Do not recommend either in favor or against the determination of molecular markers for routine use	– US assessment with or without repeat FNA (Thy3a on repeat sample requires multidisciplinary team discussion)
FN/SFN, high-risk indeterminate lesion, Neoplasm possible (BSRTC IV, TIR 3B, Thy 3f-suspected follicular neoplasm)	– Molecular testing may be used after consideration of clinical and sonographic features – Surgery if molecular testing is either not performed or inconclusive	– Surgery for most thyroid lesions – Close clinical follow-up in a minority of cases with favorable clinical and US features (only after multidisciplinary consultation and discussion with the patient)	– Diagnostic hemithyroidectomy
Suspicious for malignancy (BSRTC V, TIR 4, Thy 4)	– Surgery similar to that of malignant cytology depending on clinical risk factors, sonographic features, patient preference, and possibly results of mutational testing (if performed)	– Surgery – Repeat FNA in cases with inadequate cellularity or in those that need additional techniques for a better characterization	– Diagnostic hemithyroidectomy
Malignant (BSRTC VI, TIR 5, Thy 5)	– Surgery	– Surgery (differentiated thyroid carcinoma) – Further diagnostic work-up before surgical intervention (anaplastic thyroid carcinoma, metastatic lesions, and thyroid lymphoma)	– Therapy appropriate to tumor type, usually surgery for papillary or medullary thyroid carcinomas

Note *ATA* American Thyroid Association, *AACE/ACE/AME* American Association of Clinical Endocrinologist/American College of Endocrinology/Associazione Medici Endocrinologi, *BTA* British Thyroid Association, *BSRTC* Bethesda System for Reporting Thyroid Cytopathology, *TIR* 2014 Italian consensus for the classification and reporting of thyroid cytology [50], *Thy* 2016 UK Royal College of Pathologists guidance on the reporting of thyroid cytology specimens [51], *AUS/FLUS* atypia/follicular lesions of undetermined significance, *FN/SFN* Follicular Neoplasm or Suspicious for a Follicular Neoplasm

Nondiagnostic

The estimated malignancy rate of nodules with nondiagnostic FNA results is 5–10% [52]. Since the rate is low but not negligible, FNA should be repeated with US guidance [2, 3, 52]. The malignancy risk of nodules with nondiagnostic FNA results may be estimated using US features [41, 49]. The current guidelines generally recommend repeat FNA for initially nondiagnostic nodules because repeat FNA often provides diagnostic cytology results. However, the management of a nodule with repeatedly nondiagnostic FNA results can be a matter of debate. The ATA recommends considering close observation or surgery for nodules with no high suspicion US pattern and recommends surgery for nodules with high suspicion US pattern. The AACE/ACE/AME guideline recommends core needle biopsy or surgery in solid nodules and US follow-up in partially cystic nodules (Table 6.2).

Benign, Nonmalignant, Nonneoplastic

The estimated malignancy rate of nodules with benign cytological results is 3.7% according to a meta-analysis based on surgical diagnosis [53], and 1–2% based on repeat FNA results or long-term follow-up [49, 54–56]. The false negative rate of an initial benign FNA result is relatively high (11.3–56.6%) for thyroid nodules with suspicious US features [41, 42, 49, 56–58]. Therefore, current guidelines [2, 3, 7, 8] recommend that nodules with high suspicion or high-risk US pattern should undergo repeat FNA after the initial benign FNA results (Table 6.2).

Atypia/Follicular Lesions of Undetermined Significance, Low-Risk Indeterminate Lesion, Neoplasm Possible (Atypia)

The risk of malignancy for thyroid nodules with cytological results of atypia/follicular lesions of undetermined significance (AUS/FLUS) is estimated to be 10–30% when the noninvasive follicular thyroid neoplasm with papillary-like nuclear features is considered as malignancy [50]. The reported malignancy risk of AUS/FLUS nodules ranges approximately 27–34% according to systematic review and meta-analysis studies [59, 60]. The risk for malignancy of AUS/FLUS nodules with suspicious US features is much higher, and is reported to be as high as approximately 60–80% [44, 45, 49]. Therefore, US feature should be considered for the management of AUS/FLUS nodules and current guidelines recommend considering US features for determining the management of AUS/FLUS nodules (Table 6.2). Although guidelines recommend repeat FNA for the management of nodules with the initial AUS/FLUS result, the management strategy is still under debate and surveillance or diagnostic surgery may be considered depending on clinical risk factors, US features, and molecular test results (if performed).

Follicular Neoplasm or Suspicious for Follicular Neoplasm, High-Risk Indeterminate Lesion, Neoplasm Possible (Follicular Neoplasm)

The US features of follicular adenomas and carcinomas overlap substantially, and there is insufficient data regarding the malignancy risk stratification of these nodules based on US features. Diagnostic surgery is generally recommended for the nodules with follicular neoplasm or suspicious for follicular neoplasm cytology results. However, close follow-up or molecular testing may be considered instead of immediate surgery depending on clinical and US features.

Suspicious for Malignancy or Malignant

The role of US features is unclear in nodules with suspicious for malignancy or malignant FNA results. Surgical treatment is recommended for most of these nodules except for rare nodules with suspected anaplastic carcinoma, metastatic tumors, and thyroid lymphoma.

Role of US in Preoperative Staging of Thyroid Cancer

US Evaluation of Extrathyroidal Tumor Extension

Extrathyroidal extension (ETE) of the primary thyroid cancer is associated with a poor clinical outcome. ETE increases the risk of recurrence [61] and decreases the overall survival [62] in patients with differentiated thyroid cancers. ETE was classified as minimal (pT3) or extensive (pT4a) by the American Joint Committee on Cancer Staging (AJCC) system (seventh edition) [63]. The clinical outcome is worse in the patients with extensive ETE than in those with minimal ETE [64]. The recently updated AJCC system (eighth edition) considered gross (macroscopic) ETE alone for T3 staging, thus removing minor (microscopic) ETE from the T3 staging criteria [65]. Although gross ETE in differentiated thyroid cancer increases the disease persistence/recurrence and decreases the survival [61, 64, 66], the prognostic impact of microscopic ETE is controversial [67, 68], and the agreement among pathologists regarding identification of minimal ETE is poor [69].

Currently, the presence and the degree of ETE are essentially considered to decide on the biopsy, surgical extent, and postoperative risk stratification. However, the US prediction of ETE shows a wide range of diagnostic values and the US diagnostic criteria for ETE is somewhat subjective and has not been established yet. Direct tumor invasion of the muscles or other organs around the thyroid gland is a reliable hallmark of the gross ETE. Clinically significant tumor invasion of the trachea may be ultrasonographically suspected in the presence of tumor abutment of the trachea at an obtuse angle; tumor invasion of the recurrent laryngeal nerve may be suspected in a subcapsular tumor if there is a loss of intervening normal parenchyma in the direction of the recurrent laryngeal nerve [70]. However, US has limited ability to evaluate deep structures and enhanced CT or MRI is required for the accurate evaluation of the tumor extent when invasion of the trachea or recurrent laryngeal nerve is suspected on US. The presence of capsular abutment, contour bulging, and loss of the echogenic thyroid border may be suggestive of ETE [71], which may be mostly microscopic if there is no obvious gross tumor invasion of the adjacent perithyroidal tissue and organs.

US Diagnosis of Cervical Lymph Node Metastasis

Lymph node metastases have been reported approximately up to 50–60% of patients with papillary thyroid carcinomas (PTC) [72–75], and clinically apparent lymph node metastases are present in 22–29% of patients with PTC [75–77]. Preoperative diagnosis of clinically apparent and macroscopic metastatic lymph nodes is crucial for surgical planning in patients with thyroid cancer. Preoperative US could detect lymph node or soft-tissue metastases undetected on physical examination in approximately 40% of patients and US has been regarded as the most important tool for the diagnosis of lymph node metastasis in patients with thyroid cancer [78]. Current guidelines [2–8, 79] recommend neck US as the first-line imaging modality for the preoperative evaluation of neck lymph nodes in patients with thyroid carcinoma. However, US has several limitations: it is operator-dependent and is not able to evaluate retropharyngeal and upper mediastinal lymph nodes, and the lower level 6 lymph nodes in some patients. The diagnostic sensitivity of US for lymph node metastasis has been reported to be insufficient, especially in the central compartment [73, 79], and this low sensitivity may be explained by the presence of the overlying thyroid gland in the central neck and nodal micrometastases (less than 2 mm), which are mostly undetected on US. However, microscopic metastatic nodes have no significant association with the risk of recurrence [80, 81], and most of the microscopic metastatic nodes undetected on imaging may have little clinical significance [82].

During the past two decades, benign lymph nodes have been consistently reported to have an ovoid shape with a fat hilum or hilar vascularity on US [79]. The US features of calcification, cystic change, abnormal vascularity (peripheral or diffuse/chaotic), and hyperechogenicity in cervical lymph nodes are highly specific and predictive (approximately >90%) for metastatic lymph nodes [83, 84] (Fig. 6.3). Intranodal microcalcifications manifesting as punctate hyperechoic foci are a highly specific US feature of metastatic lymph nodes [79, 83, 84]. Since metastatic lymph nodes occasionally show nodal macrocalcifications, they should be considered as suspicious metastatic lymph nodes in patients with thyroid cancer [8]. Cystic nodal metastasis usually manifests as a lymph node with focal cystic changes; however, a metastatic lymph node may manifest as an entirely cystic mass that mimics a developmental cystic lesion. While benign lymph nodes may display a hilar-patterned flow radiating out from the hilum into the nodal periphery, a malignant tumor in the lymph node interrupts the normal flow, and as the tumor grows within the lymph node, the normal hilar vascular pattern becomes distorted and disorganized; hence, abnormal (peripheral or chaotic) flow signals may be visualized on color or power Doppler US [79, 83, 84]. Although the presence of an abnormal vascular flow signal is indicative of a pathologic lymph node, absence of flow signal can be commonly found in both benign lymph nodes and metastatic nodes. Except for the central hilar stripe, benign lymph nodes show uniform hypoechogenicity similar to those of the neck muscles. Lymph nodes involved by a metastatic tumor may appear hyperechoic (focal or diffuse). However, the enlarged hilum of a benign reactive lymph node, fatty metaplasia of lymph nodes, and ectopic thyroid tissue

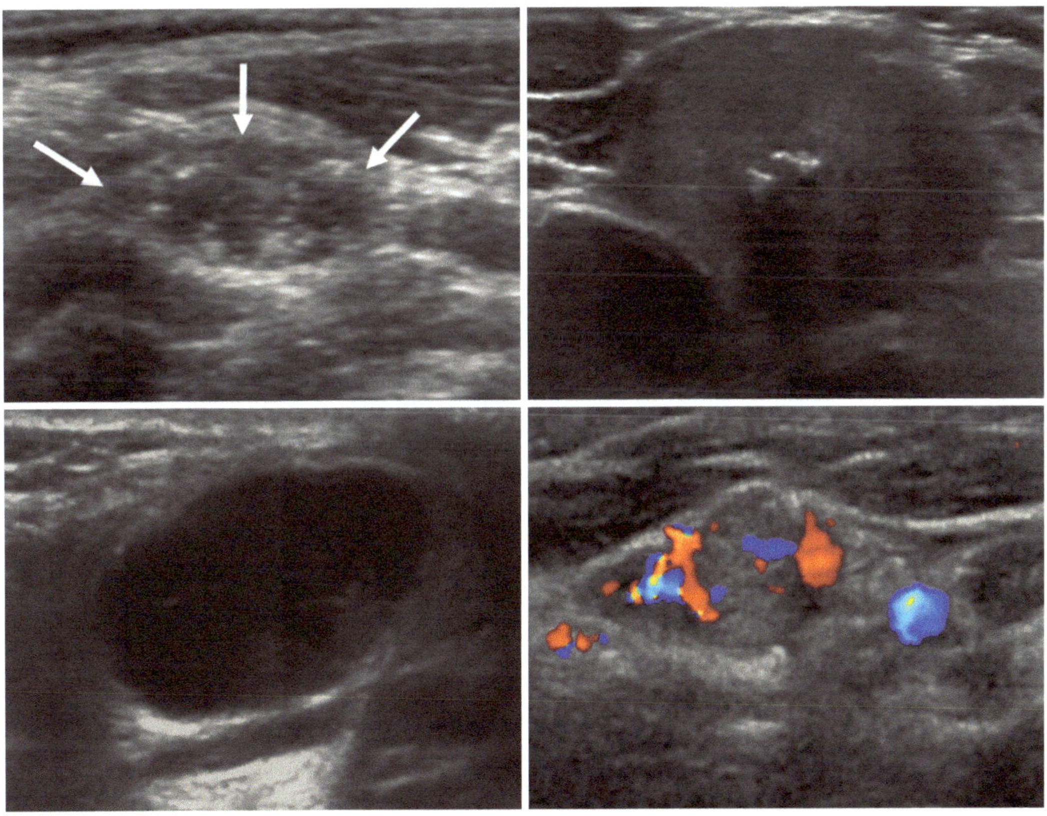

Fig. 6.3 US features of suspicious lymph nodes. (**a**) Multiple microcalcifications (arrows). (**b**) Macrocalcifications and mild hyperechogenicity. (**c**) Cystic nodal change. (**d**) Hyperechogenicity and abnormal hypervascularity. Diagnosis: metastatic papillary carcinoma (**a**–**d**)

Table 6.3 US-based risk stratification of cervical lymph nodes

Classification	ETA	Classification	KSThR
Suspicious for malignancy	At least one of the following characteristics – Microcalcifications – Partially cystic appearance – Peripheral or diffusely increased vascularization – Hyperechogenicity	Suspicious	At least one of the following characteristics – Calcifications (micro/macro) – Cystic change – Hyperechogenicity (focal or diffuse) – Abnormal vascularity (peripheral or diffuse)
Indeterminate	Absence of a hilum and at least one of the following characteristics – Round shape – Increased short axis, ≥8 mm in level II, ≥5 mm in levels III and IV – Increased central vascularity	Indeterminate	Loss of central hilar echo and absence of central hilar vascularity without any suspicious feature
Normal	Presence of hilum Ovoid shape and normal size Absent or present hilar vascularity No other suspicious signs	Benign	Presence of central hilar echo or central hilar vascularity without any suspicious feature

Note. *ETA* European Thyroid Association, *KSThR* Korean Society of Thyroid Radiology. Adapted from the ETA and KSThR guidelines [3, 8]

showing homogeneous hyperechogenicity may mimic hyperechoic metastatic lymph nodes. The size criteria, round shape, and loss of the hyperechoic hilum of lymph nodes are less specific US criteria for the diagnosis of metastatic lymph nodes. If a larger size criterion is adopted, it may be more specific but less sensitive for lymph node metastasis [85]. Malignant lymph nodes tend to be rounder; hence round lymph nodes and a Steinkamp's ratio (L/S, ratio of longer to shorter diameters) <2.0 may be considered the criteria for lymph node metastasis [86]. The loss of the hyperechoic hilar fat may be manifested by tumor involvement of normal hilum. However, US features of round nodal shape and loss of hyperechoic hilum are not specific for metastatic lymph nodes because these features are frequently present in benign lymph nodes [83, 84]. As the US features of round shape and loss of the hyperechoic hilum are less specific, the nodal size should be considered in these lymph nodes as a US diagnostic criterion for metastatic lymph nodes [83, 84].

The ATA guidelines suggest the following as the US features for metastatic lymph nodes: enlargement, loss of the fatty hilum, rounded as opposed to an oval shape, hyperechogenicity, cystic change, calcifications, and peripheral vascularity [2]. The European Thyroid Association (ETA) guidelines and KSThR recommendations suggest a 3-tier classification system for cervical lymph nodes: suspicious malignancy, indeterminate, and normal or benign [8, 84] (Table 6.3).

Fine-Needle Aspiration Cytology and Washout Thyroglobulin (Tg) Measurement for Cervical Lymph Node

Preoperative neck US has a role in the selection of abnormal lymph nodes that require confirmation using FNA. For the confirmation of metastatic lymph nodes, current guidelines [2–4, 7, 8] recommend US-guided FNA cytology and measurement of thyroglobulin (Tg) in the needle washout (FNA-Tg). Regarding the FNA criteria for cervical lymph nodes in the preoperative evaluation of thyroid carcinoma, the ATA guidelines recommend that US-guided FNA of sonographically suspicious lymph nodes with the smallest diameter ≥8–10 mm should be performed to confirm malignancy if it would change the management [2]. KTA/KSThR guideline recommends FNA for suspicious lymph nodes with the smallest diameter >3–5 mm and indeterminate lymph nodes with the smallest diameter >5 mm for surgical planning in patients with suspected or proven thyroid cancer [7, 8]. The benefit of surgical treatment or US surveillance of small volume nodal metastasis (4–7 mm size in short diameter, approximately equivalent to 6–14 mm size in maximal diameter) detected on US is not clearly demonstrated and is controversial in patients with thyroid carcinoma preoperatively.

The addition of FNA-Tg increases the sensitivity of FNA cytology in the diagnosis of lymph node metastasis from a primary differentiated thyroid cancer. The sensitivity of FNA cytology is not very high (70–85%); it has a false-negative rate of 6–8% and an inadequacy rate of 5–10% [87, 88]. Meanwhile, the overall sensitivity and specificity of FNA-Tg are 95% and 94.5%, respectively, and the diagnostic accuracy of FNA-Tg is lower in patients before than in those after thyroidectomy, according to a meta-analysis [87]. FNA-Tg is useful, especially in cystic lymph nodes, in which FNA cytology is frequently inadequate [88]. Although FNA-Tg is simple and increases the diagnostic accuracy for metastatic lymph nodes, its interpretation may be difficult and there are still many associated diagnostic issues, including methodological standardization, cutoff level, and accuracy in patients with high serum Tg or positive circulating anti-Tg antibodies. False positive results may occur in central neck lymph nodes, preoperative patients with high serum Tg [88, 89], and ectopic thyroid tissue mimicking metastatic lymph node; the influence of other components in the solution may also lead to false positive results [88]. False negative results may occur in the tall-cell or oncocytic variant of PTC [90, 91], undifferentiated/poorly differentiated carcinoma [90], and medullary thyroid carcinoma [92].

Role of US in Postoperative Surveillance

Neck US has an essential role in the detection of thyroid-bed recurrence or persistent/recurrent metastatic lymph nodes in the postoperative management of patients with thyroid cancer. Neck US with measurement of the serum Tg concentration allows reclassification in patients with differentiated thyroid cancer treated with total thyroidectomy and radioiodine remnant ablation, based on the individualized response to therapy [2, 84]. Persistent/recurrent metastatic nodes can be detected by US in patients with low or undetectable serum Tg levels when they have positive serum Tg autoantibodies or small volume metastatic nodes. Neck US allows sensitive detection of suspicious persistent/recurrent tumor, and a combination of FNA cytology and FNA-Tg is required for the confirmative diagnosis of persistent/recurrent tumor. Although suspicious US features of lymph nodes are highly suggestive of metastatic nodes, benign postoperative lesions may mimic the US features of recurrent tumors after thyroidectomy for thyroid cancer, which include remnant thyroidal tissue, postoperative fibrosis, chronic granulomatous lesions, suture granuloma, strap muscle with a nodular contour, reactive lymph nodes, and traumatic neuroma [93, 94].

Two recent studies have reported that small volume persistent/recurrent nodal lesions tend to be stable without progression to structural disease [95, 96]. They argued that surgery at the time of progression to structural disease was also successful without any evidence of local invasion or distant metastases. In addition, surgical removal of persistent tumors may achieve biochemical remission in only a limited number of patients [97]. Therefore, as surgery has a low efficacy in recurrent disease and recurrent nodes are less aggressive in nature, small volume recurrent nodal lesions may be managed by active surveillance [2, 84]. In this regard, FNA should be considered for the lymph nodes if a positive result on FNA cytology would change the management or if the nodes threaten any surrounding vital structures [2]. At present, most current international guidelines recommend a conservative approach of active surveillance without FNA for small suspicious recurrent lesions.

The ATA guideline recommends FNA cytology and FNA-Tg for the suspicious lymph nodes ≥8–10 mm in the smallest diameter if a positive result would change management [2]. The European Thyroid Association (ETA) guidelines recommend FNA cytology and FNA-Tg for suspicious and indeterminate lymph nodes ≥5–7 mm (smallest diameter) with consideration of the stage and the histology of the disease, size, and location of the lymph nodes, and serum Tg levels; FNA is also recommended for suspicious thyroid-bed lesions that are growing or >10 mm [84]. Similarly, the KTA/KSThR guidelines recommend FNA cytology and FNA-Tg for suspicious or indeterminate lymph nodes with the smallest diameter >8–10 mm [7, 8]; FNA may be performed for the smaller lymph nodes, if there is a risk of invasion of any adjacent vital organs by the suspicious lymph nodes or if less invasive non-surgical treatments, such as image-guided ablation (ethanol or radiofrequency), are considered [8].

Regarding the postoperative follow-up, ATA guideline recommends a postoperative neck US at 6–12 months and periodically thereafter, depending on the patient's risk for recurrent disease and the Tg status [2]. The ETA guideline recommends neck US 6–12 months after thyroid surgery (total thyroidectomy or lobectomy) and at the time of ablation in specific patients. The long-term follow-up protocol after the US at 6–12 months is determined according to the patients' risk for tumor recurrence [84].

Future Investigation

Most international society guidelines have a consensus that the US-based risk stratification system should be clinically feasible and effective for the diagnosis and management of thyroid nodules. Although the proposed risk stratification systems have similar US criteria and size cutoff for FNA, there are some differences in the sensitivity and specificity of FNA criteria for the diagnosis of thyroid cancer. The clinically feasible and effective US risk stratification system needs to be standardized in the future. Further investigations are required to determine whether the computer supported, elaborate risk stratification system could be a more accurate and clinically feasible tool than the current familiar US pattern-based systems [36, 98]. Most current international guidelines suggest more potentiated roles of US in the management of thyroid nodules after FNA, and agree that US has an essential role in preoperative staging and postoperative surveillance in patients with thyroid cancer. However, there are also several debatable issues regarding the roles of US in the diagnosis and management of thyroid cancer, which could be further resolved and converged toward the personalized management of patients with thyroid cancer in the future.

References

1. Vaccarella S, Dal Maso L, Laversanne M, Bray F, Plummer M, Franceschi S. The impact of diagnostic changes on the rise in thyroid cancer incidence: a population-based study in selected high-resource countries. Thyroid. 2015;25:1127–36. https://doi.org/10.1089/thy.2015.0116.
2. Haugen BR, Alexander EK, Bible KC, Doherty GM, Mandel SJ, Nikiforov YE, et al. 2015 American thyroid association management guidelines for adult patients with thyroid nodules and differentiated thyroid cancer: the American thyroid association guidelines task force on thyroid nodules and differentiated thyroid cancer. Thyroid. 2016;26(1):1–133. https://doi.org/10.1089/thy.2015.0020.
3. Gharib H, Papini E, Garber JR, Duick DS, Harrell RM, Hegedus L, et al. American Association of Clinical Endocrinologists, American College of Endocrinology, and Associazione Medici Endocrinologi Medical Guidelines for clinical practice for the diagnosis and management of thyroid nodules--2016 update. Endocr Pract. 2016;22(5):622–39. https://doi.org/10.4158/EP161208.GL.
4. Perros P, Boelaert K, Colley S, Evans C, Evans RM, Gerrard Ba G, et al. Guidelines for the management of thyroid cancer. Clin Endocrinol. 2014;81(Suppl 1):1–122. https://doi.org/10.1111/cen.12515.

5. Mitchell AL, Gandhi A, Scott-Coombes D, Perros P. Management of thyroid cancer: United Kingdom National Multidisciplinary Guidelines. J Laryngol Otol. 2016;130(S2):S150–60. https://doi.org/10.1017/S0022215116000578.
6. National Comprehensive Cancer Network. 2014 Practice Guidelines in Oncology-Thyroid Carcinoma v.2. http://www.nccn.org/. Accessed 18 May 2015.
7. Yi KH, Lee EK, Kang HC, Koh Y, Kim SW, Kim IJ, et al. 2016 revised Korean thyroid association management guidelines for patients with thyroid nodules and thyroid cancer. Int J Thyroidol. 2016;9:59–126. https://doi.org/10.11106/ijt.2016.9.2.59.
8. Shin JH, Baek JH, Chung J, Ha EJ, Kim JH, Lee YH, et al. Ultrasonography diagnosis and imaging-based management of thyroid nodules: revised Korean Society of Thyroid Radiology Consensus Statement and Recommendations. Korean J Radiol. 2016;17(3):370–95. https://doi.org/10.3348/kjr.2016.17.3.370.
9. Tessler FN, Middleton WD, Grant EG, Hoang JK, Berland LL, Teefey SA, et al. ACR thyroid imaging, reporting and data system (TI-RADS): white paper of the ACR TI-RADS Committee. J Am Coll Radiol. 2017;14(5):587–95. https://doi.org/10.1016/j.jacr.2017.01.046.
10. Russ G, Bonnema SJ, Erdogan MF, Durante C, Ngu R, Leenhardt L. European Thyroid Association Guidelines for ultrasound malignancy risk stratification of thyroid nodules in adults: the EU-TIRADS. Eur Thyroid J. 2017;6:225–37. https://doi.org/10.1159/000478927.
11. Brito JP, Gionfriddo MR, Al Nofal A, Boehmer KR, Leppin AL, Reading C, et al. The accuracy of thyroid nodule ultrasound to predict thyroid cancer: systematic review and meta-analysis. J Clin Endocrinol Metab. 2014;99(4):1253–63. https://doi.org/10.1210/jc.2013-2928.
12. Campanella P, Ianni F, Rota CA, Corsello SM, Pontecorvi A. Quantification of cancer risk of each clinical and ultrasonographic suspicious feature of thyroid nodules: a systematic review and meta-analysis. Eur J Endocrinol. 2014;170(5):R203–11. https://doi.org/10.1530/EJE-13-0995.
13. Remonti LR, Kramer CK, Leitao CB, Pinto LC, Gross JL. Thyroid ultrasound features and risk of carcinoma: a systematic review and meta-analysis of observational studies. Thyroid. 2015;25(5):538–50. https://doi.org/10.1089/thy.2014.0353.
14. Moon WJ, Jung SL, Lee JH, Na DG, Baek JH, Lee YH, et al. Benign and malignant thyroid nodules: US differentiation--multicenter retrospective study. Radiology. 2008;247(3):762–70. https://doi.org/10.1148/radiol.2473070944.
15. Ha EJ, Moon WJ, Na DG, Lee YH, Choi N, Kim SJ, et al. A multicenter prospective validation study for the Korean Thyroid Imaging Reporting and Data System in patients with thyroid nodules. Korean J Radiol. 2016;17(5):811–21. https://doi.org/10.3348/kjr.2016.17.5.811.
16. Na DG, Baek JH, Sung JY, Kim JH, Kim JK, Choi YJ, et al. Thyroid imaging reporting and data system risk stratification of thyroid nodules: categorization based on solidity and echogenicity. Thyroid. 2016;26(4):562–72. https://doi.org/10.1089/thy.2015.0460.
17. Middleton WD, Teefey SA, Reading CC, Langer JE, Beland MD, Szabunio MM, Desser TS. Multiinstitutional analysis of thyroid nodule risk stratification using the American College of Radiology Thyroid Imaging Reporting and Data System. AJR Am J Roentgenol. 2017;12:1–11. https://doi.org/10.2214/AJR.16.17613.
18. Andrioli M, Carzaniga C, Persani L. Standardized ultrasound report for thyroid nodules: the Endocrinologist's viewpoint. Eur Thyroid J. 2013;2(1):37–48. https://doi.org/10.1159/000347144.
19. Su HK, Dos Reis LL, Lupo MA, Milas M, Orloff LA, Langer JE, et al. Striving toward standardization of reporting of ultrasound features of thyroid nodules and lymph nodes: a multidisciplinary consensus statement. Thyroid. 2014;24(9):1341–9. https://doi.org/10.1089/thy.2014.0110.
20. Grant EG, Tessler FN, Hoang JK, Langer JE, Beland MD, Berland LL, et al. Thyroid ultrasound reporting lexicon: white paper of the ACR thyroid imaging, reporting and data system (TIRADS) Committee. J Am Coll Radiol. 2015;12(12 Pt A):1272–9. https://doi.org/10.1016/j.jacr.2015.07.011.20.
21. Moon HJ, Kwak JY, Kim EK, Kim MJ. A taller-than-wide shape in thyroid nodules in transverse and longitudinal ultrasonographic planes and the prediction of malignancy. Thyroid. 2011;21(11):1249–53. https://doi.org/10.1089/thy.2010.0372.
22. Beland MD, Kwon L, Delellis RA, Cronan JJ, Grant EG. Nonshadowing echogenic foci in thyroid nodules: are certain appearances enough to avoid thyroid biopsy? J Ultrasound Med. 2011;30(6):753–60.
23. Malhi H, Beland MD, Cen SY, Allgood E, Daley K, Martin SE, et al. Echogenic foci in thyroid nodules: significance of posterior acoustic artifacts. AJR Am J Roentgenol. 2014;203(6):1310 6. https://doi.org/10.2214/AJR.13.11934.
24. Lu Z, Mu Y, Zhu H, Luo Y, Kong Q, Dou J, et al. Clinical value of using ultrasound to assess calcification patterns in thyroid nodules. World J Surg. 2011;35(1):122–7. https://doi.org/10.1007/s00268-010-0827-3.
25. Na DG, Kim DS, Kim SJ, Ryoo JW, Jung SL. Thyroid nodules with isolated macrocalcification: malignancy risk and diagnostic efficacy of fine-needle aspiration and core needle biopsy. Ultrasonography. 2016;35(3):212–9. https://doi.org/10.14366/usg.15074.
26. Reading CC, Charboneau JW, Hay ID, Sebo TJ. Sonography of thyroid nodules: a "classic pattern" diagnostic approach. Ultrasound Q. 2005;21:157–65.
27. Moon HJ, Kwak JY, Kim MJ, Son EJ, Kim EK. Can vascularity at power Doppler US help predict thyroid

malignancy? Radiology. 2010;255(1):260–9. https://doi.org/10.1148/radiol.09091284.
28. Ma JJ, Ding H, Xu BH, Xu C, Song LJ, Huang BJ, et al. Diagnostic performances of various gray-scale, color Doppler, and contrast-enhanced ultrasonography findings in predicting malignant thyroid nodules. Thyroid. 2014;24(2):355–63. https://doi.org/10.1089/thy.2013.0150.
29. Papini E, Guglielmi R, Bianchini A, Crescenzi A, Taccogna S, Nardi F, et al. Risk of malignancy in nonpalpable thyroid nodules: predictive value of ultrasound and color-Doppler features. J Clin Endocrinol Metab. 2002;87(5):1941–6.
30. Shin JJ, Caragacianu D, Randolph GW. Impact of thyroid nodule size on prevalence and post-test probability of malignancy: a systematic review. Laryngoscope. 2015;125(1):263–72. https://doi.org/10.1002/lary.24784.
31. Kamran SC, Marqusee E, Kim MI, Frates MC, Ritner J, Peters H, et al. Thyroid nodule size and prediction of cancer. J Clin Endocrinol Metab. 2013;98:564–70. https://doi.org/10.1210/jc.2012-2968.
32. Cavallo A, Johnson DN, White MG, Siddiqui S, Antic T, Mathew M, et al. Thyroid nodule size at ultrasound as a predictor of malignancy and final pathologic size. Thyroid. 2017;27(5):641–50. https://doi.org/10.1089/thy.2016.0336.
33. Singh Ospina N, Maraka S, Espinosa DeYcaza A, O'Keeffe D, Brito JP, Gionfriddo MR, et al. Diagnostic accuracy of thyroid nodule growth to predict malignancy in thyroid nodules with benign cytology: systematic review and meta-analysis. Clin Endocrinol. 2016;85(1):122–31. https://doi.org/10.1111/cen.12975.
34. Yoon JH, Lee HS, Kim EK, Moon HJ, Kwak JY. Malignancy risk stratification of thyroid nodules: comparison between the thyroid imaging reporting and data system and the 2014 American Thyroid Association Management Guidelines. Radiology. 2016;278(3):917–24. https://doi.org/10.1148/radiol.2015150056.
35. Ha EJ, Na DG, Baek JH, Sung JY, Kim JH, Kang SY. US fine-needle aspiration biopsy for thyroid malignancy: diagnostic performance of seven society guidelines applied to 2000 thyroid nodules. Radiology. 2018;287(3):893–900. https://doi.org/10.1148/radiol.2018171074.
36. Choi YJ, Baek JH, Baek SH, Shim WH, Lee KD, Lee HS, et al. Web-based malignancy risk estimation for thyroid nodules using ultrasonography characteristics: development and validation of a predictive model. Thyroid. 2015;25(12):1306–12. https://doi.org/10.1089/thy.2015.0188.
37. Ito Y, Miyauchi A, Inoue H, Fukushima M, Kihara M, Higashiyama T, et al. An observational trial for papillary thyroid microcarcinoma in Japanese patients. World J Surg. 2010;34(1):28–35. https://doi.org/10.1007/s00268-009-0303-0.
38. Ito Y, Miyauchi A, Kihara M, Higashiyama T, Kobayashi K, Miya A. Patient age is significantly related to the progression of papillary microcarcinoma of the thyroid under observation. Thyroid. 2014;24(1):27–34. https://doi.org/10.1089/thy.2013.0367.
39. Brito JP, Ito Y, Miyauchi A, Tuttle RM. A clinical framework to facilitate risk stratification when considering an active surveillance alternative to immediate biopsy and surgery in papillary microcarcinoma. Thyroid. 2016;26:144–9. https://doi.org/10.1089/thy.2015.0178.
40. Moon HJ, Kim EK, Yoon JH, Kwak JY. Malignancy risk stratification in thyroid nodules with nondiagnostic results at cytologic examination: combination of thyroid imaging reporting and data system and the Bethesda System. Radiology. 2015;274(1):287–95. https://doi.org/10.1148/radiol.14140359.
41. Kwak JY, Koo H, Youk JH, Kim MJ, Moon HJ, Son EJ, Kim EK. Value of US correlation of a thyroid nodule with initially benign cytologic results. Radiology. 2010;254(1):292–300. https://doi.org/10.1148/radiol.2541090460.
42. Ha EJ, Baek JH, Lee JH, Song DE, Kim JK, Shong YK, Hong SJ. Sonographically suspicious thyroid nodules with initially benign cytologic results: the role of a core needle biopsy. Thyroid. 2013;23(6):703–8. https://doi.org/10.1089/thy.2012.0426.
43. Rosário PW, Calsolari MR. What is the best criterion for repetition of fine-needle aspiration in thyroid nodules with initially benign cytology? Thyroid. 2015;25(10):1115–20. https://doi.org/10.1089/thy.2015.0253.
44. Jeong SH, Hong HS, Lee EH, Cha JG, Park JS, Kwak JJ. Outcome of thyroid nodules characterized as atypia of undetermined significance or follicular lesion of undetermined significance and correlation with ultrasound features and BRAF(V600E) mutation analysis. AJR Am J Roentgenol. 2013;201(6):W854–60. https://doi.org/10.2214/AJR.12.9901.
45. Rosario PW. Thyroid nodules with atypia or follicular lesions of undetermined significance (Bethesda category III): importance of ultrasonography and cytological subcategory. Thyroid. 2014;24(7):1115–20. https://doi.org/10.1089/thy.2013.0650.
46. Maia FF, Matos PS, Pavin EJ, Zantut-Wittmann DE. Thyroid imaging reporting and data system score combined with Bethesda system for malignancy risk stratification in thyroid nodules with indeterminate results on cytology. Clin Endocrinol. 2015;82(3):439–44. https://doi.org/10.1111/cen.12525.
47. Chng CL, Kurzawinski TR, Beale T. Value of sonographic features in predicting malignancy in thyroid nodules diagnosed as follicular neoplasm on cytology. Clin Endocrinol. 2015;83(5):711–6. https://doi.org/10.1111/cen.12692.
48. Kuru B, Atmaca A, Tarim IA, Kefeli M, Topgul K, Yoruker S, et al. Risk factors associated with malignancy and with triage to surgery in thyroid nodules classified as Bethesda category III (AUS/FLUS). Eur J Surg Oncol. 2016;42(1):87–93. https://doi.org/10.1016/j.ejso.2015.09.026.

49. Hong MJ, Na DG, Baek JH, Sung JY, Kim JH. Cytology-ultrasonography (CU) risk stratification scoring system based on fine-needle aspiration cytology and the Korean-thyroid imaging reporting and data system (K-TIRADS). Thyroid. 2017;27(7):953–9. https://doi.org/10.1089/thy.2016.0603.
50. Nardi F, Basolo F, Crescenzi A, Fadda G, Frasoldati A, Orlandi F, et al. Italian consensus for the classification and reporting of thyroid cytology. J Endocrinol Investig. 2014;37(6):593–9. https://doi.org/10.1007/s40618-014-0062-0.
51. The Royal College of Pathologists. Guidance on the Reporting of Thyroid Cytology Specimens. London. 2016. https://www.rcpath.org/resourceLibrary/g089-guidancereportingthyroidcytology-jan16.html. Accessed 24 April 2017.
52. Cibas ES, Ali SZ. The 2017 Bethesda system for reporting thyroid cytopathology. Thyroid. 2017;27(11):1341–6. https://doi.org/10.1089/thy.2017.0500.
53. Bongiovanni M, Spitale A, Faquin WC, Mazzucchelli L, Baloch ZW. The Bethesda system for reporting thyroid cytopathology: a meta-analysis. Acta Cytol. 2012;56:333–9. https://doi.org/10.1159/000339959.
54. Chehade JM, Silverberg AB, Kim J, Case C, Mooradian AD. Role of repeated fine-needle aspiration of thyroid nodules with benign cytologic features. Endocr Pract. 2001;7:237–43.
55. Orlandi A, Puscar A, Capriata E, Fideleff H. Repeated fine needle aspiration of the thyroid in benign nodular thyroid disease: critical evaluation of long-term follow-up. Thyroid. 2005;15:274–8.
56. Shin JH, Han BK, Ko K, Choe YH, Oh YL. Value of repeat ultrasound-guided fine-needle aspiration in nodules with benign cytological diagnosis. Acta Radiol. 2006;47:469–73.
57. Chernyavsky VS, Shanker BA, Davidov T, Crystal JS, Eng O, Ibrahim K, et al. Is one benign fine needle aspiration enough? Ann Surg Oncol. 2012;19:1472–6. https://doi.org/10.1245/s10434-011-2079-3.
58. Kim SY, Han KH, Moon HJ, Kwak JY, Chung WY, Kim EK. Thyroid nodules with benign findings at cytologic examination: results of long-term follow-up with US. Radiology. 2014;271:272–81. https://doi.org/10.1148/radiol.13131334.
59. Kholová I, Ludvíková M. Thyroid atypia of undetermined significance or follicular lesion of undetermined significance: an indispensable Bethesda 2010 diagnostic category or waste garbage? Acta Cytol. 2014;58(4):319–29. https://doi.org/10.1159/000366498.
60. Straccia P, Rossi ED, Bizzarro T, Brunelli C, Cianfrini F, Damiani D, et al. A meta-analytic review of the Bethesda system for reporting thyroid cytopathology: has the rate of malignancy in indeterminate lesions been underestimated? Cancer Cytopathol. 2015;123(12):713–22. https://doi.org/10.1002/cncy.21605.
61. Radowsky JS, Howard RS, Burch HB, Stojadinovic A. Impact of degree of extrathyroidal extension of disease on papillary thyroid cancer outcome. Thyroid. 2014;24:241–4. https://doi.org/10.1089/thy.2012.0567.
62. Youngwirth LM, Adam MA, Scheri RP, Roman SA, Sosa JA. Extrathyroidal extension is associated with compromised survival in patients with thyroid cancer. Thyroid. 2017;27(5):626–31. https://doi.org/10.1089/thy.2016.0132.
63. Greene FL, Page DL, Fleming ID, Fritz AG, Balch CM, Haller DG, et al. AJCC cancer staging handbook: TNM classification of malignant tumors. 7th ed. New York: Springer; 2002.
64. Ito Y, Tomoda C, Uruno T, Takamura Y, Miya A, Kobayashi K, et al. Prognostic significance of extrathyroid extension of papillary thyroid carcinoma: massive but not minimal extension affects the relapse-free survival. World J Surg. 2006;30:780–6.
65. Edge SB, Greene FL, Byrd DR, Brookland RK, Washington MK, Gershenwald JE, et al. AJCC cancer staging handbook: TNM classification of malignant tumors. 8th ed. New York: Springer; 2017.
66. Andersen PE, Kinsella J, Loree TR, Shaha AR, Shah JP. Differentiated carcinoma of the thyroid with extrathyroidal extension. Am J Surg. 1995;170(5):467–70.
67. Nixon IJ, Ganly I, Patel S, Palmer FL, Whitcher MM, Tuttle RM, Shaha AR, Shah JP. The impact of microscopic extrathyroid extension on outcome in patients with clinical T1 and T2 well-differentiated thyroid cancer. Surgery. 2011;150(6):1242–9. https://doi.org/10.1016/j.surg.2011.09.007.
68. Hay ID, Johnson TR, Thompson GB, Sebo TJ, Reinalda MS. Minimal extrathyroid extension in papillary thyroid carcinoma does not result in increased rates of either cause-specific mortality or postoperative tumor recurrence. Surgery. 2016;159:11–9. https://doi.org/10.1016/j.surg.2015.05.046.
69. Su HK, Wenig BM, Haser GC, et al. Inter-observer variation in the pathologic identification of minimal extrathyroidal extension in papillary thyroid carcinoma. Thyroid. 2016;26:512–7. https://doi.org/10.1089/thy.2015.0508.
70. Ito Y, Miyauchi A, Oda H, Kobayashi K, Kihara M, Miya A. Revisiting low-risk thyroid papillary micro carcinomas resected without observation: was immediate surgery necessary? World J Surg. 2016;40:523–8. https://doi.org/10.1007/s00268-015-3184-4.
71. Kamaya A, Tahvildari AM, Patel BN, Willmann JK, Jeffrey RB, Desser TS. Sonographic detection of extracapsular extension in papillary thyroid cancer. J Ultrasound Med. 2015;34:2225–30. https://doi.org/10.7863/ultra.15.02006.
72. Scheumann GF, Gimm O, Wegener G, Hundeshagen H, Dralle H. Prognostic significance and surgical management of locoregional lymph node metastases in papillary thyroid cancer. World J Surg. 1994;18(4):559–67.
73. Mulla M, Schulte KM. Central cervical lymph node metastases in papillary thyroid cancer: a systematic review of imaging guided and prophylactic removal of the central compartment. Clin

Endocrinol. 2012;76:131–6. https://doi.org/10.1111/j.1365-2265.2011.04162.
74. Qubain SW, Nakano S, Baba M, Takao S, Aikou T. Distribution of lymph node micrometastasis in pN0 well-differentiated thyroid carcinoma. Surgery. 2002;131(3):249–56.
75. Cranshaw IM, Carnaille B. Micrometastases in thyroid cancer. An important finding? Surg Oncol. 2008;17(3):253–8. https://doi.org/10.1016/j.suronc.2008.04.005.
76. Bardet S, Malville E, Rame JP, Babin E, Samama G, De Raucourt D, et al. Macroscopic lymph-node involvement and neck dissection predict lymph-node recurrence in papillary thyroid carcinoma. Eur J Endocrinol. 2008;158(4):551–60. https://doi.org/10.1530/EJE-07-0603.
77. Gemsenjäger E, Perren A, Seifert B, Schüler G, Schweizer I, Heitz PU. Lymph node surgery in papillary thyroid carcinoma. J Am Coll Surg. 2003;197(2):182–90.
78. Kouvaraki MA, Shapiro SE, Fornage BD, et al. Role of preoperative ultrasonography in the surgical management of patients with thyroid cancer. Surgery. 2003;134(6):946–54. discussion 954–5
79. Yeh MW, Bauer AJ, Bernet VA, et al. American thyroid association statement on preoperative imaging for thyroid cancer surgery. Thyroid. 2015;25(1):3–14. https://doi.org/10.1089/thy.2014.0096.
80. Wada N, Duh QY, Sugino K, Iwasaki H, Kameyama K, Mimura T, et al. Lymph node metastasis from 259 papillary thyroid microcarcinomas: frequency, pattern of occurrence and recurrence, and optimal strategy for neck dissection. Ann Surg. 2003;237(3):399–407.
81. Ito Y, Tomoda C, Uruno T, Takamura Y, Miya A, Kobayashi K, et al. Preoperative ultrasonographic examination for lymph node metastasis: usefulness when designing lymph node dissection for papillary microcarcinoma of the thyroid. World J Surg. 2004;28:498–501.
82. Randolph GW, Duh QY, Heller KS, LiVolsi VA, Mandel SJ, Steward DL, et al. The prognostic significance of nodal metastases from papillary thyroid carcinoma can be stratified based on the size and number of metastatic lymph nodes, as well as the presence of extranodal extension. Thyroid. 2012;22:1144–52. https://doi.org/10.1089/thy.2012.0043.
83. Leboulleux S, Girard E, Rose M, et al. Ultrasound criteria of malignancy for cervical lymph nodes in patients followed up for differentiated thyroid cancer. J Clin Endocrinol Metab. 2007;92(9):3590–4.
84. Leenhardt L, Erdogan MF, Hegedus L, et al. European thyroid association guidelines for cervical ultrasound scan and ultrasound-guided techniques in the postoperative management of patients with thyroid cancer. Eur Thyroid J. 2013;2(3):147–59. https://doi.org/10.1159/000354537.
85. Van den Brekel M, Castelijns JA, Snow GB. The size of lymph nodes in the neck on sonograms as a radiologic criterion for metastasis: how reliable is it? Am J Neuroradiol. 1998;19(4):695–700.
86. Steinkamp H, Cornehl M, Hosten N, Pegios W, Vogl T, Felix R. Cervical lymphadenopathy: ratio of long-to short-axis diameter as a predictor of malignancy. Br J Radiol. 1995;68(807):266–70.
87. Grani G, Fumarola A. Thyroglobulin in lymph node fine-needle aspiration washout: a systematic review and meta-analysis of diagnostic accuracy. J Clin Endocrinol Metab. 2014;99(6):1970–82. https://doi.org/10.1210/jc.2014-1098.
88. Torres MR, Nóbrega Neto SH, Rosas RJ, Martins AL, Ramos AL, da Cruz TR. Thyroglobulin in the washout fluid of lymph-node biopsy: what is its role in the follow-up of differentiated thyroid carcinoma? Thyroid. 2014;24(1):7–18. https://doi.org/10.1089/thy.2013.0244.
89. Pak K, Suh S, Hong H, Cheon GJ, Hahn SK, Kang KW, et al. Diagnostic values of thyroglobulin measurement in fine-needle aspiration of lymph nodes in patients with thyroid cancer. Endocrine. 2015;49(1):70–7. https://doi.org/10.1007/s12020-014-0410.
90. Baloch ZW, Barroeta JE, Walsh J, Gupta PK, Livolsi VA, Langer JE, et al. Utility of thyroglobulin measurement in fine-needle aspiration biopsy specimens of lymph nodes in the diagnosis of recurrent thyroid carcinoma. Cytojournal. 2008;5:1. https://doi.org/10.1186/1742-6413-5-1.
91. Borel AL, Boizel R, Faure P, Barbe G, Boutonnat J, Sturm N, et al. Significance of low levels of thyroglobulin in fine needle aspirates from cervical lymph nodes of patients with a history of differentiated thyroid cancer. Eur J Endocrinol. 2008;158(5):691–8. https://doi.org/10.1530/EJE-07-0749.
92. Baldini E, Sorrenti S, Di Gioia C, De Vito C, Antonelli A, Gnessi L, et al. Cervical lymph node metastases from thyroid cancer: does thyroglobulin and calcitonin measurement in fine needle aspirates improve the diagnostic value of cytology? BMC Clin Pathol. 2013;13:7. https://doi.org/10.1186/1472-6890-13-7.
93. Shin JH, Han BK, Ko EY, Kang SS. Sonographic findings in the surgical bed after thyroidectomy: comparison of recurrent tumors and nonrecurrent lesions. J Ultrasound Med. 2007;26:1359–66.
94. Chua WY, Langer JE, Jones LP. Surveillance neck sonography after thyroidectomy for papillary thyroid carcinoma: pitfalls in the diagnosis of locally recurrent and metastatic disease. J Ultrasound Med. 2017;36(7):1511–30. https://doi.org/10.7863/ultra.16.08086.
95. Rondeau G, Fish S, Hann LE, Fagin JA, Tuttle RM. Ultrasonographically detected small thyroid bed nodules identified after total thyroidectomy for differentiated thyroid cancer seldom show clinically significant structural progression. Thyroid. 2011;21(8):845–53. https://doi.org/10.1089/thy.2011.0011.
96. Robenshtok E, Fish S, Bach A, Dominguez JM, Shaha A, Tuttle RM. Suspicious cervical lymph nodes detected after thyroidectomy for papillary thyroid cancer usually remain stable over years in properly selected patients. J Clin Endocrinol

Metab. 2012;97(8):2706–13. https://doi.org/10.1210/jc.2012-1553.

97. Al-Saif O, Farrar WB, Bloomston M, Porter K, Ringel MD, Kloos RT. Long-term efficacy of lymph node reoperation for persistent papillary thyroid cancer. J Clin Endocrinol Metab. 2010;95(5):2187–94. https://doi.org/10.1210/jc.2010-0063.

98. Choi YJ, Baek JH, Park HS, Shim WH, Kim TY, Shong YK, et al. A computer-aided diagnosis system using artificial intelligence for the diagnosis and characterization of thyroid nodules on ultrasound: initial clinical assessment. Thyroid. 2017;27(4):546–52. https://doi.org/10.1089/thy.2016.0372.

Part III

Initial Thyroid Surgery

7 The 21st Century Endocrine Surgeon

Nadine R. Caron, Tracy S. Wang, Cord Sturgeon, and Orlo H. Clark

Introduction

Surgeons who treat patients with thyroid cancer and other endocrine diseases have varied clinical backgrounds. Their training or clinical practice may be based in general surgery, otolaryngology, head and neck surgery, surgical oncology, urology (for adrenal tumors), or endocrine surgery. Regardless of the title and background, a surgeon specializing in endocrine disease has a role and responsibility far beyond the operating room. This chapter examines the specialist endocrine surgeon in the context of thyroid and other endocrine surgery.

Historically, endocrine disease was a prominent aspect of the general surgeon's practice. Indeed, some of the greatest names in the history of surgery have left their mark within endocrine surgery. General surgeons including Kocher, Halsted, Lahey, Mayo, Crile, and Cope played pivotal roles in the development of the surgical treatment of endocrine disease [1, 2]. Before the role of iodine deficiency in the epidemiology of endemic goiter was understood, this was a common disease treated with thyroidectomy performed by general surgeons [3]. Before the 1940s, when therapeutic radioiodine and antithyroid medications were first introduced, surgery was also the only available treatment for hyperthyroid states such as diffuse goiter (Graves' disease), toxic multinodular goiter (Plummer's disease), and toxic adenomas [2]. Although Billroth and Kocher (surgeons of the late nineteenth and early twentieth centuries) were among the first surgeons to perform a high volume of endocrine (thyroid) procedures [2] (Fig. 7.1), it was not until the 1950s that surgeons in several countries embraced the philosophy that an understanding of the physiology, embryology, and pathology of the endocrine system was a vital companion to technical expertise in the operating room. Realizing that advances in knowledge and skill would accompany increased clinical experience, these early "endocrine surgeons" focused their practice on endocrine surgery as a separate subspecialty within general surgery [2].

In the United States (US) this relatively informal stance changed with the establishment of the

N. R. Caron (✉)
Department of Surgery, University of British Columbia, Prince George, BC, Canada
e-mail: caronn@unbc.ca

T. S. Wang
Department of Surgery, Section of Endocrine Surgery, Medical College of Wisconsin, Milwaukee, WI, USA
e-mail: tswang@mcw.edu

C. Sturgeon
Department of Surgery, Section of Endocrine Surgery, Northwestern University, Chicago, IL, USA
e-mail: cord.sturgeon@nm.org

O. H. Clark
Department of Surgery, University of California, San Francisco, San Francisco, CA, USA

U. K. Mallick et al. (eds.), *Practical Management of Thyroid Cancer*,
https://doi.org/10.1007/978-3-319-91725-2_7

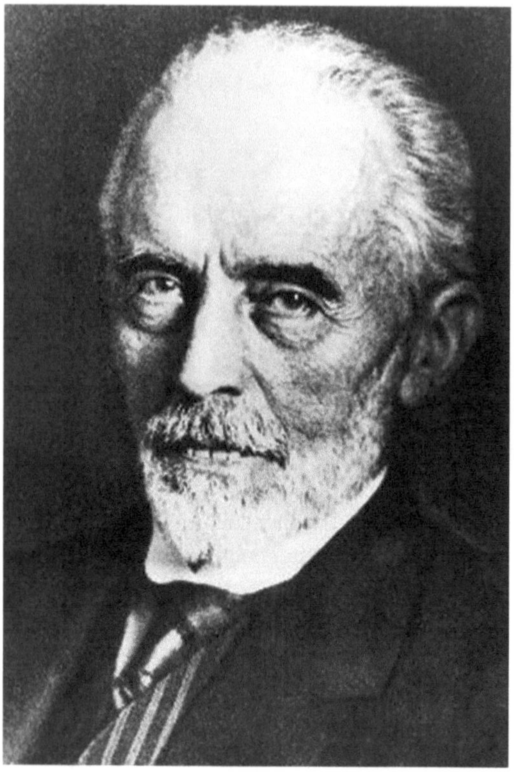

Fig. 7.1 Theodore Emil Kocher (1841–1917); a pioneer "endocrine" surgeon. (Reproduced with permission from Welbourn R. Highlights from Endocrine Surgical History. World J Surg 1996;20:603–12)

American Association of Endocrine Surgeons (AAES) in 1980, a specialty organization whose mission is 'the advancement of the science and art of endocrine surgery and maintenance of high standards in the practice of endocrine surgery.' The AAES defined endocrine surgery as the 'discipline of surgical management of endocrine disorders…of the neck and abdomen'. Today, the "specialist endocrine surgeon" is defined not only by the scope of the surgeon's clinical practice but also by the breadth of training and the depth of understanding of the biologic basis of disease. Academic endocrine surgeons also advance the knowledge of surgical endocrinology through clinical and basic science research, educating trainees (including medical students, surgical residents, and endocrine surgery fellows), and collaborating with their peers.

Exponential growth in medical knowledge and technology has fueled the demand for advanced knowledge and skills for every disease process that general surgeons treat, regardless of what subspecialty umbrella it falls under. This advanced level of expertise is becoming increasingly difficult for a general surgeon to obtain and maintain. This chapter will evaluate endocrine surgery training, analyze clinical practice profiles of those practicing endocrine surgery in the US, and describe professional aspects of endocrine surgery.

Training in Endocrine Surgery: Obtaining the Skills and Knowledge

Two opportunities for endocrine surgery training now exist: surgical residency and endocrine surgery fellowship training. The baseline level of training for thyroid and parathyroid surgery is received in surgical residency and is a mandatory component of general surgery and otolaryngology programs, while adrenal surgery is a component of general surgery and urology program; training in the surgical management of gastrointestinal neuroendocrine tumors, such as pancreas and carcinoid tumors, is primarily only received in general surgery residency programs. For general surgeons, fellowship training in endocrine surgery has become formalized in recent years. In 2005, the AAES ratified a formal fellowship curriculum, designed to ensure comparable high-quality training across different institutions and programs in North America. In 2013, the AAES then established a formal accreditation process for these endocrine surgery fellowship programs.

General Surgery Residency Training

The Accreditation Council for Graduate Medical Education (ACGME) Residency Review Committee (RRC) for Surgery requires that a standard general surgery residency program provides the training to enable its graduates to perform endocrine surgery safely and with appropriate indications, preoperative preparation and postoperative care [4, 5].

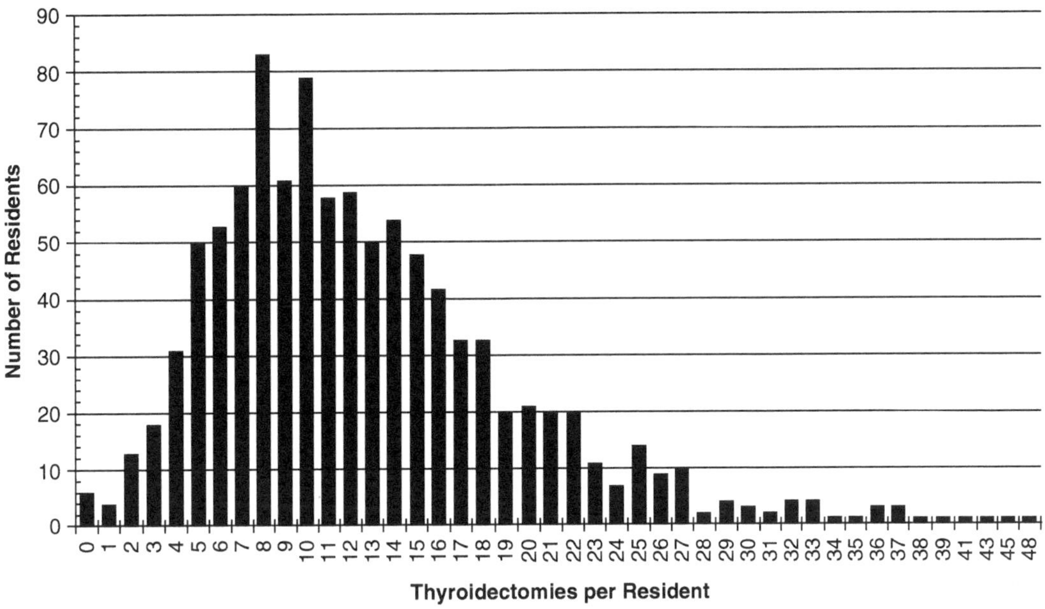

Fig. 7.2 Distribution of thyroidectomies performed by residents (1993–1994). (Reproduced from Harness K, Organ CH Jr, Thompson NW.) Operative experience of U.S. general surgery residents in thyroid and parathyroid disease. Surgery. 1995 Dec;118(6):1065. Copyright 1995, with permission from Elsevier)

In a study from several decades ago, Harness et al. compared the operative experience of graduating general surgery residents in the US between 1986–1987 and 1993–1994 to characterize the baseline level of training general surgery residents had received for thyroid, parathyroid, and adrenal surgery [5]. They found extremely varied levels of experience for the three most common endocrine organs (Fig. 7.2) [1, 5]. The average total number of thyroidectomies performed during residency ranged from 10.8 (1986–1987) to 15.2 (1998–1999). Despite the limited experience with thyroidectomy, it still made up an average of two thirds of the total operative endocrine experience in residency [5]. The average number of parathyroidectomies ranged from 4.1 to 5.1 per year, and even fewer adrenalectomies (0.98 per year) were performed [5, 6]. In a follow-up study that compared the operative experience between 1994–1995 and 2003–2004, the authors found that the average number of endocrine procedures performed by general surgery residents over the five years of residency were 15.6 ± 8.8 thyroidectomies, 6.9 ± 5.4 parathyroidectomies, and 1.5 ± 1.7 adrenalectomies. For adrenal and neuroendocrine pancreas procedures, the modal response was zero [7]. These studies questioned whether the relatively small volume of cases performed by general surgery residents, without additional fellowship training, provided adequate exposure to the broad array of endocrine disorders that surgeons may encounter in an active clinical practice. Less common clinical entities such as large substernal goiters, invasive malignancies, large distorting neoplasms, locally recurrent tumors, ectopic parathyroid glands and anaplastic or medullary thyroid cancer all add complexity and difficulty to thyroid operations and are unlikely to have been encountered to any great degree during residency training. It is probable that experience with the cervical lymph node dissections often required for appropriate treatment of patients with thyroid cancer is equally limited, although no data, to our knowledge, are currently available.

Since residency remains the endpoint in training for most surgeons who perform thyroidectomies and other endocrine procedures, it is important to consider how many operative procedures should be performed during residency for a trainee to be considered competent and qualified. The RRC for general surgery in the US categorizes and defines the minimum number of operations required during residency. For residents graduating in the 2017–2018 academic year the requirement for number of endocrine operations performed during residency will be 15. The minimum number of operations for the head and neck category will be 25, but this criterion can be fulfilled by non-endocrine operations such as neck exploration for trauma, carotid endarterectomy, and lymph node resections [5]. The endocrine requirements do not specify criteria for each specific endocrine gland (thyroid, parathyroid, adrenal or endocrine pancreas) or for specific disease processes (benign or malignant). Strictly from an accreditation point of view, the average general surgery resident in the US easily meets the current caseload criteria for endocrine surgery training; however, when the ACGME requirements were established, they did not take into consideration the range of pathology treated within surgical endocrinology.

Some residents receive appreciable experience in endocrine surgery during their residency. Harness et al. found that the maximum number of thyroid operations (either partial or complete thyroidectomies) performed by a single resident was 102 [5]. The maximum number of parathyroidectomies and adrenalectomies performed were 60 and 15, respectively [5, 6]. Zarebczan et al. reviewed similarly reviewed records from the RRC between 2004 and 2008, and found that the average endocrine case volume of general surgery residents increased by approximately 15%. Specifically, thyroidectomies increased from a mean of 17.9 to 21.8 procedures ($p = 0.007$) [8]. These studies also highlighted a significant discrepancy in average endocrine case volumes among residents of different programs; indeed, some residents will perform more thyroid operations in their residency than many general surgeons will in their entire career [1, 5, 9]. This variability suggests that the level of skill, knowledge, and understanding of endocrine diseases to achieve the successful practice of endocrine surgery within a general surgery career can be acceptable for many residents, and even exceptional for some, whereas minimal experience in residency coupled with an occasional thyroidectomy in practice is not an optimal situation. Although there is an increasing volume of literature supporting the relationship between surgeon case-specific volume and patient outcomes, evidence-derived recommendations for minimum training volumes do not exist. Because of the large variation in exposure to endocrine operations between residency programs and among general surgery practices, carefully controlled studies are needed to shed light on this controversial issue.

Some residency programs and residents have difficulty meeting the RRC minimum standards for training in endocrine surgery. Although the mean values from the Harness study could be influenced by case volume outliers, the modal values for thyroidectomy (8 to 10 cases per graduating resident) and parathyroidectomy (2 to 3 per graduating resident) continue to reflect a concerning paucity of exposure [5]. A limited residency case volume is likely indicative of a limited endocrine practice of the faculty members within such programs.

Despite an increasing number of graduates of endocrine surgery fellowship programs, there remains a relative paucity of fellowship-trained endocrine surgeons as faculty at most general surgery residency programs. A study of the 268 general surgery residency programs in the US from 1993–1994 discovered that only 70 programs (26%) had an endocrine surgeon (defined as a member of the AAES) on staff [4]. This proved to be an important factor. Those programs with an endocrine surgeon had greater numbers of thyroidectomies, parathyroidectomies, and overall endocrine cases than those without one. In addition, residents from programs with an endocrine surgeon tended to score higher on the endocrine section of the qualifying examination of the American Board of Surgery [4]. The presence of an endocrine surgeon on the teaching faculty did not affect the residents' exposure to uncommon endocrine procedures, such as those involving the endocrine pancreas [4]. This is likely due to the lack of power to detect such a difference, as the overall number of these cases is low. As part of a more recent study of the endocrine surgery job market, Shin et al. surveyed the Chairs of Surgery at 100 medical institutions. Of the 41 respondents, 23 reported an increase in the number of endocrine surgeons over the past decade (median increase from 1 to 2), 12 had the same number of endocrine surgeons, while 3 centers reported not having a specific specialist endocrine surgeon [10].

There are other advantages to having an endocrine surgeon on the teaching faculty beyond the operative volume. Endocrine surgeons tend to operate on a large number of patients with endocrine disease, and often with more complicated disease, thereby increasing both the breadth and depth of the resident's exposure. This provides additional training in the clinic and operating room and helps create an appreciation of the challenge and complexity of these cases. Cheadle et al. demonstrated an increase in the volume and complexity of chief resident cases when sub-specialty faculty from other areas of general surgery joined the department [11]. New faculty members specializing in surgical oncology, hepatobiliary, colorectal, and vascular surgery developed major referral practices that exposed residents to a wider, more challenging range of cases in their fields [11]. The greater volume and complexity of a surgical referral center may be accompanied by an increased multidisciplinary involvement of colleagues in radiology, nuclear medicine, pathology, and endocrinology and this also contributes to the residents' clinical exposure.

An Australian study of complications from total thyroidectomy demonstrated that appropriately trained general surgeons performed this operation with complication rates comparable to their endocrine surgeon counterparts, despite the significant difference in practice volume (146 versus 2–16 thyroidectomies per year) [12]. The general surgeons were former trainees in an endocrine surgery specialty unit during their residencies and at the time of their graduation were thought to be proficient in thyroid surgery. This study suggests that well-trained general surgeons who are safe and proficient in endocrine surgery at the completion of their residency can provide this safe and proficient endocrine surgery care as community-based surgeons.

Perhaps the most important influence an endocrine surgeon has in a general surgery training program is on the recruitment of future endocrine surgeons by exposing residents to the opportunities in the field. Endocrine surgeons may serve as mentors and role models for medical students and residents who have an interest in this field of surgery. Many will develop such an interest because of their mentorship. A survey of senior surgeons at regional and national surgical societies found that their role models were the number one influence on their choice of career specialty [13]. A separate survey found that two thirds of general surgery graduates chose the same career as their mentor [14]. In a recent survey by Solórzano et al. of endocrine surgery fellows and those in practice fewer than seven years, outside of clinical interest, a mentor within endocrine surgery was cited as the main reason for pursuing endocrine surgery as a specialty [15]. With the declining number of medical students pursuing careers in surgery and the high attrition rates of those who begin general surgery programs [16], the general surgery profession and all its specialties need more role models to encourage and support young prospective surgeons [17, 18].

General surgery residency programs should provide adequate experience in thyroid surgery so that their graduates can perform uncomplicated thyroid operations with minimal morbidity [18–20]. With a solid foundation of training, and by staying current with treatment and guidelines, these graduates can continue to safely and effectively treat most surgical endocrine diseases. Due to the complexity of some surgical endocrine disease, there will continue to be a role for advanced fellowship training. As with any disease, it will always be necessary for general surgeons to recognize their personal and institutional limitations and appropriately refer patients to colleagues or institutions with the capacity to manage complex endocrine surgical disease with the best outcomes [19].

Endocrine Surgery Fellowship Training

Although most surgeons in the US who perform endocrine operations do so in the context of a broad general surgery practice, many believe that additional training in endocrine surgery is required for those who will serve as experts in the field. Endocrine surgery fellowships add clinical, operative, and research experiences onto the standard training obtained in surgical residency. Furthermore, surgical endocrinology fellowship does not merely involve the acquisition of technical skills. The additional clinical experience of a fellowship program builds an in-depth knowledge in the areas of diagnosis, natural history, treatment options, preoperative preparation, operative technique, postoperative care and short- and long-term surveillance of endocrine surgical patients. Perhaps most importantly, fellows master the identification and management of surgical complications in patients with a broad range of endocrine disorders, and initiate the practice of lifelong self-evaluation and process improvement.

Endocrine surgery fellowship is comprehensive and multidisciplinary. The underpinnings of endocrine surgery fellowship are a firm understanding of endocrine biology and pathophysiology. During fellowship, the educational goal is competency in both the operative and non-operative components of surgical endocrinology. For this reason, the clinical curriculum of a fellowship program includes the acquisition of skills such as neck ultrasonography, fine-needle aspiration biopsy, and laryngoscopy. The clinical experience should include non-operative rotations in endocrinology, pathology, radiology, and nuclear medicine.

Endocrine surgery fellowships should also include a research component – basic science, clinical, or both. Regardless of the type of research, development of the associated investigative and knowledge translation skills is a vital tool that the graduating endocrine surgeon takes from their fellowship to their professional practice. The contributions from original research are one of the yardsticks by which academic surgeons are measured. More importantly, such contributions are mandatory for the continued improvement in patient care, because advances and innovations in technique and knowledge are the products of these research efforts. In addition to the increased volume and depth of clinical experience, the research element of an endocrine surgery fellowship also differentiates it from the residency training on which they are building.

In 2005, the Education and Research Committee of the AAES developed a formal fellowship curriculum, ratified by the AAES Executive Council, and revised in 2013. This was done in response to the emergence of fellowships in endocrine surgery at high-volume academic centers and the desire to ensure consistent, high-quality training across the different programs. In 2013, the AAES established a formal fellowship accreditation process and committee to provide oversight to existing programs, requiring an endocrine surgery fellowship program to "offer exposure to management of the thyroid, parathyroid, adrenal, and neuroendocrine tumors of the pancreas and GI tract". Guidelines for clinical and technical requirements are also provided, and include recommendations for exposure to cervical ultrasound and biopsy, laryngoscopy, and research and scholarly activities. At this time, there are 24 AAES-accredited fellowship programs in North America.

With the range and depth of clinical and research experience an endocrine fellowship program can provide, it is possible to visualize how one begins to make the transformation from general surgery graduate to specialized endocrine surgeon.

Clinical Practice: Maintaining and Expanding Knowledge

Surgeons who perform endocrine surgery must ensure that they maintain their level of practice at an acceptable standard, regardless of whether they have additional fellowship training or not. The maintenance of these standards should include a critical self-appraisal of patient outcomes as they relate to clinical decision-making, timing and accuracy of diagnosis, indications for and choice of operation, postoperative follow-up care and adjuvant treatment. Since medicine is a dynamic profession, this clinical competency must reflect past training and experience while incorporating any changes in clinical practice guidelines and treatment modalities. Any surgeon caring for patients with endocrine disorders must remain up to date on the advances in the multidisciplinary care (operative and non-operative) that these diseases require. The specialist surgeon should play an active role in the development of these advances, in the creation of the guidelines within which they are used, and in the promotion of the multidisciplinary approach.

Maintenance of Technical Surgical Skills: The Volume–Outcome Relationship

Perhaps the most widely quoted perspective for the role that specialist surgeons play in treating endocrine diseases stems from studies correlating surgical and hospital volume to patient outcomes. Low surgeon case-volume has been associated with higher complication rates in studies involving a vast array of specialties such as vascular, pediatric, colorectal, pancreatic, and endocrine surgery [21–27]. These studies suggest that surgeons who perform either a greater number of specific procedures or who dedicate a greater percentage of their overall practice to a specific procedure have better outcomes than surgeons whose practice is less active or focused. This association has held true with respect to mortality rates, complication rates, successful cure rates, length of hospital stay and healthcare charges in several studies, and endocrine surgery is no exception. In fact, some of the earliest accounts of thyroid surgery provide the best anecdotal evidence for the relationship between surgeon volume and patient outcomes; Theodor Kocher had a mortality rate of nearly 13% after his first 100 thyroid surgeries but by the end of his career and approximately 5000 thyroid surgeries, his overall mortality rate was 0.5% [28].

Two of the earliest studies examining the relationship between volume and outcomes in endocrine surgery utilized state-wide discharge databases in the US. Chen et al. [29] used the Maryland inpatient discharge database to evaluate the state's experience with parathyroidectomy between 1990 and 1994. Their study confirmed the high cure rates and low morbidity and mortality rates associated with specialist surgeons that have been reported in previous studies. Database limitations did not permit the evaluation of cure rates or complication rates of the patients whose operations were performed outside of the high volume center, but the analysis did show a significantly longer length of stay at these other hospitals (3.1 versus 1.3 days). The authors speculated that length of stay may be a proxy for operative complications, but although plausible, this is an assumption that has been both supported and criticized in the literature on surgical outcomes. Sosa et al. used hospital discharge data from nonfederal acute care hospitals in Maryland to compare the results of endocrine surgeons with those of lower volume surgeons over a six-year period [25]. Overall, nearly two-thirds of surgeons performed <1 thyroidectomy per year, on average, with a median number of thyroidectomies of 25 (range 4–98). On both unadjusted and adjusted analyses, the highest volume surgeons had the lowest complication rate ($p < 0.001$) and the shortest hospital length-of-stay ($p < 0.05$).

Subsequent population-based studies also have demonstrated this association across thyroidectomy, parathyroidectomy, and adrenalectomy [30–36]. In a study of patients undergoing parathyroidectomy in the state of California, of the 17,082 procedures performed, hospital volume was divided into quintile: very low (1–4 per year), low (5–9), medium (10–19), high (20–49), and very high (≥50). Over the 9-year period of the study (1999–2008), the proportion of parathyroidectomies performed at very-high volume hospitals increased from 6.4% to 20.5% and corresponded to a decrease in overall complication rates over time. In particular, rates of reoperation for primary hyperparathyroidism, while rare, were significantly higher at very-low volume hospitals (6.5%), compared to very high-volume

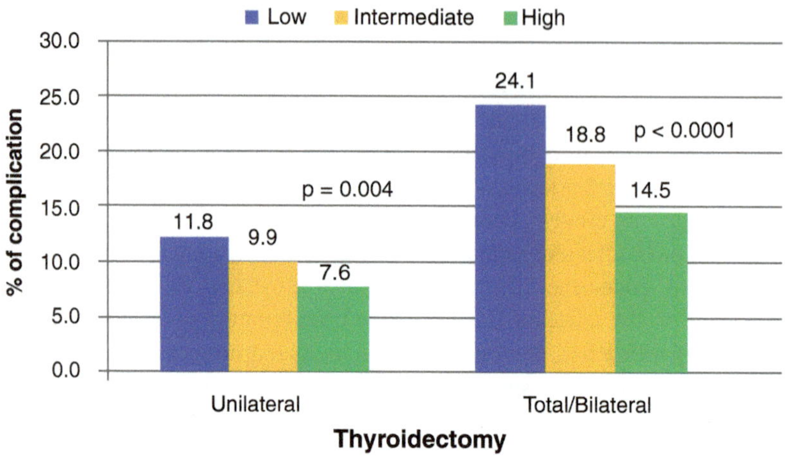

Fig. 7.3 Risk of complication by surgeon volume and type of thyroidectomy. Low surgeon volume is >10 thyroidectomies per year; intermediate, 10–99 thyroidectomies per year; and high, >99 thyroidectomies per year. (Reproduced from Hauch A, Al-Qurayshi Z, Randolph G, Kandil E. Total thyroidectomy is associated with increased risk of complications for low- and high-volume surgeons. Ann Surg Oncol 2014;21:3844–52, with permission from Springer)

hospitals (0.14%; $p < 0.001$) [34]. In a study of 3144 adrenalectomies evaluated in the Healthcare Cost and Utilization Project Nationwide Inpatient Sample (HCUP-NIS), surgeon volume was determined based on the annual number of adrenal procedures, with high-volume surgeons defined as ≥4 per year. On adjusted multivariate analysis, surgeon volume was an independent predictor of decreased complications (odds ratio = 1.5, $p < 0.01$) and shorter length-of-stay (1.0 day difference, $p < 0.001$) [35].

Individual surgeon and individual hospital annual thyroid surgery volumes were evaluated in a study of 871,644 patients from HCUP-NIS (1993–2008). Surgeon thresholds for volume were defined as: very low (≤3 cases per year), low (4–9), intermediate (9–23), and high (>23); a higher threshold for surgeon volume (i.e. >100 cases) was not used, as this was found to represent only surgeons in the 98th percentile for volume. Hospital thresholds for volume were defined as: very low (≤25 cases per year), low (26–42), intermediate (43–76), and high (>76). High-volume surgeons had a lower incidence of endocrine-specific complications, such as recurrent laryngeal nerve injury (OR = 0.7; $p = 0.024$) and hypocalcemia (OR = 0.07; $p = 0.002$). After adjustment for surgeon volume, there was no relationship between hospital volume and postoperative morbidity [33]. Hauch et al. performed a review of data from the National Inpatient Sample and compared patients who underwent total thyroidectomy or thyroid lobectomy (unilateral thyroidectomy) between 2003 and 2009. Of the 62,722 procedures included, 50.2% were performed by low-volume (defined as <10 thyroidectomies per year) surgeons, compared to only 5% by high-volume (>99 thyroidectomies per year) surgeons (Fig. 7.3). On univariate analysis, a greater number of complications occurred after procedures performed by low-volume surgeons (3492; 55%) and intermediate-volume surgeons (2577; 41%), compared to high-volume surgeons (211; 4%; $p = 0.0001$) (Tables 7.1 and 7.2) [37].

Despite these studies suggesting that increased surgical volume is associated with better clinical outcome, the majority of endocrine surgery is still performed by non-specialty trained surgeons, and the optimal threshold for a "high-volume surgeon" is debated. A study by Saunders et al. evaluated surgeons based on the number of endocrine

Table 7.1 Potential indications for referral to a specialist surgeon[a]

Recurrent disease: reoperative procedures
Anaplastic thyroid cancer
Medullary thyroid cancer
Multiple endocrine neoplasia syndromes
Advanced malignancies
Nodal metastases requiring central or lateral neck dissection
T4 primary tumor
Aerodigestive tract invasion
Recurrent laryngeal nerve paralysis
Goiters
WHO classification, stage III, possibly stage II
Substernal goiters
Graves' disease
Patient factors that increase complexity or difficulty of procedure
Comorbidities that add significant technical challenges
Pre-existing recurrent laryngeal nerve injury
Coexisting endocrine diseases, i.e. goiter and hyperparathyroidism
Significant radiation exposure in childhood or adololescence
Pediatric thyroid surgery
Patient request for endocrine surgeon

[a]Indications may be based on technical challenge of required surgical procedure or anticipated complexity of multidisciplinary care

cases they performed and the percentage of each surgeon's practice that was endocrine in nature [9]. Surgeons whose endocrine experience comprised 25% or less of their practice performed 78% of all parathyroidectomies, 94% of all adrenalectomies, and 82% of all thyroidectomies (Fig. 7.4) completed in the US in the years 1988–2000 [9]. Surgeons for whom endocrine procedures comprised 75% or more of their practice performed only 5% of all parathyroidectomies, 3% of all adrenalectomies, and 3% of all thyroidectomies in this same time period. In a study of thyroidectomies, 78.6% of surgeons who perform these procedures did fewer than ten thyroid operations per year (Fig. 7.5) [25]. A recent study sought to determine the optimal number of total thyroidectomies per surgeon per year that would be associated with the lowest risk of complications. Utilizing HCUP-NIS data from 16,954 patients who underwent total thyroidectomy between 1998 and 2009, the median annual surgeon volume was 7 cases (range, 1–157). An endocrine-specific (recurrent laryngeal nerve injury or hypoparathyroidism) complication was reported in 366 (2%) patients. After adjustment

Table 7.2 Weighted odds ratio of postoperative complication by type of thyroidectomy, overall and stratified by surgeon volume

		Unadjusted			Adjusted[a]		
Surgeon volume	Procedure	uOR	95 % CI	p	aOR	95 % CI	p
Overall	Unilateral	Reference			Reference		
	Total/complete	2.19	2.042–2.349	<0.0001	2.154	1.987–2.334	<0.0001
Low[b]	Unilateral	Reference			Reference		
	Total/complete	2.368	2.178–2.576	<0.0001	2.368	2.142–2.618	<0.0001
Intermediate[c]	Unilateral	Reference			Reference		
	Total/complete	2.109	1.892–2.351	<0.0001	1.914	1.706–2.148	<0.0001
High[d]	Unilateral	Reference			Reference		
	Total/complete	2.066	1.530–2.789	<0.0001	1.824	1.458–2.281	<0.0001

uOR unadjusted odds ratio, *aOR* adjusted odds ratio, *CI* confidence interval

Reproduced with permission from Hauch A, Al-Qurayshi Z, Randolph G, Kandil E. Total thyroidectomy is associated with increased risk of complications for low- and high-volume surgeons. Ann Surg Oncol 2014;21:3844-52

[a]Adjusted for age, gender, race, household income, type of insurance, primary diagnosis, obesity, inpatient death, neck dissection. Charlson index, hospital geographic region, hospital bed size, and hospital volume

[b]Low surgeon volume is <10 thyroidectomies/year

[c]Intermediate surgeon volume is 10–99 thyroidectomies/year

[d]High surgeon volume is >99 thyroidectomies/year

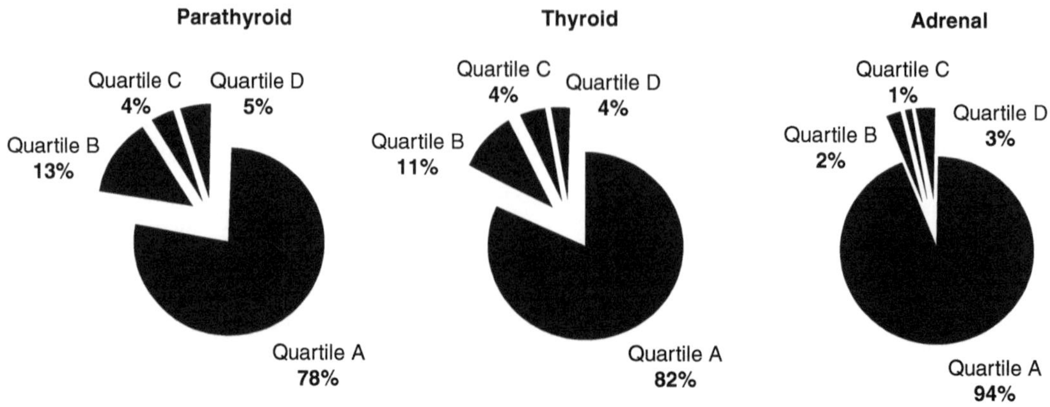

Fig. 7.4 Contribution of individual surgeon quartiles to the total number of patients who underwent operation (calculated on percentage of practice calculation: quartile A: 0–25%; quartile B: 26–50%; quartile C: 51–75%; quartile D: 76–100%). (Reproduced from Saunders BD, Nainess RM, Dimick JB, et al. Who performs endocrine operations in the United States? Surgery. 2003 Dec; 134(6):928. Copyright 2003, with permission from Elsevier)

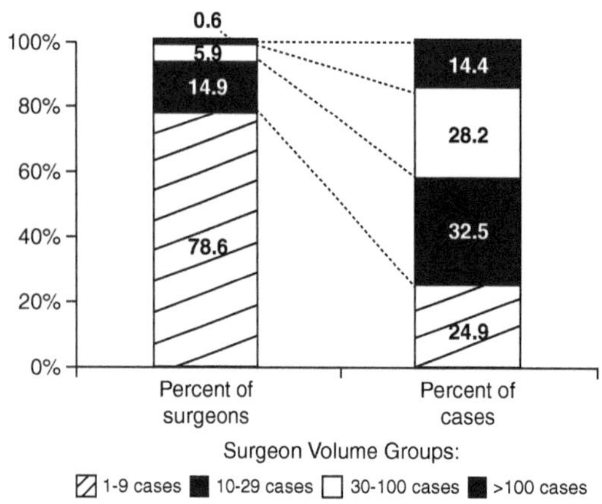

Fig. 7.5 Summary of the distribution of thyroid surgeons and cases by the four surgeon volume groups. (Reproduced with permission from Sosa JA, Bowman HM, Tielsch JM, Powe NR, Gordon TA, Udelsman R. The importance of surgeon experience for clinical and economic outcomes from thyroidectomy. Ann Surg 1998;228:320–30)

for patient demographics, clinicopathologic data, and hospital type and volume, increasing surgeon volume was associated with a lower risk of complications ($p < 0.001$). Furthermore, on logistic regression model analysis, a threshold of 26 total thyroidectomies per year was found to be associated with decreasing odds of a postoperative complication. This is the first study to objectively define a threshold for a high-volume thyroid surgeon [36].

Maintenance of Surgical Decision-Making

Integral to surgical success and often entwined in the volume–outcome relationship is the ability of the surgeon to use clinical information, interpret diagnostic studies, and employ good judgment in regard to perioperative and intraoperative decision making. How the operative approach and other treatments should be modified for each individual patient are challenging aspects of endocrine surgery that are taught in residency, refined in fellowship and remain a dynamic challenge in clinical practice.

Maintenance of "Points of Good Practice"

Postoperative management and surveillance of the patient with thyroid cancer demands a full understanding of the disease process and the indications for elements such as postoperative radioiodine ablation, thyroid-stimulating hormone (TSH) suppression, and the clinical, radiological, and biochemical monitoring of the patient for recurrent disease. Surgeons operating on the thyroid gland must be active in these treatment decisions and not simply perform the role of "technician." Patients benefit from being treated by specialists who engage in the complete care of the patient.

Kumar et al. assessed the degree to which "points of good practice" were met by groups of specialists with an interest in thyroid cancer compared to physicians and surgeons outside of a specialist clinic setting [38]. The sub-specialist group included endocrine surgeons, endocrinologists, and oncologists. The points of good practice evaluated were defined in conservative terms to highlight patterns of practice that departed from acceptable standards based on review of the literature and national guidelines. Ninety percent of specialist surgeons performed the extent of surgery that was deemed appropriate, but only 62% in the non-specialist setting met such treatment recommendations. The recommended approach to rising thyroglobulin levels and the use of radioiodine were achieved more commonly in the specialist clinics than outside of them, and this difference was statistically significant. This study highlights a volume–outcome relationship by comparing important aspects in the clinical treatment of thyroid cancer, rather than comparing surgical outcome. Overall, patients received more comprehensive, complete care in specialist clinics than in non-specialist environments [38].

Conclusion: The Endocrine Surgeon

The endocrine surgeon provides clinical expertise in the management of endocrine disease. This clinical role extends beyond the operating theater to ensure provision of quality preoperative preparation, postoperative care, and long-term follow-up. Academic endocrine surgeons may conduct clinical research, basic science research, or both, and through their contributions to the fields of surgical endocrinology they continue to improve the care and outcomes of patients with endocrine disease. Through extensive professional experience and research, endocrine surgery specialists formulate treatment recommendations and guidelines that improve the safety and efficacy of endocrine surgery. Specialist surgeons provide tertiary care for the more complex and challenging cases, while also treating a broad range of general endocrine diseases. With surgery being a central component of thyroid cancer treatment (and many other endocrine diseases), endocrine surgeons must occupy a central role in the multidisciplinary approach to these diseases.

Endocrine surgeons are not meant to replace general surgeons. Rather, they extend the ability of general surgery to care for patients with complex endocrine disease. The endocrine surgeon should provide leadership in the academic, clinical, and administrative domains to promote and protect the discipline of endocrine surgery. Moreover, adequate exposure of general surgery residents to endocrine surgery should be ensured. The endocrine surgeon serves as educator, mentor, and role model for surgical trainees. Specialist surgeons serving on surgical faculties enhance the clinical experience of residents in terms of the volume and the breadth of clinical exposure to ensure that the graduates have developed competency in endocrine surgery.

References

1. Harness JK. Presidential address: interdisciplinary care - the future of endocrine surgery. Surgery. 2000;128:873–80.
2. Welbourn R. Highlights from endocrine surgical history. World J Surg. 1996;20:603–12.
3. Harness JK, van Heerden JA, Lennquist S, et al. Future of thyroid surgery and training surgeons to

meet the expectations of 2000 and beyond. World J Surg. 2000;24:976–82.
4. Prinz RA. Endocrine surgical training--some ABC measures. Surgery. 1996;120:905–12.
5. Harness JK, Organ CH Jr, Thompson NW. Operative experience of U.S. general surgery residents in thyroid and parathyroid disease. Surgery. 1995;118: 1063–70.
6. Harness JK, Organ CH Jr, Thompson NW. Operative experience of U.S. general surgery residents with diseases of the adrenal glands, endocrine pancreas, and other less common endocrine organs. World J Surg. 1996;20:885–90. discussion 90–1
7. Le D, Karmali S, Harness JK, Sheppard BC. An update: the operative experience in adrenal, pancreatic, and other less common endocrine diseases of U.S. general surgery residents. World J Surg. 2008;32:232–6.
8. Zarebczan B, McDonald R, Rajamanickam V, Leverson G, Chen H, Sippel RS. Training our future endocrine surgeons: a look at the endocrine surgery operative experience of U.S. surgical residents. Surgery. 2010;148:1075–80. discussion 80–1
9. Saunders BD, Wainess RM, Dimick JB, Doherty GM, Upchurch GR, Gauger PG. Who performs endocrine operations in the United States? Surgery. 2003;134:924–31.
10. Shin JJ, Milas M, Mitchell J, Berber E, Gutnick J, Siperstein A. The endocrine surgery job market: a survey of fellows, department chairs, and surgery recruiters. J Surg Educ. 2013;70:377–83.
11. Cheadle WG, Franklin GA, Richardson JD, Polk HC Jr. Broad-based general surgery training is a model of continued utility for the future. Ann Surg. 2004;239:627–32. discussion 32–6
12. Reeve TS, Curtin A, Fingleton L, et al. Can total thyroidectomy be performed as safely by general surgeons in provincial centers as by surgeons in specialized endocrine surgical units? Making the case for surgical training. Arch Surg. 1994;129:834–6.
13. Ko CY, Whang EE, Karamanoukian R, Longmire WP, McFadden DW. What is the best method of surgical training? A report of America's leading senior surgeons. Arch Surg. 1998;133:900–5.
14. Thakur A, Fedorka P, Ko C, Buchmiller-Crair TL, Atkinson JB, Fonkalsrud EW. Impact of mentor guidance in surgical career selection. J Pediatr Surg. 2001;36:1802–4.
15. Solorzano CC, Sosa JA, Lechner SC, Lew JI, Roman SA. Endocrine surgery: where are we today? A national survey of young endocrine surgeons. Surgery. 2010;147:536–41.
16. Wolfson PJ, Robeson MR, Veloski JJ. Medical students who enter general surgery residency programs: a follow-up between 1972 and 1986. Am J Surg. 1991;162:491–4.
17. Kwakwa F, Biester TW, Ritchie WP Jr, Jonasson O. Career pathways of graduates of general surgery residency programs: an analysis of graduates from 1983 to 1990. J Am Coll Surg. 2002;194:48–53.
18. Neumayer L. Mentoring: the VA experience. Am J Surg. 2003;186:417–9.
19. Pasieka JL. The surgeon as a prognostic factor in endocrine surgical diseases. Surg Oncol Clin N Am. 2000;9:13–20. v–vi
20. Pasieka JL, Rotstein LE. Consensus conference on well-differentiated thyroid cancer: a summary. Can J Surg. 1993;36:298–301.
21. Feasby TE, Quan H, Ghali WA. Hospital and surgeon determinants of carotid endarterectomy outcomes. Arch Neurol. 2002;59:1877–81.
22. Pearce WH, Parker MA, Feinglass J, Ujiki M, Manheim LM. The importance of surgeon volume and training in outcomes for vascular surgical procedures. J Vasc Surg. 1999;29:768–76. discussion 77–8
23. Pranikoff T, Campbell BT, Travis J, Hirschl RB. Differences in outcome with subspecialty care: pyloromyotomy in North Carolina. J Pediatr Surg. 2002;37:352–6.
24. Porter GA, Soskolne CL, Yakimets WW, Newman SC. Surgeon-related factors and outcome in rectal cancer. Ann Surg. 1998;227:157–67.
25. Sosa JA, Bowman HM, Tielsch JM, Powe NR, Gordon TA, Udelsman R. The importance of surgeon experience for clinical and economic outcomes from thyroidectomy. Ann Surg. 1998;228:320–30.
26. Birkmeyer JD, Stukel TA, Siewers AE, Goodney PP, Wennberg DE, Lucas FL. Surgeon volume and operative mortality in the United States. N Engl J Med. 2003;349:2117–27.
27. Bachmann MO, Alderson D, Peters TJ, et al. Influence of specialization on the management and outcome of patients with pancreatic cancer. Br J Surg. 2003;90:171–7.
28. Sakorafas GH. Historical evolution of thyroid surgery: from the ancient times to the dawn of the 21st century. World J Surg. 2010;34:1793–804.
29. Chen H, Zeiger MA, Gordon TA, Udelsman R. Parathyroidectomy in Maryland: effects of an endocrine center. Surgery. 1996;120:948–52. discussion 52–3
30. Stavrakis AI, Ituarte PH, Ko CY, Yeh MW. Surgeon volume as a predictor of outcomes in inpatient and outpatient endocrine surgery. Surgery. 2007;142:887–99. discussion 99
31. Boudourakis LD, Wang TS, Roman SA, Desai R, Sosa JA. Evolution of the surgeon-volume, patient-outcome relationship. Ann Surg. 2009;250: 159–65.
32. Kandil E, Noureldine SI, Abbas A, Tufano RP. The impact of surgical volume on patient outcomes fol-

lowing thyroid surgery. Surgery. 2013;154:1346–52. discussion 52–3
33. Loyo M, Tufano RP, Gourin CG. National trends in thyroid surgery and the effect of volume on short-term outcomes. Laryngoscope. 2013;123:2056–63.
34. Abdulla AG, Ituarte PH, Harari A, Wu JX, Yeh MW. Trends in the frequency and quality of parathyroid surgery: analysis of 17,082 cases over 10 years. Ann Surg. 2015;261:746–50.
35. Park HS, Roman SA, Sosa JA. Outcomes from 3144 adrenalectomies in the United States: which matters more, surgeon volume or specialty? Arch Surg. 2009;144:1060–7.
36. Adam MA, Thomas S, Youngwirth L, et al. Is there a minimum number of thyroidectomies a surgeon should perform to optimize patient outcomes? Ann Surg. 2017;265:402–7.
37. Hauch A, Al-Qurayshi Z, Randolph G, Kandil E. Total thyroidectomy is associated with increased risk of complications for low- and high-volume surgeons. Ann Surg Oncol. 2014;21:3844–52.
38. Kumar H, Daykin J, Holder R, Watkinson JC, Sheppard MC, Franklyn JA. An audit of management of differentiated thyroid cancer in specialist and non-specialist clinic settings. Clin Endocrinol. 2001;54: 719–23.

8 Management of Cervical Lymph Nodes in Differentiated Thyroid Cancer

Hiro Ishii, Dae S. Kim, and John C. Watkinson

Introduction

The majority of patients with differentiated thyroid cancer (DTC) have papillary carcinoma (PTC) (85%). These DTCs arise from thyroid follicular epithelial cells. The remaining 15% of DTCs are made up of follicular type (12%), including conventional and oncocytic (Hürthle cell) carcinomas and poorly differentiated tumours (<3%) [1]. Metastases to the regional cervical lymph nodes are relatively common and occur early on. Regional lymph node metastases can be present at the time of diagnosis in the majority of patients with papillary carcinomas and a lesser proportion of patients with follicular carcinomas [2–4]. It has been reported that the incidence of involved cervical lymph nodes in papillary carcinoma is between 20 and 50%, and up to 90% have occult disease [5–12] and it may be present even when the primary tumour is small and intrathyroidal [13]. Compared with adults, children present more often with lymph node and/or disseminated lung disease [14]. Approximately 5–20% of patients develop local or regional recurrence that require further treatments and 10–15% go on to develop distant metastases [15].

Although the incidence of occult neck disease is high in papillary carcinoma, its prognostic significance is unclear. This is because its natural history is not known as many patients are treated with radioactive iodine [5], and there is no rationale for elective neck dissection as there is with head and neck squamous carcinoma [16]. The prognostic factors in DTC are shown below. Physicians and surgeons have no control over patient and tumour factors but can influence the management (Table 8.1).

Table 8.1 Prognostic factors associated with thyroid cancer (adapted from Moosa et al. [17])

Patient factors	Tumor factors	Management factors
Age	Tumor size	Delay in therapy
Sex	Tumor histology	Extent of surgery
	Nodal metastases (in elderly patients)	Experience of the surgeon
	Local invasion	Thyroid hormone therapy
	Distant metastases	Treatment with postoperative radioiodine
No control	*No control*	*Control*

H. Ishii (✉) · D. S. Kim
Department of Head and Neck, ENT Surgery, St. George's Hospital, London, UK
e-mail: Dae.Kim@stgeorges.nhs.uk

J. C. Watkinson
Department of Surgery, Great Ormond Street Hospital, London, UK
e-mail: john.watkinson@uhb.nhs.uk

U. K. Mallick et al. (eds.), *Practical Management of Thyroid Cancer*,
https://doi.org/10.1007/978-3-319-91725-2_8

The presence of palpable regional cervical lymphadenopathy is a poor prognosis in elderly patients, and in those with bilateral and mediastinal disease [5]. A study of the Surveillance, Epidemiology and End Results (SEER) database found that lymph node metastases, age >45 years, distant metastases and large tumour size predicted significantly poorer overall survival outcome in a multivariate analysis [18]. All-cause survival at 14 years was 82% for PTC without lymph node metastases and 79% with nodal metastases ($p < 0.05$). Another study concluded that cervical lymph node metastases conferred an independent risk of decreased survival, but only in patients with follicular cancer and patients with papillary cancer >45 years [19].

A recent comprehensive analysis of the National Cancer and SEER databases showed a small but significantly increased risk of death for patients <45 years with lymph node metastases compared with similar patients without involved lymph nodes. It was found that having incrementally more metastatic lymph nodes; up to six involved nodes conferred additional mortality risk in this age group [20].

Involved cervical lymph nodes present even when the primary tumour is small and intrathyroidal, such as microcarcinomas [13]. Papillary microcarcinomas make up 30% of all DTCs and are in part responsible for the rise in incidence of thyroid cancer in many countries over the last few years [21]. Lymph node involvement in patients with papillary microcarcinoma is relatively common, between 12.3 and 50%, with the true incidence depending on how intensely the patient is investigated [22]. The incidence of micrometastases (<2 mm) may be up to 90%, depending on the sensitivity of the detection method [23, 24]. However, the clinical implications of micrometastases are likely less significant compared to macrometastases.

Follicular carcinoma usually metastasizes by the blood route and lymph node metastases are seen in only 1–8% of patients [25]. It is the more aggressive, widely invasive follicular carcinomas that tend to spread, not only locoregionally but also to distant sites, and they are associated with a worse prognosis.

Table 8.2 The main controversies in the management of cervical lymph nodes in patients with differentiated thyroid cancer

• Assessment and staging
• Surgical management and extent of neck dissection
• Management of invasive and recurrent disease
• Mode of follow-up

The main controversies in the management of cervical lymph nodes in differentiated thyroid cancer are listed in Table 8.2.

Lymph Nodes

There are 500 lymph nodes in the body and of these, 200 are in the head and neck region [26]. In the lateral compartment of the neck, these lymph nodes are divided into a superficial lymph node system (Waldeyer's external ring) and a deep system (the cervical lymph nodes proper). These cervical lymph nodes proper are further divided into levels I to V [27, 28] and within the central compartment of the neck there is an anterior visceral compartment group (level VI) and a group within the upper anterior mediastinum (level VII).

Superficial Lymph Node System (Waldeyer's External Ring)

The lymphatic drainage of head and neck tissue is divided into superficial and deep systems and usually, but not always, the passage of lymph is lateralized and sequential and follows a predefined route from superficial to deep. The superficial nodal system, which drains the superficial tissues, consists of two circles of nodes, one in the head and the other in the neck. In the head, the nodes are situated around the skull base and are known as the occipital, postauricular, parotid or preauricular and then buccal or facial nodes. They are in continuity with the superficial nodes in the upper neck consisting of the superficial cervical, sub-mandibular, and submental nodes, along with the anterior cervical nodes. These latter nodes are situated along the external jugular vein and the anterior jugular veins, respectively. This superficial system receives drainage from the skin and underlying tissues of the scalp, eyelids and face, along with Waldeyer's internal ring (lymphatic oropharyngeal tissue consisting of the pharyngeal, tubal, and lingual tonsils), nasal sinuses, and oral cavity.

Deep System (Cervical Lymph Nodes Proper)

The deeper fascial structures of the head and neck drain either directly into the deep cervical lymph nodes or through the superficial system first and then into the deep system. These superficial nodes have already been described. The deep cervical lymph nodes proper (Fig. 8.1) consist of the junctional nodes, the upper, middle, and lower cervical nodal groups which are situated along the internal jugular vein, the spinal accessory group which accompanies the accessory nerve in the posterior triangle, the nuchal nodes, the visceral nodes in the midline of the neck, and nodes in the upper mediastinum. The junctional nodes represent the confluence of nodes at the junction of the posterior part of the submandibular triangle with the retropharyngeal nodes where they meet at the junction of the upper and middle deep cervical nodes.

In general, the passage of lymph within these systems has been well documented using lymphography and follows a sequential pattern from superficial to deep, and from the upper to lower parts of the neck [26]. These lower confluent vessels form into a jugular trunk which on the right side ends at the junction of the jugular vein, the brachiocephalic vein or joins the right lymphatic duct. On the left side, the trunk will usually join the thoracic duct as it arches behind the lower part of the carotid sheath and in front of the subclavian artery to enter the junction of the internal jugular vein with the brachiocephalic vein.

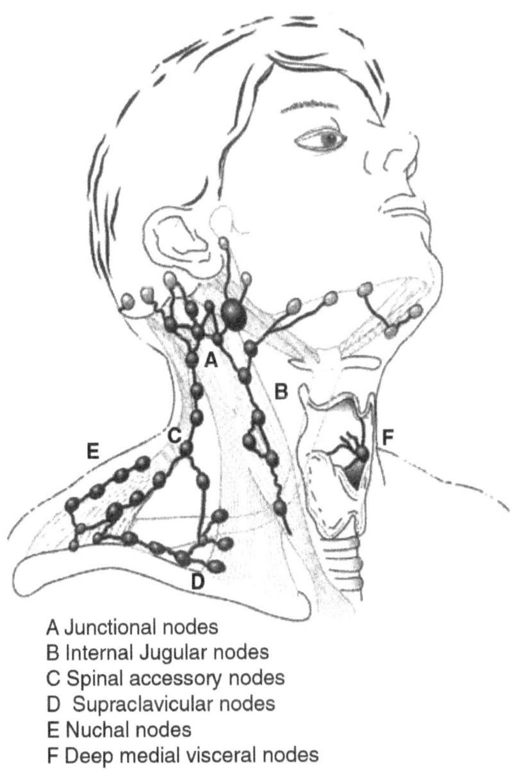

Fig. 8.1 The Deep Cervical Lymph Nodes. (From Watkinson JC, Gaze MN and Wilson JA. Stell & Maran's Head & Neck Surgery, page 200, Butterworth Heinemann 2000. Reproduced by permission of Hodder Arnold)

Lymph Node Levels

Level I: Submental and Submandibular Groups

This consists of the submental group of lymph nodes within the triangle bounded by the anterior belly of digastric and hyoid bone, and the submandibular group of nodes bounded by the posterior belly of digastric and body of the mandible.

Level II: Upper Jugular Group

This consists of the lymph nodes located around the upper third of the internal jugular vein and adjacent spinal accessory nodes extending from the skull base down to the level of the carotid bifurcation where the digastric muscle crosses the internal jugular vein. This point relates to level of the hyoid bone on a computed tomographic (CT) scan. It contains the junctional and sometimes the jugulodigastric nodes. Level II is further subdivided into level IIA, which is in front of the accessory nerve, and level IIB, which is behind. This is known as Suarez's triangle and contains Suarez's fat pad [29].

Level III: Middle Jugular Group

This consists of lymph nodes located around the middle third of the internal jugular vein extending from the carotid bifurcation superiorly (bottom of level II) down to the upper part of the cricoid cartilage (seen on a CT scan) and represents the level where the omohyoid muscle crosses the internal jugular vein. It usually contains the jugulo-omohyoid nodes and may contain the jugulodigastric node.

Level IV: Lower Jugular Group

This consists of lymph nodes located around the lower third of the internal jugular vein extending from the cricoid cartilage down to the clavicle inferiorly. It may contain some jugulo-omohyoid nodes.

Level V: Posterior Triangle Group

These nodes are located along the lower half of the spinal accessory nerve and the trans-verse cervical artery. Supraclavicular nodes are also included in this group. The posterior limit is the anterior border of the trapezius and the anterior border is the anterior border of sternomastoid. Level V is further subdivided into level VA above the omohyoid muscle and level VB below.

Level VI: Anterior Compartment Group (Visceral Group)

This consists of lymph nodes surrounding the midline visceral structures of the neck extending from the hyoid bone superiorly to the suprasternal notch inferiorly. The lateral border on each side is the medial border of the sternomastoid muscle. It contains the parathyroids, the pre- and para-tracheal, and the peri-laryngeal and pre-cricoid lymph nodes.

Level VII: Superior Mediastinal Group

This contains the lymph nodes in the upper anterior mediastinum as well as the thymus gland. The lymph node levels are shown in Figs. 8.2 and 8.3. These pre- and para-tracheal superior mediastinal lymph nodes above the level of the innominate

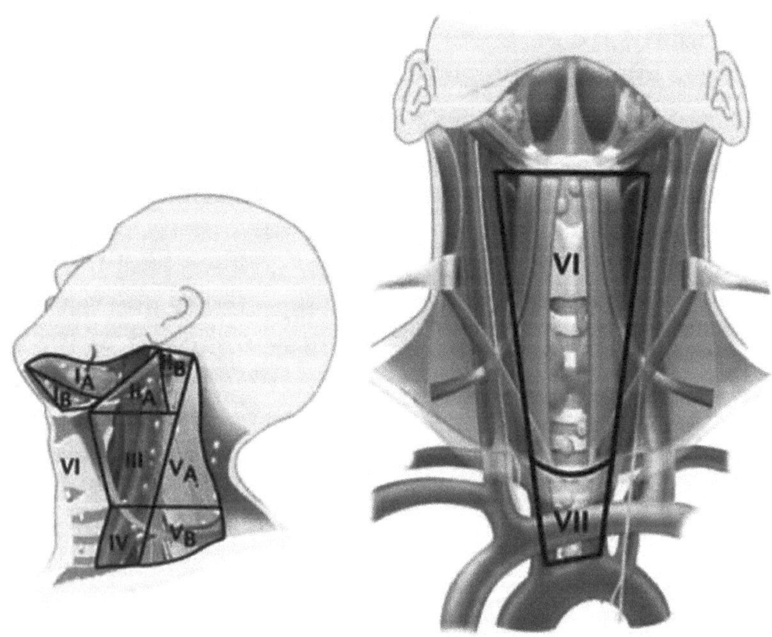

Fig. 8.2 Lymph node levels in the head and neck. (From Watkinson JC, Gaze MN and Wilson JA. Stell & Maran's Head & Neck Sugery, page 201, Butterworth Heineman 2000. Reproduced by permission of Hodder Arnold)

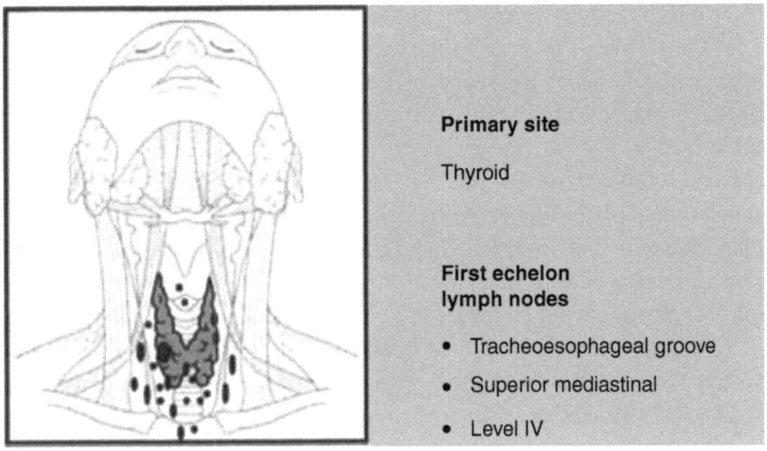

Fig. 8.3 First echelon thyroid lymph nodes. (Reprinted from Shah JP, Head and Neck Surgery & Oncology, 3rd Edition, page 358, Copyright 2003, with permission from Elsevier)

artery are typically included in the central neck dissection together with level VI nodes [30].

The above drainage patterns apply only to the non-violated neck. Once the natural history of the disease is altered, lymph node metastases can occur anywhere. This explains why the operation of selective neck dissection is only applicable in the previously untreated neck. An incision in the neck for a nodal biopsy can alter patterns of lymphatic drainage for up to 1 year following surgery. Further shunting of lymph with opening up of abnormal channels occurs when more extensive surgery and radio-therapy are undertaken, and once a malignant lymph node is palpable, there may be shunting of cells to the contralateral neck. All of these factors play a part in the management of neck disease and need to be borne in mind when assessing anatomical images following previous surgery.

Patterns of Spread

The thyroid gland contains a dense network of intrathyroidal lymphatics, which surround the thyroid follicles and facilitate direct communication across the isthmus between the two lobes of the gland. This explains the multifocality of papillary thyroid cancer and forms one of the rationales for total thyroidectomy (TTx). This intrathyroidal lymphatic network then joins collecting and draining lymphatic trunks within the subcapsular region of the gland that run alongside the extensive vascular network within the thyroid and leave the gland together with the venous drainage. This results not only in early multifocal thyroid carcinoma, but also in significant locoregional spread [5–8]. It is not uncommon to have an occult thyroid microcarcinoma with palpable neck disease [13, 22, 31], but it is uncommon to have a tumour in one lobe of the thyroid gland and contralateral neck disease without palpable unilateral neck nodes [23].

The first echelon lymph nodes of the thyroid are located within the central compartment (level VI), which then drain to the lower jugular chain (level IV) and the upper mediastinum (level VII). The most frequently involved lymph nodes are the pre-laryngeal (Delphian), that lie at the level of the cricothyroid membrane, pre-tracheal and the para-tracheal nodes [32].

The lymphatic drainage of the thyroid follows the arteries and veins that supply it. The ascending channels trace the superior thyroid artery and vein towards the jugulodigastric lymph node region, draining the upper poles. As such, metastases from the upper poles typically end up in level II and III, often without evidence of central neck disease [33]. The descending channels follow the inferior thyroid arteries. This channel follows the para-tracheal lymph nodes and continues posteriorly behind the carotid sheath, ending up at the junction of the internal jugular and subclavian veins. This is responsible for retrocarotid and inferior level IV metastases. Further drainage pathways anterior to the carotid sheath explain the frequent incidence of para-tracheal disease in patients presenting with positive lateral neck disease. The isthmus drains both in a superior and inferior direction. The superior drainage follows that of the upper poles of the thyroid gland and terminates in levels II and III. The inferior drainage follows the paths that descend towards the mediastinum [34].

Lymphatic drainage may also pass to nodes within the parapharyngeal and retropharyngeal spaces, but this tends to occur when other nodes are involved and shunting occurs, or when there has been previous treatment with either surgery or irradiation. It is very uncommon for differentiated thyroid malignancy to present with an isolated metastasis in the parapharyngeal space [35]. There are also extensive communications between the lateral cervical lymph nodes in levels II, III, and IV and the superior mediastinum via level VI.

Assessment and Staging

The majority of patients with differentiated thyroid cancer will present with a palpable nodule and/or goitre and a clinically negative neck; cN0.

The evaluation of patients with DTC involves several modalities (Table 8.3). Clinical examination of the neck has a variable reliability with inevitable false-positive and false-negative rates of around 20–30% [36]. This is compounded by the fact that many patients have micrometastases, which are often too small to palpate. The central and lateral compartments of the neck may be evaluated using the modalities listed in Table 8.3.

The range of non-pathological cervical neck nodes is from 3 mm to 3 cm, but for squamous cell carcinoma of the neck, nodes greater than a centimetre in size on CT images usually contain metastatic disease. However, for papillary thyroid cancer, the size criteria are different and metastatic nodes are usually smaller [26]. Levels I to VI should be clinically evaluated and those patients with either palpable or suspected neck disease, as well as those with proven recurrence, should be imaged anatomically. When assessing recurrent disease, it is important to evaluate both the retropharyngeal and parapharyngeal spaces with appropriate imaging modalities since patterns of drainage can be altered by previous treatment with either surgery or external beam radiotherapy.

Current American Thyroid Association (ATA) guidelines recommend pre-operative neck ultrasound (US) for the investigation of cervical (central and lateral neck compartments) lymph nodes for all patients undergoing thyroidectomy for malignant or for suspicious neck nodes. Therefore, US is becoming more important in the primary evaluation of lymph node metastases as well as in the follow-up of patients, as lymph nodes as small as 2–3 mm can now be detected when ultrasonography is performed with a high frequency probe [37]. Sonographic features suggestive of abnormal metastatic lymph nodes include enlargement, loss of the fatty hilum, a rounded rather than oval shape, hyperechogenicity, cystic change, calcifications, and peripheral vascularity (Table 8.4).

No single sonographic feature is adequately sensitive for detection of lymph nodes with metastatic thyroid cancer. However, microcalcifications have the highest specificity; any lymph nodes with microcalcifications should be consid-

Table 8.3 Modalities used to evaluate patients with differentiated thyroid cancer

• Clinical examination
• CT scan
• MRI scan
• Ultrasound scan
• Positron Emission Tomography (PET) scan

Table 8.4 Ultrasound features of lymph nodes predictive of malignant involvement

Sign	Reported sensitivity (%)	Reported specificity (%)
Microcalcifications	5–69	93–100
Cystic aspect	10–34	91–100
Peripheral vascularity	40–86	57–93
Hyperechogenicity	30–87	43–95
Round shape	37	70

Adapted from the European Thyroid Association guidelines for cervical ultrasound [38]

ered abnormal [39] (Table 7). The ATA recommend US-guided fine needle aspiration (FNA) for sonographically suspicious lymph nodes of 8–10 mm in the smallest diameter to confirm malignancy if this would change management. However, pre-operative US only identifies around half of the lymph nodes identified at surgery, due to the overlying thyroid [39].

The British Thyroid Association (BTA) [22] recommend the use of pre-operative use of cross-sectional imaging studies (computer tomography (CT), magnetic resonance imaging (MRI)) with intravenous (IV) contrast is recommended as an adjunct to US for patients with clinical suspicion for advanced disease, including invasive primary tumour, or clinically apparent multiple or bulky lymph node involvement. When cross-sectional imaging is performed, use of IV contrast is an important adjunct as it helps to delineate the anatomic relationship between the primary tumour or metastatic disease and neighbouring structures. Iodine is generally cleared within 4–8 weeks in most patients, so concern about iodine burden from IV contrast causing a clinically significant delay in subsequent whole-body scans (WBSs) or radioactive iodine (RAI) treatment after the imaging followed by surgery is generally unfounded [40]. The benefit gained from improved anatomic imaging generally outweighs any potential risk of a several week delay in RAI imaging or therapy.

The CT criteria for malignancy include cystic and haemorrhagic change, calcification, contrast enhancement, and a hypoplastic appearance [35]. Sensitivity of CT is reported to be better than US for the evaluation central and lateral compartment lymph nodes when examined together (77% vs 62%, p = 0.002), but no differences were seen between the two modalities when the central and lateral compartments were examined separately [41]. However, another study showed that combined preoperative mapping with US and CT was superior to US alone in the pre-operative detection of nodal disease, especially in the central neck [42]. MRI uses similar staging characteristics to CT with regard to malignancy but usually takes longer and is inferior to CT when imaging the chest. Routine preoperative 18 FDG-PET scanning is not recommended [40].The sensitivities of MRI and PET for the detection of cervical lymph node metastases are relatively low (30–40%) [43].

All tumours should be TNM staged. There have been some minor changes in the way lymph node are staged between the 7th and 8th edition [44, 45] of the Union for International Cancer Control—American Joint Committee on Cancer (UIC-AJCC) TNM Classification of Malignant Tumours for Thyroid Cancer. This can be seen in Table 8.5. Whilst the 8th edition of the TNM classification has been published and centres encouraged to utilise the content of this edition, the actual implementation date is set for 1st January 2018 [46]. This is to allow infrastructure changes to be made to allow accurate data collection and implementation.

Table 8.5 UIC-AJCC TNM classification of malignant tumours for thyroid cancer–the differences between the 7th and 8th Edition (changes marked with an asterisk)

7th edition	8th edition
NX—regional lymph nodes cannot be assessed	NX—regional lymph nodes cannot be assessed
N0—no regional lymph node metastasis	N0—no regional lymph node metastasis
	N0a*—one or more cytological or histologically confirmed benign lymph node
	N0b*—no radiological or clinical evidence of locoregional lymph node metastasis
N1—regional lymph node metastasis	N1—regional lymph node metastasis
N1a—metastasis to level VI	N1a*—metastasis to level VI or VII (can be unilateral or bilateral disease)
N1b—metastasis to other regional lymph nodes	N1b*—metastasis to unilateral, bilateral or contralateral lateral neck lymph nodes (levels I, II, III, IV or V) or retropharyngeal lymph nodes

Treatment Philosophy

Many patients with differentiated thyroid cancer have metastatic spread within the regional lymph nodes and for the majority, this usually represents occult disease [5–8]. Its frequency is related to histology (more common in papillary thyroid cancer) and to the size of the primary tumour.

Lymph node metastases in DTC are often multiple, and of variable size and this is one of the arguments for selective neck dissection of "at risk levels" rather than "berry picking" (selective removal of isolated lymph nodes) [23, 47]. The latter procedure has now been shown to have a less favourable prognosis than formal neck dissection [48]. The spread of disease is usually ipsilateral [23, 47], and involves progression in an orderly defined manner from level VI either laterally to levels III and IV or inferiorly into the mediastinum (level VII). Spread into level II either occurs from the superior pole of the thyroid or directly from levels III and IV. Spread into level I and the retropharyngeal and parapharyngeal spaces tends to occur when other levels are involved, or in the previously treated neck.

Many studies show that lymph node involvement is associated with a significantly higher risk of both local and regional recurrences and of distant metastases [5]. As mentioned, there does appear to be an increased risk of cancer-related mortality when lymph node metastases are extensive, bilateral, located in the mediastinum, associated with extensive primary disease, or when they occur in elderly patients [5]. Analysis of cases from the Surveillance, Epidemiology, and End Results (SEER) database indicate that lymph node metastasis is associated with increased risk of death [19, 49] particularly in patients aged >45 years [4, 18].

There is now strong evidence to support a formal selective neck/modified radical neck dissection (dissecting at least levels III, IV, and VB) in the lateral compartment for palpable or suspected disease [23, 47, 48]. This is based on the high incidence of nodal involvement, and that formal lymph node dissection facilitates accurate workup of the initial extent of the disease. Furthermore, a number of studies have shown improved outcomes with formal lymph node dissection [47] and in one series, the 20-year recurrence rate was significantly reduced after formal lymph node dissection [50]. In one study, recurrent disease after lymph node spread from papillary thyroid cancer was associated with a significant increase in the risk of death [51]. Surgery is the most effective way of treating lymph node metastases, and in particular those nodes in the so-called "coffin corners" where detection is difficult such as the retropharyngeal and parapharyngeal spaces, pre- and paratracheal grooves, and Chassaignac's triangle (Fig. 8.4).

The majority of patients have a palpable goitre and are clinically N0 in both level VI and the lateral neck compartment (levels II–V).

Current ATA and BTA guidelines recommend that for patients <45 years old, with classical unifocal papillary type cancer 1–4 cm without extrathyroidal extension and without clinical evidence of any lymph node metastases (cN0), either a TTx or a lobectomy should be performed without prophylactic central compartment neck dissection (PCCND) [22, 40].

Based on limited and imperfect data, prophylactic dissection has been suggested to improve disease-specific survival [52] and local recurrence [53–55]. Protagonists of prophylactic central compartment lymph node dissection (PCCND) also report the benefit of more accurate staging [56, 57] and its impact on the use of adjuvant radioiodine. Despite PCCND being associated with lower pre-ablation Tg concentrations and a higher rate of undetectable Tg, it is reported that the differences are not apparent at 6 months post-treatment [56, 58]. It is has been estimated that 20–31 PCCND are required to prevent one re-operation/local recurrence [53, 59]. The relative risk of loco-regional recurrence in pN1 patients with clinically uninvolved lymph nodes (cN0) is low (2%, and 4% in patients with <5 lymph node metastases) [4].

However, other studies have shown that the benefit of prophylactic central compartment node

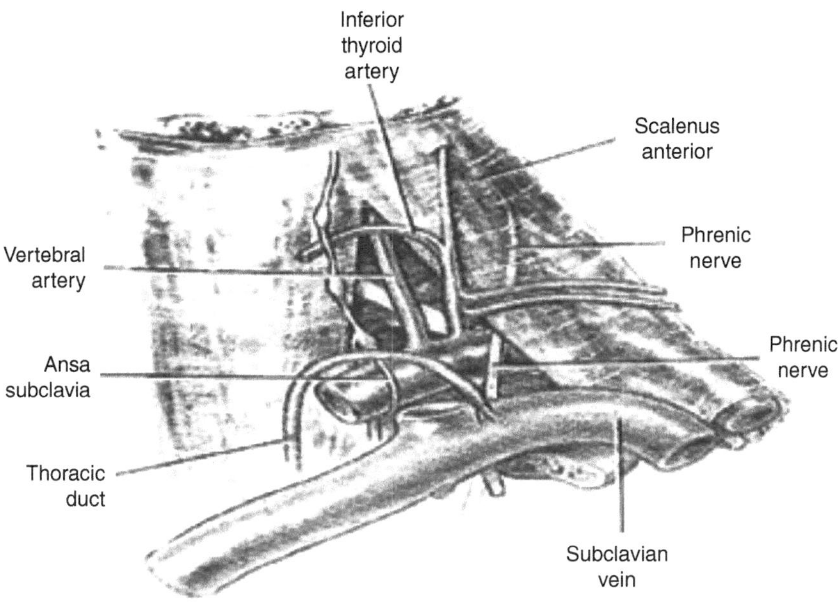

Fig. 8.4 The relationship of the prevertebral fascia to the scalene muscles and the structures over the apex of the left lung (Chaissaignac's triangle). (Reproduced from Last RJ, Anatomy Regional and Applied, 6th edn, London: Churchill Livingstone, 1978, page 377)

surgery in terms of improved disease-specific survival [52] or recurrence-free survival is not proven [60–63]. This is taken further by other authors who show prophylactic dissection does not improve long-term patient outcome, but increases the likelihood of temporary morbidity, including hypocalcemia, although prophylactic dissection may decrease the need for repeated RAI treatments [40].

Some surgeons extend the dissection to the ipsilateral supraclavicular area, thereby allowing elective dissection of the retrovascular and external part of the jugulocarotid chain, as well as the transverse superficial chain along the accessory nerve in level V [47]. This dissection is performed through a transverse incision and the operative specimen submitted to frozen section.

Lymph node dissection in the central compartment is associated with an increased risk of temporary but not permanent hypoparathyroidism compared with TTx alone [64]. A systematic review and meta analysis has compared short term (<5 years) loco-regional recurrence and surgical complications in patients undergoing TTx alone with those treated by TTx and PCCND [64]. This identified a possible 35% reduction in the risk of loco-regional recurrence in patients treated with prophylactic node surgery but the impact of increased use of radioiodine remnant ablation (RRA) and selection bias on this reduction in risk is unclear. Another meta-analysis failed to identify significant differences in the rates of loco-regional recurrence or of permanent complications in patients undergoing PCCND for PTC compared to patients undergoing TTx alone [59]. The only prospective randomised controlled trial investigating the risks and benefits of TTx with or without PCCND in patients with cN0 PTC was performed in 2015 [65]. The authors reported no difference in outcomes between the groups at five years follow-up. Those treated with TTx (n = 88) alone were found to have required higher number of ^{131}I courses (p = 0.002). Those that underwent TTx and PCCND (n = 93) were found to have a higher prevalence of permanent hypoparathyroidism (p = 0.02). In their cohort of patients who underwent TTx and PCCND, the authors discovered that almost 50% had micrometastases in the central compartment. However, analyses of the pre-operative features, including BRAF mutations, were not able to predict their presence. Moreover, being aware of their presence did not affect the final 5 year follow-up outcome.

In a personal series of 363 total thyroidectomies from 1993 to 2003 (of whom 147 had a routine level VI neck dissection for differentiated thyroid cancer), the incidence of temporary and permanent hypoparathyroidism was 19% and 1.9%, respectively. In those patients having lobectomy or TTx for malignancy (n = 353), the incidence of temporary and permanent recurrent laryngeal nerve palsy was 1.4% and 0.9%, respectively. The wound infection rate was 0.9% and hematoma rate 1.4%.

Current ATA and BTA guidelines do not feature the use of sentinel lymph node biopsy (SLNB) [22, 40]. However, it has been used to assess nodal metastases. This involves intraoperative surgical mapping of the first echelon lymph nodes using an injection of 1% isosulfan blue dye or the use of 99mTc-colloid into the thyroid nodule.

A meta-analysis [66] of fourteen studies in 2008 concluded that the use of 99mTc-colloid had a sentinel node detection rate of 96% (95% CI, 91–99%; $p < 0.05\%$ vs blue dye) and use of blue dye had a detection rate of 83% (95% CI, 79–87%). A more recent systematic review [67] in 2016 demonstrated a high false negative rate (25.4%) of sentinel lymph node biopsy despite only including studies utilising 99mTc. Their recommendation is to abandon sentinel lymph node biopsies that are performed alone and to convert to a technique that guides lymph node dissection based on radioactivity rather than sentinel node status to allow better staging and selection of patients for post-operative RAI.

How then should we manage our patients? Several different types of lymph node dissection may be done in patients with differentiated thyroid carcinoma (Table 8.6). Previously, unilateral PCCND used to be performed for those undergoing unilateral lobectomy. However, it has been shown that unilateral PCCND does not provide an advantage in reducing morbidity over bilateral PCCND or post RRA Tg levels. Neither does it lower Tg levels when compared with TTx alone post RRA. Bilateral PCCND does identify bilateral lymph node metastases in 13–50% and is the 'preferable' option for accurate staging. As such, unilateral PCCND is not recommended by the BTA [22]. For a suspected or proven malignancy when a TTx is being performed, this procedure is carried out bilaterally.

Table 8.6 Neck dissections performed for differentiated thyroid carcinomas

• Level VI neck dissection
• Level VII neck dissection
• Selective neck dissection (usually levels II_A–V_B; or levels III and IV, levels III–V_B, or levels IV–V_B)
• Modified radical neck dissection (type 1) preserving the accessory nerve (levels I–V dissected)
• Modified radical neck dissection (type 2) preserving the accessory nerve and the internal jugular vein (levels I–V dissected)
• Modified radical neck dissection (type 3) preserving the accessory nerve, internal jugular vein, and sternomastoid muscle (levels I–V dissected). Sometimes called a comprehensive neck dissection
• Radical neck dissection (levels I–V dissected). The accessory nerve, internal jugular vein, and sternomastoid muscle are all sacrificed
• Extended radical neck dissection (levels I–V dissected). This involves a radical neck dissection with sacrifice of other structures such as external skin, digastric muscle, etc.

The evidence for PCCND compared to no PCCND in patients with a cN0 neck, but deemed high risk on the basis of one or more of the following (adverse histological sub type, age ≥45 years, multifocal, tumours greater than 4 cm in diameter, extra-thyroidal extension) is unclear [68–70]. In these cases, personalised decision plans are recommended. The ATA provides weak evidence for PCCND (ipsilateral or bilateral) for patients with papillary thyroid carcinoma with clinically uninvolved central neck lymph nodes (cN0) who have advanced primary tumours (T3 or T4) or clinically involved lateral neck nodes, or if the information will be used to plan further steps in therapy. However, as mentioned above, the BTA do not recommend unilateral PCCND: if PCCND is considered, this should be bilateral.

Large nodules in the isthmus (T3/T4 lesions) require bilateral dissection.

The removal of cN0 level VI lymph nodes detects a substantial number of patients with pN1 disease; however, the direct effect of this on long-term outcome is small at best [59, 64]. The information from PCCND must be used cautiously for staging information. Since microscopic nodal positivity occurs frequently, prophylactic dissection often converts patients from clinical N0 to pathologic N1a, upstaging many patients over age 45 from AJCC stage I to stage III [40].

At the time of surgery for near-total or TTx, levels II, III, and IV should be palpated. If there is any suggestion of metastatic spread, a frozen section should be performed and the presence of metastatic disease indicates the need for an elective selective dissection of the lateral neck compartment. Frozen section has high sensitivity and specificity for detection of papillary thyroid carcinoma [71]. If the lateral nodes are suspicious pre-operatively, or malignancy confirmed on frozen section at the time of thyroidectomy, a therapeutic central and selective lateral neck dissection (levels IIa–Vb) is recommended, preserving the accessory nerve, sternocleidomastoid muscle and internal jugular vein [22, 40]. This compartmental node dissection may reduce the risk of recurrence and possibly mortality [40].

There is confusion in the literature about which levels should be routinely dissected. The previous ATA Consensus Statement (2012) [72] on the rationale for lateral neck dissection declared that prophylactic lateral neck dissection was unwarranted. However, more recent studies have reported that prophylactic lateral neck dissection (levels III and IV) yields node positive disease in 8–23% of patients [73, 74]; an increased risk of involvement of lateral neck nodes by tumour was associated with positive central compartment nodes on multivariate analysis. A further study reported that patients who had previously undergone TTx and PCCND had a 6% lateral neck node recurrence rate at 5 years follow-up [75]. Current ATA guidelines state that prophylactic lateral neck dissection in patients with no evidence of central compartment lymph node metastases, is not recommended [40]. The BTA guidelines state that the advantages of prophylactic lateral neck dissection compared to no prophylactic lateral neck dissection in patients with central compartment lymph involvement is unclear.

One study has shown that in the presence of palpable disease, nodal involvement is at a single level in 39% of cases, while 14% of cases involved four or more levels [76]. Patients with lateral neck node metastases and no evidence of central neck node involvement on pre-operative imaging are high risk (80%) for histological evidence of level VI node metastases [22].

The majority of surgeons will always dissect at least levels III and IV [76, 77] (Professor J. Shah, personal communication; Professor C. O'Brien, personal communication) and some also routinely dissect levels IIA to VB (Professor P. Gullane, personal communication). In the presence of gross disease in level IIA, level IIB should be dissected as recurrent disease at this site is difficult to treat surgically (Professor J. Shah, personal communication). The author's preference for palpable neck disease is to dissect at least levels IIA to VB (below the accessory nerve) with preservation of the sternomastoid muscle, internal jugular vein, and the accessory nerve [78]. This falls just short of a modified radical neck dis-section type three (comprehensive neck dis-section) since level I is not usually routinely dissected, although in one series, approximately 12% of cases had disease at this level [23]. This procedure may be extended to include level I, and then one or other of the accessory nerve, internal jugular vein, or sternomastoid muscle may need to be sacrificed for more advanced disease (modified or radical neck dissection). However, the BTA recommend that in the absence of clear indications, dissection of levels I, IIb and Va is not recommended. Overt disease in the central compartment discovered prior to/at surgery should be treated by a therapeutic level VI/VII node dissection [22].

Treatment of lymph node metastases for follicular carcinoma is treated in a similar way to the papillary cancer, although there seems little justification to perform a level VI neck dissection in the N0 neck as the chance of occult disease is less than 20%. If there is preoperative or intraoperative suspicion of nodal disease, FNAC or frozen section should be performed prior to therapeutic node dissection.

Patients with papillary microcarcinoma who present with cervical node metastases require TTx and therapeutic lymph node dissection of the involved nodal compartment/s as with papillary thyroid carcinoma >T1a [22]. Although PCCND may not reduce the short term risk of local recurrence, this should be considered in patients with tumours that are multifocal, pT3 and with extra-thyroidal spread [22].

Surgical Management

A level VI neck dissection can be done through a formal thyroid incision and simply involves an extended TTx with removal of the soft tissue bearing areas of level VI that contains the lymph nodes. The parathyroid glands are preserved together with the recurrent laryngeal nerves and external branches of the superior laryngeal nerves. The dissection may be facilitated by the use of operating loupes and can be extended using the cervical approach to remove the lymph node bearing areas of level VII down to the brachiocephalic vein [51]. This is usually facilitated by cervical thymectomy. For extensive disease with possible vascular involvement, a formal approach to the mediastinum is required using either a limited or full sternotomy.

The incision for a standard selective lateral compartment neck dissection is usually best done with an extended thyroid incision (thyroid utility: Fig. 8.5). This facilitates formal access to levels II to V (Figs. 8.6 and 8.7). Further access to levels II to IV can be achieved either by lifting sternomastoid up to dissect beneath the muscle or (in the author's preference) by dividing the sternomastoid at its lower end and elevating it up to improve the exposure. Access to level VII can easily be achieved with a cervical approach (Fig. 8.8). The accessory nerve is formally identified in the posterior triangle at Erb's point (which is 1 cm above where the greater auricular nerve winds around the posterior border of sternomastoid) and in the untreated neck there is no need to dissect above the nerve. Lymph node bearing tissue of the posterior triangle below the accessory nerve (essentially level VB) is removed together with tissue in levels IIA, III, and IV to include the omohyoid muscle. Special care is taken to access Chassaignac's triangle, which lies behind the posterior part of the lower end of the

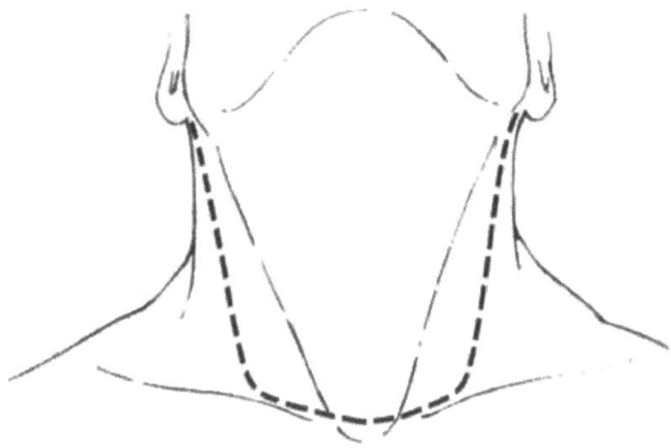

Fig. 8.5 Standard thyroidectomy incision with bilateral thyroid utility extensions. A "W"plasty can be incorporated at the upper end of the utility incision in order to achieve a better scar

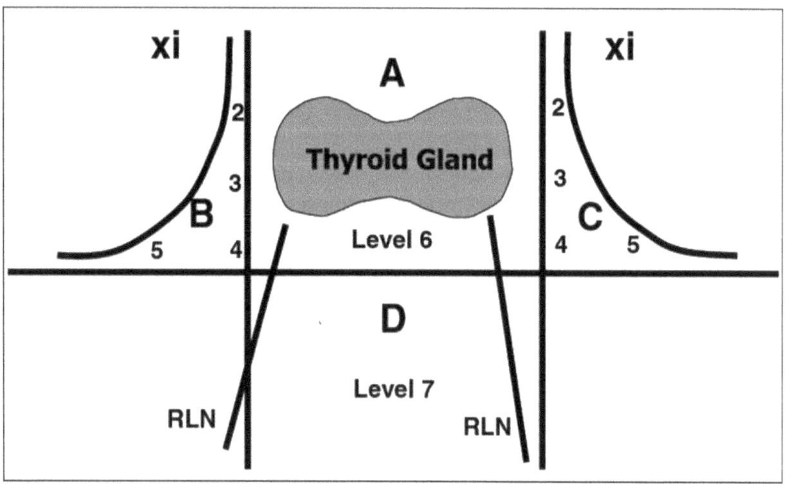

Fig. 8.6 Schematic outline of central compartment dissection and a lateral neck dissection, dissecting levels II, III, IV, and V below the accessory nerve. *RLN* recurrent laryngeal nerve

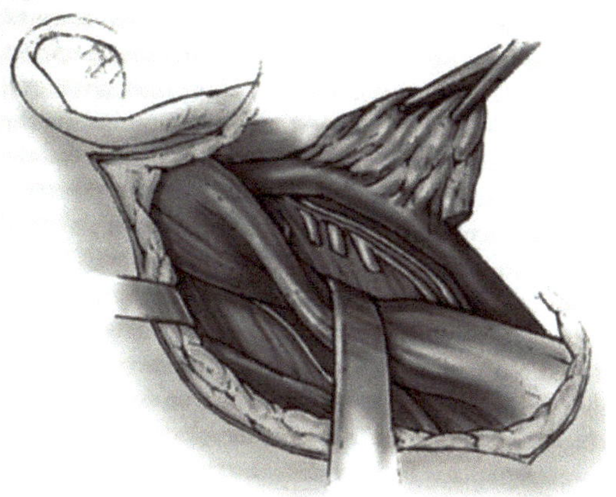

Fig. 8.7 As part of a selective neck dissection, the lymph node bearing tissue of level V is removed followed by access to levels II, III, and IV obtained by either retracting or dividing the sternomastoid muscle. The internal jugular vein and accessory nerve are also preserved. The cervical plexus is usually divided. (Reproduced with permission from Johnson JT and Gluckman JL (eds), Carcinoma of the Thyroid, Oxford: Isis Medical Media, 1999, page 79)

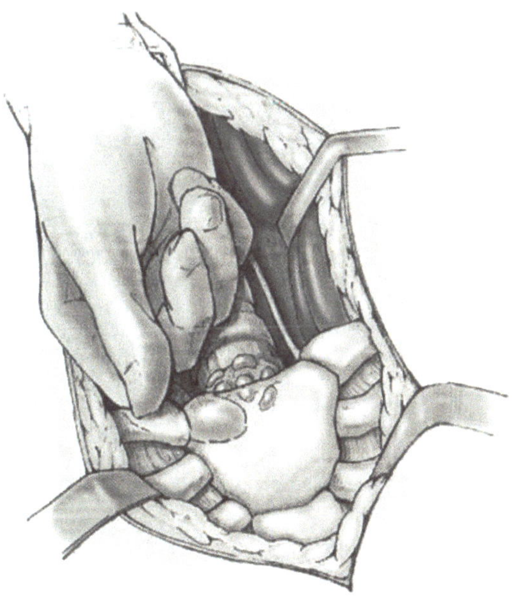

Fig. 8.8 During a formal total thyroidectomy with level VI neck dissection, access to level VII can usually be achieved by a cervical approach. (Reproduced with permission from Johnson JT and Gluckman JL (eds), Carcinoma of the Thyroid, Oxford: Isis Medical Media, 1999, page 78)

internal jugular vein (Fig. 8.4) and which often contains occult metastases from differentiated thyroid cancer.

The dissection proceeds in an upward and medial direction clearing levels IIA to VB with every attempt made to preserve the sensory branches of the cervical plexus, although it is difficult to carry out an adequate selective neck dissection without sometimes dividing some or all of these branches. This is the author's practice and the technique of routinely taking the cervical plexus with a selective neck dissection is well described [79]. For more extensive disease, level I may have to be dissected and one or all of the internal jugular vein, sternomastoid muscle, and accessory nerve sacrificed (modified radical or radical neck dissection). Very occasionally, other structures have to be removed (i.e. the digastric muscle, external skin) and this is an extended radical neck dissection. The areas dissected and key steps of a selective neck dissection (levels IIA–VB) are shown in Figs. 8.9, 8.10, 8.11, 8.12, 8.13, 8.14, and 8.15. In a personal series of 77 neck dissections (Table. 8.7), the hematoma and infection rates were 0.8%. One patient had an accessory nerve palsy (the nerve was deliberately divided), and another had a chyle leak which required re-exploration.

The key steps for performing a selective neck dissection in differentiated thyroid carcinoma are shown in Table 8.8.

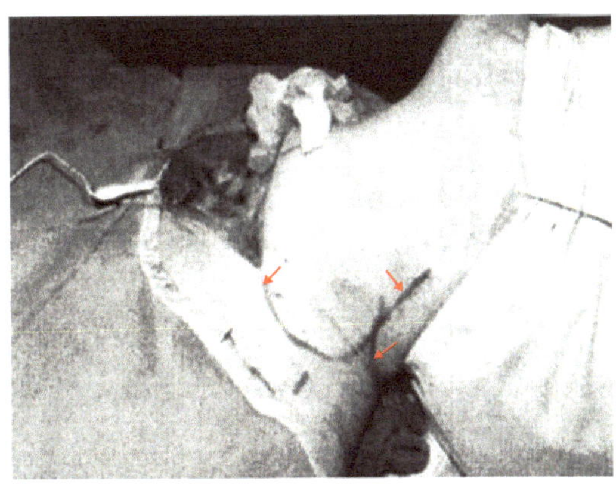

Fig. 8.9 Lateral utility incision marked out on the skin

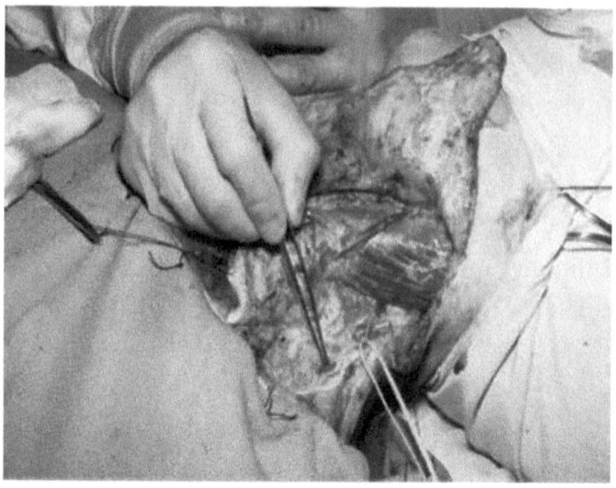

Fig. 8.10 Posterior triangle identified with the accessory nerve having been isolated with a sloop

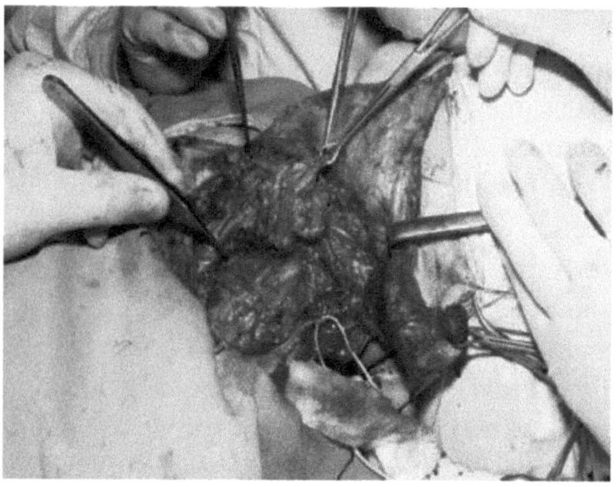

Fig. 8.11 The sternomastoid muscle has been divided and retracted superiorly. The accessory nerve is identified with a sloop and the lymphoid bearing tissue in level V below the nerve is removed; the dissection is carried forward to remove the lymph node bearing area in level IV together with the scalene nodes behind the lower end of the internal jugular vein (Chaissaignac's triangle–this area is being pointed to with a pair of forceps)

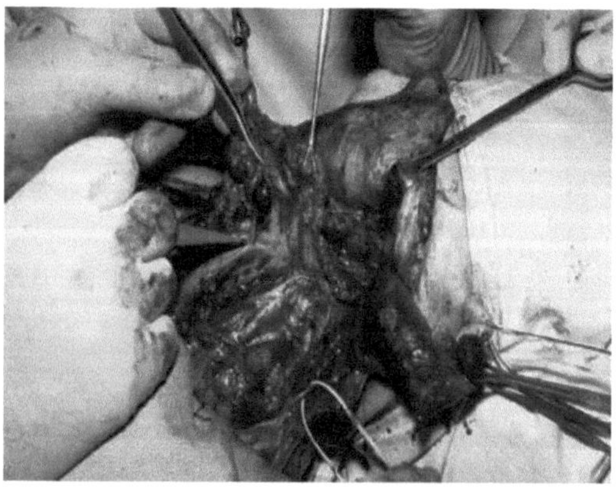

Fig. 8.12 The dissection is continued superiorly removing the lymph node bearing tissue in levels III and IIA. The mass is dissected from the internal jugular vein

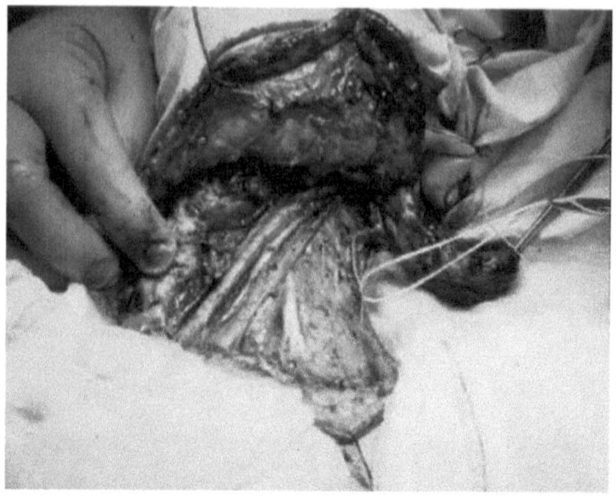

Fig. 8.13 The dissection is completed showing from lateral to medial, the divided lower end of the sternomastoid muscle, accessory nerve with a sloop around it, the brachial plexus, Chaissaignac's triangle, the internal jugular vein, the vagus nerve and the common carotid artery. The author's index finger is retracting the trachea medially and the recurrent laryngeal nerve can be seen between it and the common carotid

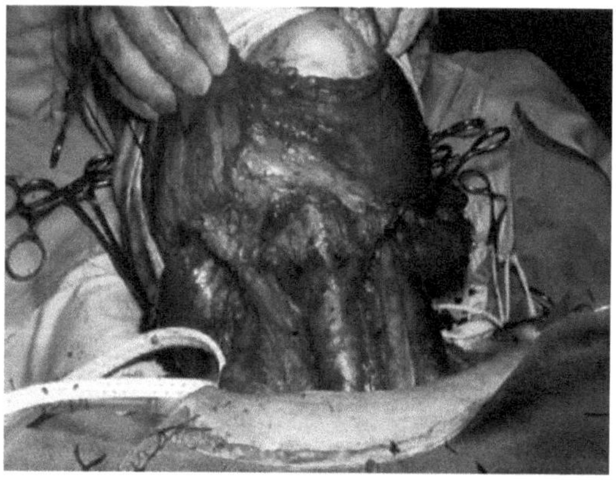

Fig. 8.14 Final result following total thyroidectomy and bilateral selective neck dissection (levels IIA–VB)

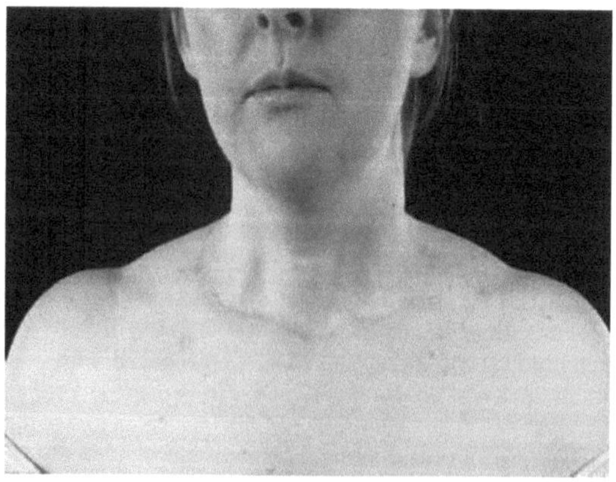

Fig. 8.15 Final result following total thyroidectomy and bilateral selective neck dissection in the same patient

Table 8.7 Author's (JCW) personal series of patients undergoing lateral neck dissection for differentiated thyroid cancer

Extended radical neck dissection	3
Radical neck dissection	3
Modified radical neck dissection	17
Selective neck dissection levels II–V	44
Selective neck dissection levels III–V	6
Selective neck dissection levels II–IV	4
Total	77

Table 8.8 The key steps for performing a selective neck dissection in patients with differentiated thyroid carcinoma

• Adequate incision
• Identify levels II, III, IV, and V
• Clearly identify the accessory nerve
• Deal with the sternomastoid muscle
• Dissect corners one and two
• Preserve the internal jugular vein, phrenic nerve and brachial plexus
• Access Chassaignac's triangle
• Finally dissect levels II_A–V_B

Table 8.9 The major complications of neck dissections performed for differentiated thyroid carcinoma

• Temporary and permanent hypoparathyroidism
• Bleeding
• Chyle leak
• Nerve injury
• Wound infection
• Poor scar

Complications

Complications relating to neck dissection for differentiated thyroid cancer can be divided into early, intermediate and late, local and general. Important complications of neck dissection are listed in Table 8.9. Although bleeding is uncommon following neck dissection, it can be dramatic. It is usually either reactionary or secondary and tends to occur in the first 6 h following surgery. It can be kept to a minimum by meticulous technique, doubly ligating or ligating and transfixing named vessels and with the routine use of drains. Significant bleeding requires return to theatre.

A chyle leak can occur when operating on the left side of the neck. The thoracic duct is particularly vulnerable when dissecting Chassaignac's triangle. Low volume leaks may be treated conservatively using a low fat diet and low suction drainage. It may be possible to inject a sclerosant into the wound (such as tetracycline or talc) to promote a seal. For those leaks that are of high volume (greater than 500 ml a day) or for those that do not settle conservatively, surgical re-exploration is required. This can be done through the neck by reopening the wound when the duct is identified and ligated. The use of loupes can facilitate the dissection. Alternatively the thoracic duct can be ligated in the chest by a thoracic surgeon. For those leaks that are high volume, early exploration is advisable rather than adopting a conservative approach. Damage to the jugular lymph ducts can give rise to lymphatic leaks, which generally settle conservatively. This can occur bilaterally. A chyle leak from the right lower neck is very uncommon but can occur. Seromas occur later on in the postoperative period (usually following drain removal) and are generally treated conservatively. Some, however, may require aspiration.

Nerve Injury

There are several nerves that are at risk during the performance of a neck dissection (Table 8.10). The accessory nerve should be identified early on as part of the neck dissection. Probably the best way to find it is at Erb's point, which is one centimeter above where the greater auricular nerve winds round the posterior border of the sternomastoid. Once identified, it can be isolated with a sloop, and the dissection proceeds caudal to the nerve. In a certain proportion of cases, the main nerve supply to trapezius comes from the contribution to the accessory nerve from the cervical plexus. In addition, preservation of the nerve does not guarantee it functions postoperatively, presumably due to devascularization. Damage to the phrenic nerve and brachial plexus can be avoided by clear identification of the prevertebral fascia and not allowing the dissection to proceed below that structure. The vagus is identified in the carotid sheath and should not be damaged unless it is invaded by tumour. The same applies to the hypoglossal nerve.

Table 8.10 The nerves at risk during neck dissection for differentiated thyroid carcinoma

• Accessory nerve
• Hypoglossal nerve
• Vagus nerve
• Phrenic nerve
• Brachial plexus
• Cervical plexus
Level VI neck dissection only
• Recurrent laryngeal nerve
• External branch of the superior laryngeal nerve

It is extremely difficult to carry out a proper neck dissection without damaging branches of the cervical plexus, and this includes the greater auricular nerve. While it may be possible in some cases to preserve these nerves, given the need for oncological clearance, and removal of all involved lymph nodes, it is better to sacrifice them since this results in minimal morbidity (loss of sensation over the side of neck and shoulder).

In general, incisions in the neck that are correctly placed heal well. Like fine wine, scars mature but if they are wrongly sited they can have disastrous results. One of the problems with using a thyroid utility incision is that in the upper posterior neck, there is a lack of platysma so that some of the scars can become hyper-trophic. This can be kept to a minimum by meticulous surgical technique, a two-layer closure, keeping the sutures in for 7–10 days, and incorporating a "W" plasty in the upper end of the incision. Generally the scar (particularly in women) can be hidden within the hairline but when patients are unhappy with the final result, scar revision may be performed.

The use of triamcinolone given subcutaneously can help. Alternatively, a different incision can be used which involves a higher than usual collar thyroidectomy incision that is simply extended across the posterior triangle without any significant upward extension. This is particularly useful when access only to levels III, VI, and VB is required.

The Difficult Neck

In patients with differentiated thyroid cancer, the management of the neck can be difficult for several reasons. Patients can be difficult to examine and assess, as well as being difficult to operate on and follow up. Necks can be difficult to examine and assess because of either obesity or previous treatment with surgery or irradiation. Difficult necks to operate on include those with extensive disease, bilateral disease, those with mediastinal extension and residual and recurrent disease following previous treatment. All the above situations can be difficult to follow up. Where there is any difficulty arising regarding clinical assessment, anatomical imaging is mandatory.

Follow-up

The majority of necks are followed up routinely by clinical examination. The thyroid bed is examined along with the central compartment and both lateral neck compartments. Previous surgery can alter patterns of lymphatic drainage, so it is not uncommon that lymph nodes may be detected after treatment. Some are benign and regress over time but those patients whose lesions persist, or who are at high risk of recurrence or have an elevated thyroglobulin will need further investigation. Any mass arising suspicion requires a FNA with or without US guidance and other relevant follow on investigations [22].

Supra-physiological doses of levothyroxine are used to reduce the risk of recurrence [80–82]. Evidence from a meta-analysis supports the efficacy of thyroid stimulating hormone (TSH) suppression in preventing recurrences [83]. The BTA recommend that patients who were not in need of radio-iodine remnant ablation therapy do not require TSH suppression [22].

A baseline postoperative serum thyroglobulin (Tg) should be checked, preferably no earlier than 6 weeks after surgery [22], then this should be monitored every 6–12 months or more frequently for high risk patients. Ideally, Tg should be measured longitudinally with serum anti-Tg [40]. In the presence of a truly positive elevated Tg, recurrent disease is assessed with whole-body ^{131}I scanning and anatomical imaging with either CT or US.

The ATA recommend neck US to evaluate the thyroid bed and the central and lateral neck compartments at 6–12 months after surgery and then periodically, depending on the patients' risk for recurrence and Tg status. If an abnormal lymph node (≥8–10 mm) is detected, a FNA should be performed with Tg measurement [40]. If a suspicious lymph node measuring <8 mm is found, serial USs and future consideration for FNA if any change is seen can be considered. For patients who have a difficult neck to examine with a negative ^{131}I scan and raised Tg level, a [18] FDG-PET scan should be performed [40].

Recurrent disease in the treated neck should be dealt with, where possible, with further surgery. However, if there is low volume recurrent/persistent disease in the neck, which is not progressive, the BTA suggest active surveillance instead of further surgery. If a formal neck dissection has not been previously performed, then this should be completed. If it has been done, local resection suffices with recourse then to further treatment with RAI and consideration for external beam radiotherapy (EBRT) when residual macroscopic disease is present. EBRT can be also utilised if there is progressive disease that is unamenable to surgery and unresponsive to ^{131}I therapy [22].

Patients with unifocal papillary microcarcinoma and no other risk factors (i.e. those who have only undergone lobectomy) have a risk of dying of thyroid cancer similar to that of the general population and have a risk of recurrence of <2.5% and a risk of distant metastases of <0.4% [84]. Given that for the general population the lifetime risk of developing any cancer is about 33% and the risk of dying from any cancer 28% the benefits of screening for recurrence, are unlikely to outweigh the disadvantages [85].

Conclusion

The majority of patients with differentiated thyroid cancer have papillary carcinoma and most will be treated by thyroidectomy. Regional metastases to the cervical lymph nodes are relatively common, occur early on and are more frequent in children. The incidence of palpable neck metastases in papillary carcinoma is between 20 and 50% and up to 90% have occult disease. The first echelon lymph nodes for drainage occur commonly in levels III, IV, VB, VI, and VII and in the untreated neck, patterns of lymph node drainage occur in a recognized, predictable, and systematic manner so as to facilitate selective neck surgery.

There is no role for prophylactic central compartment or lateral compartment dissection in the cN0 neck. Patients with overt lateral neck node disease will have clinical/radiological evidence of nodal disease in the central compartment in 80% of cases. Therefore, as well as a selective neck dissection of levels II to VB, a level VI/VII should be considered. There is no role of the historical "berry picking" of lymph node.

Key Points

- The majority of patients with differentiated thyroid cancer have papillary carcinoma and most are treated by TTx.
- Metastases to the regional cervical lymph nodes are relatively common and occur early on, irrespective of size of tumour.
- The incidence of palpable neck metastases in papillary carcinoma is between 20-50% and up to 90% have occult disease.
- In the untreated neck, patterns of lymph node drainage occur in a recognized and systematic manner facilitating selective neck surgery.
- There is no role for prophylactic central or lateral compartment dissection in the cN0 neck.
- When there is palpable (or suspected) disease within the lateral neck compartment, a selective neck dissection of levels II to VB should be performed as well as consideration of central compartment dissection (levels VI/VII).
- Selective neck surgery for differentiated thyroid cancer can be performed with low morbidity.
- There is no role for "berry picking"
- Follow-up is for life and is a dynamic process of risk assessment.

References

1. Aschebrook-Kilfoy B, Ward MH, Sabra MM, Devesa SS. Thyroid cancer incidence patterns in the United States by histologic type, 1992-2006. Thyroid. 2011;21(2):125–34. https://doi.org/10.1089/thy.2010.0021.
2. Kouvaraki MA, Shapiro SE, Fornage BD, et al. Role of preoperative ultrasonography in the surgical management of patients with thyroid cancer. Surgery. 2003;134(6):946–54. https://doi.org/10.1016/S0039.
3. Hughes DT, White ML, Miller BS, Gauger PG, Burney RE, Doherty GM. Influence of prophylactic central lymph node dissection on postoperative thyroglobulin levels and radioiodine treatment in papillary thyroid cancer. Surgery. 2010;148(6):1100–6. https://doi.org/10.1016/j.surg.2010.09.019.
4. Randolph GW, Duh Q-Y, Heller KS, et al. The prognostic significance of nodal metastases from papillary thyroid carcinoma can be stratified based on the size and number of metastatic lymph nodes, as well as the presence of extranodal extension. Thyroid. 2012;22(11):1144–52. https://doi.org/10.1089/thy.2012.0043.
5. Mazzaferri EL, Kloos RT. Clinical review 128: current approaches to primary therapy for papillary and follicular thyroid cancer. J Clin Endocrinol Metab. 2001;86(4):1447–63. https://doi.org/10.1210/jcem.86.4.7407.
6. Grebe SK, Hay ID. Thyroid cancer nodal metastases: biologic significance and therapeutic considerations. Surg Oncol Clin N Am. 1996;5(1):43–63.
7. Noguchi S, Noguchi A, Murakami N. Papillary carcinoma of the thyroid. II. Value of prophylactic lymph node excision. Cancer. 1970;26(5):1061–4.
8. Attie JN, Khafif RA, Steckler RM. Elective neck dissection in papillary carcinoma of the thyroid. Am J Surg. 1971;122(4):464–71.
9. Nam-Goong IS, Kim HY, Gong G, et al. Ultrasonography-guided fine-needle aspiration of thyroid incidentaloma: correlation with pathological findings. Clin Endocrinol. 2004;60(1):21–8.
10. Chow S-M, Law SCK, Chan JKC, Au S-K, Yau S, Lau W-H. Papillary microcarcinoma of the thyroid-prognostic significance of lymph node metastasis and multifocality. Cancer. 2003;98(1):31–40. https://doi.org/10.1002/cncr.11442.
11. Scheumann GF, Gimm O, Wegener G, Hundeshagen H, Dralle H. Prognostic significance and surgical management of locoregional lymph node metastases in papillary thyroid cancer. World J Surg. 1994;18(4):559–67.
12. Ito Y, Uruno T, Nakano K, et al. An observation trial without surgical treatment in patients with papillary microcarcinoma of the thyroid. Thyroid. 2003;13(4):381–7. https://doi.org/10.1089/105072503321669875.
13. Hay ID, Grant CS, van Heerden JA, Goellner JR, Ebersold JR, Bergstralh EJ. Papillary thyroid microcarcinoma: a study of 535 cases observed in a 50-year period. Surgery. 1992;112(6):1139–46.
14. Verburg FA, van Santen H, Luster M. Pediatric papillary thyroid cancer: current management challenges. Onco Targets Ther. 2016;10:165–75. https://doi.org/10.2147/OTT.S100512.
15. Mitchell AL, Gandhi A, Scott-Coombes D, Perros P. Management of thyroid cancer: United Kingdom National Multidisciplinary Guidelines. J Laryngol Otol. 2016;130(S2):S150–60. https://doi.org/10.1017/S0022215116000578.
16. Mastronikolis NS, Fitzgerald D, Owen C, Neary Z, Glaholm J, Watkinson JC. The management of squamous cell carcinoma of the neck. The Birmingham UK experience. Eur J Surg Oncol. 2005;31(5):461–6. https://doi.org/10.1016/j.ejso.2005.01.015.
17. Moosa M, Mazzaferri EL. Management of thyroid neoplasms. In: Cummings C, Fredrickson J, Harker LA, Krause CJ, Richardson MA, Schuller DE, editors. Otolaryngology head and neck surgery. 3rd ed. Stuttgart: Thieme Medical; 1998. p. 2480–518.
18. Podnos YD, Smith D, Wagman LD, Ellenhorn JDI. The implication of lymph node metastasis on survival in patients with well-differentiated thyroid cancer. Am Surg. 2005;71(9):731–4.
19. Zaydfudim V, Feurer ID, Griffin MR, Phay JE. The impact of lymph node involvement on survival in patients with papillary and follicular thyroid carcinoma. Surgery. 2008;144(6):1070–8. https://doi.org/10.1016/j.surg.2008.08.034.
20. Adam MA, Pura J, Goffredo P, et al. Presence and number of lymph node metastases are associated with compromised survival for patients younger than age 45 years with papillary thyroid cancer. J Clin Oncol. 2015;33(21):2370–5. https://doi.org/10.1200/JCO.2014.59.8391.
21. Bajaj Y, De M, Thompson A. Fine needle aspiration cytology in diagnosis and management of thyroid disease. J Laryngol Otol. 2006;120(6):467–9. https://doi.org/10.1017/S0022215106000703.
22. Perros P, Boelaert K, Colley S, et al. Guidelines for the management of thyroid cancer. Clin Endocrinol. 2014;81:1–122. https://doi.org/10.1111/cen.12515.
23. Qubain SW, Nakano S, Baba M, Takao S, Aikou T. Distribution of lymph node micrometastasis in pN0 well-differentiated thyroid carcinoma. Surgery. 2002;131(3):249–56.
24. Arturi F, Russo D, Giuffrida D, et al. Early diagnosis by genetic analysis of differentiated thyroid cancer metastases in small lymph nodes. J Clin Endocrinol Metab. 1997;82(5):1638. https://doi.org/10.1210/jcem.82.5.4062.
25. Roh MH, Jo VY, Stelow EB, et al. The predictive value of the fine-needle aspiration diagnosis "suspicious for a follicular neoplasm, hurthle cell type" in patients with hashimoto thyroiditis. Am J Clin Pathol. 2011;135(1):139–45. https://doi.org/10.1309/AJCP0RW2WMDUAKGK.
26. Watkinson J, Gaze M, Wilson J. Metastatic neck disease. In: Stell and Maran's head and neck surgery.

4th ed. Oxford: Butterworth Heinemann; 2000. p. 197–214.
27. Shah JP, Strong E, Spiro RH, Vikram B. Surgical grand rounds. Neck dissection: current status and future possibilities. Clin Bull. 1981;11(1): 25–33.
28. Shah J. Head and neck: surgery and oncology. In: Head and neck: surgery and oncology. 3rd ed. Edinburgh: Mosby; 2003. p. 353–94.
29. Gavilán J, Gavilán C, Herranz J. Functional neck dissection: three decades of controversy. Ann Otol Rhinol Laryngol. 1992;101(4):339–41. https://doi.org/10.1177/000348949210100409.
30. Robbins KT, Shaha AR, Medina JE, et al. Consensus statement on the classification and terminology of neck dissection. Arch Otolaryngol Neck Surg. 2008;134(5):536. https://doi.org/10.1001/archotol.134.5.536.
31. Baudin E, Travagli JP, Ropers J, et al. Microcarcinoma of the thyroid gland: the Gustave-Roussy Institute experience. Cancer. 1998;83(3):553–9.
32. Asimakopoulos P, Nixon IJ, Shaha AR. Differentiated and medullary thyroid cancer: surgical management of cervical lymph nodes. Clin Oncol. 2017;29(5):283–9. https://doi.org/10.1016/j.clon.2017.01.001.
33. Park JH, Lee YS, Kim BW, Chang H-S, Park CS. Skip lateral neck node metastases in papillary thyroid carcinoma. World J Surg. 2012;36(4):743–7. https://doi.org/10.1007/s00268-012-1476-5.
34. Likhterov I, Dos Reis L, Urken M. Central compartment management in patients with papillary thyroid cancer presenting with metastatic disease to the lateral neck: anatomic pathways of lymphatic spread. Head Neck. 2017;39(5):853–9. https://doi.org/10.1002/hed.24568.
35. Thomas G, Pandey M, Jayasree K, et al. Parapharyngeal metastasis from papillary microcarcinoma of thyroid: report of a case diagnosed by peroral fine needle aspiration. Br J Oral Maxillofac Surg. 2002;40(3):229–31. https://doi.org/10.1054/bjom.2001.0754.
36. Ali S, Tiwari RM, Snow GB. False-positive and false-negative neck nodes. Head Neck Surg. 1985;8(2):78–82.
37. Frasoldati A, Pesenti M, Gallo M, Caroggio A, Salvo D, Valcavi R. Diagnosis of neck recurrences in patients with differentiated thyroid carcinoma. Cancer. 2003;97(1):90–6. https://doi.org/10.1002/cncr.11031.
38. Leenhardt L, Erdogan MF, Hegedus L, et al. 2013 European thyroid association guidelines for cervical ultrasound scan and ultrasound-guided techniques in the postoperative management of patients with thyroid cancer. Eur Thyroid J. 2013;2(3):147–59. https://doi.org/10.1159/000354537.
39. Leboulleux S, Girard E, Rose M, et al. Ultrasound criteria of malignancy for cervical lymph nodes in patients followed up for differentiated thyroid cancer. J Clin Endocrinol Metab. 2007;92(9):3590–4. https://doi.org/10.1210/jc.2007-0444.
40. Haugen BR, Alexander EK, Bible KC, et al. 2015 American Thyroid Association Management Guidelines for adult patients with thyroid nodules and differentiated thyroid cancer: The American Thyroid Association Guidelines Task Force on thyroid nodules and differentiated thyroid cancer. Thyroid. 2016;26(1):1–133. https://doi.org/10.1089/thy.2015.0020.
41. Ahn JE, Lee JH, Yi JS, et al. Diagnostic accuracy of CT and ultrasonography for evaluating metastatic cervical lymph nodes in patients with thyroid cancer. World J Surg. 2008;32(7):1552–8. https://doi.org/10.1007/s00268-008-9588-7.
42. Choi JS, Kim J, Kwak JY, Kim MJ, Chang HS, Kim E-K. Preoperative staging of papillary thyroid carcinoma: comparison of ultrasound imaging and CT. Am J Roentgenol. 2009;193(3):871–8. https://doi.org/10.2214/AJR.09.2386.
43. Jeong H-S, Baek C-H, Son Y-I, et al. Integrated 18F-FDG PET/CT for the initial evaluation of cervical node level of patients with papillary thyroid carcinoma: comparison with ultrasound and contrast-enhanced CT. Clin Endocrinol. 2006;65(3):402–7. https://doi.org/10.1111/j.1365-2265.2006.02612.x.
44. UICC. Head and neck tumours, thyroid gland. In: UICC–AJCC, editor. TNM classification of malignant tumours. 7th ed. New York: Wiley; 2009. p. 62.
45. Brierley J, Gospodarowicz M, Wittekind C. In: Brierley JD, Gospodarowicz M, Wittekind C, eds. TNM classification of malignant tumours. 8th ed. Oxford: Wiley-Blackwell; 2016.
46. Tuttle RM, Haugen B, Perrier ND. Updated American joint committee on cancer/tumor-node-metastasis staging system for differentiated and anaplastic thyroid cancer (eighth edition): what changed and why? Thyroid. 2017;27(6):751–6. https://doi.org/10.1089/thy.2017.0102.
47. Schlumberger M, Pacini F. Initial treatment. In: Thyroid tumours. 2nd ed. Paris: Editions Nucleon; 2003. p. 127–46.
48. Rhys E, Pracy J, Vini L, A Hern, Harmer C. Selective neck dissection or simple nodal excision in the management of cervical metastases from differentiated carcinoma of the thyroid. 5th International Conference on Head and Neck Cancer. San Francisco; 2000. p. 67.
49. Yang L, Shen W, Sakamoto N. Population-based study evaluating and predicting the probability of death resulting from thyroid cancer and other causes among patients with thyroid cancer. J Clin Oncol. 2013;31(4):468–74. https://doi.org/10.1200/JCO.2012.42.4457.
50. Hay ID, Bergstralh EJ, Grant CS, et al. Impact of primary surgery on outcome in 300 patients with pathologic tumor-node-metastasis stage III papillary thyroid carcinoma treated at one institution from 1940 through 1989. Surgery. 1999;126(6):1173–81.
51. Vassilopoulou-Sellin R, Schultz PN, Haynie TP. Clinical outcome of patients with papillary thyroid carcinoma who have recurrence after initial radioactive iodine therapy.

Cancer. 1996;78(3):493–501. https://doi.org/10.1002/(SICI)1097-0142(19960801)78:3<493::AID-CNCR17>3.0.CO;2-U.
52. Barczyński M, Konturek A, Stopa M, Nowak W. Prophylactic central neck dissection for papillary thyroid cancer. Br J Surg. 2013;100(3):410–8. https://doi.org/10.1002/bjs.8985.
53. Popadich A, Levin O, Lee JC, et al. A multicenter cohort study of total thyroidectomy and routine central lymph node dissection for cN0 papillary thyroid cancer. Surgery. 2011;150(6):1048–57. https://doi.org/10.1016/j.surg.2011.09.003.
54. Hartl DM, Mamelle E, Borget I, Leboulleux S, Mirghani H, Schlumberger M. Influence of prophylactic neck dissection on rate of retreatment for papillary thyroid carcinoma. World J Surg. 2013;37(8):1951–8. https://doi.org/10.1007/s00268-013-2089-3.
55. Sywak M, Cornford L, Roach P, Stalberg P, Sidhu S, Delbridge L. Routine ipsilateral level VI lymphadenectomy reduces postoperative thyroglobulin levels in papillary thyroid cancer. Surgery. 2006;140(6):1000–5. https://doi.org/10.1016/j.surg.2006.08.001.
56. Wang TS, Evans DB, Fareau GG, Carroll T, Yen TW. Effect of prophylactic central compartment neck dissection on serum thyroglobulin and recommendations for adjuvant radioactive iodine in patients with differentiated thyroid cancer. Ann Surg Oncol. 2012;19(13):4217–22. https://doi.org/10.1245/s10434-012-2594-x.
57. Hartl DM, Leboulleux S, Al Ghuzlan A, et al. Optimization of staging of the neck with prophylactic central and lateral neck dissection for papillary thyroid carcinoma. Ann Surg. 2012;255(4):777–83. https://doi.org/10.1097/SLA.0b013e31824b7b68.
58. Lang BH-H, Wong KP, Wan KY, Lo CY. Impact of routine unilateral central neck dissection on preablative and postablative stimulated thyroglobulin levels after total thyroidectomy in papillary thyroid carcinoma. Ann Surg Oncol. 2012;19(1):60–7. https://doi.org/10.1245/s10434-011-1833-x.
59. Wang TS, Cheung K, Farrokhyar F, Roman SA, Sosa JA. A meta-analysis of the effect of prophylactic central compartment neck dissection on locoregional recurrence rates in patients with papillary thyroid cancer. Ann Surg Oncol. 2013;20(11):3477–83. https://doi.org/10.1245/s10434-013-3125-0.
60. Pelizzo MR, Boschin IM, Toniato A, et al. Papillary thyroid carcinoma: 35-year outcome and prognostic factors in 1858 patients. Clin Nucl Med. 2007;32(6):440–4. https://doi.org/10.1097/RLU.0b013e31805375ca.
61. Moo T-A, McGill J, Allendorf J, Lee J, Fahey T, Zarnegar R. Impact of prophylactic central neck lymph node dissection on early recurrence in papillary thyroid carcinoma. World J Surg. 2010;34(6):1187–91. https://doi.org/10.1007/s00268-010-0418-3.
62. Moreno MA, Edeiken-Monroe BS, Siegel ER, Sherman SI, Clayman GL. In papillary thyroid cancer, preoperative central neck ultrasound detects only macroscopic surgical disease, but negative findings predict excellent long-term regional control and survival. Thyroid. 2012;22(4):347–55. https://doi.org/10.1089/thy.2011.0121.
63. Zuniga S, Sanabria A. Prophylactic central neck dissection in stage N0 papillary thyroid carcinoma. Arch Otolaryngol Neck Surg. 2009;135(11):1087. https://doi.org/10.1001/archoto.2009.163.
64. Lang BH-H, Ng S-H, Lau LLH, Cowling BJ, Wong KP, Wan KY. A systematic review and meta-analysis of prophylactic central neck dissection on short-term locoregional recurrence in papillary thyroid carcinoma after total thyroidectomy. Thyroid. 2013;23(9):1087–98. https://doi.org/10.1089/thy.2012.0608.
65. Viola D, Materazzi G, Valerio L, et al. Prophylactic central compartment lymph node dissection in papillary thyroid carcinoma: clinical implications derived from the first prospective randomized controlled single institution study. J Clin Endocrinol Metab. 2015;100(4):1316–24. https://doi.org/10.1210/jc.2014-3825.
66. Raijmakers PGHM, Paul MA, Lips P. Sentinel node detection in patients with thyroid carcinoma: a meta-analysis. World J Surg. 2008;32(9):1961–7. https://doi.org/10.1007/s00268-008-9657-y.
67. Portinari M, Carcoforo P. Radioguided sentinel lymph node biopsy in patients with papillary thyroid carcinoma. Gland Surg. 2016;5(6):591–602. https://doi.org/10.21037/gs.2016.11.08.
68. Baek S-K, Jung K-Y, Kang S-M, et al. Clinical risk factors associated with cervical lymph node recurrence in papillary thyroid carcinoma. Thyroid. 2010;20(2):147–52. https://doi.org/10.1089/thy.2008.0243.
69. Ito Y, Kudo T, Kobayashi K, Miya A, Ichihara K, Miyauchi A. Prognostic factors for recurrence of papillary thyroid carcinoma in the lymph nodes, lung, and bone: analysis of 5,768 patients with average 10-year follow-up. World J Surg. 2012;36(6):1274–8. https://doi.org/10.1007/s00268-012-1423-5.
70. Nixon IJ, Ganly I, Patel SG, et al. Observation of clinically negative central compartment lymph nodes in papillary thyroid carcinoma. Surgery. 2013;154(6):1166–73. https://doi.org/10.1016/j.surg.2013.04.035.
71. Olson MT, Clark DP, Erozan YS, Ali SZ. Spectrum of risk of malignancy in subcategories of "atypia of undetermined significance". Acta Cytol. 2011;55(6):518–25. https://doi.org/10.1159/000333232.
72. Stack BC, Ferris RL, Goldenberg D, et al. American thyroid association consensus review and statement regarding the anatomy, terminology, and rationale for lateral neck dissection in differentiated thyroid cancer. Thyroid. 2012;22(5):501–8. https://doi.org/10.1089/thy.2011.0312.
73. Van Hove C, Perry KA, Spight DH, et al. Predictors of technical skill acquisition among resident trainees

in a laparoscopic skills education program. World J Surg. 2008;32(9):1917–21. https://doi.org/10.1007/s00268-008-9643-4.
74. Castagna MG, Tala Jury HP, Cipri C, et al. The use of ultrasensitive thyroglobulin assays reduces but does not abolish the need for TSH stimulation in patients with differentiated thyroid carcinoma. J Endocrinol Investig. 2011;34(8):e219–23. https://doi.org/10.3275/7571.
75. Pacini F, Schlumberger M, Dralle H, et al. European consensus for the management of patients with differentiated thyroid carcinoma of the follicular epithelium. Eur J Endocrinol. 2006;154(6):787–803. https://doi.org/10.1530/eje.1.02158.
76. Pingpank JF, Sasson AR, Hanlon AL, Friedman CD, Ridge JA. Tumor above the spinal accessory nerve in papillary thyroid cancer that involves lateral neck nodes: a common occurrence. Arch Otolaryngol Head Neck Surg. 2002;128(11):1275–8.
77. British Thyroid Association and Royal College of Physicians. Guidelines for the management of thyroid cancer in adults. 2002.
78. Watkinson J, Gaze M, Wilson J. Thyroid. Tumours of the thyroid and parathyroid glands. In: Stell and Maran's head and neck surgery. 4th ed. Oxford: Butterworth Heinemann; 2000. p. 459–85.
79. Zaja J, Gluckman J. Lymphadenectomy for thyroid cancer. In: Carcinoma of the thyroid. Oxford: Isis Medical Media; 1999. p. 75–80.
80. Brabant G. Thyrotropin suppressive therapy in thyroid carcinoma: what are the targets? J Clin Endocrinol Metab. 2008;93(4):1167–9. https://doi.org/10.1210/jc.2007-2228.
81. Cooper DS, Doherty GM, Haugen BR, et al. Revised American thyroid association management guidelines for patients with thyroid nodules and differentiated thyroid cancer. Thyroid. 2009;19(11):1167–214. https://doi.org/10.1089/thy.2009.0110.
82. Jonklaas J, Sarlis NJ, Litofsky D, et al. Outcomes of patients with differentiated thyroid carcinoma following initial therapy. Thyroid. 2006;16(12):1229–42. https://doi.org/10.1089/thy.2006.16.1229.
83. McGriff NJ, Csako G, Gourgiotis L, Lori CG, Pucino F, Sarlis NJ. Effects of thyroid hormone suppression therapy on adverse clinical outcomes in thyroid cancer. Ann Med. 2002;34(7-8):554–64.
84. Mernagh P, Suebwongpat A, Silverberg J, Weston A. Cost-effectiveness of using recombinant human thyroid-stimulating hormone before radioiodine ablation for thyroid cancer: the Canadian perspective. Value Health. 2010;13(2):180–7. https://doi.org/10.1111/j.1524-4733.2009.00650.x.
85. Luster M, Lippi F, Jarzab B, et al. rhTSH-aided radioiodine ablation and treatment of differentiated thyroid carcinoma: a comprehensive review. Endocr Relat Cancer. 2005;12(1):49–64. https://doi.org/10.1677/erc.1.00830.

Advances in Thyroid Surgery

9

Sara L. Richer, Dipti Kamani,
and Gregory W. Randolph

Thyroid surgery has come a long way from the revolutionary nineteenth century days of Kocher and Bilroth. The original thyroid surgeries were bloody, involved a long incision and centered on patient survival of the procedure. Today, thyroid surgery is focused not only on the disease outcomes, but also on patient safety and satisfaction. With advances in technology and greater understanding of the anatomy of the thyroid gland and surrounding structures, surgeons have more tools at their disposal for thyroid procedures. These advances in thyroid surgery have focused on voice and cosmetic outcomes.

Galen was the first to identify the Recurrent Laryngeal nerve (RLN) after recognizing aphonia as a complication of vagal nerve section. Since the time of early thyroidectomy, surgeons have known about the importance of RLN preservation. However, more recently, more subtle voice changes that occur after thyroid surgery have raised awareness of endocrine surgeons. Rate of RLN paralysis after thyroidectomy have been reported to be 9.8%, ranging from 0 to 18.6% [1]. On a recent review of post-thyroidectomy voice changes, patients were found to have changes in average fundamental frequency, shimmer and maximum phonation time in the early (less than 3 months) postoperative period. Patients undergoing total thyroidectomy and male patients more commonly had early voice impairments [2]. Approximately 1 in 10 patients has temporary laryngeal nerve injury after surgery and longer lasting voice complaints are present in up to 1 in 25 patients [1].

In 2013, the American Academy of Otolaryngology-Head and Neck Surgery published guidelines for voice optimization during thyroid surgery [3]. These guidelines stressed the importance of identification and protection of the RLN during thyroid surgery. These guidelines also include several recommendations for pre and postoperative management of voice when the decision for thyroidectomy has been made. Preoperative documentation of the assessment of the patient's voice was recommended. Visualization of the vocal cords preoperatively was recommended in the case of impaired voice or those with thyroid cancer, suspected extra

S. L. Richer
Northeast Medical Group, Yale New Haven Health, New Haven, CT, USA

D. Kamani
Division of Thyroid and Parathyroid Endocrine Surgery, Department of Otolaryngology – Head and Neck Surgery, Massachusetts Eye and Ear Infirmary, Harvard Medical School, Boston, MA, USA

G. W. Randolph (✉)
Division of Thyroid and Parathyroid Endocrine Surgery, Department of Otolaryngology – Head and Neck Surgery, Massachusetts Eye and Ear Infirmary, Harvard Medical School, Boston, MA, USA

Thyroid Surgery Oncology, Harvard Medical School, Boston, MA, USA

Department of Surgery, Endocrine Surgery Service, Massachusetts General Hospital, Boston, MA, USA
e-mail: gregory_randolph@meei.harvard.edu

U. K. Mallick et al. (eds.), *Practical Management of Thyroid Cancer*,
https://doi.org/10.1007/978-3-319-91725-2_9

thyroidal extension, or prior neck surgery. Postoperatively, visualization of the vocal cords should be performed by a qualified physician if there is voice impairment after surgery. Also, the importance of pre-operative communication with the patient regarding possible adverse vocal outcomes was stressed. These guidelines highlight the importance of management of patient expectations regarding voice. Current technological advances in thyroid surgery such as intraoperative neural monitoring (IONM) and its recent developments and remote access thyroid surgery are discussed in this chapter.

Intraoperative Neural Monitoring [IONM]

Intraoperative neural monitoring [IONM], introduced in 1990s has been increasingly recognized as an adjunct in thyroid surgery [4]. Recent studies show that IONM is used by 53% of general surgeons and 65% of otolaryngologists performing thyroid surgery in the United States with even higher rates in German surgeons [5–7]. Current IONM relies on endotracheal tube-based surface electrodes which provide audio and visual waveform information on the evoked potential of the nerve. The basic setup has been well described previously [8] and involves a multi-channel EMG system, EMG display, electrodes on an endotracheal tube and handheld stimulation electrodes.

Before embarking on a neural monitoring program, it is important to understand the team approach required between the surgeon and anesthesiologist [9, 10]. The endotracheal tube position is critical for proper neural monitoring, therefore, the anesthesiologist must understand the proper tube placement and use of non-paralytic agents in anesthesia for accurate nerve monitoring. The surgeon must also be aware of the importance of the role of vagal stimulation in the IONM of the RLN. The presurgical suprathreshold vagal nerve stimulation is vital for verification of the IONM system. It is only after a positive signal from the ipsilateral vagus nerve that the surgeon can trust a negative response. The postsurgical suprathreshold vagus stimulation is crucial for accurate prognosis of postoperative RLN function. If only the RLN is stimulated at the end of the procedure, an injury distal to the site of stimulation will not be detected and an unexpected postoperative RLN paralysis may be present.

IONM provides several benefits: (1) Intraoperative RLN mapping, (2) aids in intraoperative management by providing insight into pathological states of the RLN (3) improves prognostication of postoperative nerve function. (4) Aids in predissection identification of Non recurrent laryngeal nerve (NRLN) (5) Helps in Detection of RLN branches (6) can be utilized as a teaching tool.

Intraoperative Mapping of RLN

As an adjunct in visual nerve identification, the IONM is used to map out the nerve in the paratracheal region. The nerve is then visually identified through directed dissection from the neural mapping. Once the nerve is identified, the IONM is used to aid intraoperative management by tracing the nerve and possible branches though intermittent stimulation of neural and adjacent non-neural tissue.

Insight into Pathologic States of the RLN

When electrophysiologic stimulation of a RLN invaded by malignancy reveals significant partial EMG activity despite preoperative VCP, the surgeon becomes aware of the functional consequences of resecting such a nerve. Even in the setting of preoperative VCP, additional dysphagia and aspiration to some extent may occur postoperatively after resection of such a nerve, the patient should be informed accordingly. Sometimes, surgical management of RLN invaded by tumor can be impacted by intraoperative EMG activity [11] (Fig. 9.1).

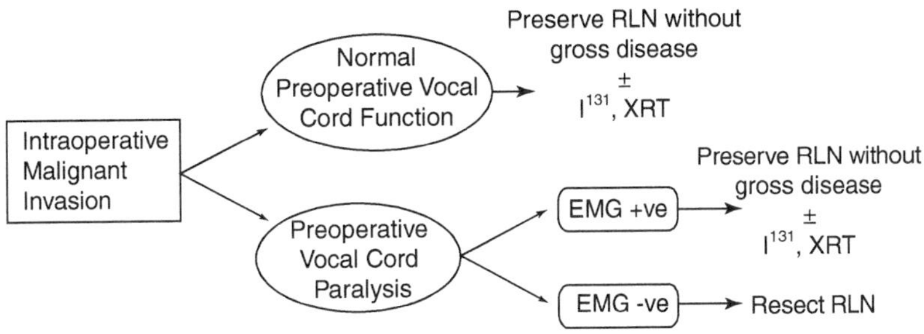

Fig. 9.1 Intraoperative management of invaded nerves based on preoperative VC function and EMG info

Aforementioned, slight but noteworthy implications of resection of invaded nerves are understood by the unique insight into the nuances of functional status of pathological nerves, provided only by IONM. Such functional information cannot be obtained by visual identification of the nerve alone.

Prognostication of Neural Function as it Relates to Intraoperative Injury

The most significant application of IONM comes from its ability of intraoperative prediction of postoperative neural function. Without IONM, visual identification and inspection of the nerve is the only available tool to determine postoperative functionality of nerve. A nerve injured by blunt trauma or stretching may appear visually intact but postoperatively may not function normally. In such cases structural integrity does not stipulate a normal postoperative functionality. Current literature shows that approximately only 10% of all injured nerves are detected by visual identification [12–14].

Contrary to this, IONM data in literature suggests that EMG testing of the vagus-RLN system after thyroid surgery is a highly precise neural function test and has negative predictive value of over 95%. However, positive predictive value is lower and can be quite variable and is related to how presumptive loss of signal (LOS) is evaluated with respect to equipment troubleshooting. Universal and accurate definition of LOS and a better knowledge of normative neural monitoring parameters will greatly augment prognostic function of IONM.

LOS is defined as no or low (i.e. 100 μV or less) electromyography response after initial satisfactory electrophysiologic response. It is critical to understand the management of an intraoperative LOS when using the IONM system, as LOS can indicate a neural injury or a monitoring system issue. When LOS occurs, the first step is the assessment of the laryngeal twitch with vagal stimulation on that side. If the twitch is present, it indicates that there is an issue with the recording side of the IONM system and should be corrected. This may require endotracheal tube repositioning maneuvers or correction of the interface of the monitoring system. If the laryngeal twitch is absent and the contralateral vagal stimulation is present, a neural injury should be considered (Fig. 9.2) [8]. After establishing that the LOS is due to a definite neural injury, retrograde testing of the affected RLN to identify injured nerve segment should be performed to help provide treatment and learning opportunities. The retrograde testing should proceed proximally after commencing at the laryngeal entry point. Consideration of postponement of the surgery on contralateral side in the setting of neural related LOS is an utmost application of neural prognostication by IONM.

The prognostic information obtained from the IONM can help prevent bilateral vocal cord paralysis as well as localize the site of nerve damage. In a study with over 1000 nerves at risk, Intraoperative nerve monitoring of the RLN was found to provide real-time information regarding neurophysiologic function of the RLN and predict immediate postoperative vocal cord palsy. The study found reliability of the RLN function when a cutoff of 200 μV was used [11].

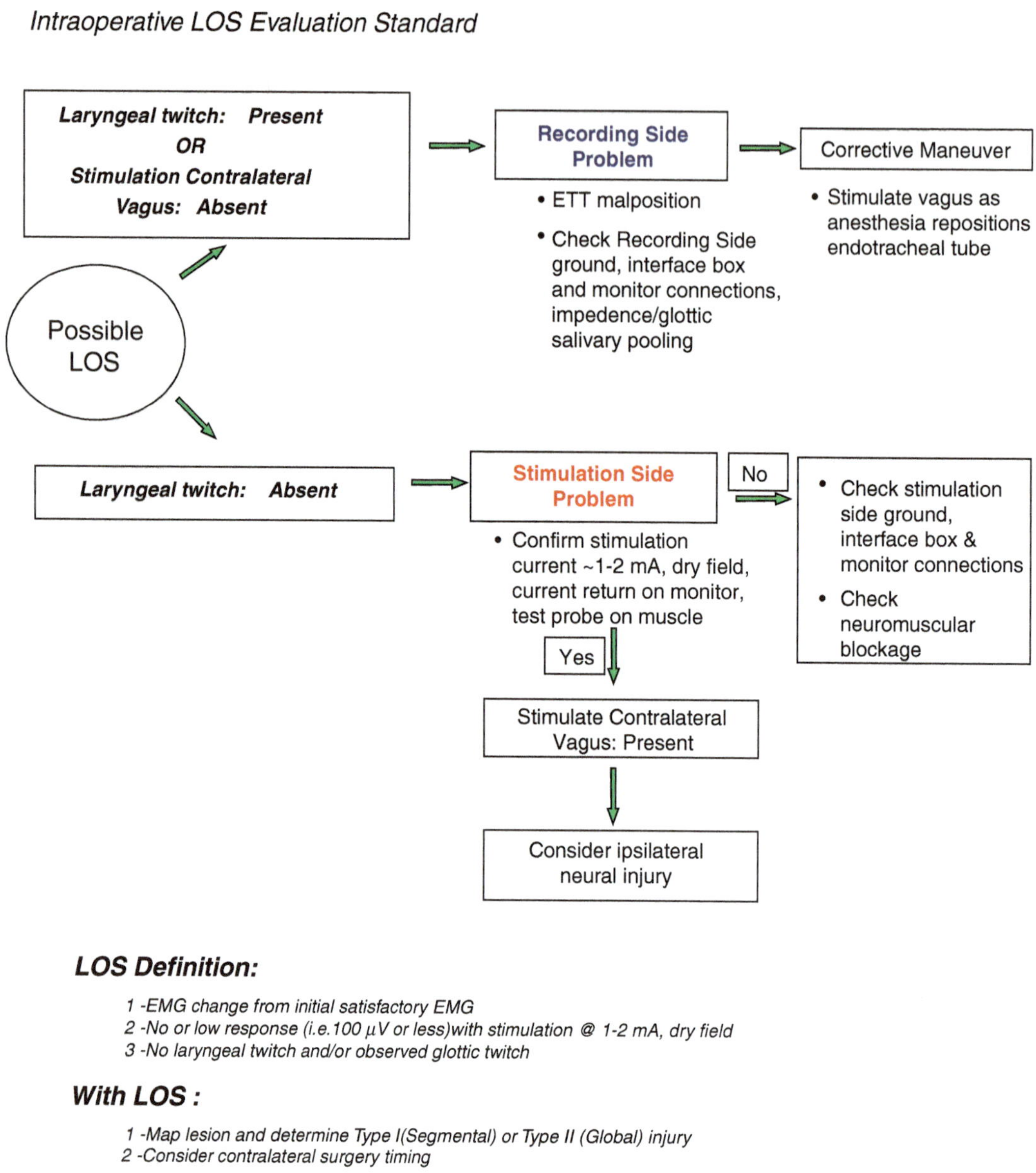

Fig. 9.2 Intraoperative LOS evaluation standard

IONM and NRLN Identification

Non-recurrent laryngeal nerve [NRLN] is an anatomic variant, more commonly occurring on the right side, a right sided NRLN is reported in the literature to be present in 0.5–1% of cases [15]. Left-sided NRLN is extremely rare and is associated with situs invertus, only a few cases [0.04%] of left side NRLN are reported in the literature. Given its unexpected anatomical course, NRLN is at a higher risk for injury during thyroidectomy. IONM can be of benefit to assist in the recognition of a NRLN. The NRLN can be identified by the presence of a positive EMG response with stimulation of the vagus nerve at the level of the superior border of the thyroid cartilage along with

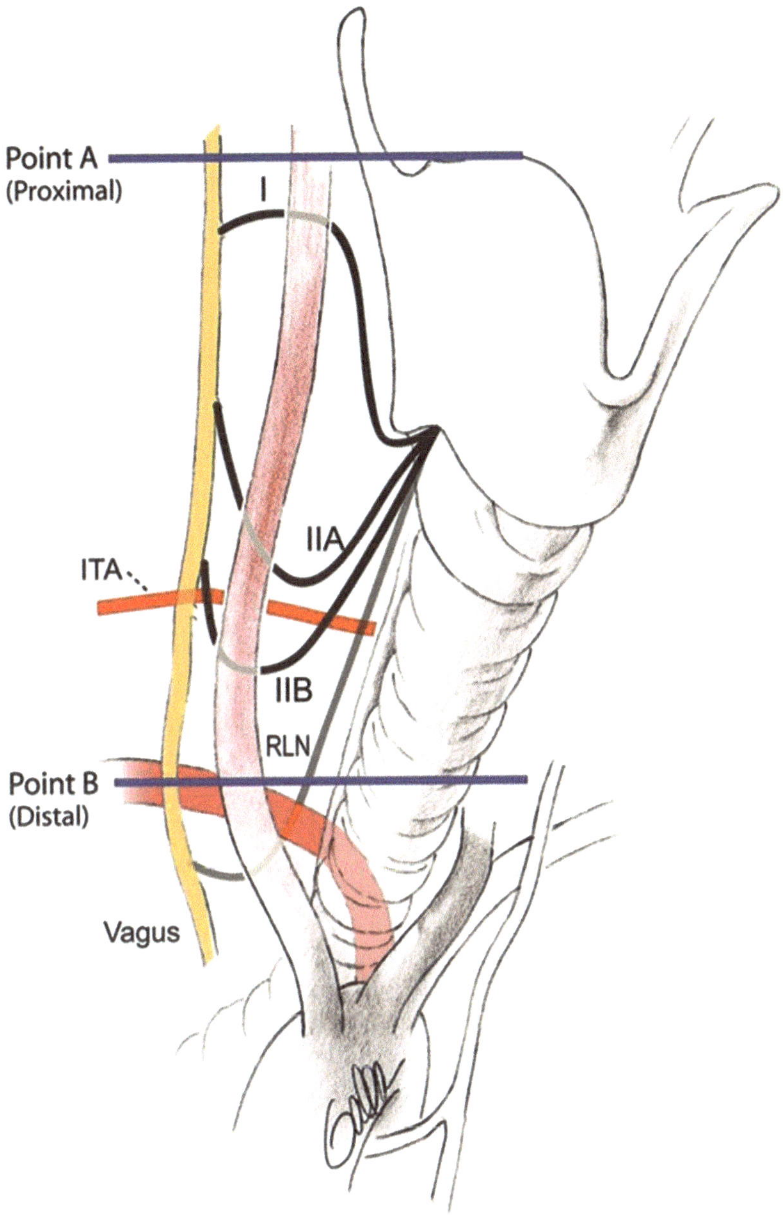

Fig. 9.3 Anatomical types of NRLN (I, IIA and IIB) and The proximal [A] and distal [B] points of vagal stimulation for detection on NRLN using IONM–point A: at the level of Superior border of thyroid cartilage and point B: at the level of inferior border of 4th tracheal ring. *ITA* inferior thyroid artery, *RLN* recurrent laryngeal nerve, *NRLN* non-recurrent laryngeal

the absence of EMG response to the distal vagal stimulation, at the level of the inferior border of the fourth tracheal ring [16] (Fig. 9.3). Whereas, preoperative identification of NRLN [through imaging studies] may be challenging, IONM can serve as a useful tool to prevent inadvertent damage of the NRLN by recognition of this anatomic variant prior to the surgical dissection in the lateral thyroid region. Routine use of IONM may improve the rate of NRLN identification [17].

IONM and RLN Branches

The RLN has been shown to branch 34–43% of the time in surgical specimens [18]. The motor fibers to the intrinsic muscles of the larynx are contained within the anterior branch with the posterior branch providing sensory function only. Therefore, if a posterior branch is visualized and the anterior branch is not recognized, RLN palsy may result from visual identification alone. The

IONM provides the ability to track specifically the motor fibers of the RLN for preservation of postoperative function.

IONM as a Teaching Tool

Another benefit of use of IONM is as a teaching tool during thyroidectomy. A study reported that the use of the IONM allowed residents and fellows in training to perform a safe operation with the acceptably low RLN paralysis rates of experienced surgeons [19]. The use of IONM has also been shown by some authors to aid in early visualization of the RLN [20]. Also, if used during surgical training, the learning curve of IONM for the surgeon who is being trained can be enhanced.

The safety of IONM has been reviewed and the consensus is that IONM is safe [9]. The stimulation intensity of 1mA for the RLN with a supramaximal stimulation of 2 mA are used only to localize the vagus or RLN [8]. Critics cite the lack of evidence of decrease in paralysis rates with IONM. However, Dralle has shown the rates of paralysis are lower with IONM and to reach statistical significance, a researcher would require 9 million patients per arm before proving a significant lowering of the RLN paralysis rate if typical rates of paralysis are used [21]. Although some surgeons choose to selectively use the IONM during potentially challenging cases, a challenging case is not always identifiable preoperatively and many high volume surgeons use the IONM routinely [7].

In 2010, the international standards of Intraoperative RLN monitoring were published [8]. As neural monitoring has gained acceptance as an adjunct to the gold standard of visual identification of the RLN, these guidelines sought to provide uniformity in application of and results from IONM. The guidelines are especially focused on the standards of equipment setup as well as standards for loss of signal evaluation and problem solving. In addition, the guidelines highlight areas that need further evaluation as the applications of IONM are advanced in thyroidectomy.

Continuous Intraoperative Neuromonitoring [CIONM]

The original intraoperative neuromonitoring formats were designed to stimulate the RLN intermittently, thus allowing the nerve to be at risk of injury in between the stimulations. The continuous vagal monitoring is designed to prevent adverse maneuvers from causing permanent nerve injury by eliciting and recording continuous electrophysiologic responses from the vagus nerves. CIONM was introduced in 2007 and uses the IONM system equipment with the addition of a stimulation electrode on the vagus nerve for the duration of the operation (Fig. 9.4) [22].

The continuous monitoring involves delivering a low current, repetitive pulsed stimulation during the surgical maneuvers. The low level, 1mA stimulation of the vagus nerve every 6 s has been found to be safe. There have not been reported vasovagal symptoms such as cardiac arrhythmias or bradycardia, bronchospasm or gastrointestinal effects from the continuous monitoring of the vagus nerve [23, 24].

CIONM requires placement of the electrode on the vagus nerve. Several electrodes have been introduced by various manufacturers. The time required to place the electrode is minimal in experienced hands. The vagus nerve most often courses medial and posterior to the internal jugular vein and common carotid artery [25]. Therefore, with lateral retraction of the strap muscles and medial retraction of the thyroid, the carotid sheath can be

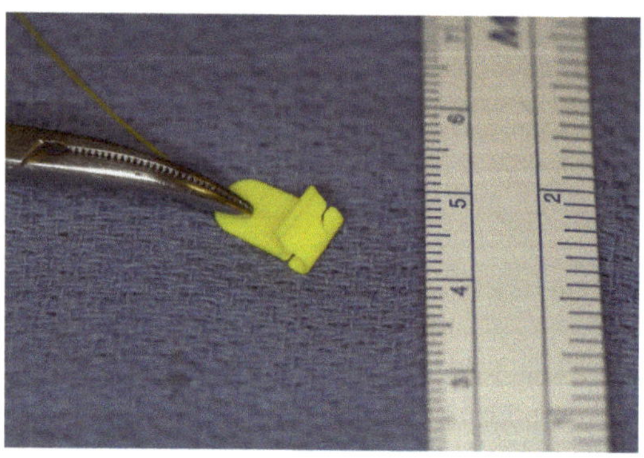

Fig. 9.4 APS electrode used for continuous IONM

entered and an electrode is placed on the vagus nerve for continuous monitoring.

Continuous vagal monitoring has been proven to be effective in the modification of surgical maneuvers to prevent LOS as well as RLN paralysis [26]. "Combined events" defined as EMG changes in amplitude (50% decrease from baseline) and latency (110% increase from baseline) proceed postoperative vocal fold palsy and can be reversed in 80% of cases in release of the maneuver [27]. CIONM provides real-time uninterrupted nerve monitoring and thereby provides opportunity to recognize impending nerve injury and reversal of associated surgical maneuver to avoid permanent injury and consequently overcomes the limitation of the traditional IONM which can only identify nerve damage after the damage is completed. CIONM has been found to provide better nerve protection than intermittent IONM with permanent RLN paralysis rates of 0% [28].

As with all IONM systems, the surgeon must be familiar in the interpretation of the EMG amplitude and latency. It has been suggested that CIONM should only be used by surgeons who are well trained in IONM [9].

External Branch of the Superior Laryngeal Nerve [EBSLN] Monitoring

The famous opera singer, Amelia Galli-Curci could no longer sing in her upper range or sustain notes after removal of a large goiter in 1935 due to presumed damage to the EBSLN [29]. A branch of the vagus nerve, the EBSLN supplies motor fibers to the cricothyroid muscle which functions to tilt and tense the vocal cord. The EBSLN is recognized as a important factor in voice projection and pitch which is important to not only singers, but also to professional voice users [30–32]. It has been suggested that the EBSLN injury can occur in up to 58% of patients [33] and is believed to be the most commonly underestimated morbidity associated with thyroid surgery [34]. Patients with EBSLN injury may complain of vocal fatigue, hoarseness, volume changes with projection and loss of upper vocal pitch [32, 35–37]. Therefore, preservation of the EBSLN is gaining recognition as a factor influencing patient's postoperative satisfaction.

The EBSLN is at greatest risk for injury during superior pole dissection. The EBSLN tracks dorsal to the superior thyroid artery and superficial to the inferior pharyngeal constrictor muscle as it travels medially to innervate the cricothyroid muscle [34]. The nerve is contained within the sternothyroid-laryngeal triangle, also known as Jolle's space which is bounded by the inferior pharyngeal constrictor and cricothyroid muscle medially, anteriorly by the sternothyroid muscle and laterally by the superior thyroid pole [38]. The laryngeal head of the sternothyroid muscle is a landmark for the course of the EBSLN along the inferior constrictor.

Cernea, known for the classification of the EBSLN found that the EBSLN is at highest risk of injury with large goiters [39] which was then confirmed by other authors who found the nerve lies inferior to the thyroid pole in 50% of goiters weighing more than 100 g [40]. However, in up to 20% of patients, the EBSLN cannot be visually identified because of its sub fascial course [41]. Neural monitoring has been shown to facilitate identification of EBSLN and quantifiable EMG response can be observed in 100% of cases [42]. Therefore, nerve monitor can be used to monitor the EBSLN as well as the RLN.

In 2013, the International Neural Monitoring Group published guidelines for EBSLN neuromonitoring during thyroid and parathyroid surgery [34]. The importance of assessment of cricothyroid twitch as well as EMG activity is stressed in these guidelines. Normative values of electrophysiological parameters obtained by EBSLN stimulations have been published [42, 43].

In an international survey of IONM use for identification of the EBSLN, only 26.3% of low volume surgeons vs 68.4% of high volume surgeons used the IONM for EBSLN [44] although 93% of respondents thought the monitoring was necessary in professional voice users. As the importance of vocal outcomes after thyroidectomy continue to be recognized, it is likely that the more and more surgeons will increasingly monitor the EBSLN.

The actual rate of EBSLN injury is unknown as it is not associated with obvious signs that can be readily identified on laryngeal exam. Laryngeal exam findings include posterior glottic rotation, inferior vocal cord positioning and bowing of the vocal cord on the side EBSLN is injured [33, 45]. Unlike RLN injury, glottic closure is not affected by EBSLN injury. EMG loss is the only way to truly know if the EBSLN is paralyzed [46]. Although a muscle-nerve-muscle anastomosis with a nerve conduit has shown promise and speech therapy to prevent or treat muscle tension dysphonia has been employed, there are no easy ways to treat EBSLN injury [35], therefore, prevention is the best strategy. It is important to note that injury to the cricothyroid muscle can cause the same symptoms and the post-surgical inflammation of the cricothyroid muscle is also a proposed transient cause of similar symptoms. Therefore, even with EBSLN preservation, patients should be counseled on transient vocal changes. As the importance of EBSLN preservation is increasing in not only singers but in all patients, the nerve is still known as the "nerve of Galli-Curci" [47].

Remote Access Surgery

Marketing strategies such as minimally invasive or scarless surgery have also promoted new directions in thyroid surgery. Remote access surgery avoids the anterior cervical scar completely and conceals the scar in a remote location. The remote access techniques rely on endoscopic or robotic technology. In the 1990s, as endoscopic surgery became commonplace among all surgical specialties, the search for an approach for endoscopic thyroidectomy began. One of the key driving forces was the avoidance of a neck scar due to cultural aspects in Southeast Asia [48]. The first endoscopic thyroidectomy was performed by Huscher in 1997 [49]. The initial remote access thyroidectomies were performed via chest, transaxillary or bilateral axillo-breast approaches. The introduction of the robotic thyroidectomy in 2009 also used an axillary approach [50]. These were largely abandoned in the West due to the substantial dissection, inpatient care and drains required.

The robotic facelift thyroidectomy sought to overcome the disadvantages of the other approaches with removal of the thyroid through a postauricular modified facelift incision [51]. The extent of dissection with this technique is believed to be 38% less than with the robotic axillary thyroidectomy [51]. As with other remote access approaches, not all thyroidectomy patients are candidates for the robotic facelift thyroidectomy. The criteria for robotic facelift thyroidectomy includes American Society of Anesthesiologists class 1 or 2, no prior neck surgery, no prior neck irradiation, no morbid obesity [BMI <40], unilateral surgery, nodule size <4 cm, and no evidence of lymphadenopathy thyroiditis, extra thyroidal disease or substernal extension [52].

Transoral endoscopic thyroidectomy by a vestibular approach is more novel approach [53, 54]. This approach, developed in Germany, is the shortest distance to the thyroid gland. This technique utilizes a natural orifice for a truly scarless technique; however, this approach can put hypoglossal, lingual and mental nerves at risk. Antibiotic prophylaxis is routinely employed to prevent infection [55]. As with other remote access techniques, the approach requires surgeon experience and appropriate instrumentation. Although one of the most recent techniques, it continues to be developed.

It is important to note that the remote access approaches cannot be considered to be minimally invasive approaches. Extensive dissection must be carried out to access the neck, the operative times are longer, and structures which are not typically at risk during conventional thyroidectomy may be encountered. As the neck is a difficult area for remote access, these procedures should only be performed at highly specialized centers after the safety of the procedure is proven. As patients drive the interest in concealing surgical scars, the remote access procedures will likely continue to evolve in a subset of the population requiring thyroid surgery.

The current thyroidectomy, an elegant operation with all of the technical advances, has come a long way from the early years. The thyroidectomy of today is a safe operation. Increasing use of IONM systems as well as a focus on patient satisfaction has brought further advances. Surgeons will certainly continue to pioneer new advances in thyroid surgery in this century and beyond.

References

1. Jeannon JP, Orabi AA, Bruch GA, Abdalsalam HA, Simo R. Diagnosis of recurrent laryngeal nerve palsy after thyroidectomy: a systematic review. Int J Clin Pract. 2009;63(4):624–9.
2. Lang BH, Wong CK, Ma EP. A systematic review and meta-analysis on acoustic voice parameters after uncomplicated thyroidectomy. Laryngoscope. 2016;126(2):528–37.
3. Chandrasekhar SS, Randolph GW, Seidman MD, Rosenfeld RM, Angelos P, Barkmeier-Kraemer J, et al. Clinical practice guideline: improving voice outcomes after thyroid surgery. Otolaryngol Head Neck Surg. 2013;148(6 Suppl):S1–37.
4. Lamade W, Meyding-Lamade U, Hund E, Senninger N, Herfarth C. Transtracheal monitoring of the recurrent laryngeal nerve. Prototype of a new tube. Chirurg. 1997;68(2):193–5.
5. Angeli V, Llodra J, Rong JX, Satoh K, Ishii S, Shimizu T, et al. Dyslipidemia associated with atherosclerotic disease systemically alters dendritic cell mobilization. Immunity. 2004;21(4):561–74.
6. Singer MC, Rosenfeld RM, Sundaram K. Laryngeal nerve monitoring: current utilization among head and neck surgeons. Otolaryngol Head Neck Surg. 2012;146(6):895–9.
7. Sturgeon C, Sturgeon T, Angelos P. Neuromonitoring in thyroid surgery: attitudes, usage patterns, and predictors of use among endocrine surgeons. World J Surg. 2009;33(3):417–25.
8. Randolph GW, Dralle H, Abdullah H, Barczynski M, Bellantone R, Brauckhoff M, et al. Electrophysiologic recurrent laryngeal nerve monitoring during thyroid and parathyroid surgery: international standards guideline statement. Laryngoscope. 2011;121(Suppl 1):S1–16.
9. Dionigi G, Chiang FY, Dralle H, Boni L, Rausei S, Rovera F, et al. Safety of neural monitoring in thyroid surgery. Int J Surg. 2013;11(Suppl 1):S120–6.
10. Macias AA, Eappen S, Malikin I, Goldfarb J, Kujawa S, Konowitz PM, et al. Successful intraoperative electrophysiologic monitoring of the recurrent laryngeal nerve, a multidisciplinary approach: The Massachusetts eye and ear infirmary monitoring collaborative protocol with experience in over 3000 cases. Head Neck. 2016;38:1487–94.
11. Kamani D, Darr EA, Randolph GW. Electrophysiologic monitoring characteristics of the recurrent laryngeal nerve preoperatively paralyzed or invaded with malignancy. Otolaryngol Head Neck Surg. 2013;149(5):682–8.
12. Bergenfelz A, Jansson S, Kristoffersson A, Martensson H, Reihner E, Wallin G, et al. Complications to thyroid surgery: results as reported in a database from a multicenter audit comprising 3,660 patients. Langenbeck's Arch Surg. 2008; 393(5):667–73.
13. Patow CA, Norton JA, Brennan MF. Vocal cord paralysis and reoperative parathyroidectomy. A prospective study. Ann Surg. 1986;203(3):282–5.
14. Bergenfelz A, Jansson S, Mårtensson H, Reihnér E, Wallin G, Kristoffersson A, et al. Scandinavian quality register for thyroid and parathyroid surgery: audit of surgery for primary hyperparathyroidism. Langenbeck's Arch Surg. 2007;392(4):445–51.
15. Henry JF, Audiffret J, Denizot A, Plan M. The nonrecurrent inferior laryngeal nerve: review of 33 cases, including two on the left side. Surgery. 1988;104(6):977–84.
16. Brauckhoff M, Machens A, Sekulla C, Lorenz K, Dralle H. Latencies shorter than 3.5 ms after vagus nerve stimulation signify a nonrecurrent inferior laryngeal nerve before dissection. Ann Surg. 2011;253(6):1172–7.
17. Kandil E, Anwar MA, Bamford J, Aslam R, Randolph GW. Electrophysiological identification of nonrecurrent laryngeal nerves. Laryngoscope. 2016;127(9):2189–93.
18. Kandil E, Abdel Khalek M, Aslam R, Friedlander P, Bellows CF, Slakey D. Recurrent laryngeal nerve: significance of the anterior extralaryngeal branch. Surgery. 2011;149(6):820–4.
19. Alesina PF, Hinrichs J, Meier B, Cho EY, Bolli M, Walz MK. Intraoperative neuromonitoring for surgical training in thyroid surgery: its routine use allows a safe operation instead of lack of experienced mentoring. World J Surg. 2014;38(3):592–8.
20. Sundaram K. Teaching RLN dissection to residents in head and neck endocrine surgery. J Head Neck Surg. 2012;3(1):5–7.
21. Dralle H, Sekulla C, Haerting J, Timmermann W, Neumann HJ, Kruse E, et al. Risk factors of paralysis and functional outcome after recurrent laryngeal nerve monitoring in thyroid surgery. Surgery. 2004;136(6):1310–22.
22. Ulmer C, Koch KP, Seimer A, Molnar V, Meyding-Lamade U, Thon KP, et al. Real-time monitoring of the recurrent laryngeal nerve: an observational clinical trial. Surgery. 2008;143(3):359–65.
23. Schneider R, Randolph GW, Sekulla C, Phelan E, Thanh PN, Bucher M, et al. Continuous intraoperative vagus nerve stimulation for identification of imminent recurrent laryngeal nerve injury. Head Neck. 2013;35(11):1591–8.
24. Schneider R, Przybyl J, Pliquett U, Hermann M, Wehner M, Pietsch UC, et al. A new vagal anchor electrode for real-time monitoring of the recurrent laryngeal nerve. Am J Surg. 2010;199(4):507–14.

25. Dionigi G, Chiang FY, Rausei S, Wu CW, Boni L, Lee KW, et al. Surgical anatomy and neurophysiology of the vagus nerve [VN] for standardised intraoperative neuromonitoring [IONM] of the inferior laryngeal nerve [ILN] during thyroidectomy. Langenbeck's Arch Surg. 2010;395(7):893–9.
26. Phelan E, Schneider R, Lorenz K, Dralle H, Kamani D, Potenza A, et al. Continuous vagal IONM prevents recurrent laryngeal nerve paralysis by revealing initial EMG changes of impending neuropraxic injury: a prospective, multicenter study. Laryngoscope. 2014;124(6):1498–505.
27. Schneider R, Lorenz K, Machens A, Thanh PN, Randolph GW, Dralle H. The recurrent and superior laryngeal nerves. Bern: Springer; 2016.
28. Schneider R, Sekulla C, Machens A, Lorenz K, Nguyen Thanh P, Dralle H. Postoperative vocal fold palsy in patients undergoing thyroid surgery with continuous or intermittent nerve monitoring. Br J Surg. 2015;102(11):1380–7.
29. Marchese-Ragona R, Restivo DA, Mylonakis I, Ottaviano G, Martini A, Sataloff RT, et al. The superior laryngeal nerve injury of a famous soprano, Amelita Galli-Curci. Acta Otorhinolaryngol Ital. 2013;33(1):67–71.
30. Crookes PF, Recabaren JA. Injury to the superior laryngeal branch of the vagus during thyroidectomy: lesson or myth? Ann Surg. 2001;233(4):588–93.
31. Kark AE, Kissin MW, Auerbach R, Meikle M. Voice changes after thyroidectomy: role of the external laryngeal nerve. Br Med J (Clin Res Ed). 1984;289(6456):1412–5.
32. Randolph GW, Sritharan N, Song P, Franco R Jr, Kamani D, Woodson G. Thyroidectomy in the professional singer-neural monitored surgical outcomes. Thyroid. 2015;25(6):665–71.
33. Teitelbaum BJ, Wenig BL. Superior laryngeal nerve injury from thyroid surgery. Head Neck. 1995;17(1):36–40.
34. Barczynski M, Randolph GW, Cernea CR, Dralle H, Dionigi G, Alesina PF, et al. External branch of the superior laryngeal nerve monitoring during thyroid and parathyroid surgery: international neural monitoring study group standards guideline statement. Laryngoscope. 2013;123(Suppl 4):S1–14.
35. Dursun G, Sataloff RT, Spiegel JR, Mandel S, Heuer RJ, Rosen DC. Superior laryngeal nerve paresis and paralysis. J Voice. 1996;10(2):206–11.
36. Eckley CA, Sataloff RT, Hawkshaw M, Spiegel JR, Mandel S. Voice range in superior laryngeal nerve paresis and paralysis. J Voice. 1998;12(3):340–8.
37. Robinson JL, Mandel S, Sataloff RT. Objective voice measures in nonsinging patients with unilateral superior laryngeal nerve paresis. J Voice. 2005;19(4):665–7.
38. Moosman DA, DeWeese MS. The external laryngeal nerve as related to thyroidectomy. Surg Gynecol Obstet. 1968;127(5):1011–6.
39. Cernea CR, Ferraz AR, Nishio S, Dutra A Jr, Hojaij FC, dos Santos LR. Surgical anatomy of the external branch of the superior laryngeal nerve. Head Neck. 1992;14(5):380–3.
40. Aina EN, Hisham AN. External laryngeal nerve in thyroid surgery: recognition and surgical implications. ANZ J Surg. 2001;71(4):212–4.
41. Lennquist S, Cahlin C, Smeds S. The superior laryngeal nerve in thyroid surgery. Surgery. 1987;102(6):999–1008.
42. Darr EA, Tufano RP, Ozdemir S, Kamani D, Hurwitz S, Randolph G. Superior laryngeal nerve quantitative intraoperative monitoring is possible in all thyroid surgeries. Laryngoscope. 2014;124(4): 1035–41.
43. Potenza AS, Phelan EA, Cernea CR, Slough CM, Kamani DV, Darr A, et al. Normative intra-operative electrophysiologic waveform analysis of superior laryngeal nerve external branch and recurrent laryngeal nerve in patients undergoing thyroid surgery. World J Surg. 2013;37(10):2336–42.
44. Barczynski M, Randolph GW, Cernea C. International survey on the identification and neural monitoring of the EBSLN during thyroidectomy. Laryngoscope. 2016;126(1):285–91.
45. Bevan K, Griffiths MV, Morgan MH. Cricothyroid muscle paralysis: its recognition and diagnosis. J Laryngol Otol. 1989;103(2):191–5.
46. Tolley NS, Chaidas K, Bergenfelz A. The recurrent and superior laryngeal nerves. Bern: Springer; 2016.
47. Souba WFM, Jurkovich GJ, et al. ACS surgery: principles and practice. 6th ed. Hamilton: BC Decker Inc; 2007.
48. Wilhelm T, Harlaar JJ, Kerver A, Kleinrensink GJ, Benhidjeb T. Surgical anatomy of the floor of the oral cavity and the cervical spaces as a rationale for trans-oral, minimal-invasive endoscopic surgical procedures: results of anatomical studies. Eur Arch Otorhinolaryngol. 2010;267(8):1285–90.
49. Huscher CS, Chiodini S, Napolitano C, Recher A. Endoscopic right thyroid lobectomy. Surg Endosc. 1997;11(8):877.
50. Kang SW, Jeong JJ, Yun JS, Sung TY, Lee SC, Lee YS, et al. Robot-assisted endoscopic surgery for thyroid cancer: experience with the first 100 patients. Surg Endosc. 2009;23(11):2399–406.
51. Terris DJ, Singer MC. Qualitative and quantitative differences between 2 robotic thyroidectomy techniques. Otolaryngol Head Neck Surg. 2012;147(1):20–5.
52. Chaung KDW. Thyroid and parathyroid diseases: medical and surgical management. New York: Thieme; 2016.
53. Inabnet WB, Suh H, Fernandez-Ranvier G. Transoral endoscopic thyroidectomy vestibular approach with intraoperative nerve monitoring. Surg Endosc. 2016;31(7):3030.
54. Cai C, Huang Y, Zhang T, Chai L, Wang G, Shi L, et al. Anatomical study of surgical approaches for minimally invasive transoral thyroidectomy: eMIT and TOPP. Minim Invasive Ther Allied Technol. 2015;24(6):340–4.
55. Witzel K, Hellinger A, Kaminski C, Benhidjeb T. Endoscopic thyroidectomy: the transoral approach. Gland Surg. 2016;5(3):336–41.

Part IV

Non Surgical Management of Differentiated Thyroid Cancer

10 Risk Stratification and Current Management of Low Risk Thyroid Cancer

Sana A. Ghaznavi and R. Michael Tuttle

Introduction

Initial and dynamic risk stratification has become a fundamental component in the management of thyroid cancer over the last ten years. This is a dramatic departure from the one size fits all management approach that was previously applied to all but the most low risk papillary thyroid cancers. For many years, nearly every patient with thyroid cancer was treated with total thyroidectomy and radioactive iodine remnant ablation. But with improved risk stratification and understanding of the natural history of disease, most international thyroid cancer guidelines now endorse an individualized approach to the management of thyroid cancer, including the selective use of radioactive iodine and surgery less than total thyroidectomy in appropriately chosen patients [1, 2].

While most chapters on risk assessment in thyroid cancer focus primarily on the risk of disease specific mortality, it is important to recognize that there are many risks that can be predicted that would be helpful in the management of patients with thyroid cancer. Obviously, risk stratification with regard to the likelihood of structural disease recurrence is a very important clinical outcome and is now included in most international thyroid cancer guidelines [1, 2]. However, the general concept of risk stratification can be applied to a wide variety of other clinical endpoints that provide insights into clinical management. For example, the likelihood that a tumor will or will not respond to radioactive iodine is an important factor in making decisions with regard to adjuvant therapy or treatment of known metastatic disease. Likewise, the likelihood that a particular therapy is going to render a patient disease free also provides meaningful information regarding the potential benefits of further surgery, additional radioactive iodine, or systemic therapy. Therefore, in addition to using risk stratification to help us understand the risk of recurrence and disease specific mortality, we apply these risk stratification concepts to all aspects of care in thyroid cancer in order to help clinicians and patients better understand the risk-benefit ratio for any planned treatment or surveillance strategy.

As our management recommendations become more individualized, it is critical that clinicians understand and routinely implement risk stratification in their daily practice. Without appropriate risk stratification, high risk patients may be undertreated or conversely low risk patients may be over treated. Furthermore, it is important to view risk stratification as a dynamic process in which the risk of recurrence and disease-related death may vary over time based on the biologic behavior of a specific tumor and

S. A. Ghaznavi · R. M. Tuttle (✉)
Department of Medicine, Memorial Sloan Kettering Cancer Center, New York, NY, USA
e-mail: tuttlem@mskcc.org

U. K. Mallick et al. (eds.), *Practical Management of Thyroid Cancer*,
https://doi.org/10.1007/978-3-319-91725-2_10

an individual patient's response to therapy. For example, a patient initially stratified as high risk of recurrence in whom there has been an excellent response to therapy for many years may not require the same intensive follow up strategy as another patient with similar initial risk stratification but with an incomplete response to prior therapy. In this chapter, we will review our approach to risk stratification, focusing primarily on the initial systems that we use to risk stratify patients with regard to their individualized risk of disease specific mortality and structural disease recurrence. We will also briefly review how risk assessment should be modified over time so that the type and intensity of follow-up testing can be tailored to updated risk assessments.

Estimating the Risk of Disease Specific Mortality

Over the years, multiple risk stratification systems have been developed and validated to allow clinicians to risk stratify patients' risk of disease specific mortality based on common variables such as age at diagnosis, tumor size, the presence or absence of gross extrathyroidal extension, and the presence or absence of distant metastases [3]. Acknowledging the strong prognostic significance of complete tumor resection, the MACIS staging system also included the completeness of tumor resection as a key variable [4]. Other staging systems have included the presence or absence of lymph node metastases, but this variable appears to have the greatest prognostic significance for disease specific mortality in older patients and does not appear to be a primary predictor of death in younger patients [5, 6].

It is important to note that the information required for appropriate initial risk stratification often includes data beyond that included in the pathology report. Multiple preoperative, intraoperative, and postoperative findings can have a direct impact on initial staging [7]. For example, preoperative findings of hoarseness or stridor, the presence of clinically palpable lymphadenopathy, the presence of distant metastasis, and the results of FDG PET scanning (if performed), could provide very important information that would impact risk stratification. Even more importantly, critical intraoperative findings such as the presence or absence of gross extrathyroidal extension, and the completeness of surgical resection, may not be immediately apparent on the pathology report. Postoperatively, while the pathology report contains valuable information for risk stratification, other data such as molecular profiling, postoperative serum thyroglobulin, and possibly even postoperative imaging may also significantly impact risk stratification. Therefore, it is imperative that the clinician doing the postoperative risk stratification has access to complete and accurate preoperative, intraoperative, and postoperative data.

Even though no single staging system has been shown to be superior to the others, the most commonly used staging systems for disease specific mortality are the American Joint Committee on Cancer/Union for International Cancer Control (AJCC/UICC) staging and the MACIS (metastasis, age, completeness of resection, invasion, size) system [4, 8]. Both of these staging systems provide valuable initial guidance as to the likelihood of dying from thyroid cancer, however, the proportion of variance explained (a statistical measure of how well a staging system can predict the outcome of interest) by both of these systems is only about 30% [9, 10]. This indicates that variables beyond those used in initial risk stratification can have a significant impact on an individual patient's risk of dying from thyroid cancer. Therefore, clinicians must modify their initial risk estimates over time as new data becomes available. Nonetheless, these staging systems do provide a reasonable guide to risk stratification that can be used to plan initial management and follow-up.

In 2017, an updated (eighth) edition of the AJCC/UICC staging system was published with plans for implementation by all United States tumor registries and hospitals beginning January 2018 [8]. While preserving the basic framework of the seventh edition staging system, the eighth edition has several modifications that have a significant impact on risk stratification (see Fig. 10.1). Not surprisingly, these changes reclassify many patients into lower risk stages. For example, older patients with only minor extrathyroidal extension or cervical lymph node metastasis (no matter how few or how small) were

Key changes in the AJCC/UICC 8th edition staging system for differentiated thyroid cancer

- The age cut off used for staging was increased from 45 to 55 years of age at diagnosis
- Minor extrathyroidal extension detected only on histologic examination was removed from the definition of T3 disease, and therefore, no longer contributes to T category or overall stage
- The presence of metastatic cervical lymphadenopathy (N1) no longer upstages a patient to stage III disease. If the patient is >/= 55 years of age, N1 disease is stage II. Patients < 55 years of age with N1 disease are stage I.
- Gross extrathyroidal extension that involves only the strap muscles (sternohyoid, sternothyroid, thyrohyoid, or omohyoid muscles) is classified as T3b disease. In patients less than 55 years of age, gross extrathyroidal extension involving only the strap muscles will continue to be stage I and in the older patients will be classified as stage II. This is in contrast to gross extra thyroid extension involving other major structures of the neck (T4a) or invading prevertebral fascia or encasing the carotid artery or mediastinal vessels (T4b), which would be classified as either stage III or stage IVa in older patients, respectively.

Fig. 10.1 Key changes in AJCC/UICC eighth edition staging system for differentiated thyroid cancer

previously classified as AJCC stage III. However, multiple studies now show that minor extrathyroidal extension and cervical lymph node metastasis, even in older patients, does not convey a risk high enough to justify stage III grouping [5, 6, 11]. Rather, staging these tumors as either stage I or stage II depending on the other clinical factors and patient age is far more appropriate.

However, it is important to recognize that the stage I category in younger patients (<55 years old at diagnosis) will now include a broad range of patients from very low risk patients that would almost certainly be cured by thyroid lobectomy to higher risk patients that may require more aggressive upfront and ongoing therapy. For example, a 54-year-old man with a poorly differentiated thyroid cancer would be classified as stage I disease in the absence of distant metastasis. However, because the vast majority of patients classified as stage I will be at very low risk of dying from thyroid cancer, moving a small number of higher risk patients into this category should have little effect on the expected excellent survival rate seen in the entire group [12, 13]. Additional risk stratification of these patients with respect to their risk of persistent or recurrent disease will ensure an individualized approach that is appropriate in this setting.

The revised AJCC staging criteria were analyzed and validated on a cohort of patients from Memorial Sloan-Kettering Cancer Center with good success [14]. The eighth edition staging system was validated at Samsung Medical Center in Korea [15]. This study showed that nearly 40% of patients moved to a lower stage upon reclassification to eighth edition staging. The proportion of patients in stage I and stage II increased from 62% to 81% and from 2% to 16%, respectively. Even more importantly, the proportion of patients classified as stage III decreased from 28% to 2%. Despite these major changes in classification, the eighth edition demonstrated a 10-year cancer specific survival of 99% in stage I patients, 94% in stage II patients, 80% in stage III patients, and 66% in stage IV patients. More recently, two additional studies have been published that provide further validation to the 8th edition risk stratification system [16, 17]. Taken together, these data indicate that despite moving many patients into lower risk categories, the eighth edition AJCC staging system provides a meaningful initial risk stratification of patients with differentiated thyroid cancer.

Estimating the Risk of Structural Disease Recurrence

As noted above, the vast majority of differentiated thyroid cancer patients will be classified as having a low risk of dying from thyroid cancer based on their initial clinical presentation. However, despite having a low risk of disease specific mortality, these patients can have a risk of structural disease recurrence that can range from 1 to 55% [1]. Therefore, initial management should be based both on assessment of the risk of disease specific mortality and also on the risk of structural disease recurrence.

To this end, most of the major international guidelines have developed staging systems that use initial clinical variables to predict the risk of recurrent/persistent disease. As originally conceived, the American Thyroid Association risk of recurrence staging system classified patients as low, intermediate, or high risk of recurrence [18]. The low risk category included only classic papillary thyroid cancers confined to the thyroid, while the high risk category included those patients with gross extra thyroid extension and distant metastases. All other patients were arbitrarily assigned intermediate risk classification. In the 2015 American Thyroid Association guidelines, the low risk category was expanded to include not only intrathyroidal classic papillary thyroid cancers, but also patients with fewer than 5 cervical micro-metastases, encapsulated follicular variant of papillary thyroid cancer, and follicular thyroid cancer with capsular invasion and/or minimal vascular invasion (see Table 10.1) [1]. Furthermore, the high risk category was expanded to include patients with metastatic cervical lymph nodes greater than 3 cm in largest dimension or with follicular thyroid cancer with extensive vascular invasion.

It is important to note that some of the features that qualify a patient as high risk in the ATA staging system may not be confidently assessed in the immediate postoperative period. For example, the thyroglobulin value that would be suggestive of distant metastasis is probably best determined about 6 weeks after thyroidectomy as it takes time for thyroglobulin to be cleared from the body [19]. Likewise, the presence of distant metastasis may not be appreciated until imaging

Table 10.1 ATA 2009 risk stratification system with proposed modifications

ATA low risk	Papillary thyroid cancer (with all of the following) • No local or distant metastases • All macroscopic tumor has been resected • No tumor invasion of loco-regional tissues or structures • The tumor does not have aggressive histology (e.g., tall cell, hobnail variant, columnar cell carcinoma) • If ^{131}I is given, there are no RAI avid metastatic foci outside the thyroid bed on the first post-treatment whole-body RAI scan • No vascular invasion • Clinical N0 or ≤5 pathologic N1 micrometastases (<0.2 cm in largest dimension)[a] Intrathyroidal, encapsulated follicular variant of papillary thyroid cancer[a] Intrathyroidal, well differentiated follicular thyroid cancer with capsular invasion and no or minimal (<4 foci) vascular invasion[a] Intrathyroidal, papillary microcarcinoma, unifocal or multifocal, including BRAF^{V600E} mutated (if known)[a]
ATA intermediate risk	Microscopic invasion of tumor into the perithyroidal soft tissues RAI avid metastatic foci in the neck on the first post-treatment whole-body RAI scan Papillary thyroid cancer with vascular invasion Aggressive histology (e.g., tall cell, hobnail variant, columnar cell carcinoma) Clinical N1 or >5 pathologic N1 with all involved lymph nodes <3 cm in largest dimension[a] Multifocal papillary microcarcinoma with extrathyroidal extension and *BRAF*^{V600E} mutated (if known)[a]
ATA high risk	Macroscopic invasion of tumor into the perithyroidal soft tissues (gross ETE) Incomplete tumor resection Distant metastases Post-operative serum thyroglobulin suggestive of distant metastases Pathologic N1 with any metastatic lymph node ≥3 in largest dimension[a] Follicular thyroid cancer with extensive vascular invasion (>4 foci of vascular invasion)[a]

[a]Proposed modifications, not present in the original 2009 initial risk stratification system

studies are done postoperatively either as part of routine radioactive iodine therapy or in response to a thyroglobulin that is inappropriately elevated 6 weeks after surgery. Therefore, just as with the AJCC staging system, the initial ATA risk of recurrence classification should utilize all pre-operative, intra-operative, and post-operative data obtained within the first 3–4 months of follow-up.

Even though the ATA strongly recommends the use of low, intermediate, and high risk of recurrence categories in clinical practice, they also recognize that individual risk may be better understood as a continuum than as discrete categories (Fig. 10.2) [1]. As can be seen from Fig. 10.2, the risk of structural disease recurrence can vary from as low as 1–2% to as high as 40–50% depending on the specific clinical features present for each case. This risk continuum is particularly important for the intermediate risk patients as this category can include patients with a risk of recurrence that ranges between 10 and 40%.

Modifying Initial Risk Estimates Over Time

While the initial risk estimates that relate to disease specific survival and structural disease recurrence are helpful starting points, they need to be adjusted over time in order to remain clinically relevant. As new data is accumulated during follow-up, the various risk estimates can either be increased or decreased depending on the individual patients' disease biology and their response to previous therapies. In order to facilitate classification and communication with regard to current disease status, the ATA guidelines recommend describing the patient's clinical status as either excellent, biochemical incomplete, structural incomplete, or indeterminate. While

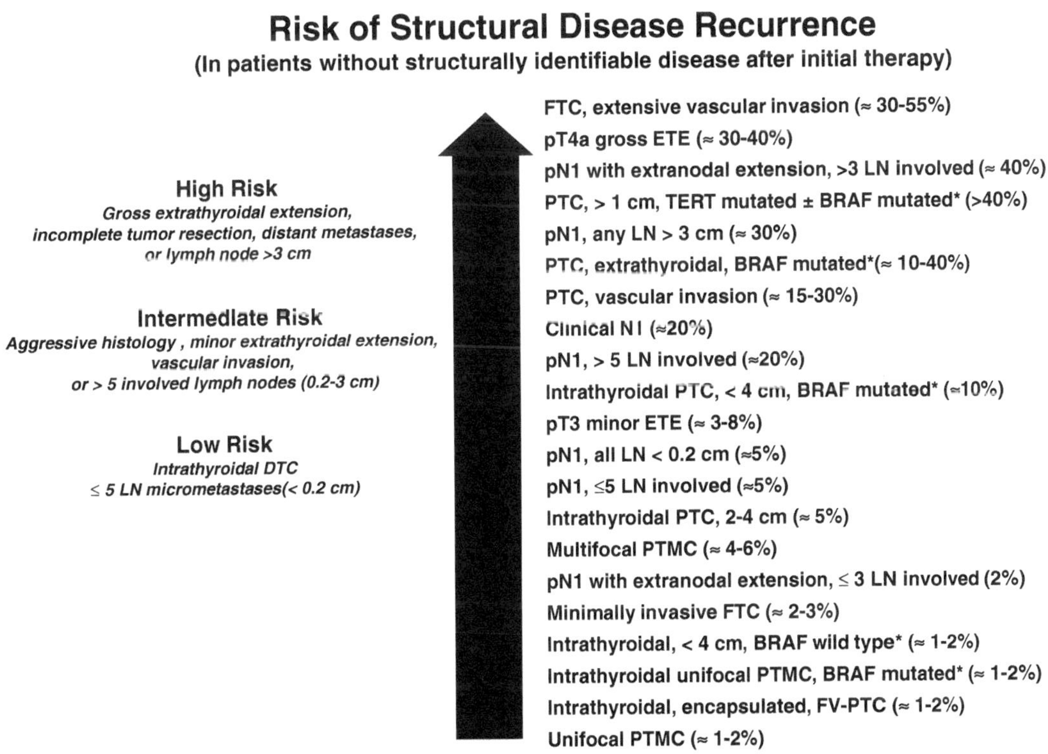

Fig. 10.2 Risk of structural disease recurrence in patients without structurally identifiable disease after initial therapy. *FTC* follicular thyroid cancer, *FV* follicular variant, *LN* lymph node, *PTMC* papillary thyroid microcarcinoma, *PTC* papillary thyroid cancer

Table 10.2 Clinical implications of response to therapy reclassification in patients with differentiated thyroid cancer treated with total thyroidectomy and RAI remnant ablation

Category	Definitions[a]	Clinical outcomes	Management implications
Excellent response	Negative imaging *and either* Suppressed Tg <0.2 ng/mL[a] *or* TSH stimulated Tg <1 ng/mL[a]	1–4% recurrence <1% disease specific death	An excellent response to therapy should lead to an early decrease in the intensity and frequency of follow up and the degree of TSH suppression
Biochemical incomplete response	Negative imaging *and* Suppressed Tg >1 ng/mL[a] *or* Stimulated Tg >10 ng/mL[a] *or* Rising Anti-Tg Ab levels	At least 30% spontaneously evolve to NED 20% achieve NED after additional therapy 20% develop structural disease <1% disease specific death	If associated with stable or declining serum Tg values, a biochemical incomplete response should lead to continued observation with ongoing TSH suppression in most patients. Rising Tg or anti-Tg antibody values should prompt additional investigations and potentially additional therapies
Structural incomplete response	Structural or functional evidence of disease With any Tg level With or without anti-Tg antibodies	50–85% continue to have persistent disease despite additional therapy Disease specific death rates as high as 11% with loco-regional metastases and 50% with structural distant metastases	A structural incomplete response may lead to additional treatments or ongoing observation depending on multiple clinico-pathologic factors including the size, location, rate of growth, RAI avidity, ^{18}FDG avidity, and specific pathology of the structural lesions
Indeterminate response	Non-specific findings on imaging studies Faint uptake in thyroid bed on RAI scanning Non-stimulated Tg detectable, but <1 ng/mL Stimulated Tg detectable, but <10 ng/mL or Anti-Tg antibodies stable or declining in the absence of structural or functional disease	15–20% will have structural disease identified during follow-up In the remainder, the non-specific changes are either stable, or resolve <1% disease specific death	An indeterminate response should lead to continued observation with appropriate serial imaging of the non-specific lesions and serum Tg monitoring. Non-specific findings that become suspicious over time can be further evaluated with additional imaging or biopsy

NED denotes a patient as having no evidence of disease at final follow-up
[a]In the absence of anti-Tg antibodies

the precise definitions can be seen in Table 10.2, patients classified as having an excellent response have no biochemical or structural evidence of persistent or recurrent disease [1]. Patients classified as biochemical incomplete response have an abnormal suppressed or stimulated thyroglobulin value but with no corresponding structural disease that can be identified. Patients classified as structural incomplete have documented or highly suspicious structural or functional findings of persistent or recurrent thyroid cancer. Finally, the indeterminate category describes patients with nonspecific findings on imaging or low level thyroglobulin values that cannot be confidently assigned to either the excellent or incomplete categories. Over time, patients in the indeterminate category can usually be moved to one of the other three categories as additional data is obtained.

While the original response to therapy definitions were based on data from patients that had total thyroidectomy and radioactive iodine remnant ablation, the same concepts have also been applied to patients treated with lobectomy or total thyroidectomy without radioactive iodine [20]. While the basic naming system remains unchanged, it is necessary to modify the definitions slightly in order to make the categories applicable to patients that are treated with less than total thyroidectomy and radioactive iodine. For example, following lobectomy, a non-stimulated thyroglobulin less than 30 ng/mL would be considered an excellent response, as this represents about 50% of the thyroglobulin value that would be expected for a patient with an intact thyroid. Likewise, the thyroglobulin cutoff values for excellent, biochemical incomplete and indeterminate also need to be tailored to the extent of initial therapy. These proposed definitions have been validated by two different groups [20, 21].

The clinical implications of ongoing risk stratification are fairly obvious. Patients that began as ATA low or intermediate risk who have an excellent response to therapy are at extraordinarily low risk of recurrence and therefore do not require intense follow-up or TSH suppression. Once classified as an excellent response, these patients can be followed every 1 2 years with just thyroglobulin and thyroglobulin antibodies. It is likely that routine use of screening neck ultrasonography to detect recurrent disease in these patients, who have very low risk of recurrence, will identify far more false positive findings than real disease [22, 23].

The management of patients with a biochemical incomplete response will depend on the magnitude of thyroglobulin elevation and the trend in thyroglobulin values over time. Most of these patients will have suppressed thyroglobulin values less than 5–10 ng/mL and will have either stable or declining thyroglobulin values over time. These patients can be followed with observation, mild TSH suppression and serial neck ultrasonography over time. However, patients with rising thyroglobulin values over time would be candidates for additional cross-sectional and functional imaging depending on the magnitude of thyroglobulin elevation and doubling time of the thyroglobulin values. The risk of distant metastasis increases as a function of the thyroglobulin value. Therefore, patients with thyroglobulin values of more than 10–20 ng/mL on suppression should be carefully evaluated with functional and structural cross sectional imaging designed to identify common sites of distant metastasis, which would include the lungs, bones, liver, and brain.

Depending on size, location, histology, FDG avidity, and rate of progression, patients with a structural incomplete response may be candidates for either observation or intervention. Many small volume lymph node metastasis and pulmonary micrometastases remain quite stable for many years and can be followed with observation [24, 25]. However, metastatic disease that is progressive or symptomatic usually constitutes an indication for therapy. Likewise, growth of metastatic disease in a location that could cause neurovascular compromise would also be a cause for intervention.

Finally, patients with an indeterminate response are usually followed with observation over time. As new data is accumulated, patients can usually be re-classified into one of the other three categories. Only 15–20% of patients in the indeterminate category will eventually be shown to have persistent/recurrent disease [18]. The majority of patients have nonspecific findings that can be re-classified over time as a benign finding or true disease.

Using Risk Stratification to Define and Inform Management Decisions in Low Risk Thyroid Cancer

As we continue to see a dramatic increase in the diagnosis of low risk thyroid cancer, it is imperative that clinicians understand how to recognize low risk thyroid cancer and modify traditional approaches to the management of intermediate and high risk thyroid cancer in a way that is appropriate for these patients. As described above, the classic low risk patients would be risk stratified as AJCC stage I and ATA low risk of recurrence. The expected outcomes would be a disease specific mortality rate of less than 1% and a structural disease recurrence rate of 2–3% in cohorts treated with total thyroidectomy with or without radioactive iodine ablation [18, 20]. If lobectomy was selected as the initial treatment, the overall disease specific survival remains more than 99% but the structural disease recurrence rate is slightly higher at 5–7% [20]. Importantly, disease recurrence is usually identified easily with either a change in thyroglobulin or structural abnormalities found on the ultrasound. This early detection of recurrent/persistent disease allows for additional effective therapy when necessary and thus results in a disease specific mortality rate of less than 1%, even in the few patients who have structural disease identified during follow-up, regardless of their initial therapy. As will be described in more detail in the following chapter, excellent outcomes are also seen in very low risk thyroid cancer patients followed with observation alone.

From a practical standpoint, risk stratification begins as soon as a diagnosis of thyroid cancer is made. If the patient is classified as having a very low risk of recurrence, for example, due to a papillary microcarcinoma that appears to be confined to the thyroid, then an observational management approach is considered. In this case, full staging information is not known because the exact histology of the small lesion cannot be definitively determined by cytology and small volume disease either in the contralateral lobe or surrounding cervical lymph nodes cannot be definitively ruled out. Nonetheless, with appropriate patient selection, these patients can be followed with observation without TSH suppression.

Similarly, in low risk patients that are being considered for a thyroid lobectomy, several important histological features cannot be known until after postoperative histological examination. Hence, there is always a small chance that after thyroid lobectomy the tumor could be determined to be a poorly differentiated thyroid cancer or to have extensive vascular invasion, in which case consideration for completion thyroidectomy and possibly radioactive iodine would be warranted. But just as with papillary microcarcinomas, with careful preoperative evaluation, we seldom need to do an immediate completion thyroidectomy. We have routinely offered thyroid lobectomy as the definitive initial operation in patients that appear to have 1–4 cm intrathyroidal differentiated thyroid cancers without evidence of extrathyroidal extension, significant cervical lymph node metastasis, or distant metastasis. Conversely, unless the patient is motivated to limit surgery to thyroid lobectomy, the presence of multiple significant nodules in the contralateral lobe or ultrasonographic findings of Hashimoto's thyroiditis would favor total thyroidectomy in order to facilitate follow-up.

Although the presence of antithyroglobulin antibodies can complicate follow up, the antibody level usually declines significantly during the first year following total thyroidectomy [26]. While it is true that after lobectomy antithyroglobulin antibody levels usually remain unabated, these patients have a low risk of recurrence; the few recurrences that do occur are almost exclusively seen in the neck, making observation with serial ultrasonography a reasonable and effective management approach, even if thyroglobulin values cannot be accurately determined.

Radioactive iodine ablation is seldom mandated in these low risk thyroid cancer patients as their outcomes with regard to both recurrence and overall survival is already excellent, and radioactive iodine is unlikely to render a substantial incremental benefit. However, occasionally radioactive iodine scanning or an ablative dose of 30 mCi of radioactive iodine may be used to facilitate staging and follow up depending on the specifics of an individual case. Likewise, TSH suppressive therapy is not required but rather a TSH goal of 0.5–2.0 mU/L is considered optimal.

The types and intensity of follow-up have not been well defined in these low risk patients. We generally follow thyroglobulin and thyroglobulin antibodies every 6–12 months. Ultrasonography is performed about 12 months after initial therapy and then less frequently after that. There is no convincing data that routine use of ultrasound, in an effort to find minimal residual disease, is beneficial in these low risk patients. If anything, excessive testing in these patients is more likely to yield false positive results than true disease given their low risk of recurrence [22].

In patients treated with lobectomy, a completion thyroidectomy is usually recommended if the serum thyroglobulin values consistently increase over time or if significant structural abnormalities are identified in the contralateral lobe or in cervical lymph nodes. Following total thyroidectomy, radioactive iodine can be considered if the postsurgical thyroglobulin is higher than anticipated (greater than about 5 ng/mL), if the thyroglobulin continues to rise over time, or if structural abnormalities are identified on follow-up ultrasonography.

References

1. Haugen B, Alexander E, Bible K, Doherty G, Mandel S, Nikiforov Y, et al. 2015 American thyroid association management guidelines for adult patients with thyroid nodules and differentiated thyroid cancer. Thyroid. 2016;26(1):1–133.
2. Perros P, Colley S, Boelaert K, Evans C, Evans RM, Gerrard GE, et al. British Medical Association: guidelines for the management of thyroid cancer. Clin Endocrinol. 2014;81:1–122.
3. Momesso D, Tuttle RM. Update on differentiated thyroid cancer staging. Endocrinol Metab Clin N Am. 2014;43:401–21.
4. Hay ID, Bergstralh EJ, Goellner JR, Ebersold JR, Grant CS. Predicting outcome in papillary thyroid carcinoma: development of a reliable prognostic scoring system in a cohort of 1779 patients surgically treated at one institution during 1940 through 1989. Surgery. 1993;114(6):1050–7.
5. Adam M, Pura J, Goffredo P, Dinan M, Reed S, Scheri R, et al. Presence and number of lymph node metastases are associated with compromised survival for patients younger than age 45 years with papillary thyroid cancer. J Clin Oncol. 2015;33(21):2370–5.
6. Nixon I, Wang L, Palmer F, Tuttle RM, Shaha A, Shah J, et al. The impact of nodal status on outcome in older patients with papillary thyroid cancer. Surgery. 2014;156(1):137–46.
7. Carty SE, Doherty GM, Inabnet WB, Pasieka JL, Randolph GW, Shaha AR, et al. American Thyroid Association statement on the essential elements of interdisciplinary communication of perioperative information for patients undergoing thyroid cancer surgery. Thyroid. 2012;22(4):395–9.
8. Tuttle M, Morris LF, Haugen B, Shah J, Sosa JA, Rohren E, Subramaniam RM, Hunt JL, Perrier ND. In: Amin MB, Edge SB, Greene F, Byrd D, Brookland RK, Washington MK, Gershenwald JE, Compton CC, Hess KR, Sullivan DC, Jessup JM, Brierley J, Gaspar LE, Schilsky RL, Balch CM, Winchester DP, Asare EA, Madera M, Gress DM, Meyer LR, editors. AJCC cancer staging manual. 8th ed. New York: Springer; 2017. p. 873–87.
9. D'Avanzo A, Ituarte P, Treseler P, Kebebew E, Wu J, Wong M, et al. Prognostic scoring systems in patients with follicular thyroid cancer: a comparison of different staging systems in predicting the patient outcome. Thyroid. 2014;14(6):453–8.
10. Brierley JD, Panzarella T, Tsang RW, Gospodarowicz MK, O'Sullivan B. A comparison of different staging systems predictability of patient outcome: thyroid cancer as an example. Cancer. 1997;79(12): 2414–23.
11. Nixon I, Ganly I, Snehal P, et al. The impact of microscopic extra thyroid extension on outcome in patients with clinical T1 and T2 well differentiated thyroid cancer. Surgery. 2011;150(6):1242–9.
12. Nixon IJ, Wang LY, Migliacci JC, Eskander A, Campbell MJ, Aniss A, et al. An international multi-institutional validation of age 55 years as a cutoff for risk stratification in the AJCC/UICC staging system for well-differentiated thyroid cancer. Thyroid. 2016;26(3):373–80.
13. Ganly I, Nixon I, Wang LY, Palmer F, Migliacci JC, Aniss A. Survival from differentiated thyroid cancer: what has age got to do with it? Thyroid. 2015;25(10):1106–14.
14. Tuttle M, Morris LF, Haugen B, Shah J, Sosa JA, Rohren E, Subramaniam RM, Hunt JL, Perrier ND. In: Amin MB, Edge SB, Greene F, Byrd D, Brookland RK, Washington MK, Gershenwald JE, Compton CC, Hess KR, Sullivan DC, Jessup JM, Brierley J, Gaspar LE, Schilsky RL, Balch CM, Winchester DP, Asare EA, Madera M, Gress DM, Meyer LR, editors. AJCC cancer staging manual. 8th ed. New York: Springer; 2017. p. 885.Figure 73.3, disease-specific survival: all patients, MSKCC data, 8th Edition.
15. Kim T, Kim YN, Kim HI, Park SY, Choe J, Kim J, et al. Prognostic value of the eight edition AJCC TNM classification for differentiated thyroid carcinoma. Oral Oncol. 2017;71:81–6.
16. Pontius LN, Oyekunle T, Thomas S, Stang M, Scheri R, Roman S, et al. Projecting survival in papillary thyroid cancer: a comparison of the 7th and 8th editions of the AJCC/UICC staging systems in two contemporary national patient cohorts. Thyroid. 2017;27(11):1408–16. https://doi.org/10.1089/thy.2017.0306.
17. Kim M, Kim WG, Oh H, Park S, Kwon H, Song D, et al. Comparison of the seventh and eighth editions of the American joint committee on cancer/union for international cancer control tumor-node-metastasis

staging system for differentiated thyroid cancer. Thyroid. 2017;27(9):1149–55.
18. Tuttle RM, Tala H, Shah J, Leboeuf R, Ghossein R, Gonen M, et al. Estimating risk of recurrence in differentiated thyroid cancer after total thyroidectomy and radioactive iodine remnant ablation: using response to therapy variables to modify the initial risk estimates predicted by the new American thyroid association staging system. Thyroid. 2010;20(12):1341–9.
19. Hocevar M, Auersperg M, Stanovnik L. The dynamics of serum thyroglobulin elimination from the body after thyroid surgery. Eur J Surg Oncol. 1997;23(3):208–10.
20. Momesso DP, Vaisman F, Yang SP, Bulzico DA, Corbo R, Vaisman M, Tuttle RM. Dynamic risk stratification in patients with differentiated thyroid cancer treated without radioactive iodine. J Clin Endocrinol Metab. 2016;101(7):2692–700.
21. Park S, Kim WG, Song E, Oh H, Kim M, Kwon H, et al. Dynamic risk stratification for predicting recurrence in patients with differentiated thyroid cancer treated without radioactive iodine remnant ablation therapy. Thyroid. 2017;27(4):524–30.
22. Yang S, Bach A, Tuttle RM, Fish S. Serial neck ultrasound is more likely to identify false-positive abnormalities than clinically significant disease in low-risk papillary thyroid cancer patients. Endocr Pract. 2015;21(12):1372–9.
23. Yang S, Bach A, Tuttle RM, Fish S. Frequent screening with serial neck ultrasound is more likely to identify false-positive abnormalities than clinically significant disease in the surveillance of intermediate risk papillary thyroid cancer patients without suspicious findings on follow-up ultrasound evaluation. J Clin Endocrinol Metab. 2015;100(4):1561–7.
24. Robenshtok E, Fish S, Bach A, Dominguez J, Shaha A, Tuttle RM. Suspicious cervical lymph nodes detected after thyroidectomy for papillary thyroid cancer usually remain stable over years in properly selected patients. J Clin Endocrinol Metab. 2012;97(8):2706–13.
25. Sabra M, Ghossein R, Tuttle RM. Time course and predictors of structural disease progression in pulmonary metastases arising from follicular cell-derived thyroid cancer. Thyroid. 2016;26(4):518–24.
26. Chiovato L, Latrofa F, Braverman LE, Pacini F, Capezzone M, Masserini L, et al. Disappearance of humoural thyroid autoimmunity after complete removal of thyroid antigens. Ann Intern Med. 2003;139(5 Pt 1):346–51.

Management of Low-Risk Papillary Thyroid Carcinoma and Papillary Microcarcinoma: The Japanese Experience

11

Yasuhiro Ito and Akira Miyauchi

Introduction

In Western countries, therapeutic strategy for papillary thyroid carcinoma (PTC) has been rather stereotypical: total thyroidectomy with or without lymph node dissection, radioactive iodine (RAI) ablation, thyroid-stimulating hormone (TSH) suppression and postoperative thyroglobulin (Tg) monitoring. In Japan, however, hemithyroidectomy has been extensively performed for PTCs except for high-risk ones. Instead, regional lymph nodes have been extensively dissected and even though it is prophylactic, level VI and ipsilateral level II–IV dissection were almost routine surgical procedures for PTC in most Japanese institutes.

There are two reasons for the traditional Japanese therapeutic strategics for PTC. In Japan, the use of RAI is significantly limited based on legal restraints. However, this is not the main reason; the other is more important: surgeons knew that surgery for PTC generally results in an excellent prognosis, with some exceptions due to aggressive clinicopathological features, even though total thyroidectomy and RAI ablation are not performed.

The Japanese guidelines issued by the Japan Association of Endocrine Surgeons (JAES)/Japanese Society of Thyroid Surgery (JSTS) strongly recommend aggressive therapy for PTCs with high-risk features, but they also do not recommend overtreatment for PTC without these features. The second edition of the JAES/JSTS guidelines, which are scheduled to be published in 2017, classify PTCs ≤2 cm without significant extrathyroid extension (Ex), clinical node metastasis (N), or distant metastasis at diagnosis (M) as low-risk, and among them, PTCs ≤1 cm (i.e., low-risk papillary microcarcinomas [PMCs]) are classified as very low-risk [1] (Table 11.1).

According to the same guidelines, high-risk cases are PTCs with one or more of the following five characteristics: (1) M1, (2) T >4 cm, (3) Ex-positive, (4) N >3 cm, and (5) extranodal

Table 11.1 Risk classification of PTC based on the JAES/JSTS guidelines [1]

Risk classification	Variable
Very low	T ≤1 cm, N0M0Ex-negative[a]
Low	1 cm < T ≤2 cm, N0M0Ex-negative
Intermediate	PTC that do not belong to the very-low, low or high-risk categories
High	PTC with one or more of the following features: 1. M1 2. T >4 cm 3. Ex-positive N >3 cm 4. Extranodal tumor extension-positive

[a]Ex: extrathyroid extension corresponding to T4a or T4b

Y. Ito (✉) · A. Miyauchi
Department of Surgery, Kuma Hospital, Kobe, Japan
e-mail: ito01@kuma-h.or.jp

U. K. Mallick et al. (eds.), *Practical Management of Thyroid Cancer*,
https://doi.org/10.1007/978-3-319-91725-2_11

tumor extension-positive. Intermediate-risk cases are PTCs that do not belong to the very-low, low and high-risk categories. The guidelines encourage physicians to select therapeutic strategies suitable for each risk factor, e.g., limited thyroidectomy for low-risk patients and active surveillance for very-low-risk patients.

In this chapter, active surveillance of very-low-risk PTCs and surgical designs for low-risk PTCs based on Japanese data are introduced.

Therapeutic Strategy for Very-Low-Risk PTC (Low-Risk PMC) Patients

Background and History

PMCs are frequently detected in autopsy studies as latent PMCs, and latent PMCs measuring 3–10 mm (the size detectable by ultrasound) were found in 0.5–5.2% of autopsy studies [2]. Takebe et al. reported that thyroid carcinoma was detected in 3.5% of otherwise healthy women aged ≥30 years on screening by ultrasound and ultrasound-guided fine needle aspiration biopsy (FNAB) [3]. They also showed that 85% of these were small carcinomas measuring ≤15 mm. The incidences of thyroid cancer at autopsy studies and the incidence revealed by this screening study are in accord with each other.

Based on the much higher incidence of latent thyroid carcinomas in autopsy studies and that of small thyroid carcinomas revealed in a mass screening by ultrasound compared to the prevalence of clinical thyroid carcinoma (3.1 in 100,000 Japanese women being reported at that time), Akira Miyauchi at Kuma Hospital in Kobe, Japan hypothesized that most PMCs do not grow or grow very slowly and that immediate surgical treatment for all PMCs might result in more harm than good. He also speculated that active surveillance alone could identify PMCs that showing progression, and that performing rescue surgeries for such PMCs after slight progression is identified might manage the disease successfully.

Based on these considerations, Dr. Miyauchi proposed an active surveillance clinical trial for low-risk PMCs at a meeting of Kuma Hospital physicians. After the approval of the other physicians was confirmed, the active surveillance study at Kuma Hospital started in 1993 [4]. The Cancer Institute Hospital (CIH, Tokyo, Japan) also initiated an active surveillance program for low-risk PMC under a similar concept in 1995, and promising data have been published from these two institutions.

Changes in the Incidence of PTC and the Mortality Rate

Changes in the incidence and mortality of PTC over time have been reported in many countries, such as the United States, Korea, Italy, France, England and Scotland, Australia, and Nordic countries [5–8]. In the United States, the incidence of thyroid carcinoma increased by 2.4-fold and 2.9-fold between 1973 and 2002 and between 1975 and 2009, respectively [5, 6]. In Korea, the increase in the incidence was much greater at 15-fold between 1993 and 2011 [7]. The increased incidence was definitely due to the increased detection of small PTCs on ultrasound and ultrasound-guided FNAB.

Interestingly, in all of the above-cited countries, the rate of mortality from thyroid carcinoma did not change. These data suggest that many harmless small carcinomas were surgically treated—which may have done more harm than good without improvement in the patients' survival—and they significantly support the validity of an active surveillance strategy for low-risk PMC.

Complications of Surgery for Low-Risk PMC

It is true that surgery for low-risk PMC is not difficult from the standpoint of surgical technique. However, Oda et al. reported that at Kuma Hospital, permanent vocal cord paralysis induced by recurrent laryngeal nerve injury and permanent hypoparathyroidism occurred in 0.2% and 1.6% of patients who underwent surgery for low-risk PMC [9]. Kuma Hospital is a center for patients with thyroid disease and also a high-volume center for thyroid surgery, but this cannot provide a zero-incidence of unfavorable complications, as indicated above. If these patients with nerve injury and hypoparathyroidism had not been surgically treated, their complications would have been avoided. Moreover, the incidences of the complications would be higher when non-experts perform the surgery.

Contraindications for the Active Surveillance of PMC

Contraindications for the active surveillance of PMC are summarized in Table 11.2. There are two groups of contraindications: clinicopathologically high-risk features, and features that are unsuitable for active surveillance (and it is unclear whether the feature is biologically aggressive). The presence of clinical distant metastasis (M) (although very rare) and clinical node metastasis (N) on imaging studies at diagnosis is a sign of a high-risk case. Recurrent laryngeal nerve paralysis of the ipsilateral side of a tumor located in the course of the recurrent laryngeal nerve is also a sign of an aggressive feature. Although rare, cases suspected of aggressive histological types on cytology such as poorly differentiated carcinoma and tall cell variant are strong candidates for immediate surgery. Cases with size enlargement or a novel appearance of lymph node metastasis should be immediately operated, because they are confirmed to be oncologically aggressive.

Table 11.2 Contraindications for active surveillance of PMC

Type	Contraindications
Clinically high-risk features	1. Clinical distant metastasis-positive (very rare) or clinical lymph node metastasis-positive 2. Signs or symptoms of invasion to the recurrent laryngeal nerve or trachea 3. High-grade malignancy on cytology (very rare) 4. Cases showing progression signs during active surveillance
A feature unsuitable for active surveillance, and it is unclear whether it is clinically aggressive	Tumors sticking to the trachea or located in the course of the recurrent laryngeal nerve

Invasion to the trachea is not easy to diagnose. Our data showed that the angle formed by the tracheal and tumor surfaces is useful for the evaluation of the tracheal invasion of a PMC (Fig. 11.1) [10]. PMC with an obtuse angle is a candidate for immediate surgery, because 24% of these cases (measuring 7–10 mm) showed a significant invasion to the trachea requiring the resection of a partial layer or the full thickness of the trachea, whereas no significant invasion to the trachea was observed in PMCs with an acute angle.

Recurrent laryngeal nerve invasion is evaluated based on whether the normal rim of the thyroid is present between the tumor and the course of nerve. In 9% of the cases in our study [10] with no normal rim between the tumor and the course of the nerve, a significant nerve invasion requiring partial layer dissection or segmental resection of the nerve with reconstruction of the resected nerve was necessary. Physicians should

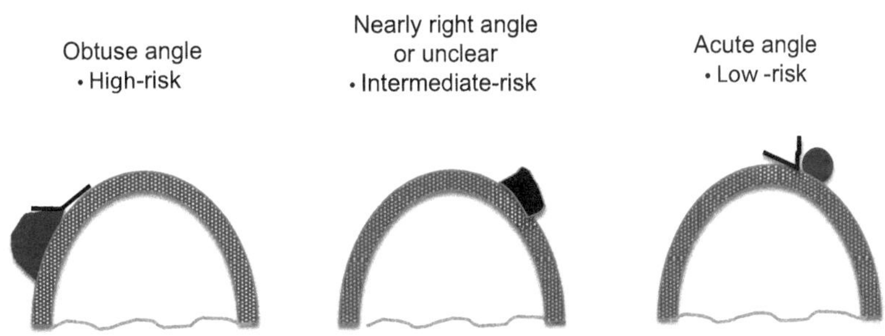

Fig. 11.1 Risk classifications of tracheal invasion of PMC based on the angle formed by the tracheal and tumor surfaces

carefully evaluate the risk of invasion to the trachea and the recurrent laryngeal nerve based on ultrasound and a CT scan in order to determine whether a patient can be monitored under active surveillance or should undergo immediate surgery.

Tumor multiplicity and the existence of a family history of PMC do not negate the use of active surveillance, because the presence of these factors was not related to PMC progression [11]. Possible invasion to organs other than the trachea and recurrent laryngeal nerve on imaging studies is not a contraindication for active surveillance, because rescue surgery after progression for these PMC is not difficult and does not significantly affect the patients' quality of life, even though carcinoma invades organs other than the trachea and recurrent laryngeal nerve. For accurate evaluation, sometimes CT scan is also helpful before considering an active surveillance. As indicated below, PMC in pregnant women or in young female patients who may become pregnant can undergo active surveillance.

How to Perform Active Surveillance of Low-Risk PMC

Active surveillance starts from the diagnosis of suspicious nodules as PTC based on an ultrasound-guided FNAB. At Kuma Hospital, the positive predictive value (PPV) of FNAB is very high at 98%. Diagnosis based on cytology is the best strategy for PMC diagnosis. In the guidelines issued by the American Thyroid Association (ATA), a cytological diagnosis of subcentimeter nodules is not recommended when the nodules are not symptomatic or have no evidence of malignancy such as node metastasis and distant metastasis [12]. However, at Kuma Hospital, we think it better to cytologically diagnose suspicious nodules as PMC and clearly disclose a diagnosis of carcinoma to patients. This is to prevent patients from visiting other hospitals and undergoing unnecessary surgery by non-experts. We also feel that it is better to diagnose PTC and notify the patients in order to encourage them to consistently return to the hospital for follow-up. We think that regular follow-up is necessary for suspicious nodules and we have not found that this is possible without an accurate diagnosis based on cytology.

The next important step is to accurately evaluate the PMC of each patient based on imaging studies. Ultrasound is a useful tool to evaluate the location of the primary lesion and to determine whether it is N-negative. If the location of tumor is observed to be adjacent to the trachea or recurrent laryngeal nerve, a CT scan is useful for further evaluation (see the next paragraph). Physicians should decide whether a patient's PMC is suitable for active surveillance or should undergo surgical treatment. In the past, we presented the two therapy options of active surveillance and surgical treatment equally, and the patients made their choice. At present, we recommend active surveillance as the first-line management because of the accumulation of favorable data for active surveillance.

For active surveillance, the patient is asked to visit the hospital for the evaluation of their PMC by ultrasound (and CT scan, in case tumors are located in the dorsal side) 6 months from the diagnosis and once per year thereafter. If any progression signs are detected (i.e., the size of the lesion has increased by $\geq$3 mm compared to the size at the initiation of active surveillance, or the novel appearance of metastatic nodes), we recommend surgical treatment. For the diagnosis of metastasis from suspicious nodes, FNAB for the nodes and Tg measurement in the wash-out of the FNAB needle are useful [13]. Active surveillance is continued if progression signs of progression are lacking. It remains an open question how long patients should undergo an active surveillance, and therefore, at least at present, lifelong observation is recommended. In Japan, as indicated above and shown in Table 11.3, active surveillance is more economical than immediate surgery [19]. It may be better for patients to undergo an active surveillance in a single institution for their lifetime. However, all hospitals can do it, if they follow similar surveillance protocols.

Table 11.3 Active surveillance for low-risk PMC at Kuma Hospital and the Cancer Institute Hospital: results of ten studies

Kuma Hospital [11, 14–19]	Cancer Institute Hospital [20–22]
1. Of 1235 patients, 8% and 3.8% showed size enlargement and novel node metastasis, respectively, at the 10-year observation by the Kaplan-Meier method 2. Gender, multiplicity and family history do not affect the growth of PMC 3. The PMC of young patients (<40 years) are likely to progress, whereas the PMC of older patients (>60 years) are the most unlikely to grow. None of the young patients with TSH suppression showed progression 4. Only 8% of the patients showed PMC progression during pregnancy, and rescue surgery after delivery was successful 5. In Japan, the medical cost of immediate surgery was 4.1 times the cost of active surveillance 6. None of the patients who underwent a rescue surgery after the detection of progression signs showed significant recurrence or died of PTC	1. Only 7% and 1% of 300 lesions showed size enlargement and novel node metastasis, respectively during active surveillance (not a time-sequential study) 2. The TSH value was not linked to the progression of PMC during an active surveillance 3. PMC with a rich blood supply or lack of strong calcification on ultrasound are likely to grow. Rich vascularity often decreased over time 4. None of the patients who underwent surgery after the detection of progression signs showed significant recurrence or died of PTC

Outcomes of Active Surveillance for Low-Risk PMCs

Table 11.3 summarizes the findings of an active surveillance strategy for low-risk PMC at two institutions, Kuma Hospital [11, 14–19] and Tokyo's Cancer Institute Hospital [20–22]. The incidences of size enlargement and novel node metastasis were low, and importantly, none of the patients who underwent surgery after the appearance of progression signs showed significant recurrence or died of PTC. These findings are coincident between the two institutions. One important finding is that PMCs in older patients (≥60 years) are less likely to grow compared to PMCs in young patients (<40 years) [17]. This is very interesting because in clinical PTC, old age is the most important prognostic factor for the cause-specific survival (CSS) of M-negative PTC patients [22, 23].

Therefore, the relationship between growth activity and age completely differs between subclinical PMC and clinical PTC. Clinical PTCs in older patients should be carefully and extensively treated, whereas low-risk PMCs in older patients are the strongest candidate for active surveillance. Although PMCs in young patients are likely to grow, none of the patients showed significant recurrence after rescue surgery and, although the number of patients examined was not large, it was reported that TSH suppression (TSH set at low normal) may be useful for preventing growth [17], although at present, it remains unknown how long TSH suppression should be continued. Sugitani et al. showed that the serum TSH value was not related to PMC growth [21], but this may because the age of patients at CIH is generally old.

As shown in Table 11.3, among pregnant patients, only 8% (4 of 51 cases) of PMC enlarged after delivery compared to before pregnancy [18]. However, only two of these four patients underwent surgery after delivery, and the remaining two continued under active surveillance because no further progression was detected and the tumor size was actually decreased after delivery compared to before delivery. Therefore, young women with PMC who may become pregnant can also be candidates for active surveillance.

Medical costs vary from country to country, but in Japan, the total costs for immediate surgery for PMC with postoperative management for 10 years were 4.1 times the total cost of active surveillance [19]. Similar results were reported from Hong Kong [24].

The use of markers predicting the progression of PMC would contribute to the decisions regarding whether to provide active surveillance or surgery for each patient, but such markers have not yet been identified. To date, some molecular markers such as *BRAF* mutations and *TERT* mutations have been identified for predicting the prognoses of patients with clinical PTC [25, 26].

However, at present, there are no molecular markers that can be used to predict the growth of PMCs using FNAB specimens. One report showed that the cell-proliferating activity of PMCs that were resected after the appearance of progression signs (as evaluated using the Ki-67 labeling index by means of immunohistochemistry for surgical specimens) was higher than that of PMCs resected without progression signs [27]. However, the Ki-67 labeling index on FNAB specimens has not been evaluated for the prediction of the progression of PMCs. Therefore, at present, active surveillance is the only reliable method to evaluate the growth activity of PMCs.

Surgical Treatment for Low- and Very-Low-Risk PTC

Postoperative Prognosis of PTC Without "High-Risk" Features in Japan

There are a few studies from Japan regarding the postoperative prognosis of PTC without high-risk features, although the definition of high-risk features differs among the studies. Matsuzu et al. analyzed 1080 PTC patients who underwent hemithyroidectomy as an initial surgery (median follow-up period, 17.6 years). They set four risk factors: age ≥45 years, T >4 cm, Ex-positive, and N-positive [28]. The patients' outcomes are summarized in Table 11.4. Notably, patients with 0 or 1 risk factor showed excellent prognosis for distant recurrence-free survival (D-RFS) and cause-specific survival (CSS). None of these patients underwent RAI ablation, because none of the patients underwent a total thyroidectomy.

Table 11.4 Prognosis of 1080 patients with PTC who underwent hemithyroidectomy as an initial surgery [28]

	No. of risk factors			
	0	1	2	3 or 4
25-year L-RFS (%)	92.1	93.7	75.6	59.4
25-year D-RFS (%)	99.6	92.1	86.1	62.3
25-year CSS (%)	100	95.1	82.5	64.1

CSS cause-specific survival, *D-RFS* distant recurrence-free survival, *L-RFS* lymph node recurrence-free survival
Risk factors: age ≥45 years, T >4 cm, Ex-positive, and N-positive

Table 11.5 L-RFS and D-RFS of the N0M0Ex-negative PTC patients [29]

	Tumor size		
	≤2 cm	2.1–4	>4 cm
10-year L-RFS (%)	98.1	95.4	91.9
10-year D-RFS (%)	99.6	98.4	96.6

Only 5 of 3965 patients (0.1%) died of PTC
D-RFS distant recurrence-free survival, *L-RFS* lymph node recurrence-free survival

We also analyzed 3965 patients with N0M0Ex-negative PTC (median follow-up period, 10.5 years) [29]. During the follow-up, only 5 (0.1%) died of PTC. As shown in Table 11.5, their L-RFS and D-RFS were excellent. This series included 2301 patients (58%) who underwent a limited thyroidectomy such as a subtotal thyroidectomy (dissection of one lobe, isthmus and lower pole of ipsilateral lobe), lobectomy with isthmectomy, and isthmectomy. A whole body scan using 3–10 mCi of RAI was performed for 475 patients (12%), who underwent total or near total thyroidectomy, and only 19 (0.5%) underwent RAI ablation using ≥100 mCi.

Ebina et al. showed that the DFS and CSS of 967 PTCs larger than 1.0 cm without high-risk features (i.e., M1 regardless of patient age, and patients aged ≥50 years with tumor extension to the mucosa of the trachea and/or esophagus or N >3 cm) did not significantly differ between patients who underwent a total thyroidectomy and those who underwent a hemithyroidectomy (mean follow-up period, 8.3 years) [30].

Studies of the Prognosis of Low- and Very-Low-Risk PTC per the Japanese Guidelines

As shown in Table 11.1, low- and very-low-risk PTCs are defined as PTCs with T ≤2 cm N0M0 and Ex-negative in the JAES/JSTS guidelines to be published in 2017 [1]. To date, two studies investigating low- and very-low-risk PTCs per the JAES/JSTS guidelines have been published.

We showed that, in the series of 2638 T1N0M0Ex-negative PTC patients (median follow-up period, 7.6 years), the 10-year DFS rate was excellent at 97% [21]. Distant recurrence was observed in only four patients (0.4%), and only two patients (0.2%) died of PTC. In that series, only three patients underwent RAI ablation using ≥100 mCi RAI, and 1601 (61%) underwent a subtotal or more limited thyroidectomy. If recurrence to the remnant thyroid is deleted, the DFS rate did not significantly differ between the patients who underwent a total thyroidectomy and those who underwent a limited thyroidectomy.

The second study was also from our institution, Kuma Hospital (Table 11.5) [29]. The 10-year L-RFS and D-RFS rates of the T1N0M0Ex-negative PTC patients were excellent at 98.1% and 99.6%, respectively. The novel appearance of node metastasis in the lateral compartment can appear after surgery for low- and very-low-risk patients and after active surveillance for very-low-risk patients, although the incidence is very small [11]. Interestingly, the L-RFS (mostly node metastasis to the lateral compartment) of very-low-risk PTC did not differ among an active surveillance group, a surgery group with and a surgery group without prophylactic modified radical neck dissection (MND) [11].

The Extent of Thyroidectomy for Low- and Very-Low-Risk PTC Patients

Although no prospective studies have been published, based on previous studies the prognosis of low-risk and very-low-risk PTC is excellent. Therefore, the JAES/JSTS guidelines recommend hemithyroidectomy for low-risk and very-low-risk PTCs if no pathological lesions are present in the contralateral lobe [1]. The incidence of recurrence to the remnant thyroid is very low, at 1% [31], and none of the patients died of PTC after the recurrence only to the remnant thyroid [32], indicating that salvage surgery after the detection of recurrence is adequate. In our previous study [21], the prognoses of low-risk and very-low-risk patients were similar after surgery, although an active surveillance is indicated in a majority of very-low-risk patients.

RAI ablation cannot be performed and serum Tg is difficult to use as a marker of recurrence after hemithyroidectomy. However, distant recurrence of low-risk and very-low-risk PTC is very rare, as indicated above. Conversely, total thyroidectomy should be performed for cases requiring RAI ablation and close monitoring of Tg and TgAb, because the Tg-doubling time significantly affects the CSS of TgAb-negative PTC patients [33], and TgAb is a surrogate tumor marker of TgAb-positive PTC patients after total thyroidectomy [34]. At Kuma Hospital, patients with intermediate-risk PTC,which includes >2 to <4 cm N0M0Ex-negative PTC undergo total thyroidectomy, although in the JAES/JSTS guidelines [1], either total thyroidectomy or hemithyroidectomy is recommended. This is because the rate of adverse events following total thyroidectomy is not very high if experts perform the surgery.

The Extent of Lymph Node Dissection for Low-Risk and Very-Low-Risk PTC Patients

In Japan, lymph node dissection has been actively performed even though it is prophylactic. This is because the organ to which PTCs are most likely to recur is the lymph nodes, and extensive node dissection was thought to reduce the recurrence rate of PTC. In the present JAES/JSTS guidelines, routine level VI dissection is recommended for all PTC cases [1]. This is because reoperation for recurrence to level VI is difficult and may induce severe complications such as recurrent laryngeal nerve injury and permanent hypoparathyroidism. In hemithyroidectomy, level VI dissection on the contralateral side is not recommended, because the incidence of node metastasis to the contralateral level VI is not common and a completion total thyroidectomy due to recurrence becomes difficult.

It is debatable whether prophylactic modified radical neck dissection (MND, level II–IV dissection) is beneficial for patients without detectable nodal metastasis. In Japan, in the past, prophylactic level II–IV dissection was performed almost routinely because it was believed to reduce the rate of lymph node recurrence. In 2007, our institution demonstrated that the 10-year L-RFS rates of PTC patients with no or only one of the four risk factors was excellent at 95%: (1) T >3 cm, (2) Ex-positive, (3) male gender, and (4) age ≥55 years [35].

A second report showed that, although the number of enrolled patients was small (829 patients), prophylactic MND did not improve the L-RFS of the patients who had Ex-negative PTCs measuring 1.1–3.0 cm [36]. According to our most recent study, in patients with PTC ≤4 cm N0M0, although we stopped performing prophylactic MNDs in 2006, the discontinuation of prophylactic MNDs did not worsen the L-RFS of the patients (manuscript submitted). We suspect that this is due to the improvement of ultrasound's diagnostic accuracy for lymph node metastasis.

Taking all of the above-described findings into consideration, we conclude that prophylactic MND is not necessary and is even an overtreatment for patients with low-risk or very-low-risk PTC.

Summary

Based on the Japanese experience, it is apparent that low-risk and very-low-risk PTC have undergone overtreatment. Especially for very-low-risk PTC, an active surveillance strategy is more beneficial for patients than immediate surgery. Rescue surgery for very-low-risk PTC after the detection of progression signs, size enlargement and/or novel metastasis to the regional lymph nodes is not too late.

For the surgical treatment of low-risk (T ≤2 cm, N0M0Ex-negative) and very-low-risk PTC (T ≤1 cm, N0M0Ex-negative), total thyroidectomy is not mandatory or should even be avoided in consideration of the risk of recurrent laryngeal paralysis and persistent hypoparathyroidism if the lesion is solitary and no other pathological lesions were detected in the contralateral lobe. Level II–IV dissection is not necessary, because there is no evidence that prophylactic level II–IV dissection improves the L-RFS in these patients. Level VI dissection is recommended (at least, in the JAES/JSTS guidelines), but contralateral level VI dissection is not recommended for patients who undergo a hemithyroidectomy.

At Kuma Hospital, patients with intermediate-risk PTC, which includes >2 to <4 cm N0M0Ex-negative PTC, undergo total thyroidectomy, although in the JAES/JSTS guidelines either total thyroidectomy or hemithyroidectomy is recommended.

The stereotyped therapeutic strategy for PTC is not always beneficial for patients. Physicians should consider the appropriate therapy for PTC from the viewpoint of personalized medicine.

References

1. The Japanese Society of Thyroid Surgery/The Japan Association of Endocrine Surgeons. Guidelines for management of thyroid tumor. 2nd ed. Tokyo: Kanehara Press; 2017.
2. Ito Y, Miyauchi A. A therapeutic strategy for incidentally detected papillary microcarcinoma of the thyroid. Nat Clin Pract Endocrinol Metab. 2007;3:240–8.
3. Takebe K, Date M, Yamamoto Y. Mass screening for thyroid cancer with ultrasonography [in Japanese]. Karkinos. 1994;7:309–17.
4. Miyauchi A. Clinical trials of active surveillance of papillary microcarcinoma of the thyroid. World J Surg. 2016;40:516–22.
5. Davies L, Welch HG. Increasing incidence of thyroid cancer in the United States, 1973-2002. JAMA. 2006;595:2164–7.
6. Davies L, Welch HG. Current thyroid cancer trends in the United States. JAMA Otolaryngol Head Neck Surg. 2014;140:317–22.
7. Ahn HS, Kim HJ, Welch HG. Korea's thyroid-cancer "epidemic"—screening and overdiagnosis. N Engl J Med. 2014;371:1765–7.
8. Vaccarelia S, Franceschi S, Bray F, et al. Worldwide thyroid-cancer epidemic? The increasing impact of overdiagnosis. N Engl J Med. 2016;375:614–7.
9. Oda H, Miyauchi A, Ito Y, et al. Incidences of unfavorable events in the management of low-risk papillary microcarcinoma of the thyroid by active surveillance *vs*. immediate surgery. Thyroid. 2016;26:150–5.
10. Ito Y, Miyauchi A, Oda H, Kobayashi K, Kihara M, Miya A. Revisiting low-risk thyroid papillary microcarcinomas resected without observation: was immediate surgery necessary? World J Surg. 2016;40:523–8.
11. Ito Y, Miyauchi A, Inoue H, et al. An observational trial for papillary thyroid microcarcinoma in Japanese patients. World J Surg. 2010;34:28–35.

12. Haugen BR, Alexander EK, Bible KC, et al. American thyroid association management guidelines for adult patients with thyroid nodules and differentiated thyroid cancer: the American thyroid association guidelines task force on thyroid nodules and differentiated thyroid cancer. Thyroid. 2015;26:1–133.
13. Uruno T, Miyauchi A, Shimizu K, et al. Usefulness of thyroglobulin measurement in fine-needle aspiration biopsy specimens for diagnosing cervical lymph node metastasis in patients with papillary thyroid cancer. World J Surg. 2005;29:483–5.
14. Ito Y, Uruno T, Nakano K, et al. An observation trial without surgical treatment in patients with papillary microcarcinoma of the thyroid. Thyroid. 2003;13:381–7.
15. Ito Y, Tomoda C, Uruno T, et al. Papillary microcarcinoma of the thyroid: how should it be treated? World J Surg. 2004;28:1115–21.
16. Ito Y, Miyauchi A, Inoue H, et al. An observation trial for papillary thyroid microcarcinoma in Japanese patients. World J Surg. 2010;34:28–35.
17. Ito Y, Miyauchi A, Kihara M, et al. Patient age is significantly related to the progression of papillary microcarcinoma of the thyroid under observation. Thyroid. 2014;24:27–34.
18. Ito Y, Miyauchi A, Kudo T, et al. Effects of pregnancy on papillary microcarcinoma of the thyroid re-evaluated in the entire patient series at Kuma Hospital. Thyroid. 2016;26:156–60.
19. Oda H, Miyauchi A, Ito Y, et al. Comparison of the costs of active surveillance and immediate surgery in the management of low-risk papillary microcarcinoma of the thyroid. Endocr J. 2016;64(1):59–64.
20. Sugitani I, Toda K, Yamada K, et al. Three distinctly different kinds of papillary thyroid microcarcinoma should be recognized: our treatment strategies and outcomes. World J Surg. 2010;34:1222–31.
21. Sugitani I, Fujimoto Y, Yamada K. Association between thyrotropin concentration and growth of asymptomatic papillary thyroid microcarcinoma. World J Surg. 2014;38:573–8.
22. Fukuoka O, Sugitani I, Ebina A, et al. Natural history of asymptomatic papillary thyroid microcarcinoma: time-dependent changes in calcification and vascularity during active surveillance. World J Surg. 2016;40:529–37.
23. Ito Y, Kudo T, Kobayashi K, et al. Prognostic factors for recurrence of papillary thyroid carcinoma in the lymph nodes, lung, and bone: analysis of 5,768 patients with average 10-year follow-up. World J Surg. 2012;36:1274–8.
24. Lang BH, Wong CK. A cost-effectiveness comparison between early surgery and non-surgical approach for incidental papillary thyroid microcarcinoma. Eur J Endocrinol. 2016;173:367–75.
25. Xing M, Liu B, Liu X, et al. *BRAFV600E* and *TERT* promoter mutations cooperatively identify the most aggressive papillary thyroid cancer with highest recurrence. J Clin Oncol. 2014;32:2716–26.
26. Lee SE, Hwang TS, Choi YL, et al. Prognostic significance of TERT promoter mutations in papillary thyroid carcinomas in a BRAF(V600E) mutation-prevalent population. Thyroid. 2016;26:901–10.
27. Hirokawa M, Kudo T, Ota H, Suzuki A, Miyauchi A. Pathological characteristics of low-risk papillary thyroid microcarcinoma with progression during active surveillance. Endocr J. 2016;63:805–10.
28. Matsuzu K, Sugino K, Masudo K, et al. Thyroid lobectomy for papillary thyroid cancer: long-term follow-up study of 1,088 cases. World J Surg. 2014;38:68–79.
29. Ito Y, Kudo T, Kihara M, et al. Prognosis of low-risk papillary thyroid carcinoma patients: its relationship with the size of primary lesions. Endocr J. 2012;59:119–25.
30. Ebina A, Sugitani I, Fujimoto Y, et al. Risk-adapted management of papillary thyroid carcinoma according to our own risk group classification system: is thyroid lobectomy the treatment of choice for low-risk patients? Surgery. 2014;156:1579–89.
31. Ito Y, Masuoka H, Fukushima M, et al. Excellent prognosis of patients with solitary T1N0M0 papillary thyroid carcinoma who underwent thyroidectomy and elective lymph node dissection without radioiodine therapy. World J Surg. 2010;34:1285–90.
32. Ito Y, Higashiyama T, Takamura Y, et al. Prognosis of patients with papillary thyroid carcinoma showing postoperative recurrence to the central neck. World J Surg. 2011;35:767–72.
33. Miyauchi A, Kudo T, Miya A, et al. Prognostic impact of serum thyroglobulin doubling-time under thyrotropin suppression in patients with papillary thyroid carcinoma who underwent total thyroidectomy. Thyroid. 2011;21:707–16.
34. Yamada O, Miyauchi A, Ito Y, et al. Changes in serum thyroglobulin antibody levels as a dynamic prognostic factor for early recurrence of thyroglobulin antibody-positive papillary thyroid carcinoma after total thyroidectomy. Endocr J. 2014;6:961–5.
35. Ito Y, Higashiyama T, Takamura Y, et al. Risk factors for recurrence to the lymph node in papillary thyroid carcinoma patients without preoperatively detectable lateral node metastasis: validity of prophylactic modified radical neck dissection. World J Surg. 2007;31:2085–91.
36. Ito Y, Tsushima Y, Masuoka H, et al. Significance of prophylactic modified radical neck dissection for patients with low-risk papillary thyroid carcinoma measuring 1.1-3.0 cm: first report of a trial at Kuma Hospital. Surg Today. 2011;41:1486–91.

12 Radioiodine Ablation: Current Status

Furio Pacini and Maria Grazia Castagna

In the management of differentiated thyroid cancer (DTC) total thyroidectomy may be followed by the administration of Radioactive iodine (RAI) therapy. Post-surgical ablation of thyroid remnant with RAI is aimed to facilitate the early detection of recurrence based on serum thyroglobulin measurement and to obtain a post-therapy whole body scan (WBS), whose results may change the initial staging by identifying previously undiagnosed disease. In addition, RAI ablation may represent an *adjuvant therapy* by cleaning persistent microscopic foci of cancer, which can be present in the thyroid remnant especially in PTC, which is frequently multifocal, and by destroying small-volume microscopic lymph node metastases (present in up to 80% of PTC) [1, 2]. Remnant ablation after lobectomy is more difficult and a repeat administration may be required. Ablation of a large remnant may cause radiation thyroiditis with neck pain and swelling.

In past years, RAI ablation was indicated in almost every patient with a diagnosis of DTC. Nowadays, careful revision of patients' outcome has introduced the concept of risk-based selection of patients, candidates to RAI ablation [1, 2]. According to the American Thyroid Association (ATA) stratification system [1] the individual risk depends on initial prognostic indicators obtained at surgery and on results of serum Tg measurements and neck ultrasonography obtained after surgery (Table 12.1).

RAI ablation is indicated in ATA high-risk patients. In a meta-analysis of 79 studies, Sacks et al. [3] concluded that there was sufficient evidence of improve cause-specific survival associated with radioiodine ablation in AJCC TNM stage IV patients. There was also evidence of a benefit for patients aged <45 years with significant extrathyroidal extension or distant metastases. Thus, routine post-surgical ^{131}I treatment with high activity is recommended in high risk DTC patients (Table 12.1).

For patients with ATA intermediate-risk DTC, limited risk-group specific data examining RAI efficacy are available [4–9]. Aggressive variant of PTC, such as diffuse sclerosing (DSV) and tall cell (TCV) variants, have a worse prognosis that classic PTC variant [4, 5]. Patients with DSV and TCV who did not receive RAI are 4.9 and 2.1 times more likely to die compared to patients who received RAI [4]. The clinical importance of minimal extrathyroidal extension on outcome of PTC is not well established. Nixon et al., reported no significant difference in 10 year OS, DSS or RFS between the pT1/pT2 and pT3 groups (OS: 93% versus 88%, $p = 0.129$; DSS: 99% versus 100%, $p = 0.733$; RFS: 98% versus 95%, $p = 0.188$ respectively) [7]. In addition, the administration of post-operative RAI in patients with minimal extrathyroidal invasion does not

F. Pacini (✉) · M. G. Castagna
Department of Medical, Surgical and Neurological Sciences, University of Siena, Siena, Italy
e-mail: pacini8@unisi.it

U. K. Mallick et al. (eds.), *Practical Management of Thyroid Cancer*,
https://doi.org/10.1007/978-3-319-91725-2_12

Table 12.1 Post-operative administration of radioactive iodine (RAI): indication and procedures

Risk class	Indication for remnant ablation	Activity of ^{131}I when indicated	Preparation
Low risk (1) Intrathyroidal PTC without vascular invasion; (2) Intrathyroidal encapsulated follicular variant of papillary thyroid cancer or intrathyroidal well differentiated follicular cancer with capsular or minor vascular invasion (<4 vessels involved); (3) Intrathyroidal papillary microcarcinomas that are either BRAF wild type or BRAF mutated	Not routinely recommended	30 mCi	Recombinant human TSH (rhTSH)
Intermediate risk (1) Microscopic invasion of tumor into the perithyroidal soft tissues at initial surgery; (2) Aggressive histology (e.g., tall cell, hobnail variant, columnar cell carcinoma); (3) RAI-avid metastatic foci in the neck on the first post-treatment WBS; (4) PTC with vascular invasion; (5) Clinical N1 or >5 pathologic N1 with all involved lymph nodes <3 cm in largest dimension; (6) Multifocal papillary microcarcinoma with microscopic invasion of tumor into the perithyroidal soft tissues and BRAFV600E mutation (if known)	May be considered	30 mCi (if low volume central neck nodal metastases with no other known residual disease are present) 30–150 mCi (if extensive lymph node disease, multiple clinically-involved LN or suspected or documented microscopic residual disease are present)	Recombinant human TSH (rhTSH) Thyroid hormone withdrawal or recombinant human TSH (rhTSH)
High risk (1) Incomplete tumor resection; Distant metastases; (2) Postoperative serum Tg suggestive of distant metastases; (3) Pathologic N1 with any metastatic lymph node ≥3 cm in largest dimension; (4) follicular thyroid cancer with extensive vascular invasion (>4 foci of vascular invasion)	Is routinely recommended	100–150 mCi	Thyroid hormone withdrawal or recombinant human TSH (rhTSH)

impact on survival or recurrence [7]. After exclusion of aggressive variants, overall survival was better in intermediate risk patients (lymph node metastases and/or extrathyroidal invasion) treated with RAI [9]. RAI was associated with a 29% reduction in the risk of death, with a hazard ratio of 0.71. RAI improved overall survival also in patients younger than 45 years (36% reduction in risk of death with a hazard ratio of 0.64) [9]. In PTC, BRAF V600E mutation is associated with increased disease specific mortality [10] and a significantly higher risk of recurrence than BRAF wild type tumors (24.9% vs. 12.6%, $p < 0.00001$) [11]. The risk of recurrence in BRAF V600E positive tumors ranged from 11 to 40% (median 26.5%) while the risk of recurrence in BRAF wild type tumors ranged from 2 to 36% (median 9.5%) [11]. However, because BRAF V600E mutation is associated with aggressive histologic phenotypes, lymph node metastases, and extrathyroidal extension, it is difficult to determine the proportion of risk attributable to the BRAF mutation versus that attributable to the other clinicopathologic features. There are currently no sufficient data to establish whether the presence or absence of BRAFV600E mutation should dictate the need of remnant ablation in PTC. In conclusion, for patients with *ATA intermediate-risk DTC*, existing data suggest that the greatest potential benefit may be observed with adverse thyroid cancer histologies, increasing volume of nodal disease, lymph node metastases outside the central neck, and advanced patient age [1]. In the others conditions (i.e. minimal extrathyroidal invasion, microscopic lymph node metastases and intrathyroidal PTC with BRAFV600E mutation), post-operative Tg together with neck ultrasound, can be used to select intermediate patients for RAI ablation (Table 12.1).

In the ATA low-risk category, RAI ablation is not recommended because the risk of disease-specific mortality and of persistent/recurrent disease is so low, that it is unlikely that may be improved by RAI administration [1, 12]. A retrospective study by Schvartz et al. [13] assessed the effect of ^{131}I on survival in patients with pT1 or pT2 tumors without nodal or distant metastases. After a median follow-up of 10.3 years, there was no difference in overall or disease-free survival between 911 patients who received ^{131}I treatment and 387 patients who did not. Prospective data suggest that overall and disease-specific mortality are not improved by RAI treatment in stage I and II patients [14, 15]. No indication for RAI ablation is also reported in ATA guidelines [1] for low risk patients also in the presence of microscopic lymph node metastases when less than 5 lymph node were involved. Despite the rate of microscopic histological lymph node metastases can be found in as much as 62% of PTC >1 cm, the recurrence rate is only 1–6% [16]. RAI remnant ablation is unlikely to improve the outcome of papillary microcarcinoma (<1 cm, uni- or multi-focal), in absence of other higher risk features [17, 18]. In conclusion, there is little evidence to suggest that in low risk patients ^{131}I may improve disease-specific mortality and risk of recurrence, and thus ^{131}I should not be administered. The overall risk of persistent disease is 3% and is even lower when serum Tg is undetectable. In this patients category, thyroid ablation may be considered only when serum Tg values are >5–10 ng/ml, when the likelihood of finding foci of radioiodine uptake outside the thyroid bed is significant [19, 20] (Table 12.1).

Remnant ablation has been traditionally performed after thyroid hormone withdrawal to increase endogenous thyroid-stimulating hormone (TSH) to levels sufficient to induce robust RAI uptake in thyroid cells. Empirically, it is estimated that a TSH >30 mU/L is a good cut off [21], but no comparative study has ever been done to document this assumption. Since several years, the alternative way of preparation for RAI ablation is the administration of rhTSH. A prospective, multicenter, randomized study have, in fact, demonstrated that ^{131}I remnant ablation with 100 mCi is equally effective after rhTSH stimulation or thyroid hormone withdrawal [22]. In another study, ablation rates were similar with either withdrawal or preparation with rhTSH using 50 mCi of ^{131}I [23]. Recently, two randomized non inferiority trials comparing low and high activities of radioiodine, each in combination with either rhTSH or hypothyroidism, have been published [24, 25]. The majority of patients were "low risk" but patients at "intermediate risk" (with lymph node metastases or minimal extrathyroidal invasion) were also included [24, 25]. The ablation rate was similar in the groups despite the thyrotropin stimulation method used, and the authors concluded that the use of rhTSH could be sufficient for the management of low risk patients. In addition, short-term recurrence rates have been found to be similar in patients prepared with thyroid hormone withdrawal or rhTSH both in low [26, 27] and intermediate risk patients [28]. The preparation with rhTSH significantly improves quality of life [22, 29], and reduces both whole body irradiation [30, 31] and hospitalization time [32]. A recent meta-analysis confirmed the above results [33]. Nowadays, the use of rhTSH is approved for remnant ablation, with any ^{131}I activity, both in the United States and Europe.

There is no consensus regarding the optimal activity of post-thyroidectomy RAI ablation. Post-operative activity may vary from low "ablation" activities (1.1 GBq or 30 mCi) to high "treatment" (5.5 GBq or 150 mCi) activities [2, 11].

Two prospective randomized studies in very large number of patients conducted in France and in the United Kingdom, found no significant difference in the remnant ablation rate using 30 or 100 mCi of ^{131}I, either after preparation with thyroid hormone withdrawal or rhTSH [24, 25]. It is worth noting that these two studies included not only low risk patients, but also patients at intermediate risk of recurrence, including those showing minimal extrathyroidal extension of the primary tumor [25] or lymph node metastases [24, 25]. Also in this category the authors found no difference between low and high RAI activities in term of ablation success rates. This finding has been confirmed in a retrospective study including only patients at intermediate risk, treated with low or high RAI activities [28]. Concerning the issue of the follow up of patients treated with low activity of ^{131}I a prospective, randomized study comparing the rate of recurrent disease in low risk patients ablated with 30 or 100 mCi, showed that in 10 years of follow up, the rate of persistent disease was similar in both groups [34]. Also in 225 intermediate DTC patients, the final outcome was similar between patients treated with low and high activities of ^{131}I at ablation [28]. On the contrary, it has been recently reported an higher DTC-related mortality in low and high risk patients treated with low activities of ^{131}I at ablation ($\leq$2000 MBq) when patients were at least 45 years of age at diagnosis and an higher recurrence rate in older high risk patients without distant metastases [35].

Conclusion

In past years, thyroid remnant ablation was indicated in almost every patients with a diagnosis of DTC. Nowadays, careful revision of patients' outcome has introduced the concept or risk-based selection of patients as candidates for thyroid remnant ablation. According to this concept RAI ablation is recommended based on the individual recurrence risk assessed using ATA stratification system (1).

In patients with *low risk* and ATA *intermediate risk* DTC without extensive LN involvement in whom radioiodine remnant ablation is planned, preparation with rhTSH stimulation is an acceptable alternative to thyroid hormone withdrawal for achieving remnant ablation and a low administered activity of approximately of 30 mCi (1.1 GBq) is generally favored over higher administered activities [1, 11] (Table 12.1).

In patients with ATA *intermediate risk* DTC who have extensive lymph node disease (multiple clinically-involved LN) in absence of distant metastases, preparation with rhTSH stimulation may be considered as an alternative to thyroid hormone withdrawal either using low or high RAI activities [1, 11] (Table 12.1).

In patients with ATA *high risk* DTC more data from long-term outcome studies are needed, before rhTSH preparation can be recommended. When RAI is used to treat suspected or documented residual disease in ATA high risk patients, administered activities of 100–150 mCi are generally recommended [1, 11] (Table 12.1).

References

1. Haugen BR, Alexander EK, Bible KC, et al. American thyroid association management guidelines for adult patients with thyroid nodules and differentiated thyroid cancer: the American thyroid association guidelines task force on thyroid nodules and differentiated thyroid cancer. Thyroid. 2016;26(1):1–133.
2. Castagna MG, Cantara S, Pacini F. Reappraisal of the indication for radioiodine thyroid ablation in differentiated thyroid cancer patients. J Endocrinol Investig. 2016;39(10):1087–94.
3. Sacks W, Fung CH, Chang JT, et al. The effectiveness of radioactive iodine for treatment of low-risk thyroid cancer: a systematic analysis of the peer-reviewed literature from 1966 to April 2008. Thyroid. 2010;20:1235–45.
4. Kazaure HS, Roman SA, Sosa JA. Aggressive variants of papillary thyroid cancer: incidence, characteristics and predictors of survival among 43,738 patients. Ann Surg Oncol. 2012;19:1874–80.
5. Regalbuto C, Malandrino P, Frasca F, et al. The tall cell variant of papillary thyroid carcinoma: clinical and pathological features and outcomes. J Endocrinol Investig. 2013;36:249–54.
6. Radowsky JS, Howard RS, Burch HB, et al. Impact of degree of extrathyroidal extension of disease on papillary thyroid cancer outcome. Thyroid. 2014;24:241–4.
7. Nixon IJ, Ganly I, Patel S, et al. The impact of microscopic extrathyroid extension on outcome in patients with clinical T1 and T2 well-differentiated thyroid cancer. Surgery. 2011;150:1242–9.
8. Ahn D, Sohn JH, Jeon JH, et al. Clinical impact of microscopic extrathyroidal extension in patients with papillary thyroid microcarcinoma treated with hemithyroidectomy. J Endocrinol Investig. 2014;37:167–73.
9. Ruel E, Thomas S, Dinan M, et al. Adjuvant radioactive iodine therapy is associated with improved survival for patients with intermediate-risk papillary thyroid cancer. J Clin Endocrinol Metab. 2015;100:1529–36.

10. Xing M, Alzahrani AS, Carson KA, et al. Association between BRAFV600E mutation and mortality in patients with papillary thyroid cancer. JAMA. 2013;309:1493–501.
11. Tufano RP, Teixeira GV, Bishop J, et al. BRAF mutation in papillary thyroid cancer and its value in tailoring initial treatment: a systematic review and meta-analysis. Medicine (Baltimore). 2012;91:274–86.
12. Pacini F, Brianzoni E, Durante C, et al. Recommendations for post-surgical thyroid ablation in differentiated thyroid cancer: a 2015 position statement of the Italian Society of Endocrinology. J Endocrinol Investig. 2016;39:341–7.
13. Schvartz C, Bonnetain F, Dabakuyo S, et al. Impact on overall survival of radioactive iodine in low-risk differentiated thyroid cancer patients. J Clin Endocrinol Metab. 2012;97:1526–35.
14. Jonklaas J, Sarlis NJ, Litofsky D, et al. Outcomes of patients with differentiated thyroid carcinoma following initial therapy. Thyroid. 2006;16:1229–42.
15. Jonklaas J, Cooper DS, Ain KB, et al. Radioiodine therapy in patients with stage I differentiated thyroid cancer. Thyroid. 2010;20:1423–4.
16. Randolph GW, Duh QY, Heller KS, et al. The prognostic significance of nodal metastases from papillary thyroid carcinoma can be stratified based on the size and number of metastatic lymph nodes, as well as the presence of extranodal extension. Thyroid. 2012;22:1144–52.
17. Hay ID, Hutchinson ME, Gonzalez-Losada T, et al. Papillary thyroid microcarcinoma: a study of 900 cases observed in a 60 year period. Surgery. 2008;144:980–7.
18. Baudin E, Travagli JP, Ropers J, et al. Microcarcinoma of the thyroid gland: the Gustave-Roussy Institute experience. Cancer. 1998;83:553–9.
19. Webb RC, Howard RS, Stojadinovic A, et al. The utility of serum thyroglobulin measurement at the time of remnant ablation for predicting disease-free status in patients with differentiated thyroid cancer: a meta-analysis involving 3947 patients. J Clin Endocrinol Metab. 2012;97:2754–63.
20. Melo M, Costa G, Ribeiro C, et al. Stimulated thyroglobulin at recombinant human TSH-aided ablation predicts disease-free status one year later. J Clin Endocrinol Metab. 2013;98:4364–72.
21. Edmonds CJ, Hayes S, Kermode JC, et al. Measurement of serum TSH and thyroid hormones in the management and treatment of thyroid carcinoma with radioiodine. Br J Radiol. 1977;50:799–807.
22. Pacini F, Ladenson PW, Schlumberger M, et al. Radioiodine ablation of thyroid remnants after preparation with recombinant human thyrotropin in differentiated thyroid carcinoma: results of an international, randomized, controlled study. J Clin Endocrinol Metab. 2006;91:926–32.
23. Chianelli M, Todino V, Graziano F, et al. Low dose (2.0 GBq; 54 mCi) radioiodine postsurgical remnant ablation in thyroid cancer: comparison between hormone withdrawal and use of rhTSH in low risk patients. Eur J Endocrinol. 2006;160:431–6.
24. Schlumberger M, Catargi B, Borget I, et al. Strategies of radioiodine ablation in patients with low-risk thyroid cancer. NEJM. 2012;366:1663–73.
25. Mallick U, Harmer C, Yap B, et al. Ablation with low-dose radioiodine and thyrotropin alfa in thyroid cancer. NEJM. 2012;366:1674–85.
26. Tuttle RM, Brokhin M, Omry G, et al. Recombinant human TSH-assisted radioactive iodine remnant ablation achieves short-term clinical recurrence rates similar to those of traditional thyroid hormone withdrawal. J Nucl Med. 2008;49:764–70.
27. Molinaro E, Giani C, Agate L, et al. Patients with differentiated thyroid cancer who underwent radioiodine thyroid remnant ablation with low-activity 131I after either recombinant human TSH or thyroid hormone therapy withdrawal showed the same outcome after a 10-year follow-up. J Clin Endocrinol Metab. 2013;98:2693–700.
28. Castagna MG, Cevenini G, Theodoropoulou A, et al. Post-Surgical thyroid ablation with low or high radioiodine activities results in similar outcomes in intermediate risk differentiated thyroid cancer patients. Eur J Endocrinol. 2013;23–29(2013):169.
29. Taieb D, Sebag F, Cherenko M, et al. Quality of life changes and clinical outcomes in thyroid cancer patients undergoing radioiodine remnant ablation (RRA) with recombinant human TSH (rhTSH): a randomized controlled study. Clin Endocrinol. 2009;71:115–23.
30. Hanscheid H, Lassmann M, Luster M, et al. Iodine biokinetics and dosimetry in radioiodine therapy of thyroid cancer: procedures and results of a prospective international controlled study of ablation after rhTSH or hormone withdrawal. J Nucl Med. 2006;47:648–54.
31. Frigo A, Dardano A, Danese E, et al. Chromosome translocation frequency after radioiodine thyroid remnant ablation: a comparison between recombinant human thyrotropin stimulation and prolonged levothyroxine withdrawal. J Clin Endocrinol Metab. 2009;94:3472–6.
32. Borget I, Remy H, Chevalier J, et al. Length and cost of hospital stay of radioiodine ablation in thyroid cancer patients: comparison between preparation with thyroid hormone withdrawal and thyrogen. Eur J Nucl Med Mol Imaging. 2008;35:1457–63.
33. Tu J, Wang S, Huo Z, et al. Recombinant human thyrotropin-aided versus thyroid hormone withdrawal-aided radioiodine treatment for differentiated thyroid cancer after total thyroidectomy: a meta-analysis. Radiother Oncol. 2014;110:25–30.
34. Maenpaa HO, Heikkonen J, Vaalavirta L, et al. Low vs. high radioiodine activity to ablate the thyroid after thyroidectomy for cancer: a randomized study. PLoS One. 2008;3:e1885.
35. Verburg FA, Mader U, Reiners C, et al. Long term survival in DTC is worse after low-activity initial post-surgical I-131 therapy in both high and low risk patients. J Clin Endocrinol Metab. 2014;99:4487–96.

Dosimetric Approaches: Current Concepts

13

Michael Lassmann, Markus Luster, and Heribert Hänscheid

Introduction

An important step in the therapy of patients with differentiated thyroid carcinoma is, in addition to surgical resection of the thyroid gland and/or tumourous tissue, to administer high activities of the iodine isotope I-131 (radioiodine therapy, RIT). In spite of numerous treatment optimization studies, the questions, when to administer radioiodine and the dosage of the treatment activity, are still not well defined and remain a matter of ongoing scientific debate. Because of lacking evidence to establish definitive recommendations, the national and international guidelines leave it to the responsibility of the attending physician to consider when and how to administer RIT [1–3].

Individual dosimetry is one of the largely unregulated aspects of RIT, although for the technical implementation of dosimetry, standardized procedures are now available [4–7]. In everyday practice, however, RIT is rarely performed on the basis of an individual dose calculation, although this can at least be regarded as medically meaningful for some patients. In general, the treating physician is left without recommendations on how to interpret the respective results and assess the therapeutic consequences.

The following chapter provides an overview of the basic principles, procedures and clinical results of the dosimetric approaches for further individualizing radioiodine therapy of differentiated thyroid carcinoma.

M. Lassmann (✉) · H. Hänscheid
Department of Nuclear Medicine, University Hospital Würzburg, Würzburg, Germany
e-mail: lassmann_m@ukw.de

M. Luster
Department of Nuclear Medicine, University Hospital Marburg, Marburg, Germany

Dosimetric Approaches

Current guidelines still advocate the administration of fixed activities for treating patients with differentiated thyroid carcinomas [1–3]. This leads to variable therapy conditions and radiation exposures for the patients due to individual differences in radioiodine kinetics.

The administered amount of radioiodine is only one factor influencing success of treatment. Other parameters are equally or even more important in determining the radiation absorbed dose to the target tissue, such as

- the time integrated activity coefficient per volume of blood, which represents the bioavailability of the I-131 and depends on body size and renal function,
- vascularization and blood supply of the target tissue, and
- the differentiation of the target tissue, which determines I-131 uptake and the effective half-life in the target volume.

U. K. Mallick et al. (eds.), *Practical Management of Thyroid Cancer*,
https://doi.org/10.1007/978-3-319-91725-2_13

Since all these parameters show a high individual variability, it is reasonable to consider them in any attempt to optimize RIT. Some adjustment of the activity for RIT to the individual patient is possible by considering the patient's disease stage, body size and renal function. A personalized treatment, however, requires a dosimetric strategy and measurements of the patients' individual iodine biokinetics to plan and optimize RIT.

In pre-therapeutic dosimetry, the administration of a tracer activity of I-131 potentially influences the biokinetics and reduces the absorbed dose administered to the target tissue by the therapy itself [8]. For patients with newly diagnosed DTC, a small diagnostic activity of only a few MBq I-131 is sometimes administered after thyroidectomy in order to determine the thyroid remnant by the remaining iodine uptake in the neck and to estimate the necessity for further surgery. Administration of higher diagnostic I-131 activities for pre-therapeutic imaging in the context of a more precise determination of the tumor stage or measurement of the kinetics in the target tissue, however, is contraindicated at least prior to the first radioiodine therapy generally intended to ablate the thyroid remnant.

Nevertheless, an individualized, dosimetry-optimized therapy can be safely performed in DTC patients. There are two different approaches: tumor dosimetry based on measurements of iodine kinetics in malignant tissue and the determination of the blood dose as a dosimetry of the dose-limiting organ, the bone marrow.

Tumor Dosimetry

Maxon et al. [9] were the first to perform tumor dosimetry in a larger patient population, with the aim of determining the doses required for a complete remission. According to the authors, an absorbed dose of 300 Gy to the thyroid remnant should be targeted in the ablation therapy and the absorbed dose to cervical lymph node metastases should exceed 80 Gy. These findings were confirmed in several independent studies, especially in the treatment of metastases [10–13]. Maxon's approach requires the application of pre-therapeutic tumor dosimetry with measurement of the kinetics in the target volume with the aim of curing the patient with the lowest radiation exposure. This procedure should be performed with an activity that is sufficiently low to avoid a radiation induced deterioration of the kinetics in the target tissue. In this context, the use of I-124 PET is advocated as it is capable of carrying out uptake measurements with superior image quality at lower absorbed doses.

Pre-therapeutic dosimetry, if not voxel-based, requires knowledge of the activity kinetics and the mass of the target tissue. As a reliable mass estimate after thyroidectomy is difficult to obtain, dosimetry for the thyroid remnant is typically uncertain with a high probability of under-dosing the patient. The patient-tailored treatment of metastases of known mass is also not uncritical, since different metastases in the same patient may have different kinetics and the absorbed dose distribution have been reported to be heterogeneous even within individual tumors [11, 14]. Basing the amount of the therapy activity on the mean kinetics in dosimetrically detected lesions carries the risk that disregarded manifestations or even areas within the measured tumors receive insufficient absorbed doses. In order to increase the probability of a therapy success, it therefore may be more appropriate to administer more radioiodine than potentially sufficient and accept a slightly higher radiation exposure.

Blood Dosimetry

Benua et al. [15] were the first to target at the highest possible tumor doses while avoiding severe myelotoxicity. They measured the dose to the blood as a surrogate of the organ-at-risk, the red bone marrow.

According to their data, Benua suggested limiting the blood absorbed dose to 2 Gy during therapy, as, below this value, he did not observe any significant hematological problems. The proposed limit of 2 Gy blood dose seems to be, however, very conservative. A significant proportion of the patients have been reported to achieve this dose already with the application of activities in the range of 7 GBq I-131 [16, 17], which are typically used in tumor therapies. In this group of patients, no serious corresponding side effects have been observed. Even when the activity is still significantly higher, the rate of adverse events remains low [18], and only a transient myelotoxicity was observed in a study targeting at a bone marrow dose of 3 Gy [10]. A therapy limited to 2 Gy absorbed dose to the blood can therefore be considered safe. The median of the specific blood absorbed doses observed in carcinoma patients is slightly less than 0.1 Gy/GBq I-131 [19–21]. It can therefore be concluded, that the therapy activities can be increased after blood dosimetry on average by 2–3 times in comparison to the application of standard activities.

Blood dosimetry is also useful peri-therapeutically in an attempt to estimate the radiation exposure caused by the therapy. The patient exposure cannot be derived solely from the administered activity because of a large spread of the absorbed doses per unit administered activity [22] especially in patients treated under hypothyroid conditions. The blood dose, on the other hand, is a good surrogate value for the radiation exposure. The content of body water in which the iodide is distributed, and thus the I-131 concentration and consequently the absorbed dose, is somewhat higher in the blood than in the dose-relevant organs. Measurements of the exposure of various organs show that the doses are generally 10–20% below the blood absorbed doses [23].

Peri-therapeutic accurate blood-based dosimetry is time-intensive, complex for the routine, and represent a burden on the patient because of the additional blood withdrawals and on the staff due to increased radiation exposure. A single measurement of whole body activity retention allows for the estimation of the absorbed dose to the blood [24]. The accuracy of dosimetry is, of course, reduced, but still adequate for a post-therapeutic dose evaluation.

Results

Tumor Dosimetry

There are some publications reporting values on tumor absorbed doses after the administration of standard activities. De Keizer et al. [25] determined absorbed doses to tumors from the I-131 uptake after stimulation with recombinant, human thyrotropin (rhTSH) and an estimation of the tumor volume derived from radiological images. The authors found a high variability of the values with doses between 1.3 and 368 Gy. Only 5 out of 25 examined lesions received doses of more than 80 Gy. Chiesa et al. [11] calculated doses of less than 80 Gy for 17 out of 20 evaluated lesions after standard activities. Flux et al. [12] reported an evaluation of sequential SPECT images for thyroid remnants of 23 patients after ablation therapy with 3 GBq. The maximum achieved voxel doses varied between 7 and 570 Gy. Flux et al. observed a significant difference in the absorbed doses between the groups of unsuccessfully and successfully treated patients. Verburg et al. [26] found, in a retrospective analysis, that long-term survival is worse after low-activity ablation therapy in both high and low risk patients.

Two groups have reported results obtained after treatment based on pre-therapeutic dosimetry using PET with I-124. Sgouros et al. [27] conducted dosimetry at the voxel level and found considerable heterogeneity of tumor absorbed doses. Jentzen et al. [13] reported high rates of completely responding lesions after dosimetry guided therapy.

The data in the references suggest that the use of standard activities may lead to suboptimal treatments. The administered tumor absorbed doses are often too low particularly in patients in an advanced stage of disease. Patients with insufficiently treated lesions usually receive additional courses of RIT which, however, are most likely to be expected to become more and more ineffective. It has been shown, that the iodine uptake and thus the absorbed tumor doses are drastically reduced from therapy to therapy, resulting in a progressive loss of therapeutic efficacy [11, 25]. In addition, an increasing number of therapies is associated with higher recurrence and cancer related mortality rates [28].

Blood Dosimetry

Compartment model calculations suggest that the time integral of the I-131 activity concentration in the blood and thus the blood absorbed dose is a decisive parameter for the activity uptake into thyroid remnants and tumors. It is not only determined by the administered activity but also by the patient's size, sex, and kidney function. Especially during hypothyroidism, blood absorbed doses are heterogeneous due to impairment of renal function in some of the patients and the mean blood absorbed dose is lower in individuals treated in euthyroidism [19, 20]. Assessing groups of patients treated in hypothyroidism after thyroid hormone withdrawal or in euthyroidism after recombinant human TSH, Hänscheid et al. [19] found that compared to the correspondent data in the euthyroid group, the mean remnant residence time was higher in hypothyroid patients by the same factor as the blood absorbed dose. The authors suggested to target at a fixed blood absorbed dose at ablation therapy in order to provide identical uptake conditions. Verburg et al. [22] actually found a significant increase in the success rate of ablation therapy with the blood dose in a retrospective analysis. However, the concept has not yet been validated since prospective studies are missing.

Since the pioneering work of Benua et al. [15], blood dosimetry is predominantly used to estimate the maximum tolerable therapeutic activity. As has been shown in patient studies [20–22], the mean blood dose per GBq I-131 is approximately 0.1 Gy. As a consequence, most patients with metastatic diseases can receive significantly higher therapeutic activities than the typically prescribed activity of approximately 7 GBq. Much higher absorbed doses to the target tissue can be achieved which is of particular importance in patients with advanced tumor stages.

Lee et al. [29] treated patients after failure of standard fixed activity therapy with the maximum safe therapeutic activity according to the Benua approach. Of 46 patients treated, 7 showed complete and 15 partial remissions. In 19 patients the course of the disease was stabilized; only 6 patients showed progression. The conclusion of Lee et al. was that the approach of the maximum safe blood dose is an effective treatment option for patients who no longer respond to conventional standard therapy. Similar results were observed by Verburg et al. [30] in a smaller group of patients.

Dorn et al. [10] applied, in 124 patients, a slightly different dose regimen, which was supposed to ensure that a bone marrow dose of 3 Gy was not exceeded. In this study, complete remission was observed in tumors receiving absorbed doses of more than 100 Gy. No persistent bone marrow depression was observed in patients with bone marrow doses of less than 3 Gy. A retrospective single-center study compared two patient groups with empiric prescribed activity vs. dosimetry-based prescribed activity and showed an improved response rate for patients with lymph node metastases and distant metastases [14] after administration of the maximum tolerable activity, which was statistically not significant. A recent retrospective analysis by Deandreis et al. even showed a tendentially worse survival for the patients treated with a dosimetry-based approach [31]. The latter group concluded that the lack of apparent benefit from dosimetry-derived activities made the value of dosimetry questionable. In this study, however, the patients treated based on dosimetry were older (median: 10 years) and showed a greater extent of distant metastatic disease than those treated with fixed activities. Therefore, as the groups differ significantly, the lack of a significant difference between the two patient groups should not be interpreted as a proof of lacking efficacy.

Conclusions

Since radioiodine therapy of differentiated thyroid carcinoma until today is largely empirical and there are almost no prospective, randomized dosimetry-based therapy optimization trials, the superiority of the individualized approach compared to the administration of I-131 standard activities and thus a compelling medical necessity for the implementation of individual dosimetry has currently not been shown. The theoretical advantage of a tailored therapy thus has not been shown to result in improved patient-relevant outcomes.

However, there are important arguments favoring a dosimetry-based approach:

The calculation of the absorbed doses pre- or peri-therapeutically can be applied to identify patients for whom standard activities may be insufficient. The use of blood-based dosimetry allows an increase in the administered activity and thus the achievable doses in the target tissue. Another advantage of a dosimetry-based approach is to identify patients with insufficient uptake to achieve a promising tumor absorbed dose even with the maximum tolerable activity and to spare those patients further meaningless therapies.

Aspects of Physics and Methodology

Radioiodine

Radioiodine I-131 is produced during the fission of actinides in nuclear reactors and decays with 8.02 days half-life into the stable isotope Xe-131. A total energy of 971 keV is released during the nuclear transformation, of which on average 192 keV are emitted by beta and 383 keV by gamma radiation. The therapeutic effect of the I-131 is almost exclusively due to the beta radiation, which is locally absorbed within a mean range of about 0.4 mm in soft tissue.

Gamma Camera Measurements

The primary gamma transition in the disintegration of I-131 to Xe-131, which is emitted with an energy of 364.5 keV in 81.7% of the nuclear transformations, can be used for scintigraphic imaging by a gamma camera equipped with a high energy collimator. Repeated measurements under identical conditions over several days allow a determination of the temporal development of the counting rate in organs and target tissues. Usually planar scintigrams are acquired in well reproducible geometry and the net count rates induced by the activity in a target tissue r_T are assessed for each time of measurement from the counting rates in a ROI (region-of-interest) around the target volume and a region which is representative of the activity background. The time course of the net count rate is then approximated by fitting a mathematical function, usually a linear combination of exponential functions, to the data (Fig. 13.1a). Reasonable fit functions reflect the expected behavior of the activity kinetics in r_T and are ideally based on compartment model analyses.

To obtain an absolute quantification of the activity, the net count rates are divided by the sensitivity (counting rate per activity) of the gamma camera taking into account attenuation and scattering of the photon radiation within the body of the patient. An accurate quantitative measurement of the I-131 is possible with modern SPECT (Single Photon Emission Computer Tomography) cameras with integrated CT, which calculate the necessary corrections from the CT information and quantify the distribution of the activity concentration in the patient. For a dosimetry, it is often sufficient to perform only one absolute measurement with SPECT/CT, which is then used to normalize the time function of the net count rate in the planar images (Fig. 13.1b) [6].

Positron Emission Tomography (PET)

PET with the iodine isotope I-124 provides, in principle, a superior method for measuring the iodine distribution in patients (Fig. 13.2). I-124 has a half-life of 4.2 d, and emits positrons usable for PET in about 23% of the nuclear transformations. For PET, an activity of about 25 MBq I-124 is sufficient to assess the biokinetics of the iodide in the patient.

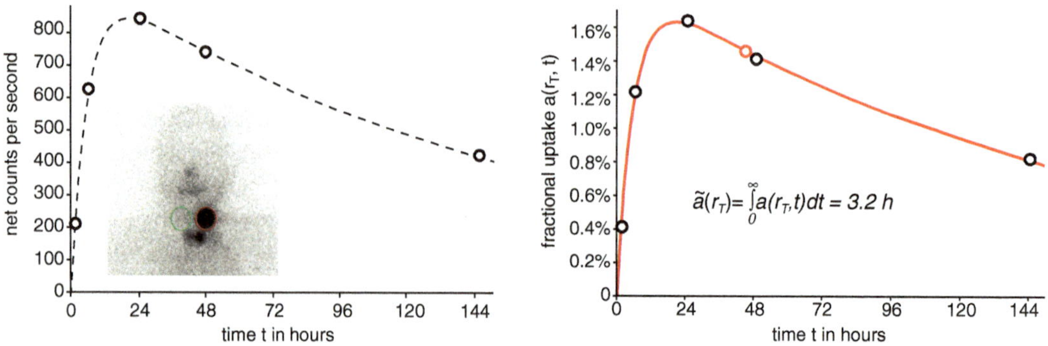

Fig. 13.1 (**a**) Net count rates (count rate differences in red and green ROIs) measured in a lymph node metastasis 2, 6, 25, 48, and 145 h after treatment with 3.5 GBq I-131 (black circles) and fit of a reasonable time function (two compartment model, dashed line). (**b**) Normalization of the data to match a quantitative SPECT/CT measurement of the fractional uptake in the lesion (1.46% at 46 h; red circle). The number of disintegrations in the target tissue r_T per unit administered activity and thus the absorbed dose is determined by the time integral of the uptake function $a(r_T,t)$ (area under the red line)

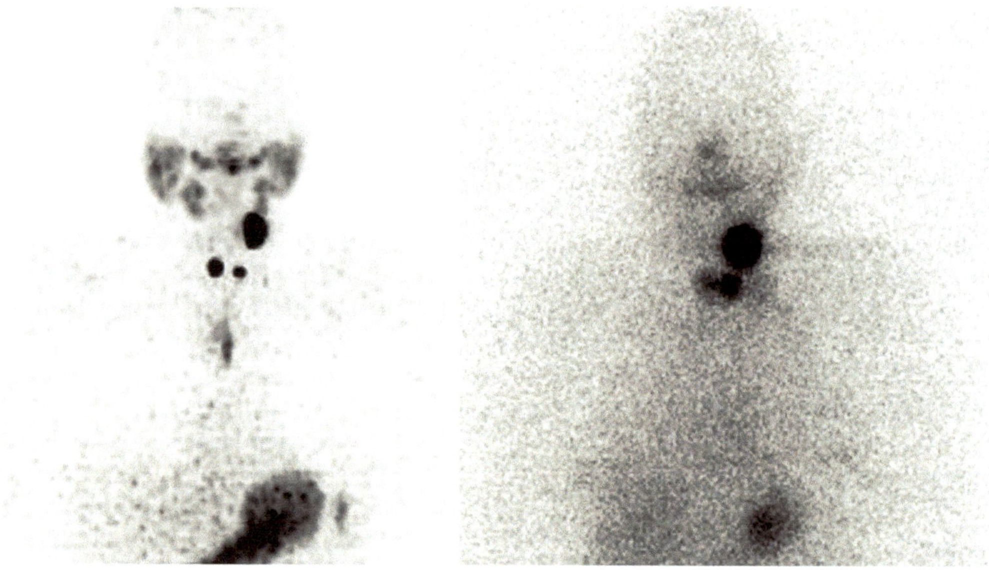

Fig. 13.2 Patient with a lymph node metastasis in PET imaging 24 h after administration of 25 MBq I-124 (left) and gamma camera imaging 5 days after therapy with 3.5 GBq I-131 (right). PET provides improved spatial resolution and activity quantification

Absorbed Dose

The success of (internal) radiation therapy is mainly determined by the energy dose $D(r_T)$ administered to the target tissue r_T. It is defined as the radiation energy E deposited per unit tissue mass $M(r_T)$, $D(r_T) = E/M(r_T)$, and is measured in the unit Gray (Gy, 1 Gy = 1 J/kg). In RIT, the absorbed dose is almost exclusively imparted by self-irradiation of the target tissue and the energy E is the product of the number of decays in $M(r_T)$ and the mean energy $\bar{E}$ deposited per disintegration. The total number of nuclear transformations in $M(r_T)$, also called time-integrated or cumulative activity, is calculated as the integral of the activity $A(r_T,t)$ in $M(r_T)$ over time t:

$$D(r_T) = \frac{\bar{E} \cdot \int_0^\infty A(r_T,t)\,dt}{M(r_T)} \quad (13.1)$$

When $A(r_T,t)$ is expressed as the product of the administered activity A_0 and the fractional activity uptake $a(r_T,t) = A(r_T,t)/A_0$ in r_T, Eq. (13.1) can be written as

$$D(r_T) = \frac{\bar{E} \cdot A_0 \cdot \int_0^\infty a(r_T,t)\,dt}{M(r_T)} = \frac{\bar{E} \cdot A_0 \cdot \tilde{a}(r_T)}{M(r_T)}, \quad (13.2)$$

where $\tilde{a}(r_T)$ is the time-integrated activity coefficient (residence time, area under the uptake function, Fig. 13.1b).

The mean energy $\bar{E}$ released in the target tissue per nuclear transformation increases with the target mass $M(r_T)$ because the fraction of energy lost by beta radiation originating at the surface of the target volume and leaving that volume decreases and more energy is imparted by gamma radiation. While the change of gamma absorption is generally of minor importance, the loss of beta energy can be considerable for small target volumes whose diameters are not much larger than the average range of the beta radiation. The fraction of beta energy absorbed within a small metastasis is reduced to 50% in a lesion with a diameter of 0.8 mm and to less than 30% for a diameter of 0.4 mm [32].

For evaluable lesions with diameters of several mm or more it is adequate to calculate the absorbed dose assuming a mean energy absorption of $\bar{E} = 2.8$ Gy·g/(MBq·d)

$$\frac{D(r_T)}{Gy} = 2.8 \cdot \frac{A_0}{MBq} \cdot \frac{\tilde{a}(r_T)}{d} \cdot \frac{g}{M(r_T)}, \quad (13.3)$$

Blood Dosimetry

For most patients, the tolerable radiation exposure in radioiodine therapy is limited by the toxicity in the critical organ, the red bone marrow, for which a reliable direct determination of the absorbed dose is not feasible. Benua et al. [16] suggested measuring the dose in the blood instead. Since the free iodide in the organism is assumed to be uniformly distributed in the readily interchangeable fraction of the body water, it can be safely assumed that the energy dose per volume of blood represents an upper estimate of the bone marrow absorbed dose.

Measurement of the blood absorbed dose per unit administered activity is feasible with low activities of about 10 MBq I-131 or with I-124. The complete assessment includes the determination of the time-integrated activity coefficients per liter of blood ã(Bl) and in the whole body ã(TB) [4] (Fig. 13.3).

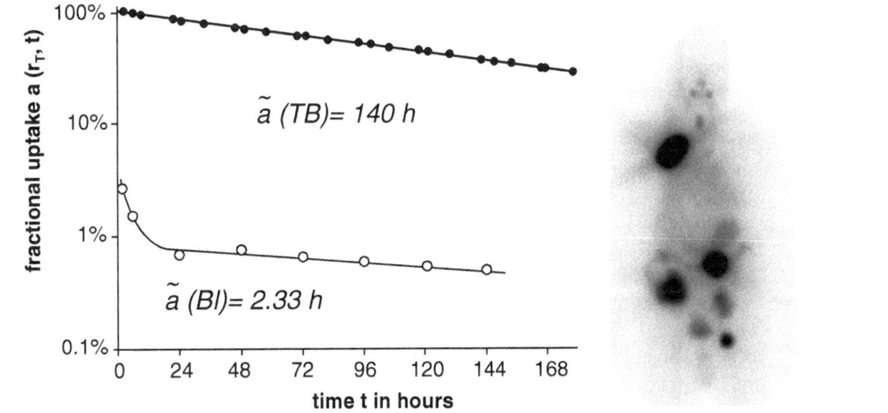

Fig. 13.3 Activity retention in the total body (filled dots) and per liter of blood (open circles) in a patient (88 kg) with large distant metastases. The gamma camera image was acquired 10 days after therapy with 5.8 GBq I-131. The blood absorbed dose was D(blood) = 2.2 Gy

The mean blood absorbed dose per unit administered I-131 activity can be calculated by:

$$\frac{D(blood)}{A_0}\cdot\frac{GBq}{Gy} = 0.108\cdot\frac{\tilde{a}(Bl)}{h} + \frac{0.0188}{(wt/kg)^{2/3}}\cdot\frac{\tilde{a}(TB)}{h}, \quad (13.4)$$

where wt is the total body mass.

In Eq. (13.4), the first addend describes the contribution of self-irradiation of the blood by beta radiation. The second addend accounts for the less important gamma contribution from activity in the total body.

References

1. Luster M, Clarke SE, Dietlein M, Lassmann M, Lind P, Oyen WJ, et al. Guidelines for radioiodine therapy of differentiated thyroid cancer. Eur J Nucl Med Mol Imaging. 2008;35(10):1941–59. https://doi.org/10.1007/s00259-008-0883-1.
2. Haugen BR, Alexander EK, Bible KC, Doherty GM, Mandel SJ, Nikiforov YE, et al. 2015 American thyroid association management guidelines for adult patients with thyroid nodules and differentiated thyroid cancer the American thyroid association guidelines task force on thyroid nodules and differentiated thyroid cancer. Thyroid. 2016;26(1):1–133. https://doi.org/10.1089/thy.2015.0020.
3. Pacini F, Schlumberger M, Dralle H, Elisei R, Smit JWA, Wiersinga W, et al. European consensus for the management of patients with differentiated thyroid carcinoma of the follicular epithelium. Eur J Endocrinol. 2006;154(6):787–803.
4. Lassmann M, Hänscheid H, Chiesa C, Hindorf C, Flux G, Luster M. EANM Dosimetry Committee series on standard operational procedures for pretherapeutic dosimetry I: blood and bone marrow dosimetry in differentiated thyroid cancer therapy. Eur J Nucl Med Mol Imaging. 2008;35(7):1405–12. https://doi.org/10.1007/s00259-008-0761-x.
5. Dewaraja YK, Ljungberg M, Green AJ, Zanzonico PB, Frey EC, Bolch WE, et al. MIRD pamphlet No. 24: guidelines for quantitative 131I SPECT in dosimetry applications. J Nucl Med. 2013;54(12):2182–8. https://doi.org/10.2967/jnumed.113.122390.
6. Dewaraja YK, Frey EC, Sgouros G, Brill AB, Roberson P, Zanzonico PB, et al. MIRD pamphlet No. 23: quantitative SPECT for patient-specific 3-dimensional dosimetry in internal radionuclide therapy. J Nucl Med. 2012;53(8):1310–25. https://doi.org/10.2967/jnumed.111.100123.
7. Siegel JA, Thomas SR, Stubbs JB, Stabin MG, Hays MT, Koral KF, et al. MIRD pamphlet no. 16: techniques for quantitative radiopharmaceutical biodistribution data acquisition and analysis for use in human radiation dose estimates. J Nucl Med. 1999;40(2):37s–61s.
8. Lassmann M, Luster M, Hanscheid H, Reiners C. Impact of ^{131}I diagnostic activities on the biokinetics of thyroid remnants. J Nucl Med. 2004;45(4):619–25.
9. Maxon HR, Thomas SR, Hertzberg VS, Kereiakes JG, Chen IW, Sperling MI, et al. Relation between effective radiation-dose and outcome of radioiodine therapy for thyroid-cancer. New Engl J Med. 1983;309(16):937–41. https://doi.org/10.1056/Nejm198310203091601.
10. Dorn R, Kopp J, Vogt H, Heidenreich P, Carroll RG, Gulec SA. Dosimetry-guided radioactive iodine treatment in patients with metastatic differentiated thyroid cancer: largest safe dose using a risk-adapted approach. J Nucl Med. 2003;44(3):451–6.
11. Chiesa C, Castellani MR, Vellani C, Orunesu E, Negri A, Azzeroni R, et al. Individualized dosimetry in the management of metastatic differentiated thyroid cancer. Q J Nucl Med Mol Imaging. 2009;53(5):546–61.
12. Flux GD, Haq M, Chittenden SJ, Buckley S, Hindorf C, Newbold K, et al. A dose-effect correlation for radioiodine ablation in differentiated thyroid cancer. Eur J Nucl Med Mol Imaging. 2010;37(2):270–5. https://doi.org/10.1007/s00259-009-1261-3.
13. Jentzen W, Hoppenbrouwers J, van Leeuwen P, van der Velden D, van de Kolk R, Poeppel TD, et al. Assessment of lesion response in the initial radioiodine treatment of differentiated thyroid cancer using I-124 PET imaging. J Nucl Med. 2014;55(11):1759–65. https://doi.org/10.2967/jnumed.114.144089.
14. Klubo-Gwiezdzinska J, Van Nostrand D, Atkins F, Burman K, Jonklaas J, Mete M, et al. Efficacy of dosimetric versus empiric prescribed activity of I-131 for therapy of differentiated thyroid cancer. J Clin Endocrinol Metabol. 2011;96(10):3217–25. https://doi.org/10.1210/jc.2011-0494.
15. Benua RS, Cicale NR, Sonenberg M, Rawson RW. The relation of radioiodine dosimetry to results and complications in the treatment of metastatic thyroid cancer. Am J Roentgenol Radium Therapy, Nucl Med. 1962;87:171–82.
16. Tuttle RM, Leboeuf R, Robbins RJ, Qualey R, Pentlow K, Larson SM, et al. Empiric radioactive iodine dosing regimens frequently exceed maximum tolerated activity levels in elderly patients with thyroid cancer. J Nucl Med. 2006;47(10):1587–91.
17. Kulkarni K, Van Nostrand D, Atkins F, Aiken M, Burman K, Wartofsky L. The relative frequency in which empiric dosages of radioiodine would potentially overtreat or undertreat patients who have metastatic well-differentiated thyroid cancer. Thyroid. 2006;16(10):1019–23. https://doi.org/10.1089/thy.2006.16.1019.
18. Menzel C, Grunwald F, Schomburg A, Palmedo H, Bender H, Spath G, et al. "High-dose" radioiodine therapy in advanced differentiated thyroid carcinoma. J Nucl Med. 1996;37(9):1496–503.

19. Hänscheid H, Lassmann M, Luster M, Thomas SR, Pacini F, Ceccarelli C, et al. Iodine biokinetics and dosimetry in radioiodine therapy of thyroid cancer: procedures and results of a prospective international controlled study of ablation after rhTSH or hormone withdrawal. J Nucl Med. 2006;47(4):648–54.
20. Hartung-Knemeyer V, Nagarajah J, Jentzen W, Ruhlmann M, Freudenberg LS, Stahl AR, et al. Pre-therapeutic blood dosimetry in patients with differentiated thyroid carcinoma using 124-iodine: predicted blood doses correlate with changes in blood cell counts after radioiodine therapy and depend on modes of TSH stimulation and number of preceding radioiodine therapies. Ann Nucl Med. 2012;26(9):723–9. https://doi.org/10.1007/s12149-012-0632-1.
21. Giostra A, Richetta E, Pasquino M, Miranti A, Cutaia C, Brusasco G, et al. Red marrow and blood dosimetry in I-131 treatment of metastatic thyroid carcinoma: pre-treatment versus in-therapy results. Phys Med Biol. 2016;61(11):4316–26. https://doi.org/10.1088/0031-9155/61/11/4316.
22. Verburg FA, Lassmann M, Mader U, Luster M, Reiners C, Hanscheid H. The absorbed dose to the blood is a better predictor of ablation success than the administered I-131 activity in thyroid cancer patients. Eur J Nucl Med Mol Imaging. 2011;38(4):673–80. https://doi.org/10.1007/s00259-010-1689-5.
23. Kolbert KS, Pentlow KS, Pearson JR, Sheikh A, Finn RD, Humm JL, et al. Prediction of absorbed dose to normal organs in thyroid cancer patients treated with I-131 by use of I-124 PET and 3-dimensional internal dosimetry software. J Nucl Med. 2007;48(1):143–9.
24. Hänscheid H, Lassmann M, Luster M, Kloos RT, Reiners C. Blood dosimetry from a single measurement of the whole body radioiodine retention in patients with differentiated thyroid carcinoma. Endocr Relat Cancer. 2009;16(4):1283–9. https://doi.org/10.1677/Erc-09-0076.
25. de Keizer B, Brans B, Hoekstra A, Zelissen PMJ, Koppeschaar HPF, Lips CJM, et al. Tumour dosimetry and response in patients with metastatic differentiated thyroid cancer using recombinant human thyrotropin before radioiodine therapy. Eur J Nucl Med Mol Imaging. 2003;30(3):367–73. https://doi.org/10.1007/s00259-002-1076-y.
26. Verburg FA, Mader U, Reiners C, Hänscheid H. Long-term survival in differentiated thyroid cancer is worse after low-activity initial post-surgical I-131 therapy in both high- and low-risk patients. J Clin Endocrinol Metabol. 2014;99(12):4487–96. https://doi.org/10.1210/jc.2014-1631.
27. Sgouros G, Kolbert KS, Sheikh A, Pentlow KS, Mun EF, Barth A, et al. Patient-specific dosimetry for I-131 thyroid cancer therapy using I-124 PET and 3-dimensional-internal dosimetry (3D-ID) software. J Nucl Med. 2004;45(8):1366–72.
28. Thies ED, Tanase K, Maeder U, Luster M, Buck AK, Hanscheid H, et al. The number of I-131 therapy courses needed to achieve complete remission is an indicator of prognosis in patients with differentiated thyroid carcinoma. Eur J Nucl Med Mol Imaging. 2014;41(12):2281–90. https://doi.org/10.1007/s00259-014-2851-2.
29. Lee JJ, Chung JK, Kim SE, Kang WJ, Park do J, Lee DS, et al. Maximal safe dose of I-131 after failure of standard fixed dose therapy in patients with differentiated thyroid carcinoma. Ann Nucl Med. 2008;22(9):727–34. https://doi.org/10.1007/s12149-007-0179-8.
30. Verburg FA, Stokkel MPM, Duren C, Verkooijen RBT, Mader U, van Isselt JW, et al. No survival difference after successful I-131 ablation between patients with initially low-risk and high-risk differentiated thyroid cancer. Eur J Nucl Med Mol Imaging. 2010;37(2):276–83. https://doi.org/10.1007/s00259-009-1315-6.
31. Deandreis D, Rubino C, Tala H, Leboulleux S, Terroir M, Baudin E, et al. Comparison of empiric versus whole body/blood clearance dosimetry-based approach to radioactive iodine treatment in patients with metastases from differentiated thyroid cancer. J Nucl Med. 2016. https://doi.org/10.2967/jnumed.116.179606.
32. Bardiès M, Chatal JF. Absorbed doses for internal radiotherapy from 22 beta-emitting radionuclides: beta dosimetry of small spheres. Phys Med Biol. 1994;39(6):961–81.

External Radiation in Differentiated Thyroid Cancer in the Era of IMRT and Modern Radiation Planning Techniques

14

James D. Brierley and Meredith E. Giuliani

Introduction

The roles of surgery and postoperative administration of radioactive iodine (RAI) in the management of differentiated thyroid cancer (DTC) are discussed in other aspects of this book. However, we know that not all patients are cured from their loco-regional disease following appropriate management with surgery and RAI. Some patients may present late with unresectable cancer particularly if the carotid artery or paravertebral space is involved. In other situations the morbid nature of the surgery required for a complete resection is prohibitive such as disease in the tracheoesophageal groove necessitating a laryngectomy or pharyngo-laryngectomy. Although RAI is used to address microscopic residual disease following surgery RAI may not be effective either because of poor distribution due to interrupted blood distribution of RAI post-surgery, or because of a relative degree of lack of differentiation of the malignant cells that no longer take up therapeutic dose of RAI, or a combination of both. In these scenarios appropriate surgery and RAI is insufficient to control the residual DTC. Recurrence DTC in the neck can result in unresectable cervical recurrence that can have a devastating effect of the patients quality of life. To prevent this occurring in many high risk situations there may be a role for additional treatment with external beam radiation (EBRT). However given the effectiveness of surgery and RAI in intermediate and high risk patients the number of patients expected to benefit from additional EBRT is small. Patients must be carefully selected to receive EBRT to balance treatment related morbidity and benefits of improved disease control. The importance of selecting high risk patients was an issue in the only randomized controlled study to investigate the role of EBRT [1].

The prognostic features that predict for local recurrence in thyroid cancer are well recognized, age and local extent being two of the most import factors. However in recent years both the extent of local invasion and the age at which that predicts for poorer prognosis has come into question so that in the recently published 8th edition of TNM [2, 3] the respective cut offs and definitions were changed. In regard to age the cut off for defining poor prognostic group was increased from 45 to 55 years of age. Similarly the definition of T3 was changed from: T3, any tumour larger than 4 cm or tumour with minimal extrathyroid extension (e.g. extension to the sternothyroid muscle or into the perithyroidal tissue), to: T3a, tumour more than 4 cm in greatest dimension, limited to the thyroid and T3b, gross extrathyroid extension only

M. E. Giuliani · J. D. Brierley (✉)
Department of Radiation Oncology, Princess Margaret Cancer Centre, University of Toronto, Toronto, ON, Canada
e-mail: James.Brierley@rmp.uhn.on.ca

U. K. Mallick et al. (eds.), *Practical Management of Thyroid Cancer*,
https://doi.org/10.1007/978-3-319-91725-2_14

into the strap muscles. The reason for downgrading the importance of minimal extrathyroid extension is because the thyroid capsule is incomplete and as the thyroid contains fibrous and adipose tissue as well as muscle tissue, so that the criteria for extrathyroid extension are uncertain and probably of no significance [4]. This is important because the entry criterial for the only randomized study on the role of EBRT was any patient irrespective of age with pathological extension beyond the thyroid capsule. Recruitment was poor and only 45 of a planned 311 patients consented, and only 26 patients received EBRT. The local failure rate in the observation group without EBRT was only 3% confirming that this group had a low risk of local recurrence risk [1]. However there have been several single institutional studies that in the era before IMRT showed a benefit in improved local control and in some improved survival in high risk patients who had ERBT compared to similar risk patient who did not.

A comprehensive literature search on the role of adjuvant EBRT identified 16 articles with a pooled population of over 5000 patients and concluded that EBRT improves local control in patients over 45 years of age with at high risk of local recurrence, this included patients with gross residual as well as microscopic residual disease [5]. In a recent review from France of 13 papers a scoring system was developed to define patients who would benefit from EBRT. Any patient who scored 6 or more points would be recommended EBRT. Being over 60 years of age, with both extrathyroidal extension and microscopic residual disease, all score two points each giving a total of 6 and thereby recommending EBRT for these patients [6].

Despite the problems associated with retrospective analyses the existing data was such that the 2009 American Thyroid Association guidelines recommend that EBRT should be considered in patients over age 45 with grossly visible extrathyroidal extension at the time of surgery and a high likelihood of postoperative microscopic residual disease [7]. The more recent 2016 American Thyroid Association guideline does not address the situation of adjuvant radiation but comments that for tumors that invade the upper aerodigestive tract, surgery combined with additional therapy such as RAI and/or EBRT is generally advised [8]. The British Thyroid Association recommends consideration of adjuvant EBRT for patients with a high risk of recurrence/progression with: (a) gross evidence of local tumour invasion at surgery with significant macroscopic residual disease, or (b) residual or recurrent tumour that fails to concentrate radioiodine, i.e. loco-regional disease where further surgery or radioiodine is ineffective or impractical [9]. Most recently the American Head and Neck Society have stated that after complete resection, EBRT may be considered in selected patients greater than 45 years old with high likelihood of microscopic residual disease and low likelihood of responding to RAI [10]. In summary therefore EBRT should be considered in patients at high risk of local recurrence and that such patients are older patients with gross extrathyroid extension at the time of surgery and a high likelihood of residual disease.

There is less uncertainty on the role of EBRT in patients who have unresectable disease as indicted above on the discussion on guidelines. The American Head and Neck society guidelines similar to the others state that EBRT is recommended for patients with gross residual or unresectable locoregional disease [10].

When EBRT is indicated IMRT techniques should be used where possible. IMRT is the delivery of high-dose, high-precision radiation to a target while minizing dose to adjacent organs at risk (OARs). There is limited data and no randomized data on the role of IMRT specifically for thyroid cancers [11] however the data from other head and neck cancers is relevant. IMRT can ensure a greater dose of radiotherapy is delivered to the targets while keeping dose to OARs to a reasonable level. In nasopharyngeal cancer this had impacts on local control [12].

The use of IMRT in nasopharyngeal cancers has made loco-regional failure unusual and distant failure the primary concern. In addition to benefits on tumor control IMRT can allow for greater sparing of OARs [13].

In IMRT in thyroid cancer dose to the mandible (osteoradionecrosis risk), the submandibular glands and parotids glands (xerostomia risk) and spinal cord as well as other OARs are critical to toxicity and overall quality of life. IMRT also facilitates the delivery of differential doses to different areas at risk. For instance in one of the first reports of the use of IMRT in the management of thyroid cancer, three distinct different dose levels where recommend, one to gross residual disease, a second to adjacent soft tissue and a third to elective nodal areas. Typicaly however at our institution we recommend only two distinct volumes, 66 Gy in 33 fraction to gross residual disease (GTV) and 56 Gy in 33 fractions to elective adjacent volume and nodal areas (CTV) (Fig. 14.1). If there is no gross residual disease but treating for potential microscopic residual disease 60 Gy in 30 fractions to the high risk areas with 54 Gy to elective nodal areas.

The oesophagus is an OAR that is responsible for a significant component of toxicity in EBRT of the thyroid bed; with both acute oesphagitis and oesophageal stenosis, requiring gastrostomy tube insertion which has been reported as high as 5% in a series of mixed non-IMRT and IMRT planned patients [14], however gastrostomy tube placement has not been required in our own experience [15]. This toxicity is because the oesophagus is frequently in the CTV to be treated especially when concern is actual or potential residual disease in the tracheosophageal groove, even the best planned IMRT can not spare the oesophagus from being irradiated. However careful delineation of appropriate CTV, the use of differential doses for high risk and elective risk areas combined with IMRT can reduce the length and volume of the oesophagus getting the maximum dose of radiation. In one series the incidence of oesophageal stenosis requiring dilatation with non-IMRT planned treatments was 12% compared with only 2% following IMRT planned treatments. It should be noted that this was a retrospective analysis with shorter follow-up for patients treated with IMRT.

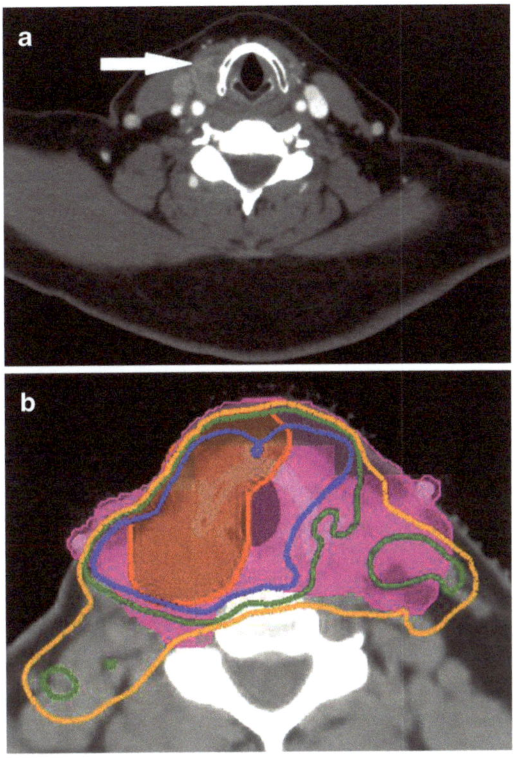

Fig. 14.1 (a) A 68 year old woman presents with a short history of shortness of breath and altered voice. She is found to have a mass in the right lobe of her thyroid and possible laryngeal involvement (see arrow on figure **a**) and right neck nodes enlarged. She underwent a thyroidectomy, the tumour was involving the cricoid and part of the cricoid was resected enblock with the tumour mass. The final pathology revealed a 4.6 cm multifocal papillary carcinoma with angioinvasion and 30% tall cell changes. The margins were involved with tumour. Twelve out of 42 lymph nodes were involved. She had 150 mCi of RAI. Post therapy scan showed uptake in the neck. (**b**) In addition, she had EBRT 66 Gy in 33 fractions the area of presumed microscopic residual disease and 56 Gy in 33 fractions to the elective nodal regions bilaterally. The red shaded area is the clinical target volume to receive 66 Gy. The purple shaded area is the volume clinical target volume to receive 56 Gy. The blue line is the 66 Gy isodose line and the green line is the 62.7 Gy isodosel ine (so that the majority of the tissue within the 66 Gy CTV will get 62.7 Gy). The orange line is the 56 Gy isodose line

Given the precise nature of IMRT treatments careful and accurate delineation of the GTV and CTV is essential. The optimal microscopic nodal volumes to be included in IMRT plans is controversial. The risk of nodal failure must be balanced with toxicity risk. As in squamous cell carcinoma of the head and neck sparing superior nodal volumes in certain circumstances is safe and reduces salivary toxicity [16].

In a retrospective review of treatment patterns in the United States between 2004 and 2011 there was a greater use of IMRT and a higher prescribed dose of radiation in tertiary referral centers than what was used in community radiation oncology centers [17]. It was also noted there was a trend to greater overall survival after IMRT but given this was a retrospective review there are many possible explanation.

In our institution the elective nodal clinical target volume includes levels III-VI, with level V and II partially included [18]. These volumes are extended to ensure a minimum of 1 cm on any gross nodal disease. We have reported our patterns of failure following IMRT using restricted elective neck volumes and found few out of field failures, Four out of 30 patients with differentiated thyroid cancer patients developed regional recurrence (one was in-field (level III) and 3 were out-of-field (all level II) [19]. Similarly others have reported in a series of 30 patients with differentiated thyroid cancer treated with IMRT that 86% or recurrences occurred in the para-oesphageal area and that the majority (58%)were marginal. When designing an IMRT plan to elective nodal coverage extent must balance the risk of regional failure, the potential salvage options and radiation related toxicity.

The role of EBRT to control the symptoms of metastatic disease is well established. Bone metastases are frequent in patients who die from thyroid cancer, it has been estimated at 42% [20]. Along with appropriate analgesia and surgery for patients with metastases in weight barring bones EBRT is an essential tool to help control pain. Not all bone metastases are widespread at presentation and unfortunately RAI is less effective in controlling bone metastases than lung metastases. Therefore an aggressive surgical approach for patients with isolated bone metastases may be considered, but because of the site of the metastases a surgical approach may not be possible. In this situation modern radiation treatment planning may enable high doses of radiotherapy to be given with the long term aim of control of the disease in that site. Small volume disease can be considered for hypofractionated high dose stereotactic body radiotherapy (SBRT) as described in more detail below (Fig. 14.2). In addition to the treatment of bone metastases SBRT can be considered in patients with oligometastastic disease with brain and lung metastases (Figs. 14.3 and 14.4).

The oligometastatic state is a situation with a limited number of metastases (general 3–5), in a limited number of organs (ideally 1) and where local ablative therapy (surgery, RT, etc) could render the person disease free for a prolonged period of time) [21]. There is growing interest in managing such patients with ablative treatment of their limited distant metastases in multiple disease sites [22]. This is a paradigm most established in isolated liver metastases from colorectal cancer [23]. The impetus for treating these individuals

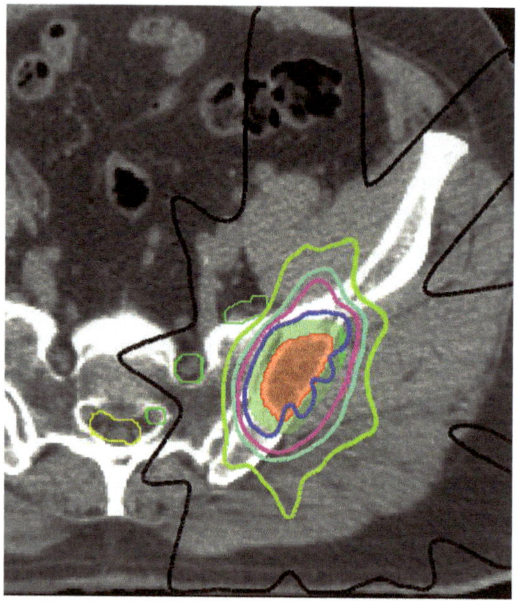

Fig. 14.2 A 72 year old man has a thyroidectomy for a 4 cm papillary carcinoma with angioinvasion. Post RAI scan show uptake in the thyroid bed and in the left pelvis. There is no evidence of any other metastases. He is given stereotactic radiotherapy 45 Gy in 5 fractions. The red shaded area is the clinical target volume (GTV). The green shaded area the planning target volume (PTV). The yellow line is the spinal canal. The lime green lines are the sacral plexus. The dark blue line is the 45 Gy isodose line (so that all the tissue with the volume described by the 45 Gy isodose line received a minimum of 45 Gy). The purple line is the 40.5 Gy isodose line. The light blue line is the 36 Gy isodose line. The yellow line is the 27 Gy isodose line. The black line is the 10 Gy isodose line

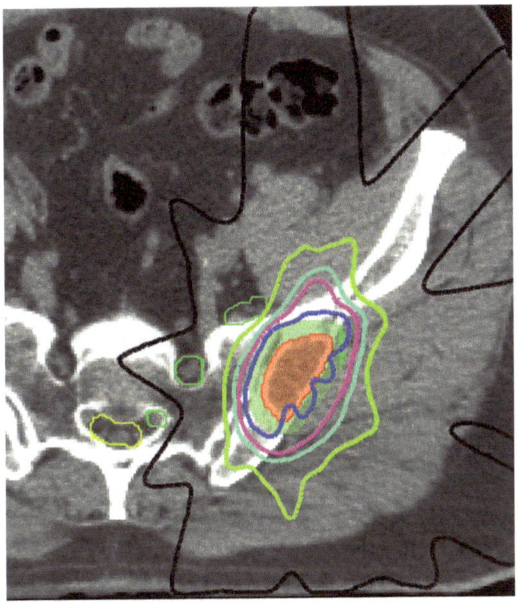

Fig. 14.3 A 51 year old man presents with a large thyroid mass with extrathyroidal extension. Surgery is performed the mass is dissected off the carotid sheath. He receives RAI and EBRT. Three years later he develops left leg weekness. An MRI reveals two lesions in his right parietal lobe and left occipital lobe. He is treated with whole brain radiation with radiosurgery boost from Gamma-Knife©. Four years later he remains free from disease. The red line is the gross target volume (CTV). The yellow line the planning target volume (PTV). The outer green line is the 12 Gy isodose line (so that all the tissue with the volume described by the 12 Gy isodose line received a minimum of 12 Gy). The inner green line is the 38 Gy isodose line

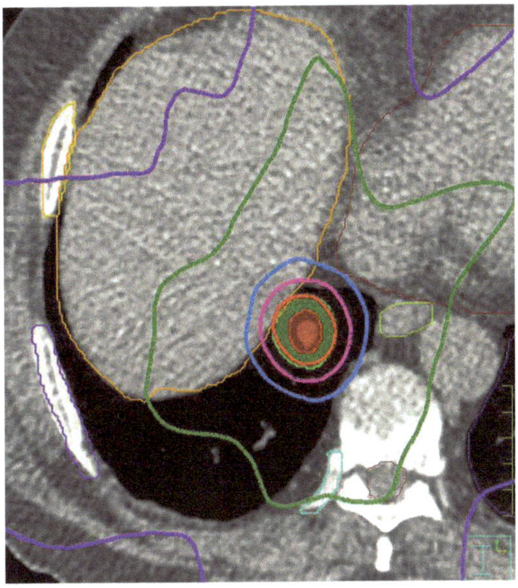

Fig. 14.4 A 69 year old woman with a previous history of thyroidectomy and RAI for a T2N1b differentiated thyroid cancer has an episode of coughing up blood. A CT scan shows a right lower lobe lung nodule. Her supressed TG is undetectable. A biopsy confirms differentiated thyroid cancer. She receives 5550 MBq of RAI, but her post therapy scan was negative. Two years later a repeat CT scan shows minimal growth in the lung nodule but no new lesions. Given the lack of appearance of any new metastases over the time period she was offered stereotactic radiotherapy and received 50 Gy in 5 fractions. The red shaded area is the internal target volume (ITV). The green shaded area is the planning target volume (PTV). The redline is the 50 Gy isodose line (so that all the tissue with the volume described by the 50 Gy isodose line received a minimum of 50 Gy). The pink line is the 35 Gy isodose line. The blue line is the 25 Gy isodose line. The green line is the 10 Gy isodose line. The dark purple line is the 5 Gy isodose line

with ablative therapy is that they may not progress to further widespread metastases, may have better quality of life and possible survival [24]. There is limited experience using such an approach in thyroid cancers but the efficacy and toxicity associated with SBRT in various body sites is well reported for other disease and can be extrapolated to thyroid cancers as this experience grows. When considering a SBRT approach in the oligometastatic setting a multi-disciplinary approach is essential to explore system options, surgical options as well as radiotherapy and other interventional options such as radiofrequency ablation. The risk and possible benefits need to be discussed with patients and where possible they should be enrolled on a clinical trial. Careful consideration needs to be given to adjacent OARs and established treatment protocols should be adhered to for specific OARs and SBRT dose/fractionations. Given the usually natural history of differentiated thyroid cancer to metastases when it does to multiple area, there may be a limited role for SBRT in oligometastatic disease but it is a treatment option that can be considered in suitable patients. It remains to be seen if however it significantly alters the natural history of the disease for these patients. Figures 14.2, 14.3, and 14.4 give examples of SBRT use in patients with oligometastatic disease.

References

1. Biermann M, Pixberg M, Riemann B, Schuck A, Heinecke A, Schmid KW, et al. Clinical outcomes of adjuvant external-beam radiotherapy for differentiated thyroid cancer - results after 874 patient-years of follow-up in the MSDS-trial. Nuklearmedizin. 2009;48(3):89–98. quiz N15
2. Brierley JD, Gospodarowicz MK, Wittekind CH. The TNM classification of malignant tumours. 8th ed. Oxford: Wiley Blackwell; 2017.
3. Amin MB, Greene FL, Edge SB, Compton CC, Gershenwald JE, Brookland RK, et al. The eighth edition AJCC cancer staging manual: continuing to build a bridge from a population-based to a more "personalized" approach to cancer staging. CA Cancer J Clin. 2017;67(2):93–9.
4. Mete O, Rotstein L, Asa SL. Controversies in thyroid pathology: thyroid capsule invasion and extrathyroidal extension. Ann Surg Oncol. 2010;17(2):386–91.
5. Fussey JM, Crunkhorn R, Tedla M, Weickert MO, Mehanna H. External beam radiotherapy in differentiated thyroid carcinoma: a systematic review. Head Neck. 2016;38(Suppl 1):E2297–305.
6. Sun XS, Sun SR, Guevara N, Marcy PY, Peyrottes I, Lassalle S, et al. Indications of external beam radiation therapy in non-anaplastic thyroid cancer and impact of innovative radiation techniques. Crit Rev Oncol. 2013;86(1):52–68.
7. Cooper DS, Doherty GM, Haugen BR, Kloos RT, Lee SL, Mandel SJ, et al. Revised American Thyroid Association management guidelines for patients with thyroid nodules and differentiated thyroid cancer. Thyroid. 2009;19(11):1167–214.
8. Haugen BR, Alexander EK, Bible KC, Doherty GM, Mandel SJ, Nikiforov YE, et al. 2015 American thyroid association management guidelines for adult patients with thyroid nodules and differentiated thyroid cancer: the American thyroid association guidelines task force on thyroid nodules and differentiated thyroid cancer. Thyroid. 2016;26(1):1–133.
9. Perros P, Boelaert K, Colley S, Evans C, Evans RM, Gerrard Ba G, et al. Guidelines for the management of thyroid cancer. Clin Endocrinol. 2014;81(Suppl 1):1–122.
10. Kiess AP, Agrawal N, Brierley JD, Duvvuri U, Ferris RL, Genden E, et al. External-beam radiotherapy for differentiated thyroid cancer locoregional control: a statement of the American Head and Neck Society. Head Neck. 2016;38(4):493–8.
11. Rosenbluth BD, Serrano V, Happersett L, Shaha AR, Tuttle RM, Narayana A, et al. Intensity-modulated radiation therapy for the treatment of nonanaplastic thyroid cancer. Int J Radiat Oncol Biol Phys. 2005;63(5):1419–26.
12. Lee N, Xia P, Fischbein NJ, Akazawa P, Akazawa C, Quivey JM. Intensity-modulated radiation therapy for head-and-neck cancer: the UCSF experience focusing on target volume delineation. Int J Radiat Oncol Biol Phys. 2003;57(1):49–60.
13. Kam MK, Leung SF, Zee B, Chau RM, Suen JJ, Mo F, et al. Prospective randomized study of intensity-modulated radiotherapy on salivary gland function in early-stage nasopharyngeal carcinoma patients. J Clin Oncol. 2007;25(31):4873–9.
14. Terezakis SA, Lee KS, Ghossein RA, Rivera M, Tuttle RM, Wolden SL, et al. Role of external beam radiotherapy in patients with advanced or recurrent non-anaplastic thyroid cancer: memorial sloan-kettering cancer center experience. Int J Radiat Oncol Biol Phys. 2009;73(3):795–801.
15. Tsang RW, Brierley JD, Simpson WJ, Panzarella T, Gospodarowicz MK, Sutcliffe SB. The effects of surgery, radioiodine and external radiation therapy on the clinical outcome of patients with differentiated thyroid cancer. Cancer. 1998;82:375–88.
16. Eisbruch A, Kim HM, Terrell JE, Marsh LH, Dawson LA, Ship JA. Xerostomia and its predictors following parotid-sparing irradiation of head-and-neck cancer. Int J Radiat Oncol Biol Phys. 2001;50(3):695–704.
17. Goffredo P, Robinson TJ, Youngwirth LM, Roman SA, Sosa JA. Intensity-modulated radiation therapy use for the localized treatment of thyroid cancer: nationwide practice patterns and outcomes. Endocrine. 2016;53(3):761–73.
18. Gregoire V, Levendag P, Ang KK, Bernier J, Braaksma M, Budach V, et al. CT-based delineation of lymph node levels and related CTVs in the node-negative neck: DAHANCA, EORTC, GORTEC, NCIC,RTOG consensus guidelines. Radiother Oncol. 2003;69(3):227–36.
19. Vulpe H, Kwan J, McNiven A, Et al. Patterns of recurrence after external beam radiotherapy for anaplastic and differentiated thyroid carcinoma. Radiother Oncol. 2016;120(Supplement 1):S80.
20. Coleman RE. Clinical features of metastatic bone disease and risk of skeletal morbidity. Clin Cancer Res. 2006;12(20 Pt 2):6243s–9s.
21. Hellman S, Weichselbaum RR. Oligometastases. J Clin Oncol. 1995;13(1):8–10.
22. Rusthoven KE, Kavanagh BD, Cardenes H, Stieber VW, Burri SH, Feigenberg SJ, et al. Multi-institutional phase I/II trial of stereotactic body radiation therapy for liver metastases. J Clin Oncol. 2009;27(10):1572–8.
23. Al Bandar MH, Kim NK. Current status and future perspectives on treatment of liver metastasis in colorectal cancer (review). Oncol Rep. 2017;37(5):2553–64.
24. Salama JK, Hasselle MD, Chmura SJ, Malik R, Mehta N, Yenice KM, et al. Stereotactic body radiotherapy for multisite extracranial oligometastases: final report of a dose escalation trial in patients with 1 to 5 sites of metastatic disease. Cancer. 2012;118(11):2962–70.

Part V

Follow Up and Longterm Management of Differentiated Thyroid Cancer

Thyroglobulin

15

Shireen Fatemi and Carole Spencer

Abbreviations

CRM-457	Certified reference material
CV	Coefficient of variation
DTC	Differentiated thyroid cancer
FNA	Fine needle aspiration
FNAB	Fine needle aspiration biopsy
FS	Functional sensitivity
HAb	Heterophile antibody
HAMA	Human anti-mouse antibody
hCG	Human chorionic gonadotropin
IMA	Immunometric assay
LC-MS/MS	Liquid chromatography tandem mass spectrometry
LOQ	Limit of quantitation
L-T4	Levothyroxine
Lx	Lobectomy
MAb	Monoclonal antibody
MCO	Manufacturer cutoff
NPV	Negative predictive value
PAb	Polyclonal antibody
PPV	Positive predictive value
PTC	Papillary thyroid cancer
PTH	Parathyroid hormone
RAI	Radioiodine
RF	Rheumatoid factor
rhTSH	Recombinant human TSH
RIA	Radioimmunoassay
Tg	Thyroglobulin
TgAb	Thyroglobulin autoantibodies
TRAb	TSH receptor antibodies
TSH	Thyroid stimulating hormone

S. Fatemi, M.D.
Kaiser Permanente, Panorama City, CA, USA
e-mail: sfatemi@kp.org

C. Spencer, Ph.D. (✉)
University of Southern California, USC Endocrine Laboratory, Pasadena, CA, USA
e-mail: cspencer@usc.edu

Thyroglobulin (Tg) Biosynthesis and Clearance

The Tg gene has been mapped to human chromosome 8q24.2–8q24.3 [1]. Tg genetic variants are not uncommon and likely play a role in the pathogenesis of autoimmune thyroid diseases [2–6], and some may be associated with increased risk for DTC [2, 3, 7–9]. Translation of the 8.7 kb mRNA transcript to form the initial 330 kDa monomeric protein is regulated by TSH, as well as the thyroid-specific transcription factors, TTF-1, TTF-2 and Pax8 [10–13]. Post-translational processing of the Tg transcript is complex, involving homodimerization and site-directed glycosylation, sulfation and folding in the Golgi complex to produce the mature 660 kDa dimeric Tg protein which undergoes chaperone-controlled transportation to the follicular lumen where hormonogenetic iodination of tyrosine residues occurs [13, 14]. Only mature Tg molecules that have an appropriate conformation can be

U. K. Mallick et al. (eds.), *Practical Management of Thyroid Cancer*,
https://doi.org/10.1007/978-3-319-91725-2_15

trafficked to the apical membrane for iodination [10, 12–16]. TSH stimulates the endocytosis of iodinated Tg from the follicular lumen before lysozomal proteolysis that releases thyroid hormones along with some undigested Tg protein into the circulation [13] (Fig. 15.1).

Critical steps involved in the post-translational modifications necessary to form mature Tg molecules may become dysregulated in thyroid tumors, resulting in the secretion of Tg molecules with abnormal carbohydrate [17, 18], sulfate [19–21] and/or iodine [22–24] composition. Since Tg epitopes are conformational [25, 26], any abnormalities in Tg sequence, tertiary structure, carbohydrate, iodine or sulfate composition, have the potential to alter the immunoreactivity of the molecule [27–34]. This Tg molecular heterogeneity also has the potential to prevent the generation of the proteotypic Tg tryptic peptide(s) necessary for LC-MS/MS detection [13, 35–39]. Heterogeneity of circulating Tg [27–32, 34], as well as differences between circulating Tg and

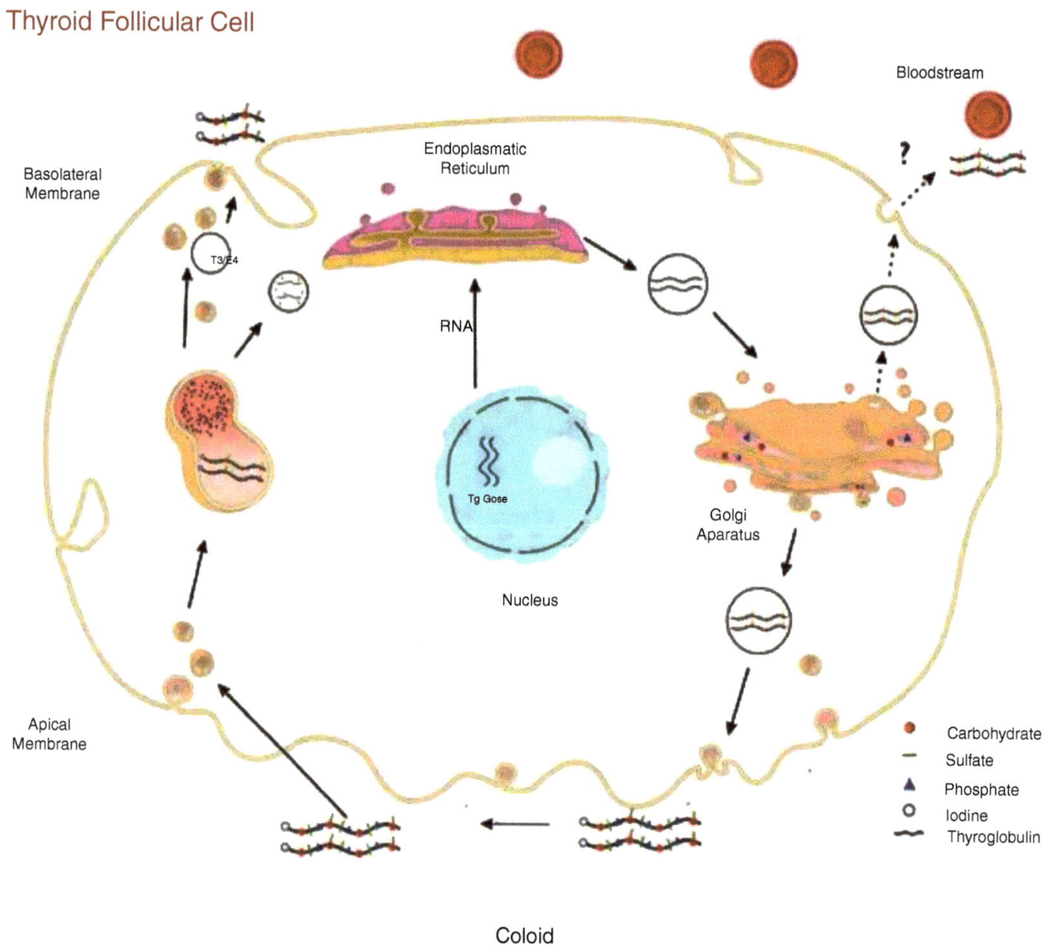

Fig. 15.1 Schematic model of synthesis and posttranslational modifications of thyroglobulin (Tg) in the follicular cell. The two 330-kDa polypeptide chains, linked by disulfide bonds, are synthesized in the endoplasmic reticulum from mRNA transcribed from the Tg gene, located on chromosome 8. Posttranslational modifications (glycation, sulfation, and phosphorylation) take place in the Golgi apparatus. Tg is then secreted into the colloid, where iodination occurs to form the thyroid hormone precursors MIT and DIT. Iodinated Tg enters the follicular cell cytoplasm by pinocytosis and combines with lysosomal vesicles containing proteolytic enzymes which lyse Tg and release the thyroid hormones into the bloodstream. Part of the remaining material is re-used by the cell from [13] with permission

the glandular Tg preparation (CRM-457) used for assay standardization [40], are reasons why up to a twofold difference in serum Tg values may be reported for the same specimen measured by different methods, even when TgAb is absent (Fig. 15.2) [30, 31, 41, 42].

As with other glycoproteins, Tg is primarily cleared from the circulation by the hepatic asialoglycoprotein receptor (ASGPR) [43–46] with a half-life approximating three days [47, 48]. Receptor-mediated clearance may be influenced by both the iodine and sialic acid composition of the Tg molecule [43, 46]. Since both iodine and sialic acid content tends to be low in the papillary morphotype (PTC), Tg molecules secreted by papillary tumors may have accelerated metabolic clearance that could lead to a disproportionally lower serum Tg relative to tumor burden [17, 20, 22, 48–54]. Indeed, preoperative serum Tg concentrations tend to be lower in papillary thyroid cancers (PTC), compared with Follicular or Hurthle Cell neoplasms [55, 56]. Tg metabolic clearance may also be altered by the presence of TgAb. Specifically, both animal and human

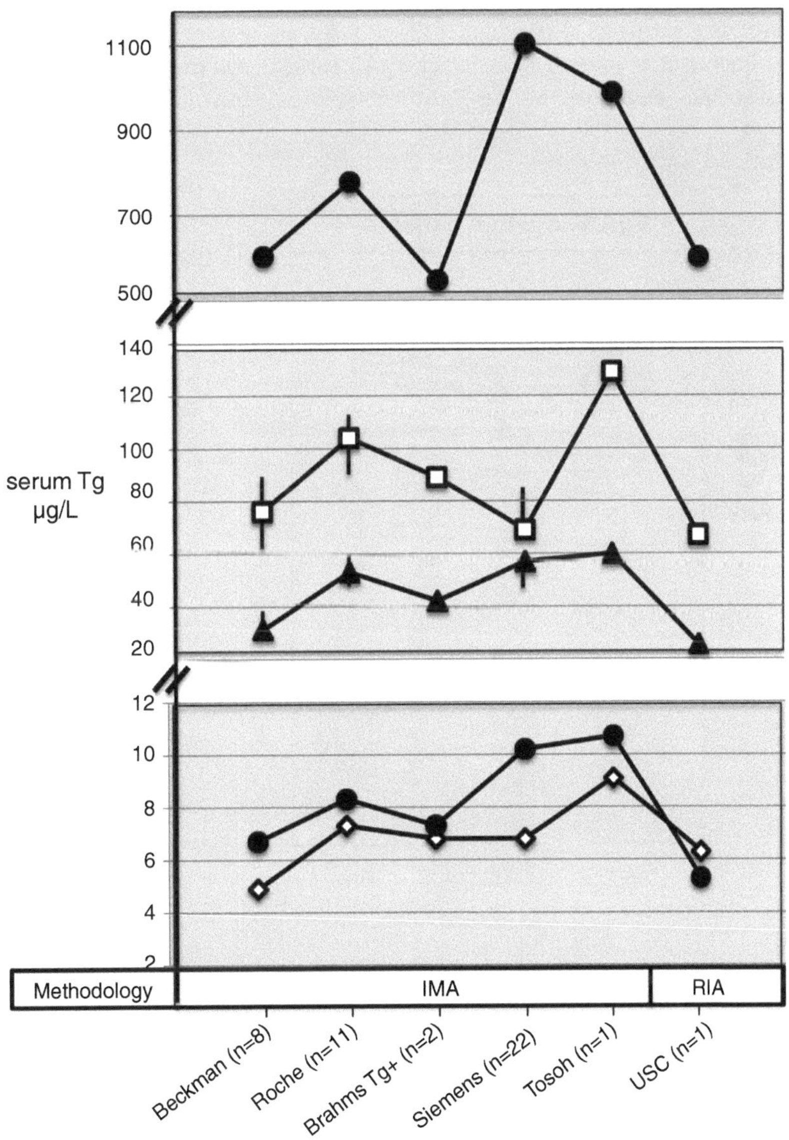

Fig. 15.2 2015–2016 Tg method comparison data from the United Kingdom National External Quality Assessment Service for Thyroglobulin Surveys. Five different TgAb-negative sera were measured by ~50 different laboratories. The percent confidence limits are shown for the three methods with sufficient participants. The data is shown with permission

studies suggest that TgAb complexing of Tg may enhance Tg metabolic clearance, perhaps because TgAb acts as a “sweeping antibody” for the hepatic ASGPR receptor to remove Tg-TgAb complexes from the circulation [46, 49, 57, 58]. Consistent with enhanced TgAb-mediated Tg clearance is the observation that TgAb-positive DTC patients with structural disease have lower serum Tg (irrespective of whether IMA, RIA or LC-MS/MS methodology is used), as compared with a comparable group of patients with structural disease and absent TgAb (Fig. 15.3b) [59]. TgAb concentrations are known to rise as disease progresses, such that the trend in TgAb can be used as a surrogate tumor-marker [25, 60–76]. It is important to investigate whether TgAb facilitates the clearance of Tg-TgAb complexes because as disease progresses and TgAb rises, a faster clearance of Tg-TgAb complexes would result in a paradoxical fall in serum Tg concentration, rendering serum Tg a misleading tumor-marker irrespective of the class of Tg method used.

Tg Measurement: Technical Issues

Tg methodology has evolved over four decades from RIA (1970s–present) to IMA (1980s–present) and most recently LC-MS/MS (2008–present). Methodological developments have been spurred by a quest for higher Tg assay sensitivity and freedom from TgAb interference. A comparison of the different classes of Tg method is shown

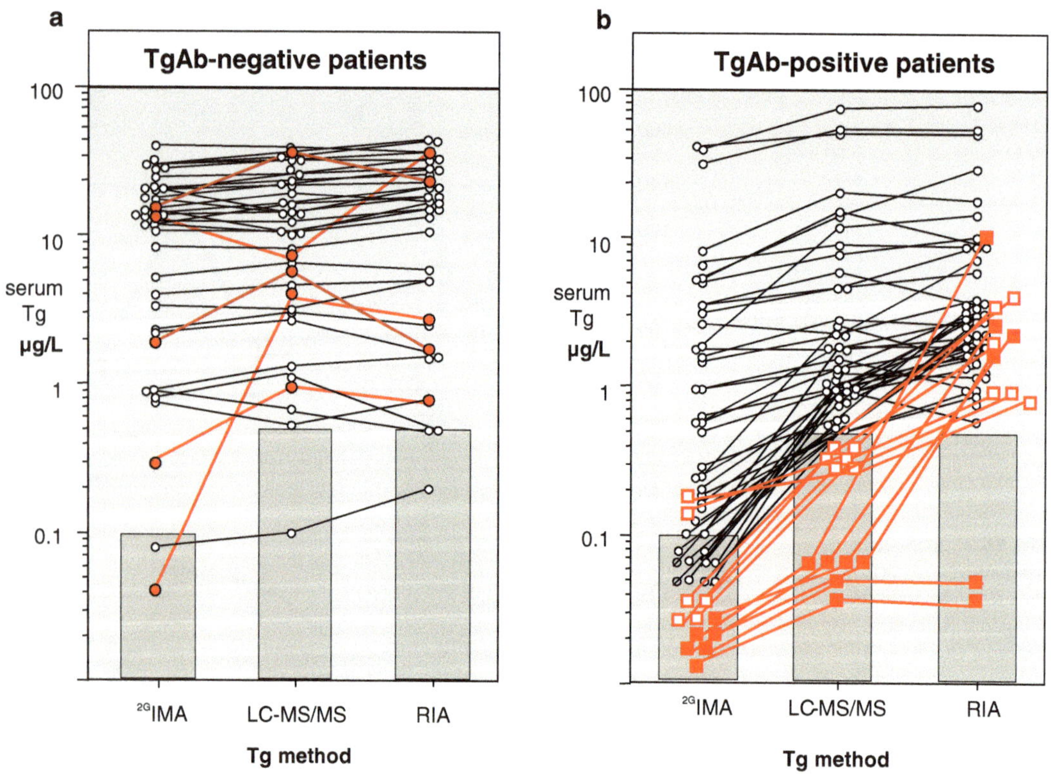

Fig. 15.3 Serum Tg was measured by the ^{2G}-Tg-IMA (Beckman), Tg-LC-MS/MS (Mayo Medical Labs) and Tg-RIA (University of Southern California) methods. The functional sensitivities of the methods are shown by dark bars. (**a**) 37 sera from TgAb-negative DTC patients with structural disease. The sera shown in red had a >30% between-method differences. (**b**) Shows the method comparison for 52 TgAb-positive DTC patients with structural disease. Sera with unequivocally undetectable Tg-LC-MS/MS values (no peak) are shown by solid red squares, whereas sera with marginally detectable Tg-LC-MS/MS values (0.3–0.5 µg/L range) are shown by open red squares. Data from [59]

Table 15.1 Classes of Tg method

Method class	Principle	Turn-around time	• Functional sensitivity (FS) • Strengths/pitfalls
Radioimmunoassay (RIA) 1973–present	Competitive/ isotopic-serum Tg and ^{125}I-labeled Tg compete for a limited quantity of polyclonal (rabbit) antibody (PAb)	Up to 6 days (cannot be fully automated)	• FS ~0.5 μg/L • PAbs have broad epitope specificities for detecting heterogeneous tumor Tgs • No HAb/HAMA[a] interferences • Resists TgAb interference
Immunometric assay (IMA) 1990–present	Non-competitive/ non-isotopic-serum Tg is first "captured" by a solid-phase monoclonal Ab (MAb) before detection by a different liquid-phase labeled MAb	Hours (can be automated)	• FS ~0.1 μg/L • MAbs have limited epitope specificities to detect heterogeneous tumor Tgs • HAb/HAMA[a] interferes (false highs) • TgAb interferes (false lows)
Liquid chromatography Tandem mass spectrometry (LC-MS/MS) 2009–present	Specimens may be concentrated and/or reduced, alkylated and digested with trypsin before target peptides are immunoaffinity enriched prior to detection by LC/MS/MS	? 1–2 days (specimen preparation difficult to automate)	• FS ~0.5 μg/L • No HAb/HAMA[a] interference • Clinically insensitive when TgAb is present • Polymorphic tumor Tg may fail to yield target peptides

[a]*HAb/HAMA* heterophile antibodies/human anti-mouse antibodies

in Table 15.1. The three classes of method have intrinsic differences in functional sensitivity (FS), specificity for detecting Tg heterogeneous serum isoforms and propensity for interference by both heterophile antibodies (HAb) and Tg autoantibodies (TgAb). Currently, most Tg testing is made using automated, IMA methods. However, because the IMA class of method is especially prone to TgAb interference, some laboratories first establish the TgAb status of the specimen (negative or positive) in order to reflex TgAb-positive sera for Tg testing by RIA or LC-MS/MS—methodologies believed to be less affected by TgAb.

Functional Sensitivity (FS)

Functional Sensitivity represents the lowest analyte concentration that can be reliably detected under conditions used in clinical practice. For Tg assays, FS is defined as the lowest Tg concentration that can be measured in human serum with 20% coefficient of variation (CV) in runs made over a 6–12 month period, using at least two different lots of reagents and two instrument calibrations [41, 65, 76–78]. Such stipulations are necessary because assay precision erodes over the long clinical intervals (6–12 months) typical for DTC monitoring, due to a myriad of variables that include changes in reagent lots [79–81]. Functional Sensitivity is a more clinically relevant indicator of Tg assay sensitivity than a limit of quantitation calculation (LOQ = 20% CV), because LOQ does not stipulate a DTC-relevant time-span for assessing precision [65, 82–85]. Another stipulation of the FS protocol [65] is that because instruments and methods are matrix-sensitive [83] precision should be assessed in the relevant test matrix (human serum) in preference to a commercial quality control material. Thus, since Tg-IMA testing is typically restricted to TgAb-negative sera, IMA precision estimates should be made in TgAb-negative human serum pools [83]. In contrast, Tg-RIA and Tg-LC-MS/MS testing is typically reserved for sera containing

TgAb, necessitating precision assessment in TgAb-positive human serum pools. Improvements in the FS of Tg methods over time has led to the adoption of a generational approach to Tg assay nomenclature, analogous to TSH [86, 87]. Tg assays with first-generation functional sensitivity (FS = 0.5–1.0 μg/L) include some IMAs, all RIAs and all LC-MS/MS methods [41, 74, 88–90]. Because first-generation assays are too insensitive to distinguish a subnormal post-thyroidectomy Tg level from the serum Tg typical of patients with an intact thyroid gland (~2–40 μg/L), first-generation assays have been typically used in conjunction with recombinant human TSH (rhTSH) stimulation [91–96]. Over the last 10 years second-generation Tg IMAs (^{2G}Tg-IMA), characterized by an order of magnitude greater functional sensitivity (FS = ≤0.10 μg/L) have become available and are now the standard of care [76]. This is because in the absence of TgAb, ^{2G}Tg-IMA has sufficient FS to monitor post-thyroidectomy subnormal basal Tg concentrations without the need for rhTSH stimulation [41, 59, 74, 76, 89, 90, 93, 97–111].

Specificity/Between-Method Tg Differences

Although most Tg methods claim standardization against the Certified Reference Preparation CRM-457 [80, 112, 113], Fig. 15.2 shows that there can be up to a twofold difference in the numeric Tg values reported for the same serum specimen when measured by different methods, even when methods claim CRM-457 standardization and TgAb is absent. The 95% confidence intervals of measurements made by laboratories using the same method shown in Fig. 15.2 indicate that this Tg variability reflects differences in method specificities for detecting heterogeneous serum Tg isoforms [30, 31, 37, 41, 42, 65, 74, 89, 114, 115]. These between-method biases far exceed the Tg biologic variability for euthyroid subjects (~16%) [79, 116]. Although some between-method variability arises from zero-matrix differences and differences between the secondary Tg standard and the CRM-457 reference, the major factor contributing to between-method variability is the heterogeneity of Tg in sera [31, 41, 89, 117–120]. This is especially the case for tumor-derived Tg that may be heterogeneous with respect to carbohydrate [17, 18], sulfate [19] and iodine [22, 23] composition, resulting in abnormal tertiary Tg molecular structures that may have altered immunoreactivity [31, 33, 41, 89, 117, 118]. Thus, because Tg epitopes are conformational [25, 26] abnormal Tgs may be detected by immunoassays differently [31, 89, 117, 118, 121]. IMA methods are especially sensitive to Tg molecular heterogeneity, because each method uses a different monoclonal antibody (MAb) pair to detect Tg in the serum sample, and in general MAbs have narrower epitope specificities for detecting abnormal Tgs than the polyclonal antibodies used for RIA methods [28, 29, 31, 80, 89, 118]. Tumor-related Tg heterogeneity is evident in Fig. 15.3a from the number of TgAb-negative patients with structural disease who displayed a greater than 30% difference in serum Tg when measured by ^{2G}IMA, LC-MS/MS and RIA [59]. These between-method biases contrast with the ~10% between-run precision (over 6–12 months) expected when using the same ^{2G}Tg-IMA consistently. The magnitude of between-method differences shown in Figs. 15.2 and 15.3 have the potential to disrupt serial Tg monitoring and negatively impact clinical management should the Tg method be changed without re-baselining the patient [41, 65, 84, 89]. Current guidelines recognize Tg between-method variability and recommend that the same Tg method (and preferably the same laboratory) be used for serial Tg monitoring of DTC patients [76]. Tg molecular heterogeneity may also impact the reliability of LC-MS/MS measurements, because tumors display a higher frequency of Tg polymorphisms than normal tissue [13, 39]. There can be a failure to generate the proteotypic Tg peptide necessary for LC-MS/MS detection either as a result of such Tg polymorphisms, or because post-translational modifications change the mass or charge of tryptic fragments [2, 8, 10, 13, 39]. Since TgAb interferes with different Tg methods to differing extents, an additional cause of between-method variability can be a failure to detect interfering TgAb (Fig. 15.4) [37, 122, 123].

Interferences with Tg Measurement

Only the physician can suspect interference with a test result and request that the laboratory perform interference checks! This is because the hallmark of interference is discordance between the test result and the clinical presentation of the patient—information not usually available to the laboratory. Failure to recognize interferences can have adverse clinical consequences [124–130]. Laboratory checks for interference include showing discordance between different manufacturers methods [131–134], re-measurement of analyte after adding reagents to block heterophile antibody (HAb) interferences [93, 134–137], performing linearity studies or precipitating immunoglobulins with polyethylene glycol (PEG) [119, 125, 131, 132, 134, 135, 138, 139]. A change in analyte concentration in response to one of these maneuvers suggests interference, but a lack of effect does not rule out interference. Interferences with Tg measurements can be classified as either non-specific or Tg-specific [140, 141].

Non-Specific Interferences

Heterophile Antibodies (HAb)

HAbs, including Human Anti-Mouse Antibodies (HAMA) and Rheumatoid Factor (RF), are human poly-specific antibodies that target animal antigens [134, 141–143] and interfere with a broad range of tests that use non-competitive IMA methodology [131, 139, 141, 144–148]. HAbs have the potential to interfere with both Tg-IMAs [70, 93, 136, 148–153] and TgAb-IMAs [154]. Typically, HAb interference causes a falsely high Tg-IMA and/or TgAb-IMA, less commonly falsely low Tg-IMA values have been reported [151]. HAbs do not affect either RIA [93, 155] or Tg-LC-MS/MS methodologies

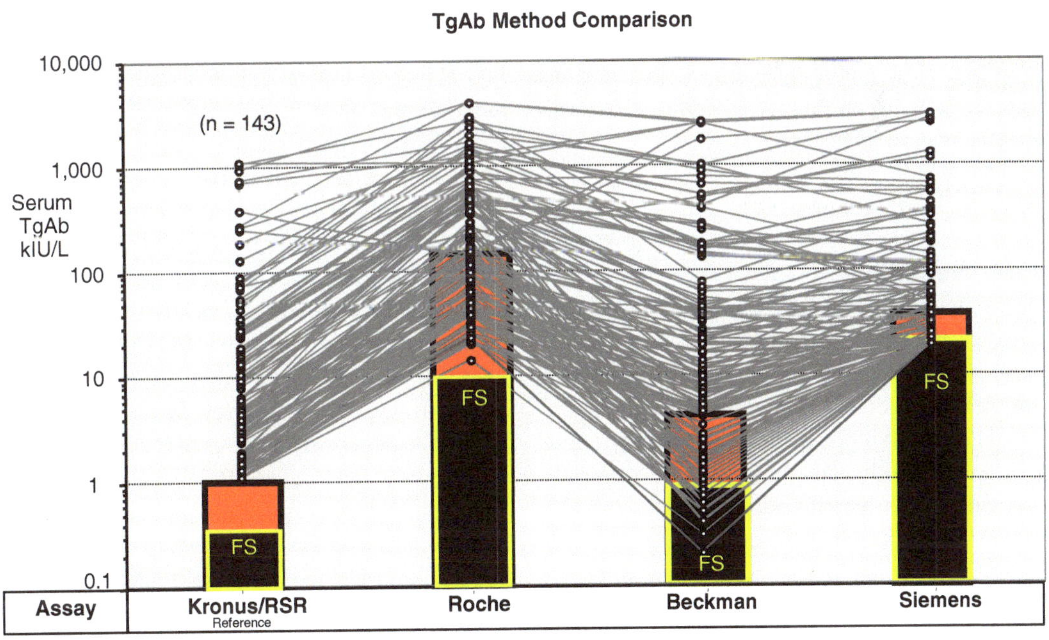

Fig. 15.4 Comparison of 143 DTC sera measured by four TgAb different methods—Kronus/RSR radioassay (reference method) versus Roche, Beckman and Siemens automated IMA tests. Red bars show the manufacturer recommended cutoffs (MCO) for TgAb-positivity of each method. Black bars denote the functional sensitivity limit of each method. All sera had TgAb above the MCO of the reference method and evidence of TgAb interference (a low ^{2G}Tg-IMA/Tg-RIA ratio). Data taken from [123]

[153]. Despite an overall HAb prevalence averaging 30–40% [155–157] manufacturers have reduced HAb interference to less than 1% by adding immunoglobulin blocker reagents to their IMA tests [93, 138, 146, 152]. However, the affinity and specificity of HAbs varies among patients and severe interference may be seen when using one manufacturer's test whereas a different manufacturer's test appears unaffected when measuring the same serum specimen. This is why the first step for investigating interference is re-measurement of the specimen with a different manufacturers method. It should be noted that patients receiving recent vaccines, blood transfusions or monoclonal antibodies (for treatment or scintigraphy), as well as veterinarians and those coming into contact with animals, are especially prone to interferences caused by induced HAbs [138, 158].

Reagent Interferences

Interference can result from antibodies targeting assay reagents. In the case of assays employing Streptavidin or Biotin methodology there can be interference from either Streptavidin [159] and/or Biotin antibodies [160]. Alternatively, exogenous high dose biotin ingestion can produce test interference in an analyte-specific, platform-specific manner [161–166].

Specific Interference

TgAb Interference

Approximately 25% of DTC patients have TgAb detected pre-operatively, or within 3 months of surgery [70, 123, 167–169]—a prevalence that is approximately double that of the general population [170]. TgAb prevalence is higher for papillary versus follicular tumors, and frequently associated with lymph node metastases [68, 70, 168, 171]. TgAb interference with Tg measurement remains the major problem limiting the clinical utility of Tg testing using any class of method. Either in-vitro mechanisms (epitope masking) [62, 89, 169, 172, 173] and/or in-vivo mechanisms (enhanced TgAb-mediated Tg clearance) could be responsible for these interferences [46, 49, 57, 58]. The propensity for TgAb interference differs between classes of Tg method (Table 15.1), as well as between methods from the same methodologic class. This in part reflects qualitative differences in the TgAb epitope specificities expressed by normal individuals versus patients with DTC, either associated with or without thyroid autoimmunity [171, 174–176]. It is clear that these patient-specific differences in TgAb specificities are maintained despite changing TgAb concentrations (Fig. 15.5). These specificity differences impact methodologic sensitivity as well as the propensity for that patient's TgAb to interfere with a Tg measurement [70, 171, 177]. These patient-related specificity differences are why no threshold TgAb concentration can preclude TgAb interference [59, 62, 65, 76, 80, 89, 122, 123, 171], and why high TgAb concentrations do not necessarily interfere, whereas low TgAb may profoundly interfere with a Tg measurement [25, 59, 62, 70, 80, 122, 123, 173, 178–181].

TgAb Methods

Tg autoantibodies predominantly belong to the IgG class of immunoglobulins, are not complement fixing, and are generally conformational [25]. Two approaches have been used to assess whether there is TgAb in the specimen causing interference with the Tg measurement. The older "Tg recovery" approach, whereby Tg is measured before and after the addition of a known amount of Tg standard, has mostly been replaced by direct quantitative TgAb tests. Current guidelines [76] mandate that a quantitative TgAb measurement be made with every Tg test, and stress that the Tg recovery approach is not a reliable method for detecting interfering TgAb [89, 173, 176]. Quantitative TgAb methods are based on RIA or non-isotopic IMA principles [89, 123, 167, 171, 174, 182–186]. Unfortunately, TgAb tests are highly variable with respect to sensitivity, specificity and the numeric values they report, despite using the same International Reference Preparation (MRC 65/93) (Fig. 15.4). In fact, there can be a 100-fold difference between the TgAb concentrations reported by different meth-

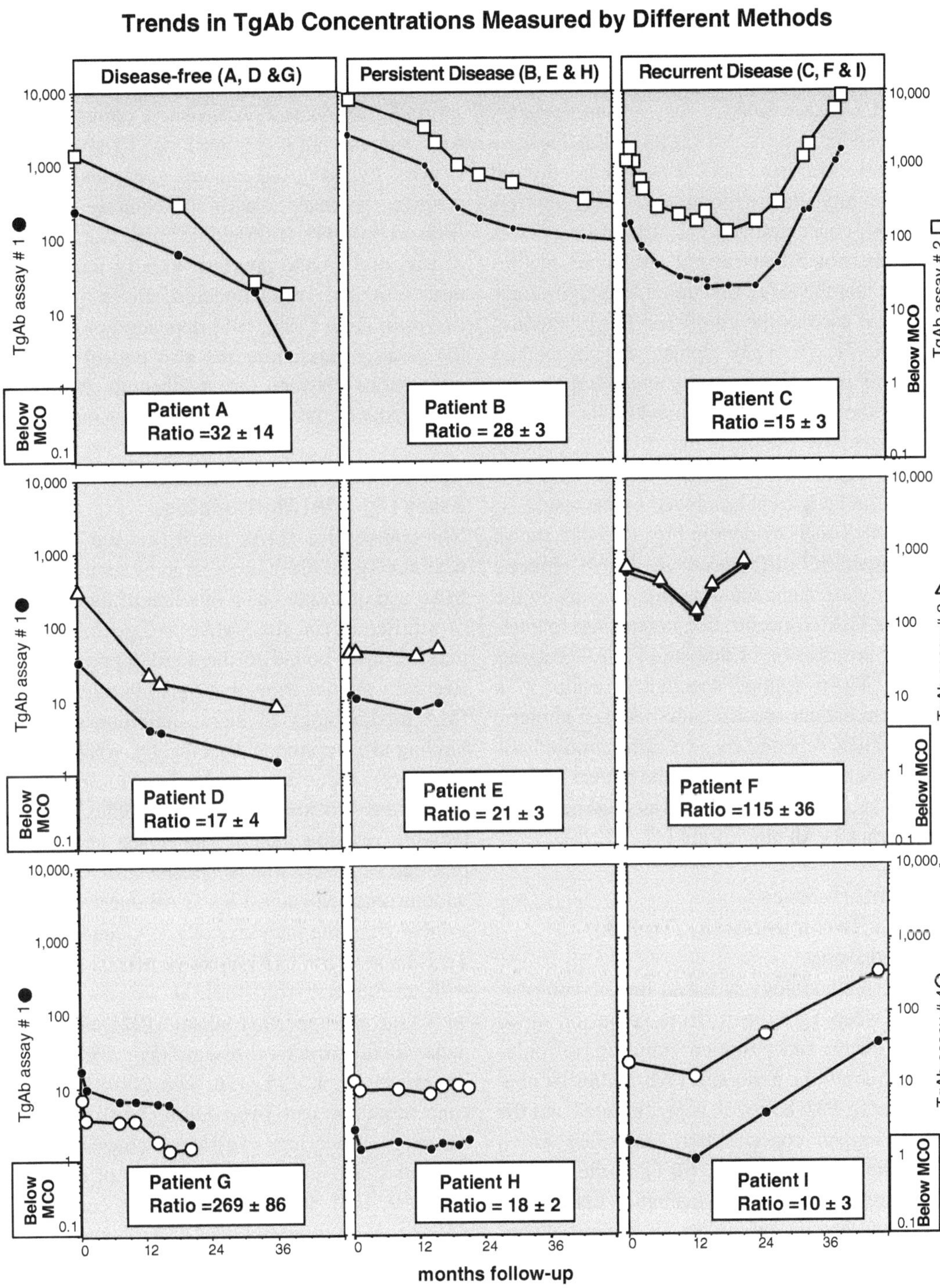

Fig. 15.5 Trends in serum TgAb measurements (ordinates) made for nine DTC patients (A–I) monitored over 1–4 year. Each specimen had TgAb measured by a reference assay (assay 1, Kronus/RSR, *solid circles*) and one of three test assays: (assay 2, Siemens Immulite, *open squares*) used for patients A–C; assay 3 (Beckman Access, *open triangles*) used for patients D–F; and (assay 4, Nichols Advantage, *open circles*) used for patients G–I. The *clear boxes* at the bottom of each patient's plot show the mean (±SD) of the ratios between test method TgAb values divided by the reference method values. Patients A, D, and G were judged disease-free after thyroidectomy (±RAI) and had a declining TgAb trend irrespective of the assay used. Patients B, E, and H had evidence of disease and maintained stable, detectable TgAb values. Patients C, F, and I had recurrences characterized by rising a TgAb trend. MCO = Manufacturer recommended cutoff for TgAb "positivity". The data were taken from [70, 212]

ods for the same serum (Figs. 15.4 and 15.5) [70, 123]. These differences decrease the reliability of TgAb detection [89, 123, 171, 183, 185–187], a problem exacerbated by manufacturer-recommended cutoffs (MCO) for TgAb "positivity" that are set for diagnosing thyroid autoimmunity and are too high to detect interfering TgAb concentrations [71, 123, 184–187]. It should be noted that current guidelines recommended that the assay functional sensitivity limit should be used as the cutoff for TgAb "positivity" [65, 71, 76, 123]. Some between-method variability relates to the purity and epitope specificity of the Tg reagent employed by the method, exacerbated by the fact that different patients produce TgAbs with different epitope specificities for the Tg reagent employed by the test [171, 176, 188]. This is evident in Fig. 15.5 that shows patient-specific differences in TgAb epitope specificity are maintained despite changes in the patient's TgAb concentration in response to treatment or progression of disease [42, 70]. Patient-specific TgAb epitope specificity results in a consistent patient-specific ratio between numeric TgAb values reported by two different methods that can be used to re-baseline the patient's TgAb trend should a change in TgAb method be necessary during TgAb monitoring [42, 70, 76].

TgAb Interference with Radioimmunoassay (Tg-RIA) Methodology

Tg-RIA methodology is based on the competition between Tg antigen (from serum or added ^{125}I-Tg tracer) and a low concentration of polyclonal (rabbit) Tg antibody (PAb). After incubation, the Tg-PAb complex is precipitated and the serum antigen concentration quantified as an inverse relationship to the ^{125}I-Tg in the precipitate. The use of a 48-h pre-incubation before adding a high specific activity ^{125}I-Tg tracer produces a maximal functional sensitivity of 0.5 μg/L for this class of method [189, 190]. The use of a high affinity PAb coupled with a species-specific second antibody can minimize the TgAb interference with the RIA method [191]. Resistance to TgAb interference is evidenced by appropriately normal Tg-RIA values for TgAb-positive euthyroid controls [89] and detectable Tg-RIA for TgAb-positive DTC patients with structural disease (Fig. 15.3b) [59]. This contrasts with IMA methods that report paradoxically undetectable serum Tg for some TgAb-positive normal euthyroid subjects [89] as well as TgAb-positive Graves' hyperthyroid patients [192] and TgAb-positive patients with structural disease (Fig. 15.3b) [89]. It should be noted that the propensity of TgAb to interfere with Tg-RIA determinations and cause underestimation [193] or overestimation [194, 195] depends not only on the assay formulation, but also patient-specific interactions between the endogenous serum Tg and TgAb and the exogenous RIA reagents [196].

TgAb Interference with Immunometric Assay (Tg-IMA) Methodology

Non-competitive IMAs use a two-site reaction whereby Tg in serum is captured by a solid-phase MAb and quantified as a function of the binding of a different (labeled) MAb to Tg from serum that becomes bound to the solid support [197]. Recovery studies show that TgAb interferes with IMA methodology by steric inhibition of MAb binding to Tg epitopes. Specifically, when the Tg epitope(s) necessary for binding to the IMA MAbs are blocked by TgAb complexing, the two-site reaction cannot take place and Tg is reported as falsely low or undetectable. Tg-IMA underestimation caused by TgAb interference is evident from the paradoxically low/undetectable Tg-IMA seen for TgAb-positive normal controls with an intact thyroid [89], as well as patients with Graves' hyperthyroidism [192] and DTC patients with structural disease (Fig. 15.3b) [25, 71, 80, 89, 123, 175, 176, 198–200]. High Tg concentrations can overwhelm TgAb binding capacity rendering Tg-IMA concentrations detectable and lessening the degree of interference [59, 123]. It follows that as Tg concentrations rise with progression of disease, more Tg is free, the influence of TgAb lessens and the discordance between Tg-IMA and Tg-RIA disappears (Fig. 15.6a) [59, 123]. Although some IMA methods claim to overcome TgAb interference by using MAbs directed against specific epitopes not involved in thyroid autoimmunity [201, 202], this approach has not proved effective in clinical practice, possibly because less restricted TgAb

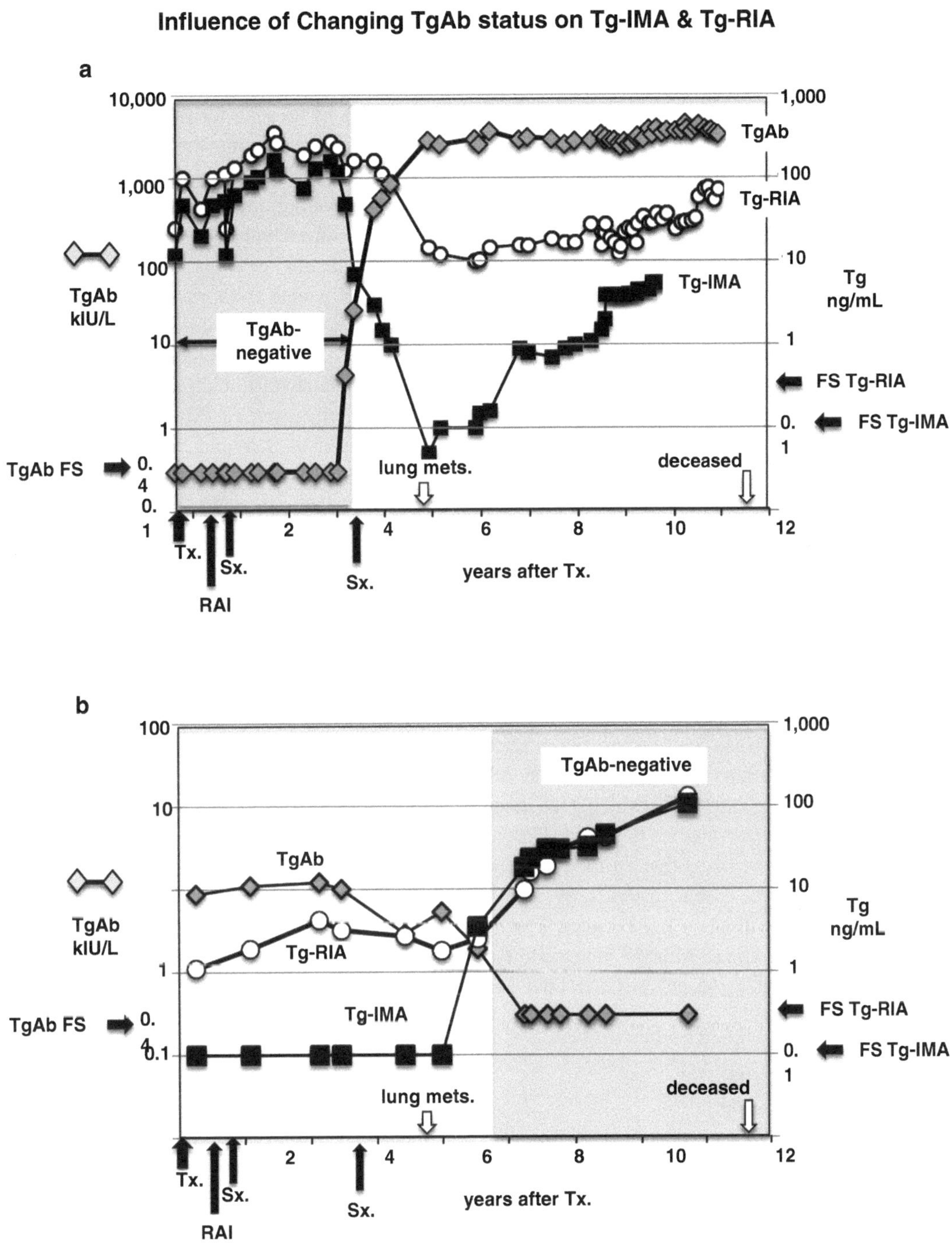

Fig. 15.6 Serial TgAb, Tg-RIA and Tg-IMA concentrations in two DTC patients with persistent/recurrent disease who underwent a change in TgAb status before death from disease-related complications. (**a**) A patient who converted from TgAb-negative to TgAb-positive. (**b**) A patient who converted from TgAb-positive to TgAb-negative

epitopes are more often associated with DTC than with autoimmune thyroid conditions [171, 175, 176, 199, 203].

TgAb Interference with Liquid Chromatography Tandem Mass Spectrometry (Tg-LC-MS/MS)

The new LC-MS/MS methods measure Tg as a Tg-specific peptide(s) generated after trypsinization of Tg-TgAb complexes in the serum specimen [39, 202, 204, 205]. Although LC-MS/MS methods currently only have first-generation functional sensitivity (FS ~0.5 μg/L) [37, 38, 114], they have the advantage of being free from HAb interferences [153]. Tg-LC-MS/MS methods were primarily developed to overcome TgAb interference and avoid falsely low/undetectable Tg-IMA results that can mask disease [37–39, 114, 204, 206, 207]. However, the diagnostic advantage of LC-MS/MS is currently questionable, given that a number of studies have now reported that over 40% of TgAb-positive patients with structural disease have paradoxically undetectable Tg-LC-MS/MS values [59, 114, 208, 209]. In fact, the most recent study concluded that Tg-LC-MS/MS offers no diagnostic advantage for detecting Tg in the presence of TgAb as compared with ^{2G}Tg-IMA [209], and confirmed another report that the higher the TgAb concentration the more likely that Tg-LC-MS/MS would be undetectable, despite disease [209, 210]. Note that an inverse relationship between TgAb concentration and Tg-LC-MS/MS detectability would be expected if TgAb enhanced in-vivo Tg clearance (see below).

In-Vitro Mechanisms for TgAb Interference

TgAb interferes with Tg measurements in a qualitative, quantitative and method-dependent manner [62, 70, 123, 172, 195, 196]. The potential for in-vitro interference is multifactorial and depends not only on the assay methodology (IMA, RIA or LC-MS/MS), but also the concentration and epitope specificity of the TgAb produced by the patient [70, 89, 180]. TgAb interference can be minimized using an RIA method that employs a PAb with broad epitope specificity to detect not only free Tg, but also Tg bound to TgAb where some epitopes may be masked by complexing. The selection of the PAb for maximal affinity for human Tg, and restricting the specificity of the second antibody reagent to precipitate selectively rabbit (not human) immunoglobulins, further minimizes TgAb interference [191]. In contrast, IMA methodology mainly detects the free Tg moiety—Tg molecules whose epitopes are not masked by TgAb complexing. Steric masking of Tg epitopes is the reason why TgAb interference with IMA methodology is always unidirectional (underestimation), and why a low Tg-IMA/Tg-RIA ratio has frequently been used to indicate TgAb interference [59, 120, 123, 167, 211, 212]. More studies are needed to determine why LC-MS/MS is undetectable in >40% of TgAb-positive patients with structural disease [59, 114, 208, 209]. Possibilities include tumor Tg polymorphisms that prevent the production of the Tg-specific tryptic peptide [2, 8, 13, 39], suboptimal trypsinization of Tg-TgAb complexes [35, 36], or Tg levels that are truly below detection because of TgAb-mediated increased clearance of Tg [46, 49, 57, 58].

In-Vivo Mechanisms for TgAb to Interference

Over past decades a number of studies have suggested that the presence of TgAb enhances Tg metabolic clearance. In 1967 Weigle et al showed increased clearance of endogenously ^{131I}-labeled Tg in rabbits after inducing TgAb by immunizing the animals with an immunogenic Tg preparation [57]. Human studies of the acute Tg and TgAb changes after sub-total thyroidectomy have also suggested that TgAb may increase Tg metabolic clearance [213]. TgAb-enhanced Tg clearance may result from TgAbs acting as "sweeper" antibodies to facilitate clearance of Tg antigen by the hepatic asialoglycoprotein receptor (ASGPR) [58, 167, 214–216]. Patients who undergo a permanent change in TgAb status (negative to positive or vice versa) that is discordant with their clinical disease status provide insights on the influence of TgAb on Tg-RIA and Tg-IMA measurements and possible effects of TgAb on Tg metabolic clearance. The patient shown in Fig. 15.6a had a de novo appearance of TgAb 2.5 years after thyroidectomy (Tx) + RAI treatment for PTC. The appearance of TgAb was associated with a steep fall in ^{2G}-Tg-IMA to undetectability, consistent with masking of Tg epitopes by TgAb complexing. There was also a slower decline in Tg-RIA to levels that remained detectable but at levels that were tenfold lower than before the TgAb appearance. Thereafter as disease progressed, TgAb remained elevated and Tg-IMA rose to parallel Tg-RIA, but at a concentration fivefold lower than for Tg-RIA. Since Tg-RIA measurements are considered less prone to TgAb interference than Tg-IMA, the declining Tg-RIA trend seen after the appearance of TgAb would be consistent with a TgAb-mediated increase in Tg metabolic clearance [59, 74, 123, 167, 217].

Tg Measurement: Clinical Utility

Over the past decade, the incidence of DTC has risen, partly because small thyroid nodules and micropapillary cancers [76, 218–220] are increasingly being detected by anatomic imaging for non-thyroidal purposes [221–224]. Most DTC patients are rendered disease-free by their initial surgery, however, ~15% experience recurrences and ~5% die from disease-related complications [202, 225–228]. In most cases, persistent/recurrent disease is detected within the first five post-operative years, although recurrences can occur decades after initial surgery necessitating life-long monitoring for recurrence [226, 227]. Current guidelines recommend a risk-stratified approach to diagnosis and treatment of DTC [76, 228–230]. Since most patients have a low pre-test probability for disease recurrence, protocols for follow-up need a high negative predictive value (NPV) to eliminate unnecessary testing, as well as a high positive predictive value (PPV) for identifying patients with persistent/recurrent disease. Biochemical testing (serum Tg+TgAb) used in conjunction with periodic ultrasound is now recognized as more sensitive for detecting disease than diagnostic ^{131}I whole body scanning [76, 230–235]. However, close physician-laboratory cooperation is necessary when interpreting Tg and TgAb measurements given the persistent technical limitations affecting these tests discussed above.

Most (~75%) DTC patients have no TgAb detected [167]. When TgAb is absent, four factors influence the interpretation of serum Tg concentrations: (1) the mass of thyroid tissue present (normal tissue + tumor); (2) The intrinsic ability of the tumor to secrete Tg; (3) the presence of any inflammation of or injury to thyroid tissue, secondary to FNAB, surgery, RAI therapy or thyroiditis; and (4) the degree of TSH receptor stimulation by TSH, hCG or TRAb [65]. TgAb interference with Tg measurement remains problematic, irrespective of the class of Tg method used (RIA, IMA or LC-MS/MS). When TgAb is present, serum Tg is a less reliable tumor marker test making the serum TgAb concentration the primary (surrogate) tumor-marker. For patients either with or without TgAb, it is the *trend* in Tg and TgAb concentrations (measured by the same methods) that has the more prognostic value than the use of fixed cutoff values to assess risk for disease [74, 76, 97, 111, 229, 233, 236–242].

Preoperative Serum Tg Measurement

Current guidelines do not recommend routine preoperative Tg testing [76, 95]. However, some believe that serum Tg measured preoperatively may indicate the tumor's intrinsic ability to secrete Tg, and thus impact the interpretation of post-operative Tg changes [243, 244]. Approximately 50% of DTC patients have an elevated preoperative serum Tg—highest with Follicular > Hurthle > Papillary tumors [55, 56]. When small tumors give rise to an elevated preoperative Tg, that tumor may be an efficient Tg secretor. In other cases the relationship between serum Tg and tumor mass suggests that the tumor, especially BRAF-positive tumors, may be a poor Tg secretor [56, 245]. When a tumor is known to be an inefficient Tg secretor, the clinical sensitivity of post-operative Tg monitoring may be decreased, necessitating an enhanced role for anatomic imaging [245, 246].

Serum Tg: First Post-Operative Year

The half-life of Tg in the circulation approximates 3 days [47, 48], such that the acute Tg release resulting from surgical injury and healing of tissue margins should largely resolve within the first six months, provided that thyroid hormone is initiated to prevent TSH stimulation [247]. However, when surgery is followed by RAI treatment there may be a slow Tg decline over subsequent years, presumably reflecting long-term radiolytic destruction of remnant tissue [248, 249]. A serum Tg measurement made as early as 6–8 weeks after thyroidectomy has been shown to have prognostic value, with the higher the serum Tg the greater the risk of persistent/recurrent disease [98, 241, 250–259]. After thyroidectomy, approximately one-gram of normal remnant tissue typically remains [202, 260]. This small thyroid remnant would be expected to produce a serum Tg approximating 1.0 μg/L, provided that TSH is not elevated [65]. Indeed, most disease-free PTC patients have ^{2G}Tg-IMA measurements below 0.5 μg/L (with TSH below 0.5 mIU/L). In the absence of disease the low Tg concentration arising from the normal remnant remains remarkably stable during long-term monitoring (Fig. 15.7) [74, 261, 262]. This is in accord with studies reporting that a serum Tg below 1.0 μg/L, 6 weeks after thyroidectomy has a 98% NPV (PPV 43%) [241]. When L-T4 therapy maintains a stable TSH, a rising trend in ^{2G}Tg-IMA concentrations that

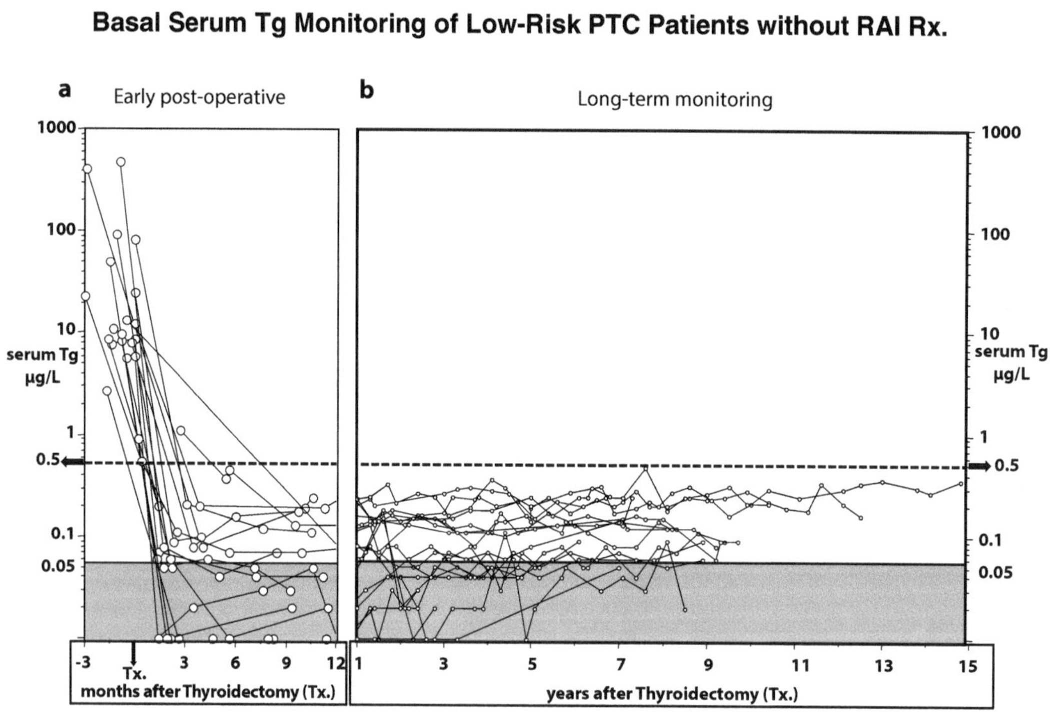

Fig. 15.7 Shows serum basal Tg^{2G}IMA measurements [Beckman Access analyses of frozen archived specimens {Spencer C, 2013 #8892}] made for 18 TgAb-negative PTC patients treated by thyroidectomy alone (no RAI treatment), maintained on long-term TSH suppression (<0.5 mIU/L), without evidence of recurrence at the end of >5 years of follow-up. (**a**) Shows that during the early post-operative phase, all patients achieved a basal serum Tg below 0.5 μg/L by 6–12 months after thyroidectomy (Tx). (**b**) Shows the stability of Tg secretion from normal remnant tissue when TSH is held constant. Data is taken from [74]

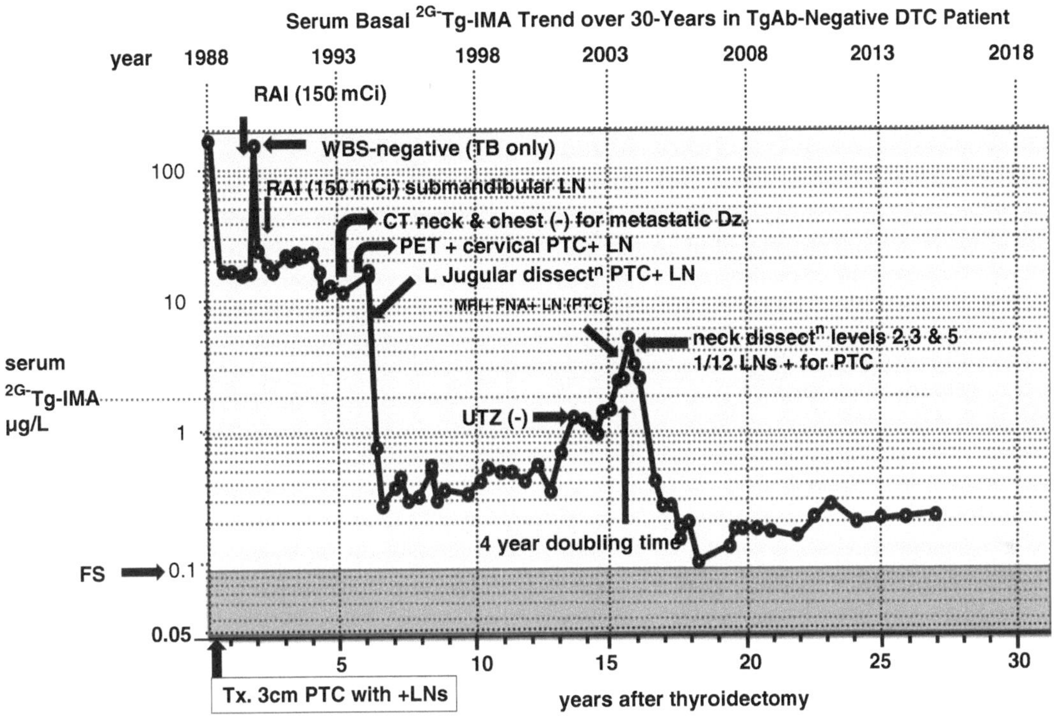

Fig. 15.8 A 30-year history of the basal Tg^{2G}IMA trend (TSH <0.5 mIU/L) in a TgAb-negative patient treated for persistent/recurrent PTC. (The data was established using frozen archived specimens). Data taken from [74]

results in a doubling of serum Tg suggests recurrent disease (Fig. 15.8). Serum Tg can still be used as a tumor marker following lobectomy provided that a mass-adjusted reference range is employed. For example, the population reference range for TgAb-negative euthyroid subjects with an intact thyroid gland is broad, approximating 3–40 µg/L [34, 41, 65, 263, 264], whereas intra-individual serum Tg variability is relatively narrow (CV ~15%) [116, 117]. It follows that after a lobectomy, a mass-adjusted reference range of 1.5–20 µg/L would be appropriate, provided TSH is not elevated, but should be lowered an additional 50% to 0.75–10 µg/L should TSH be suppressed [65, 247].

TSH-Stimulated Tg Measurements

When TSH is elevated, the degree of Tg stimulation depends on the chronicity of stimulation, with ~20-fold rise in Tg resulting from the endogenous TSH stimulation seen after thyroid hormone withdrawal, and ~tenfold Tg rise typically seen 5-days after short-term rhTSH stimulation [91, 94, 96, 265, 266]. Before sensitive ^{2G}Tg-IMA methods became available, the rhTSH-stimulation test was adopted as a standardized approach for boosting the Tg level into the detectable range of the insensitive first-generation tests [91–96]. Specifically, a 72-h rhTSH-stimulated Tg value below an arbitrary cutoff of 2.0 µg/L was adopted as a "negative" rhTSH test and shown to have a high NPV [91, 94, 98, 233, 237, 238, 240, 241, 256, 266–269]. Recombinant human TSH testing had a number of limitations. First, a negative test did not guarantee the absence of tumor [91, 266, 267] and the biases between different Tg methods (Figs. 15.2 and 15.3) made the use of the fixed numeric cut-off value of 2.0 µg/L problematic [41, 89]. Furthermore, the rhTSH dose delivered from the injection site was influenced by absorption, surface area and age of the patient [270–273]. The TSH sensitivity of tumor tissue was also a factor, with poorly differentiated tumors having blunted Tg responses to TSH [245, 246, 274, 275]. Because there is a strong correlation between the basal and rhTSH-stimulated Tg values [93, 106] it is not surprising that an undetectable (<0.10 μg/L) basal ^{2G}Tg-IMA has comparable NPV to a negative rhTSH test (<2.0 μg/L) [41, 93, 97, 101–103, 106, 108, 276, 277]. It follows that rhTSH-stimulated Tg testing provides little additional information above that of basal Tg measured by a ^{2G}Tg-IMA method [41, 76, 93, 101–103, 106, 108, 276]. Although a ^{2G}Tg-IMA below 0.1 μg/L predicts the absence of disease with a high degree of confidence [76, 93, 107, 108, 263], periodic cervical ultrasound is still recommended [76], because some lymph nodes metastases have inefficient Tg secretion associated with an undetectable ^{2G}Tg-IMA [101, 266, 269, 278, 279]. It should be noted that rhTSH stimulation testing can be useful when investigating interferences in patients who appear disease-free yet have paradoxically high basal ^{2G}Tg-IMA that appears clinically inappropriate [93]. Interference (usually from HAb/HAMA) is the most likely cause for an absent or blunted rhTSH-stimulated Tg response in a patient with a detectable basal ^{2G}Tg-IMA [93, 106, 152]. Alternatively, it should be noted that a blunted or absent rhTSH response is sometimes seen in the presence of TgAb, as would be expected if TgAb enhanced the clearance of Tg-TgAb complexes, as discussed above [57, 58, 192, 213].

TgAb-Negative Patients: Long-Term Follow-up of Basal Tg Trends

The higher the post-operative Tg the greater the risk for persistent/recurrent disease [98, 241, 251–258]. Now that ^{2G}Tg-IMA measurement has become the standard of care, subnormal basal (non-TSH stimulated) Tg can be monitored during L-T4 therapy without rhTSH stimulation [41, 76, 93, 101–103, 106, 108, 276]. The *trend* in basal Tg is now recognized as a better prognostic indicator than using a fixed Tg cutoff value or Tg "detectability" to determine disease risk [74, 76, 97, 111, 229, 233, 236–242], especially since Tg "detectability" is merely determined by assay functional sensitivity [41, 100, 101, 106, 262]. Thus, under non-elevated (≤0.5 mIU/L) TSH conditions [74, 262], the serum Tg trend reflects changes in tumor mass, with a declining Tg trend suggesting absence or regression of disease (Fig. 15.7) and a rising Tg trend being suspicious for tumor recurrence (Fig. 15.8) [74, 76, 84, 90, 97, 229, 233, 240, 248, 249, 280]. As with other tumor-markers such as calcitonin, the Tg doubling time, measured under stable, non-elevated TSH conditions, is now recognized as a prognostic marker for mortality [242, 261, 280–286]. However, between-method variability (Figs. 15.2 and 15.3) necessitates that the serum Tg trend be measured using the same method, and preferably the same laboratory [76]. One approach used to mitigate between-run imprecision and improve the reliability of assessing Tg trends has been to measure the current specimen concurrently (in the same run) with an archived specimen from that patient. Concurrent serum Tg measurement eliminates run-to-run variability and increases confidence for detecting small Tg changes [80, 82]. Figure 15.8 shows a 30-year history of serial Tg^{2G}IMA measurements made for a TgAb-negative PTC patient (T2N1M0) who had persistent/recurrent disease and in whom the post-operative serum Tg^{2G}IMA trend was monitored (during TSH suppression) using frozen archived specimens [42]. This case illustrates a number of points: (1) the high preoperative Tg (154 μg/L) suggested that serum Tg would be a sensitive post-operative tumor-marker; (2) the Tg stimulation in response to thyroid hormone withdrawal prior to the first RAI treatment suggested that the tumor was responsive to TSH and supported the efficacy for TSH suppression; (3) surgery was clearly a more effective treatment for metastatic PTC lymph nodes than RAI treatments; (4) combined imaging modalities were needed to detect disease; (5) persistent disease remained quiescent for many years during TSH suppression before an active recurrence manifested; (6) a rising trend in basal Tg^{2G}IMA (non-elevated TSH) suggested an increase in tumor mass [74, 262]; (7) the doubling of basal Tg^{2G}IMA during TSH suppression approximated 4-years—an interval indicating a good, long-term prognosis [242], and (8) the continued detection of serum Tg above the assay functional sensitivity limit 30 years after initial treatment and despite elimination of thyroid rem-

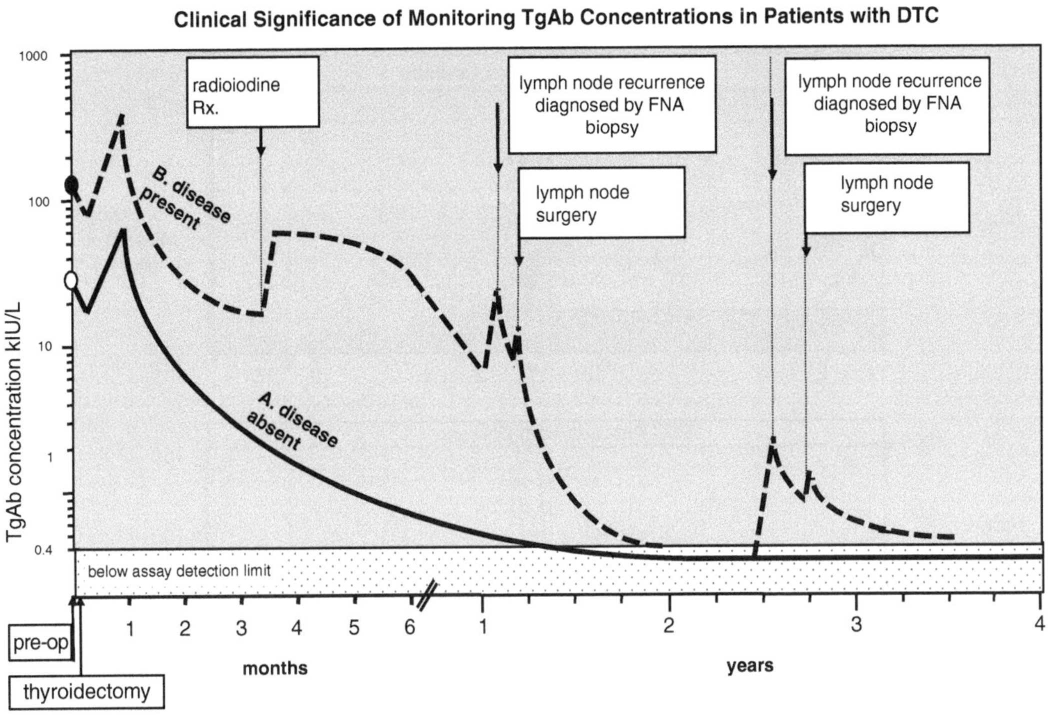

Fig. 15.9 Schematic representing changes in TgAb trends following thyroidectomy in patients rendered disease-free by surgery (pattern A) versus patients with persistent/recurrent disease (pattern B). TgAb concentrations may rise or become detectable de novo in response to an increase in Tg antigen following surgical injury, lymph node recurrence(s), lymph node resection(s) FNA biopsy of metastatic lymph nodes, or RAI treatment. Data taken from [70]

nant by two doses of RAI, suggests that disease may persist, warranting continued monitoring.

TgAb-Positive Patients: Monitor TgAb Trends as a Surrogate Tumor-Marker

The trend in serum TgAb concentrations can be used as a surrogate tumor-marker for TgAb-positive DTC patients, in whom Tg measurement may be unreliable (Figs. 15.9 and 15.10) [25, 60–76]. Because TgAb tests differ in sensitivity and specificity (Figs. 15.4 and 15.5), it is essential that the trend in TgAb concentrations be measured using the same manufacturers method and preferably the same laboratory [62, 71, 76, 80, 89, 123, 184–187, 314–317]. Studies have shown that after initial treatment (Tx ± RAI), serum TgAb progressively falls over time (months/years) when patients are disease-free. This is consistent with a decline in Tg antigen stimulation of the immune system [60, 61, 64, 67, 68, 70, 74, 76, 169, 318, 319]. The time needed for TgAb to become undetectable or fall below 10% of the initial value is related to the initial TgAb concentration, measured before or early in the post-operative period (Fig. 15.10a, b) [74]. Those patients exhibiting a TgAb decline of more than 50% by the end of the first post-operative year have been shown to have a low recurrence risk [42, 68, 75, 320, 321]. Approximately 3% of patients lose TgAb-positivity and yet still have persistent disease (Fig. 15.6b). Whereas most patients who undergo TgAb-positive to TgAb-negative conversions are disease-free and have low/undetectable Tg concentrations (<1.0 μg/L), those patients who lose TgAb-positivity despite disease typically have a detectable or rising serum Tg (Fig. 15.6b). The patient shown in Fig. 15.6b was TgAb-positive at the time of initial treatment at which time Tg-RIA was detectable and ^{2G}-Tg-IMA was undetectable. Despite extensive disease, TgAb became undetectable five years after initial treatment. The change in

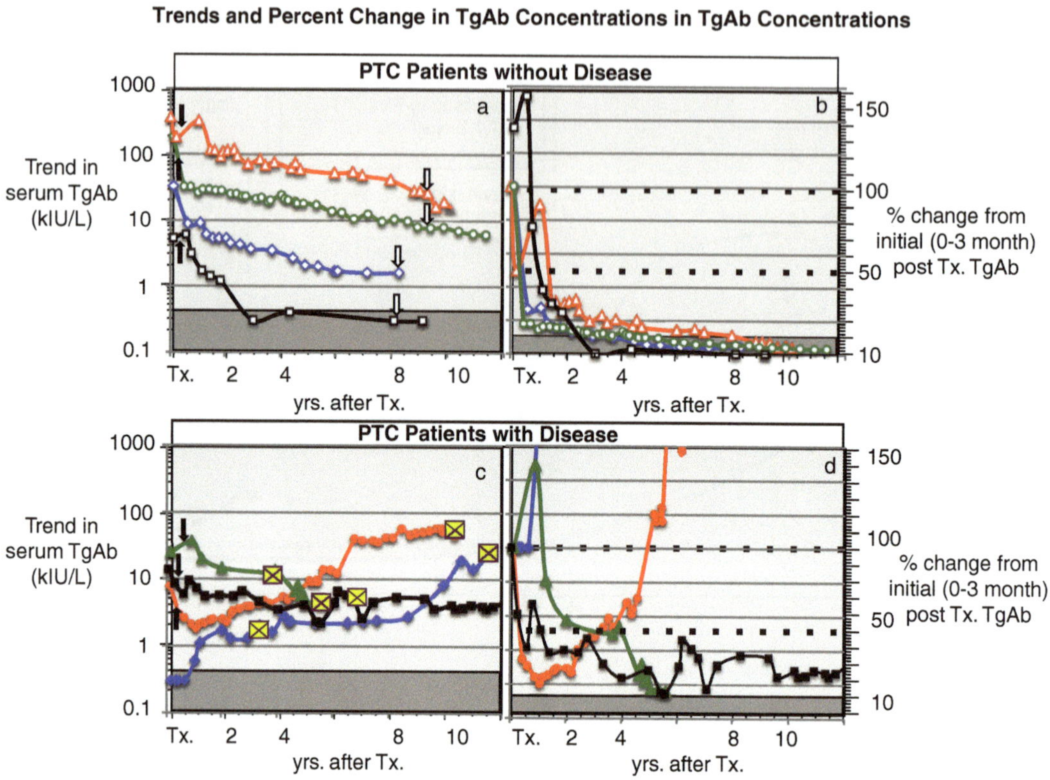

Fig. 15.10 Serial TgAb concentrations measured by the Kronus/RSR method showing how the TgAb trend (**a**, **c**) and the % change in TgAb concentrations from the initial (0–3 month) TgAb concentration (**b**, **d**) can be used as a surrogate tumor-marker. (**a**) Shows 4 PTC patients who were judged disease-free by ultrasound (open arrows). TgAb values progressively declined over time (years) to <10% of initial level. (**b**) Shows tht the higher the initial TgAb the longer it took for TgAb to fall below 10%. (**c**, **d**) Show comparative TgAb data for 4 PTC patients with persistent/recurrent disease detected during follow-up (indicated by crosses). A de novo TgAb appearance, a TgAb rise or a stable TgAb concentration that fails to fall below 10% of initial value were indicators of active disease. Data taken from [74]

TgAb status was associated with a rapid rise in Tg-IMA to parallel a steep increase in Tg-RIA with a doubling time of less than one year before death from disease-related complications [242, 261, 280–286]. This TgAb loss could reflect RAI destruction of the source (thyroid remnant tissue) of more antigenic, normally iodinated Tg, while the tumor was secreting poorly iodinated Tg molecules that were less antigenic [33] and did not stimulate the immune system. Most patients with persistent/recurrent disease exhibit only a marginal TgAb decline, or have a stable or rising TgAb that rarely falls below 10% of the initial value (Fig. 15.10c, d) [60–63, 68, 73–75, 80, 89, 123, 169, 185–187, 212, 322]. However, it should be noted that some patients maintain a low, stable TgAb concentration for many years without evidence of disease. This could reflect immune system sensitivity to Tg secreted by a small thyroid remnant or long-lived memory of plasma cells [323]. Approximately 10% of TgAb-negative patients convert to TgAb-positivity at some time in their course, emphasizing the need to measure TgAb with every Tg test [71, 76]. Because the immune system is sensitive to the Tg antigen concentration, there can be a *transient* rise or de novo appearance of TgAb in response to the acute release of Tg following thyroid surgery [324, 325], FNAB [326, 327] or more chronically (months) the radiolytic damage following RAI treatment [42, 70, 168, 247, 328–331]. However, the appearance of *permanent* TgAb-positivity after the first post-operative year typically indicates metastatic disease, as illustrated by the patient shown in Fig. 15.6a [68, 70, 167]. This appearance of permanent TgAb positivity likely reflects a change in in the heterogeneity of tumor-derived Tg (secretion of a more immunogenic Tg molecule), or a delayed recognition of tumor Tg by the immune system.

Tg Measurement in FNA Needle Washouts (FNA-Tg)

Because Tg protein is tissue-specific, the detection of Tg in non-thyroidal tissues or fluids (such as pleural fluid) indicates the presence of metastatic thyroid cancer [287]. Struma ovarii is the only (rare) condition in which the Tg in the circulation does not originate from the thyroid [288, 289]. A high concentration of Tg or parathyroid hormone (PTH) measured in the cyst fluid provides a reliable indicator of the tissue origin of a cyst (thyroid versus parathyroid, respectively), information that is critical for surgical decision-making [287, 290]. Although ultrasound characteristics are helpful for distinguishing benign reactive lymph nodes from those suspicious for malignancy, the finding of Tg in the needle washout of a lymph node biopsy has higher diagnostic accuracy than the ultrasound appearance [291–305]. The current protocol for obtaining FNA-Tg samples recommends rinsing the biopsy needle in 1.0 mL of saline and sending this specimen to the laboratory for Tg analysis. A common cutoff value used for a "positive" FNA-Tg in a thyroidectomized patient is 1.0 μg/L [295, 302, 306, 307], although this cutoff can vary by assay and institution [301, 308]. When investigating suspicious lymph nodes in patients with an intact thyroid, a higher FNA-Tg cutoff value (~35–40 μg/L) is recommended [292, 297, 307]. Although there is controversy whether TgAb interferes with FNA-Tg analyses [293, 309, 310], in a patient with a very high serum TgAb concentration there can be serum contamination of the FNA washout that may cause a falsely low/undetectable FNA-Tg due to TgAb interference when measured by an IMA method. This would occur if the expected serum dilution (~40-fold) in the wash fluid were insufficient to lower TgAb in the washout below detection. Note, the FNA needle washout procedure can also be used to detect calcitonin in neck masses of patients with primary and metastatic medullary thyroid cancer [290, 311–313], and FNA-PTH determinations may be useful for identifying parathyroid tissue [290].

Summary: Key Points

1. The tissue-specific (thyroid) origin of Tg in the circulation is why serum Tg measurement is the primary biochemical tumor-marker test for monitoring patients with DTC.
2. The biosynthetic processes necessary to make a mature 660 kDa Tg molecule are complex, and may become dysregulated in thyroid tumors leading to serum Tg heterogeneity.
3. Tg molecular abnormalities and polymorphisms may alter serum Tg detection by either immunoassay or LC-MS/MS methods, necessitating monitoring the serum Tg trend using the same method and preferably the same laboratory.
4. Second-generation Tg IMA methods (^{2G}Tg-IMA), characterized by an assay functional sensitivity ≤0.1 μg/L, have now become the standard of care, because ^{2G}Tg-IMA has sufficient FS to monitor the low basal serum Tg concentrations typically seen after thyroidectomy without the need for rhTSH stimulation.
5. Tg-IMA methodology is most prone to interference by the TgAb that is present in ~25% of DTC patients. TgAb causes falsely low/undetectable Tg-IMA values that can mask disease. In-vitro and/or in-vivo TgAb interferences with the RIA and/or LC-MS/MS classes of Tg method are also possible.
6. It is currently unclear why Tg-LC-MS/MS methods fail to detect Tg in >40% of TgAb-positive patients with structural disease. The problem could relate to tumor Tg polymorphisms, post-translational Tg modifications that change the mass or charge of tryptic fragments, or exceedingly low Tg concentrations secondary to TgAb-enhanced clearance of Tg-TgAb complexes.
7. Both serum Tg and TgAb trends should be monitored as DTC tumor-marker tests (maintaining the continuity of methods), because the TgAb status of the patient can change and may become discordant with disease status.

8. When TgAb is present and Tg measurement is unreliable, the trend in TgAb concentrations should be used as the primary tumor-marker and the trend in Tg concentrations becomes the secondary tumor-marker.

References

1. Baas FBH, Van Geurts KA, Melsert R, Pearson PL, de Vijlder JJM, Van Ommen GJB. The human thyroglobulin gene: a ploymorphic marker localized distal to c-myc on chromosome 8 band q 24. Hum Genet. 1985;69:138–43.
2. Matakidou A, Hamel N, Popat S, Henderson K, Kantemiroff T, Harmer C, et al. Risk of non-medullary thyroid cancer influenced by polymorphic variation in the thyroglobulin gene. Carcinogenesis. 2004;25(3):369–73.
3. Hishinuma A, Fukata S, Kakudo K, Murata Y, Ieiri T. High incidence of thyroid cancer in long-standing goiters with thyroglobulin mutations. Thyroid. 2005;15:1079–84.
4. Vono-Toniolo J, Rivolta CM, Targovnik HM, Medeiros-Neto G, Kopp P. Naturally occurring mutations in the thyroglobulin gene. Thyroid. 2005;15:1021–33.
5. Caputo M, Rivolta CM, Mories T, Corrales JJ, Galindo P, Gonzalez-Sarmiento R, et al. Analysis of thyroglobulin gene polymorphisms in patients with autoimmune thyroiditis. Endocrine. 2010;37(3):389–95.
6. Citterio CE, Machiavelli GA, Miras MB, Gruñeiro-Papendieck L, Lachlan K, Sobrero G, et al. New insights into thyroglobulin gene: molecular analysis of seven novel mutations associated with goiter and hypothyroidism. Mol Cell Endocrinol. 2013;365:277–91.
7. Rubio IG, Medeiros-Neto G. Mutations of the thyroglobulin gene and its relevance to thyroid disorders. Curr Opin Endocrinol Diabetes Obes. 2009;16:373–8.
8. Akdi A, Pérez G, Pastor S, Castell J, Biarnés J, Marcos R, et al. Common variants of the thyroglobulin gene are associated with differentiated thyroid cancer risk. Thyroid. 2011;21:519–25.
9. Siraj AK, Masoodi T, Bu R, Beg S, Al-Sobhi SS, Al-Dayel F, et al. Genomic profiling of thyroid cancer reveals a role for thyroglobulin in metastasis. Am J Hum Genet. 2016;98(6):1170–80.
10. van de Graaf SA, Ris-Stalpers C, Pauws E, Mendive FM, Targovnik HM, de Vijlder JJ. Up to date with human thyroglobulin. J Endocrinol. 2001;170:307–21.
11. De Felice M, Di Lauro R. Thyroid development and its disorders: genetics and molecular mechanisms. Endocr Rev. 2004;25:722–46.
12. Lin JD. Thyroglobulin and human thyroid cancer. Clin Chim Acta. 2008;388(1-2):15–21.
13. Xavier AC, Maciel RM, Vieira JG, Dias-da-Silva MR, Martins JR. Insights into the posttranslational structural heterogeneity of thyroglobulin and its role in the development, diagnosis, and management of benign and malignant thyroid diseases. Arch endocrinol metabol. 2016;60(1):66–75.
14. Arvan P, Kim PS, Kuliawat R, Prabakaran D, Muresan Z, Yoo SE, et al. Intracellular protein transport to the thyrocyte plasma membrane: potential implications for thyroid physiology. Thyroid. 1997;7:89–105.
15. Lee J, Di Jeso B, Arvan P. The cholinesterase-like domain of thyroglobulin functions as an intramolecular chaperone. J Clin Invest. 2008; 118:2950–8.
16. Di Jeso B, Ulianich L, Pacifico F, Leonardi A, Vito P, Consiglio E, et al. Folding of thyroglobulin in the calnexin/calreticulin pathway and its alteration by loss of Ca2+ from the endoplasmic reticulum. Biochem J. 2003;370:449–58.
17. Shimizu K, Nakamura K, Kobatake S, Satomura S, Maruyama M, Kameko F, et al. The clinical utility of Lens culinaris agglutinin-reactive thyroglobulin ratio in serum for distinguishing benign from malignant conditions of the thyroid. Clin Chim Acta. 2007;379:101–4.
18. Kanai T, Amakawa M, Kato R, Shimizu K, Nakamura K, Ito K, et al. Evaluation of a new method for the diagnosis of alterations of lens culinaris agglutinin binding of thyroglobulin molecules in thyroid carcinoma. Clin Chem Lab Med. 2009;47(10):1285–90.
19. Schneider AB, Dudlak D. Differential incorporation of sulfate into the chondroitin chain and complex carbohydrate chains of human thyroglobulin: studies in normal and neoplastic thyroid tissue. Endocrinology. 1989;124(1):356–62.
20. Magro G, Perissinotto D, Schiappacassi M, Goletz S, Otto A, Muller EC, et al. Proteomic and postproteomic characterization of keratan sulfate-glycanated isoforms of thyroglobulin and transferrin uniquely elaborated by papillary thyroid carcinomas. Am J Pathol. 2003;163:183–96.
21. Emoto N, Kunii YK, Ashizawa M, Oikawa S, Shimizu K, Shimonaka M, et al. Reduced sulfation of chondroitin sulfate in thyroglobulin derived from human papillary thyroid carcinomas. Cancer Sci. 2007;98:1577–81.
22. Schneider AB, Ikekubo K, Kuma K. Iodine content of serum thyroglobulin in normal individuals and patients with thyroid tumors. J Clin Endocrinol Metab. 1983;57:1251–6.
23. Saboori AM, Rose NR, Bresler HS, Vladut-Talor M, Burek CL. Iodination of human thyroglobulin (Tg) alters its immunoreactivity. 1. Iodination alters muliple epitopes of human Tg. Clin Exp Immunol. 1998;113:297–302.

24. Gerard AC, Daumerie C, Mestdagh C, Gohy S, De Burbure C, Costagliola S, et al. Correlation between the loss of thyroglobulin iodination and the expression of thyroid-specific proteins involved in iodine metabolism in thyroid carcinomas. J Clin Endocrinol Metab. 2003;88:4977–83.
25. McLachlan SM, Rapoport B. Why measure thyroglobulin autoantibodies rather than thyroid peroxidase autoantibodies. Thyroid. 2004;14:510–20.
26. Prentice L, Kiso Y, Fukuma N, Horimoto M, Petersen V, Grennan F, et al. Monoclonal thyroglobulin autoantibodies: variable region analysis and epitope recognition. J Clin Endocrinol Metab. 1995;80:977–86.
27. Kohno Y, Tarutani O, Sakata S, Nakajima H. Monoclonal antibodies to thyroglobulin elucidate differences in protein structure of thyroglobulin in healthy individuals and those with papillary adenocarcinoma. J Clin Endocrinol Metab. 1985;61:343–50.
28. de Micco C, Ruf J, Carayon P, Chrestian MA, Henry JF, Toga M. Immunohistochemical study of thyroglobulin in thyroid carcinomas with monoclonal antibodies. Cancer. 1987;59:471–6.
29. Kim PS, Dunn AD, Dunn JT. Altered immunoreactivity of thyroglobulin in thyroid disease. J Clin Endocrinol Metab. 1988;67:161–8.
30. Hufner M, Pfahl H, Bethauser H, Heilig B, Georgi P. Comparative plasma thyroglobulin measurements with three non-cross-reactive monoclonal antibodies in metastatic thyroid cancer patients. Acta Endocrinol. 1988;118:528–32.
31. Schulz R, Bethauser H, Stempka L, Heilig B, Moll A, Hufner M. Evidence for immunological differences between circulating and tissue-derived thyroglobulin in men. Eur J Clin Investig. 1989;19:459–63.
32. Saboori AM, Rose NR, Kuppers RC, Butscher WG, Bresler HS, Burek CL. Immunoreactivity of multiple molecular forms of human thyroglobulin. Clin Immunol Immunopathol. 1994;72(1):121–8.
33. Rose NR, Saboori AM, Rasooly L, Burek CL. The role of iodine in autoimmune thyroiditis. Crit Rev Immunol. 1997;17:511–7.
34. Spencer CA, Bergoglio LM, Kazarosyan M, Fatemi S, LoPresti JS. Clinical impact of thyroglobulin (Tg) and Tg autoantibody method differences on the management of patients with differentiated thyroid carcinomas. J Clin Endocrinol Metab. 2005;90(10):5566–75.
35. Saboori AM, Burek CL, Rose NR, Bresler HS, Talor M, Kuppers RC. Tryptic peptides of human thyroglobulin: I. Immunoreactivity with murine monoclonal antibodies. Clin Exp Immunol. 1994;98(3):454–8.
36. Saboori AM, Caturegli P, Rose NR, Mariotti S, Pinchera A, Burek CL. Tryptic peptides of human thyroglobulin: II. Immunoreactivity with sera from patients with thyroid diseases. Clin Exp Immunol. 1994;98(3):459–63.
37. Clarke NJ, Zhang Y, Reitz RE. A novel mass spectrometry-based assay for the accurate measurement of thyroglobulin from patient samples containing antithyroglobulin autoantibodies. J Investig Med. 2012;60(8):1157–63.
38. Kushnir MM, Rockwood AL, Roberts WL, Abraham D, Hoofnagle AN, Meikle AW. Measurement of thyroglobulin by liquid chromatography-tandem mass spectrometry in serum and plasma in the presence of antithyroglobulin autoantibodies. Clin Chem. 2013;59(6):982–90.
39. Hoofnagle AN, Roth MY. Clinical review: improving the measurement of serum thyroglobulin with mass spectrometry. J Clin Endocrinol Metab. 2013;98(4):1343–52.
40. Fenouillet E, Fayet G, Hovsepian S, Bahraoui EM, Ronin C. Immunochemical evidence for a role of complex carbohydrate chains in thyroglobulin antigenicity. J Biol Chem. 1986;261(32):15153–8.
41. Schlumberger M, Hitzel A, Toubert ME, Corone C, Troalen F, Schlageter MH, et al. Comparison of seven serum thyroglobulin assays in the follow-up of papillary and follicular thyroid cancer patients. J Clin Endocrinol Metab. 2007;92(7):2487–95.
42. Spencer C, Fatemi S. Thyroglobulin antibody (TgAb) methods - strengths, pitfalls and clinical utility for monitoring TgAb-positive patients with differentiated thyroid cancer. Best Pract Res Clin Endocrinol Metab. 2013;27:701–12.
43. Tatumi K, Suzuki Y, Sinohara H. Clearance of circulating desialylated thyroglobulins in the rat. Biochim Biophys Acta. 1979;583(4):504–11.
44. Brix K, Wirtz R, Herzog V. Paracrine interaction between hepatocytes and macrophages after extrathyroidal proteolysis of thyroglobulin. Hepatology. 1997;26:1232–40.
45. Whitley RJ, Ain KB. Thyroglobulin: a specific serum marker for the management of thyroid carcinoma. Clin Lab Med. 2004;24(1).29–47.
46. Sellitti DF, Suzuki K. Intrinsic regulation of thyroid function by thyroglobulin. Thyroid. 2014;24(4):625–38.
47. Feldt-Rasmussen U, Petersen PH, Nielsen H, Date J. Thyroglobulin of varying molecular sizes with different disappearence rates in plasma following subtotal thyroidectomy. Clin Endocrinol. 1978;9:205–14.
48. Hocevar M, Auersperg M, Stanovnik L. The dynamics of serum thyroglobulin elimination from the body after thyroid surgery. Eur J Surg Oncol. 1997;23:208–10.
49. Feldt-Rasmussen U. Serum thyroglobulin and thyroglobulin autoantibodies in thyroid disease. Allergy. 1983;38:369–87.
50. Jeevanram RK, Shah DH, Sharma SM, Ganatra RD. Disappearance rate of endogenously radioiodinated thyroglobulin and thyroxine after radioiodine treatment. Cancer. 1982;49:2281–4.
51. Ikekubo K, Pervos R, Schneider AB. Clearance of normal and tumor-related thyroglobulin from the circulation of rats: role of the terminal sialic acid residues. Metabolism. 1980;29:673–81.

52. Morell AG, Gregoriadis G, Scheinberg IH. The role of sialic acid in determining the survival of glycoproteins in the circulation. J Biol Chem. 1971;246:1461–7.
53. Sinadinovic J, Cvejic D, Savin S, Jancic-Zuguricas M, Micic JV. Altered terminal glycosylation of thyroglobulin in papillary thyroid carcinoma. Exp Clin Endocrinol. 1992;100:124–8.
54. Bastiani P, Papandreou J, Blanck O, Fenouillet E, Thibault V, Miquelis R. On the relationship between completion of N-acetllactosamine oligosaccharide units and iodine content of thyroglobulin; a reinvestigation. Endocrinology. 1995;136:4204–9.
55. Hocevar M, Auersperg M. Role of serum thyroglobulin in the pre-operative evaluation of follicular thyroid tumours. Eur J Surg Oncol. 1998;24:553–7.
56. Ericsson UB, Tegler L, Lennquist S, Christensen SB, Ståhl E, Thorell JI. Serum thyroglobulin in differentiated thyroid carcinoma. Acta Chir Scand. 1984;150:367–75.
57. Weigle WO, High GJ. The behaviour of autologous thyroglobulin in the circulation of rabbits immunized with either heterologous or altered homologous thyroglobulin. J Immunol. 1967;98:1105–14.
58. Igawa T, Haraya K, Hattori K. Sweeping antibody as a novel therapeutic antibody modality capable of eliminating soluble antigens from circulation. Immunol Rev. 2016;270(1):132–51.
59. Spencer C, Petrovic I, Fatemi S, LoPresti J. Serum thyroglobulin (Tg) monitoring of patients with differentiated thyroid cancer using sensitive (second-generation) immunometric assays can be disrupted by false-negative and false-positive serum thyroglobulin autoantibody misclassifications. J Clin Endocrinol Metab. 2014;99(12):4589–99.
60. Pacini F, Mariotti S, Formica N, Elisei R. Thyroid autoantibodies in thyroid cancer: incidence and relationship with tumor outcome. Acta Endocrinol. 1988;119:373–80.
61. Rubello D, Casara D, Girelli ME, Piccolo M, Busnardo B. Clinical meaning of circulating antithyroglobulin antibodies in differentiated thyroid cancer: a prospective study. J Nucl Med. 1992;33:1478–80.
62. Spencer CA, Takeuchi M, Kazarosyan M, Wang CC, Guttler RB, Singer PA, et al. Serum thyroglobulin autoantibodies: prevalence, influence on serum thyroglobulin measurement, and prognostic significance in patients with differentiated thyroid carcinoma. J Clin Endocrinol Metab. 1998;83(4):1121–7.
63. Chung JK, Park YJ, Kim TY, So Y, Kim SK, Park DJ, et al. Clinical significance of elevated level of serum antithyroglobulin antibody in patients with differentiated thyroid cancer after thyroid ablation. Clin Endocrinol. 2002;57:215–21.
64. Chiovato L, Latrofa F, Braverman LE, Pacini F, Capezzone M, Masserini L, et al. Disappearance of humoral thyroid autoimmunity after complete removal of thyroid antigens. Ann Intern Med. 2003;139:346–51.
65. Baloch Z, Carayon P, Conte-Devolx B, Demers LM, Feldt-Rasmussen U, Henry JF, et al. Laboratory medicine practice guidelines. Laboratory support for the diagnosis and monitoring of thyroid disease. Thyroid. 2003;13(1):3–126.
66. Küçük ON, Aras G, Kulak HA, Ibiş E. Clinical importance of anti-thyroglobulin auto-antibodies in patients with differentiated thyroid carcinoma: comparison with 99mTc-MIBI scans. Nucl Med Commun. 2006;27:873–6.
67. Thomas D, Liakos V, Vassiliou E, Hatzimarkou F, Tsatsoulis A, Kaldrimides P. Possible reasons for different pattern disappearance of thyroglobulin and thyroid peroxidase autoantibodies in patients with differentiated thyroid carcinoma following total thyroidectomy and iodine-131 ablation. J Endocrinol Investig. 2007;30:173–80.
68. Kim WG, Yoon JH, Kim WB, Kim TY, Kim EY, Kim JM, et al. Change of serum antithyroglobulin antibody levels is useful for prediction of clinical recurrence in thyroglobulin-negative patients with differentiated thyroid carcinoma. J Clin Endocrinol Metab. 2008;93(12):4683–9.
69. Feldt-Rasmussen U, Rasmussen AK. Autoimmunity in differentiated thyroid cancer: significance and related clinical problems. Hormones. 2010;9:109–17.
70. Spencer CA. Clinical utility of thyroglobulin antibody (TgAb) measurements for patients with differentiated thyroid cancers (DTC). J Clin Endocrinol Metab. 2011;96(12):3615–27.
71. Verburg FA, Luster M, Cupini C, Chiovato L, Duntas L, Elisei R, et al. Implications of thyroglobulin antibody positivity in patients with differentiated thyroid cancer: a clinical position statement. Thyroid. 2013;23(10):1211–25.
72. Hsieh CJ, Wang PW. Sequential changes of serum antithyroglobulin antibody levels are a good predictor of disease activity in thyroglobulin-negative patients with papillary thyroid carcinoma. Thyroid. 2014;24(3):488–93.
73. Feldt-Rasmussen U, Verburg FA, Luster M, Cupini C, Chiovato L, Duntas L, et al. Thyroglobulin autoantibodies as surrogate biomarkers in the management of patients with differentiated thyroid carcinoma. Curr Med Chem. 2014;21(32):3687–92.
74. Spencer C, LoPresti J, Fatemi S. How sensitive (second-generation) thyroglobulin measurement is changing paradigms for monitoring patients with differentiated thyroid cancer, in the absence or presence of thyroglobulin autoantibodies. Curr Opin Endocrinol Diabetes Obes. 2014;21(5):394–404.
75. Rosario PW, Carvalho M, Mourao GF, Calsolari MR. Comparison of antithyroglobulin antibody concentrations before and after ablation with 131I as a predictor of structural disease in differentiated thyroid carcinoma patients with undetectable basal thyroglobulin and negative neck ultrasonography. Thyroid. 2016;26(4):525–31.

76. Haugen BR, Alexander EK, Bible KC, Doherty GM, Mandel SJ, Nikiforov YE, et al. 2015 American thyroid association management guidelines for adult patients with thyroid nodules and differentiated thyroid cancer: the American thyroid association guidelines task force on thyroid nodules and differentiated thyroid cancer. Thyroid. 2016;26(1):1–133.
77. Giovanella L, Feldt-Rasmussen U, Verburg FA, Grebe SK, Plebani M, Clark PM. Thyroglobulin measurement by highly sensitive assays: focus on laboratory challenges. Clin Chem Lab Med. 2015;53(9):1301–14.
78. Rosario PW, Mourao GF, Calsolari MR. Low postoperative nonstimulated thyroglobulin as a criterion for the indication of low radioiodine activity in patients with papillary thyroid cancer of intermediate risk 'with higher risk features'. Clin Endocrinol. 2016;85(3):453–8.
79. Spencer CA, Wang CC. Thyroglobulin measurement. Techniques, clinical benefits, and pitfalls. Endocrinol Metab Clin N Am. 1995;24(4):841–63.
80. Spencer CA, Takeuchi M, Kazarosyan M. Current status and performance goals for serum thyroglobulin assays. Clin Chem. 1996;42:164–73.
81. Algeciras-Schimnich A, Bruns DE, Boyd JC, Bryant SC, La Fortune KA, Grebe SK. Failure of current laboratory protocols to detect lot-to-lot reagent differences: findings and possible solutions. Clin Chem. 2013;59:1187–94.
82. Spencer CA, Wang CC. Thyroglobulin measurement: techniques, clinical benefits and pitfalls. Endocrinol Metab Clin N Am. 1995;24:841–63.
83. Ross HA, Netea-Maier RT, Schakenraad E, Bravenboer B, Hermus AR, Sweep FC. Assay bias may invalidate decision limits and affect comparability of serum thyroglobulin assay methods: an approach to reduce interpretation differences. Clin Chim Acta. 2008;394:104–9.
84. Zucchelli G, Iervasi A, Ferdeghini M, Iervasi G. Serum thyroglobulin measurement in the follow-up of patients treated for differentiated thyroid cancer. Q J Nucl Med Mol Imaging. 2009;53:482–9.
85. Reix N, Massart C, Gasser F, Heurtault B, Agin A. Should functional sensitivity of a new thyroid stimulating hormone immunoassay be monitored routinely? The ADVIA Centaur TSH3-UL assay experience. Clin Biochem. 2012;45:1260–2.
86. Nicoloff JSC. Use and misuse of the sensitive thyrotropin assays. J Clin Endocrinol Metab. 1990;71:553–8.
87. Spencer CA, LoPresti JS, Patel A, Guttler RB, Eigen A, Shen D, et al. Applications of a new chemilunino-metric thyrotropin assay to subnormal measurement. J Clin Endocrinol Metab. 1990;70:453–60.
88. Van Herle AJ, Uller RP, Matthews NL, Brown J. Radioimmunoassay for measurement of thyroglobulin in human serum. J Clin Invest. 1973;52:1320–7.
89. Spencer CA, Bergoglio LM, Kazarosyan M, Fatemi S, Lopresti JS. Clinical impact of thyroglobulin (Tg) and Tg autoantibody method differences on the management of patients with differentiated thyroid carcinomas. J Clin Endocrinol Metab. 2005;90(10):5566–75.
90. Giovanella L, Clark P, Chiovato L, Duntas LH, Elisei R, Feldt-Rasmussen U, et al. Thyroglobulin measurement using highly sensitive assays in patients with differentiated thyroid cancer: a clinical position paper. Eur J Endocrinol. 2014;171:R33–46.
91. Haugen BR, Ladenson PW, Cooper DS, Pacini F, Reiners C, Luster M, et al. A comparison of recombinant human thyrotropin and thyroid hormone withdrawal for the detection of thyroid remnant or cancer. J Clin Endocrinol Metab. 1999;84:3877–85.
92. Pacini F, Castagna MG. Diagnostic and therapeutic use of recombinant human TSH (rhTSH) in differentiated thyroid cancer. Best Pract Res Clin Endocrinol Metab. 2008;22:1009–21.
93. Spencer CA, Fatemi S, Singer P, Nicoloff JT, LoPresti JS. Serum basal thyroglobulin measured by a 2nd generation assay correlates with the recombinant human TSH-Stimulated thyroglobulin response in patients treated for differentiated thyroid cancer. Thyroid. 2010;20:587–95.
94. Cooper DS, Doherty GM, Haugen BR, Kloos RT, Lee SL, Mandel SJ, et al. Management guidelines for patients with thyroid nodules and differentiated thyroid cancer. The American Thyroid Association Guidelines Taskforce. Thyroid. 2006;16:109–42.
95. Pacini F, Schlumberger M, Dralle H, Elisei R, Smit JW, Wiersinga W. European consensus for the management of patients with differentiated thyroid carcinoma of the follicular epithelium. Eur J Endocrinol. 2006;154:787–803.
96. Cooper DS, Doherty GM, Haugen BR, Kloos RT, Lee SL, Mandel SJ, et al. Revised American Thyroid Association management guidelines for patients with thyroid nodules and differentiated thyroid cancer. Thyroid. 2009;19:1167–24.
97. Zophel K, Wunderlich G, Smith BR. Serum thyroglobulin measurements with a high sensitivity enzyme-linked immunosorbent assay: is there a clinical benefit in patients with differentiated thyroid carcinoma? Thyroid. 2003;13:861–5.
98. Kloos RT, Mazzaferri EL. A single recombinant human thyrotropin-stimulated serum thyroglobulin measurement predicts differentiated thyroid carcinoma metastases three to five years later. J Clin Endocrinol Metab. 2005;90:5047–57.
99. Rosario PW, Borges MA, Fagundes TA, Franco AC, Purisch S. Is stimulation of thyroglobulin (Tg) useful in low-risk patients with thyroid carcinoma and undetectable Tg on thyroxin and negative neck ultrasound? Clin Endocrinol. 2005;62:121–5.
100. Iervasi A, Iervasi G, Carpi A, Zucchelli GC. Serum thyroglobulin measurement: clinical background and main methodological aspects with clinical impact. Biomed Pharmacother. 2006;60:414–24.
101. Iervasi A, Iervasi G, Ferdeghini M, Solimeo C, Bottoni A, Rossi L, et al. Clinical relevance of highly sensitive Tg assay in monitoring patients treated

for differentiated thyroid cancer. Clin Endocrinol. 2007;67(6):434–41.
102. Smallridge RC, Meek SE, Morgan MA, Gates GS, Fox TP, Grebe S, et al. Monitoring thyroglobulin in a sensitive immunoassay has comparable sensitivity to recombinant human TSH-stimulated thyroglobulin in follow-up of thyroid cancer patients. J Clin Endocrinol Metab. 2007;92:82–7.
103. Mazzaferri EL. Will highly sensitive thyroglobulin assays change the management of thyroid cancer? Clin Endocrinol. 2007;67:321–3.
104. Persoon AC, Jager PL, Sluiter WJ, Plukker JT, Wolffenbuttel BH, Links TP. A sensitive Tg assay or rhTSH stimulated Tg: what's the best in the long-term follow-up of patients with differentiated thyroid carcinoma. PLoS ONE. 2007;2:e816.
105. Giovanella L. Highly sensitive thyroglobulin measurements in differentiated thyroid carcinoma management. Clin Chem Lab Med. 2008;46(8):1067–73.
106. Spencer CA, Lopresti JS. Measuring thyroglobulin and thyroglobulin autoantibody in patients with differentiated thyroid cancer. Nat Clin Pract Endocrinol Metab. 2008;4:223–33.
107. Malandrino P, Latina A, Marescalco S, Spadaro A, Regalbuto C, Fulco RA, et al. Risk-adapted management of differentiated thyroid cancer assessed by a sensitive measurement of basal serum thyroglobulin. J Clin Endocrinol Metab. 2011;96:1703–9.
108. Chindris AM, Diehl NN, Crook JE, Fatourechi V, Smallridge RC. Undetectable sensitive serum thyroglobulin (<0.1 ng/ml) in 163 patients with follicular cell-derived thyroid cancer: results of rhTSH stimulation and neck ultrasonography and long-term biochemical and clinical follow-up. J Clin Endocrinol Metab. 2012;97(8):2714–23.
109. Trimboli P, La Torre D, Ceriani L, Condorelli E, Laurenti O, Romanelli F, et al. High sensitive thyroglobulin assay on thyroxine therapy: can it avoid stimulation test in low and high risk differentiated thyroid carcinoma patients? Horm Metab Res. 2013;45(9):664–8.
110. Giovanella L, Treglia G, Sadeghi R, Trimboli P, Ceriani L, Verburg FA. Unstimulated high-sensitive thyroglobulin in follow-up of differentiated thyroid cancer patients: a meta-analysis. J Clin Endocrinol Metab. 2014;99:440–7.
111. Giovanella L, Clark PM, Chiovato L, Duntas L, Elisei R, Feldt-Rasmussen U, et al. Thyroglobulin measurement using highly sensitive assays in patients with differentiated thyroid cancer: a clinical position paper. Eur J Endocrinol. 2014;171(2):R33–46.
112. Feldt-Rasmussen U, Profilis C, Colinet E, Black E, Bornet H, Bourdoux P, et al. Human thyroglobulin reference material (CRM 457) 1st part: assessment of homogeneity, stability and immunoreactivity. Ann Biol Clin. 1996;54:337–42.
113. Feldt-Rasmussen U, Profilis C, Colinet E, Black E, Bornet H, Bourdoux P, et al. Human thyroglobulin reference material (CRM 457) 2nd part: physico-chemical characterization and certification. Ann Biol Clin. 1996;54:343–8.
114. Netzel BC, Grebe SK, Carranza Leon BG, Castro MR, Clark PM, Hoofnagle AN, et al. Thyroglobulin (Tg) testing revisited: Tg Assays, TgAb assays, and correlation of results with clinical outcomes. J Clin Endocrinol Metab. 2015;100(8):E1074–83.
115. Kim M, Jeon MJ, Kim WG, Lee JJ, Ryu JS, Cho EJ, et al. Comparison of thyroglobulin measurements using three different immunoassay kits: a BRAMHS Tg-Plus RIA Kit, a BRAMHS hTg sensitive kryptor kit, and a Beckman Coulter ACCESS immunoassay kit. Endocrinol Metab. 2016;31:462–8.
116. Jensen E, Petersen PH, Blaabjerg O, Hegedüs L. Biological variation of thyroid autoantibodies and thyroglobulin. Clin Chem Lab Med. 2007;45:1058–64.
117. Feldt-Rasmussen U, Petersen PH, Blaabjerg O, Horder M. Long-term variability in serum thyroglobulin and thyroid related hormones in healthy subjects. Acta Endocrinol. 1980;95:328–34.
118. Heilig B, Hufner M, Dorken B, Schmidt-Gayk H. Increased heterogeneity of serum thyroglobulin in thyroid cancer patients as determined by monoclonal antibodies. Klin Wochenschr. 1986;64:776–80.
119. Ross HA, Menheere PP, Thomas CM, Mudde AH, Kouwenberg M, Wolffenbuttel BH. Interference from heterophilic antibodies in seven current TSH assays. Ann Clin Biochem. 2008;45:616–8.
120. Clark P, Franklyn J. Can we interpret serum thyroglobulin results? Ann Clin Biochem. 2012;49:313–22.
121. Fenouillet E, Fayet G, Hovsepian S, Bahraoui EM, Ronin C. Immunochemical evidence for a role of complex carbohydrate chains in thyroglobulin antigenicity. J Biol Chem. 1986;261:15153–8.
122. Cubero JM, Rodríguez-Espinosa J, Gelpi C, Estorch M, Corcoy R. Thyroglobulin autoantibody levels below the cut-off for positivity can interfere with thyroglobulin measurement. Thyroid. 2003;13:659–61.
123. Spencer C, Petrovic I, Fatemi S. Current thyroglobulin autoantibody (TgAb) assays often fail to detect interfering TgAb that can result in the reporting of falsely low/undetectable serum Tg IMA values for patients with differentiated thyroid cancer. J Clin Endocrinol Metab. 2011;96(5):1283–91.
124. Rotmensch S, Cole LA. False diagnosis and needless therapy of presumed malignant disease in women with false-positive human chorionic gonadotropin concentrations. Lancet. 2000;355:712–5.
125. Jones AM, Honour JW. Unusual results from immunoassays and the role of the clinical endocrinologist. Clin Endocrinol. 2006;64(3):234–44.
126. Ballieux BE, Weijl NI, Gelderblom H, van Pelt J, Osanto S. False-positive serum human chorionic gonadotropin (HCG) in a male patient with a malignant germ cell tumor of the testis: a case report and review of the literature. Oncologist. 2008;13(11):1149–54.

127. Henry N, Sebe P, Cussenot O. Inappropriate treatment of prostate cancer caused by heterophilic antibody interference. Nat Clin Pract Urol. 2009;6(3):164–7.
128. Georges A, Charrie A, Raynaud S, Lombard C, Corcuff JB. Thyroxin overdose due to rheumatoid factor interferences in thyroid-stimulating hormone assays. Clin Chem Lab Med. 2011;49(5):873–5.
129. Bjerner J, Bolstad N, Piehler A. Belief is only half the truth--or why screening for heterophilic antibody interference in certain assays makes double sense. Ann Clin Biochem. 2012;49(Pt 4):381–6.
130. Pishdad GR, Pishdad P, Pishdad R. The effect of glucocorticoid therapy on a falsely raised thyrotropin due to heterophilic antibodies. Thyroid. 2013;23(12):1657–8.
131. Marks V. False-positive immunoassay results: a multicenter survey of erroneous immunoassay results from assays of 74 analytes in 10 donors from 66 laboratories in seven countries. Clin Chem. 2002;48:2008–16.
132. Ellis MJ, Livesey JH. Techniques for identifying heterophile antibody interference are assay specific: study of seven analytes on two automated immunoassay analyzers. Clin Chem. 2005;51:639–41.
133. Lewandowski KC, Dabrowska K, Lewinski A. Case report: When measured free T4 and free T3 may be misleading. Interference with free thyroid hormones measurements on Roche(R) and Siemens(R) platforms. Thyroid Res. 2012;5(1):11.
134. Bolstad N, Warren DJ, Nustad K. Heterophilic antibody interference in immunometric assays. Best Pract Res Clin Endocrinol Metab. 2013;27(5):647–61.
135. Emerson JF, Ngo G, Emerson SS. Screening for interference in immunoassays. Clin Chem. 2003;49(7):1163–9.
136. Massart C, Corcuff JB, Bordenave L. False-positive results corrected by the use of heterophilic antibody-blocking reagent in thyroglobulin immunoassays. Clin Chim Acta. 2008;388:211–3.
137. Koshida S, Asanuma K, Kuribayashi K, Goto M, Tsuji N, Kobayashi D, et al. Prevalence of human anti-mouse antibodies (HAMAs) in routine examinations. Clin Chim Acta. 2010;411:391–4.
138. Ismail AA. On detecting interference from endogenous antibodies in immunoassays by doubling dilutions test. Clin Chem Lab Med. 2007;45(7):851–4.
139. Gulbahar O, Konca Degertekin C, Akturk M, Yalcin MM, Kalan I, Atikeler GF, et al. A case with immunoassay interferences in the measurement of multiple hormones. J Clin Endocrinol Metab. 2015;100(6):2147–53.
140. Klee GG. Interferences in hormone immunoassays. Clin Lab Med. 2004;24(1):1–18.
141. Sturgeon CM, Viljoen A. Analytical error and interference in immunoassay: minimizing risk. Ann Clin Biochem. 2011;48:418–32.
142. Kricka LJ. Human anti-animal antibody interference in immunological assays. Clin Chem. 1999;45:942–56.
143. Levinson SS, Miller JJ. Towards a better understanding of heterophile (and the like) antibody interference with modern immunoassays. Clin Chim Acta. 2002;325:1–15.
144. Covinsky M, Laterza O, Pfeifer JD, Farkas-Szallasi T, Scott MG. Lamda antibody to Esherichia coli produces false-positive results in multiple immunometric assays. Clin Chem. 2000;46:1157–61.
145. Bjerner J, Olsen KH, Bormer OP, Nustad K. Human heterophilic antibodies display specificity for murine IgG subclasses. Clin Biochem. 2005;38(5):465–72.
146. Preissner CM, Dodge LA, O'Kane DJ, Singh RJ, Grebe SK. Prevalence of heterophilic antibody interference in eight automated tumor marker immunoassays. Clin Chem. 2005;51:208–10.
147. Despres N, Grant AM. Antibody interference in thyroid assays: a potential for clinical misinformation. Clin Chem. 1998;44:440–54.
148. Astarita G, Gutierrez S, Kogovsek N, Mormandi E, Otero P, Calabrese C, et al. False positive in the measurement of thyroglobulin induced by rheumatoid factor. Clin Chim Acta. 2015;447:43–6.
149. Preissner CM, O'Kane DJ, Singh RJ, Morris JC, Grebe SK. Phantoms in the assay tube: heterophile antibody interferences in serum thyroglobulin assays. J Clin Endocrinol Metab. 2003;88(7):3069–74.
150. Giovanella L, Ghelfo A. Undetectable serum thyroglobulin due to negative interference of heterophile antibodies in relapsing thyroid carcinoma. Clin Chem. 2007;53:1871–2.
151. Giovanella L, Keller F, Ceriani L, Tozzoli R. Heterophile antibodies may falsely increase or decrease thyroglobulin measurement in patients with differentiated thyroid carcinoma. Clin Chem Lab Med. 2009;47:952–4.
152. Verburg FA, Wäschle K, Reiners C, Giovanella L, Lentjes EG. Heterophile antibodies rarely influence the measurement of thyroglobulin and thyroglobulin antibodies in differentiated thyroid cancer patients. Horm Metab Res. 2010;42:736–9.
153. Netzel BC, Grebe SK, Algeciras-Schimnich A. Usefulness of a thyroglobulin liquid chromatography-tandem mass spectrometry assay for evaluation of suspected heterophile interference. Clin Chem. 2014;60:1016–8.
154. Petrovic I, Mandel S, Fatemi S, LoPresti J, Spencer C. Heterophile antibodies (HAb/HAMA) interfere with automated TgAb IMA tests. Thyroid. 2016;26(S1):A120.
155. Weber TH, Käpyaho KI, Tanner P. Endogenous interference in immunoassays in clinical chemistry. A review. Scand J Clin Lab Invest. 1990;201:77–82.
156. Bjerner J, Nustad K, Norum LF, Olsen KH, Børmer OP. Immunometric assay interference: incidence and prevention. Clin Chem. 2002;48:613–21.
157. Ghosh S, Howlett M, Boag D, Malik I, Collier A. Interference in free thyroxine immunoassay. Eur J Intern Med. 2008;19:221–2.

158. Nakano K, Yasuda K, Shibuya H, Moriyama T, Kahata K, Shimizu C. Transient human anti-mouse antibody generated with immune enhancement in a carbohydrate antigen 19-9 immunoassay after surgical resection of recurrent cancer. Ann Clin Biochem. 2016;53(Pt 4):511–5.
159. Rulander NJ, Cardamone D, Senior M, Snyder PJ, Master SR. Interference from anti-streptavidin antibody. Arch Pathol Lab Med. 2013;137(8):1141–6.
160. Vos MJ, Rondeel JM, Mijnhout GS, Endert E. Immunoassay interference caused by heterophilic antibodies interacting with biotin. Clin Chem Lab Med. 2016;55:e122–6.
161. Kwok JS, Chan IH, Chan MH. Biotin interference on TSH and free thyroid hormone measurement. Pathology. 2012;44(3):278–80.
162. Wijeratne NG, Doery JC, Lu ZX. Positive and negative interference in immunoassays following biotin ingestion: a pharmacokinetic study. Pathology. 2012;44(7):674–5.
163. Elston MS, Sehgal S, Du Toit S, Yarndley T, Conaglen JV. Factitious Graves' disease due to biotin immunoassay interference-A case and review of the literature. J Clin Endocrinol Metab. 2016;101(9):3251–5.
164. Pedersen IB, Laurberg P. Biochemical hyperthyroidism in a newborn baby caused by assay interaction from biotin intake. Eur Thyroid J. 2016;5:212–5.
165. Barbesino G. Misdiagnosis of Graves' disease with apparent severe hyperthyroidism in a patient taking biotin megadoses. Thyroid. 2016;26(6):860–3.
166. Chun KY. Biotin interference in diagnostic tests. Clin Chem. 2017;63(2):619–20.
167. Spencer CA, Takeuchi M, Kazarosyan M, Wang CC, Guttler RB, Singer PA, et al. Serum thyroglobulin autoantibodies: prevalence, influence on serum thyroglobulin measurement and prognostic significance in patients with differentiated thyroid carcinoma. J Clin Endocrinol Metab. 1998;83:1121–7.
168. Kumar A, Shah DH, Shrihari U, Dandekar SR, Vijayan U, Sharma SM. Significance of antithyroglobulin autoantibodies in differentiated thyroid carcinoma. Thyroid. 1994;4:199–202.
169. Gorges R, Maniecki M, Jentzen W, Sheu SN, Mann K, Bockisch A, et al. Development and clinical impact of thyroglobulin antibodies in patients with differentiated thyroid carcinoma during the first 3 years after thyroidectomy. Eur J Endocrinol. 2005;153(1):49–55.
170. Hollowell JG, Staehling NW, Flanders WD, Hannon WH, Gunter EW, Spencer CA, et al. Serum TSH, T(4), and thyroid antibodies in the United States population (1988 to 1994): National Health and Nutrition Examination Survey (NHANES III). J Clin Endocrinol Metab. 2002;87(2):489–99.
171. Latrofa F, Ricci D, Montanelli L, Rocchi R, Piaggi P, Sisti E, et al. Thyroglobulin autoantibodies in patients with papillary thyroid carcinoma: comparison of different assays and evaluation of causes of discrepancies. J Clin Endocrinol Metab. 2012;97:3974–82.
172. Schaadt B, Feldt-Rasmussen U, Rasmussen B, Torring H, Foder B, Jorgensen K, et al. Assessment of the influence of thyroglobulin (Tg) autoantibodies and other interfering factors on the use of serum Tg as tumor marker in differentiated thyroid carcinoma. Thyroid. 1995;5:165–70.
173. Spencer CA. Recoveries cannot be used to authenticate thyroglobulin (Tg) measurements when sera contain Tg autoantibodies. Clin Chem. 1996;42(5):661–3.
174. Ericsson UB, Christensen SB, Thorell JI. A high prevalence of thyroglobulin autoantibodies in adults with and without thyroid disease as measured with a sensitive solid-phase immunosorbent radioassay. Clin Immunol Immunopathol. 1985;37:154–62.
175. Ruf J, Carayon P, Lissitzky S. Various expressions of a unique anti-human thyroglobulin antibody repertoire in normal state and autoimmune disease. Eur J Immunol. 1985;15:268–72.
176. Okosieme OE, Evans C, Moss L, Parkes AB, Premawardhana LD, Lazarus JH. Thyroglobulin antibodies in serum of patients with differentiated thyroid cancer: relationship between epitope specificities and thyroglobulin recovery. Clin Chem. 2005;51(4):729–34.
177. Latrofa F, Ricci D, Montanelli L, Piaggi P, Mazzi B, Bianchi F, et al. Thyroglobulin autoantibodies switch to immunoglobulin (Ig)G1 and IgG3 subclasses and preserve their restricted epitope pattern after 131I treatment for Graves' hyperthyroidism: the activity of autoimmune disease influences subclass distribution but not epitope pattern of autoantibodies. Clin Exp Immunol. 2014;178(3):438–46.
178. Spencer CA, Takeuchi M, Kazarosyan M. Current status and performance goals for serum thyroglobulin assays. Clin Chem. 1996;42(1):164–73.
179. Tozzoli R, Bizzaro N, Tonutti E, Pradella M, Manoni F, Vilalta D, et al. Immunoassay of antithyroid autoantibodies: high analytical variability in second generation methods. Clin Chem Lab Med. 2002;40:568–73.
180. Benvenga S, Burek CL, Talor M, Rose NR, Trimarchi F. Heterogeneity of the thyroglobulin epitopes associated with circulating thyroid hormone autoantibodies in hashimoto's thyroiditis and non-autoimmune thyroid diseases. J Endocrinol Investig. 2002;25:977–82.
181. Rosário PW, Maia FF, Fagundes TA, Vasconcelos FP, Cardoso LD, Purisch S. Antithyroglobulin antibodies in patients with differentiated thyroid carcinoma: methods of detection, interference with serum thyroglobulin measurement and clinical significance. Arq Bras Endocrinol Metabol. 2004;48:487–92.
182. Beever K, Bradbury J, Phillips D, McLachlan SM, Pegg C, Goral A, et al. Highly sensitive assays of autoantibodies to thyroglobulin and to thyroid peroxidase. Clin Chem. 1989;35:1949–54.
183. Feldt-Rasmussen U. Analytical and clinical performance goals for testing autoantibodies to thyroperoxidase, thyroglobulin and thyrotropin receptor. Clin Chem. 1996;42:160–3.

184. La'ulu SL, Slev PR, Roberts WL. Performance characteristics of 5 automated thyroglobulin autoantibody and thyroid peroxidase autoantibody assays. Clin Chim Acta. 2007;376:88–95.
185. Krahn J, Dembinski T. Thyroglobulin and anti-thyroglobulin assays in thyroid cancer monitoring. Clin Biochem. 2009;42:416–9.
186. Pickett AJ, Jones M, Evans C. Causes of discordance between thyroglobulin antibody assays. Ann Clin Biochem. 2012;49:463–7.
187. Taylor KP, Parkington D, Bradbury S, Simpson HL, Jefferies SJ, Halsall DJ. Concordance between thyroglobulin antibody assays. Ann Clin Biochem. 2011;48(Pt 4):367–9.
188. Ruf J, Henry M, DeMicco C, Carayon P. Characterization of monoclonal and autoimmune antibodies to thyroglobulin: application to clinical investigation. In: Hufner M, Reiners C, editors. Thyroglobulin and thyrolobulin antibodies in the follow-up of thyroid cancer and endemic goiter. Stuttgart: G Thieme; 1987. p. 21–30.
189. Spencer CA, Platler BW, Nicoloff JT. The effect of 125-I thyroglobulin tracer heterogeneity on serum Tg RIA measurement. Clin Chim Acta. 1985;153:105–15.
190. Spencer CA, Platler B, Guttler RB, Nicoloff JT. Heterogeneity of 125-I labelled thyroglobulin preparations. Clin Chim Acta. 1985;151:121–32.
191. Black EG, Hoffenberg R. Should one measure serum thyroglobulin in the presence of anti-thyroglobulin antibodies? Clin Endocrinol. 1983;19:597–601.
192. Mariotti S, Barbesino G, Caturegli P, Marino M, Manetti L, Pacini F, et al. Assay of thyroglobulin in serum with thyroglobulin autoantibodies: an unobtainable goal? J Clin Endocrinol Metab. 1995;80:468–72.
193. Weightman DR, Mallick UK, Fenwick JD, Perros P. Discordant serum thyroglobulin results generated by two classes of assay in patients with thyroid carcinoma: correlation with clinical outcome after 3 years of follow-up. Cancer. 2003;98(1):41–7.
194. Jahagirdar VR, Strouhal P, Holder G, Gama R, Singh BM. Thyrotoxicosis factitia masquerading as recurrent Graves' disease: endogenous antibody immunoassay interference, a pitfall for the unwary. Ann Clin Biochem. 2008;45(Pt 3):325–7.
195. Schneider AB, Pervos R. Radioimmunoassay of human thyroglobulin: effect of antithyroglobulin autoantibodies. J Clin Endocrinol Metab. 1978;47:126–37.
196. Feldt-Rasmussen U, Rasmussen AK. Serum thyroglobulin (Tg) in presence of thyroglobulin autoantibodies (TgAb). Clinical and methodological relevance of the interaction between Tg and TgAb in vivo and in vitro. J Endocrinol Investig. 1985;8:571–6.
197. Miles LEM, Hales CN. Labeled antibodies and immunological assay systems. Nature. 1968;219: 186–9.
198. Bayer MF, Kriss JP. Immunoradiometric assay for serum thyroglobulin: semiquantitative measurement of thyroglobulin in antithyroglobulin-positive sera. J Clin Endocrinol Metab. 1979;49:557–64.
199. Latrofa F, Ricci D, Grasso L, Vitti P, Masserini L, Basolo F, et al. Characterization of thyroglobulin epitopes in patients with autoimmune and non-autoimmune thyroid diseases using recombinant human monoclonal thyroglobulin autoantibodies. J Clin Endocrinol Metab. 2008;93:591–6.
200. Rahmoun MN, Bendahmane I. Anti-thyroglobulin antibodies in differentiated thyroid carcinoma patients: study of the clinical and biological parameters. Ann Endocrinol (Paris). 2014;75(1):15–8.
201. Marquet PY, Daver A, Sapin R, Bridgi B, Muratet JP, Hartmann DJ, et al. Highly sensitive immunoradiometric assay for serum thyroglobulin with minimal interference from autoantibodies. Clin Chem. 1996;42:258–62.
202. Grebe SKG. Diagnosis and management of thyroid carcinoma: a focus on serum thyroglobulin. Expert Rev Endocrinol Metab. 2009;4:25–43.
203. Haapala AM, Soppi E, Morsky P, et al. Thyroid antibodies in association with thyroid malignancy II: qualitative properties of thyroglobulin antibodies. Scand J Clin Lab Invest. 1995;55:317–22.
204. Hoofnagle AN, Becker JO, Wener MH, Heinecke JW. Quantification of thyroglobulin, a low-abundance serum protein, by immunoaffinity peptide enrichment and tandem mass spectrometry. Clin Chem. 2008;54(11):1796–804.
205. Netzel BC, Grant RP, Hoofnagle AN, Rockwood AL, Shuford CM, Grebe SK. First steps toward harmonization of LC-MS/MS thyroglobulin assays. Clin Chem. 2016;62(1):297–9.
206. Hoofnagle AN, Wener MH. The fundamental flaws of immunoassays and potential solutions using tandem mass spectrometry. J Immunol Methods. 2009;347(1-2):3–11.
207. Grebe SK. Soluble thyroid tumor markers – old and new challenges and potential solutions. N Z J Med Lab Sci. 2013;67:76–87.
208. Jindal A, Khan U. Is thyroglobulin level by liquid chromatography tandem-mass spectrometry always reliable for follow-up of DTC after thyroidectomy: a report on two patients. Thyroid. 2016;26(9):1334–5.
209. Azmat U, Porter K, Senter L, Ringel MD, Nabhan F. Thyroglobulin liquid chromatography-tandem mass spectrometry has a low sensitivity for detecting structural disease in patients with antithyroglobulin antibodies. Thyroid. 2016;27(1):74–80.
210. Petrovic I, Fatemi S, LoPresti J, Grebe SK, Algeciras-Schimnich A, Netzel BC, et al. SerumTg is frequently undetectable by mass spectrometry (Tg-MS) IN TgAb-positive differentiated thyroid cancer (DTC) patients with structural disease. Thyroid. 2015;25(S1):A251.
211. Crane MS, Strachan MW, Toft AD, Beckett GJ. Discordance in thyroglobulin measurements by radioimmunoassay and immunometric assay: a use-

ful means of identifying thyroglobulin assay interference. Ann Clin Biochem. 2013;50:421–32.
212. Spencer C, Fatemi S. Thyroglobulin antibody (TgAb) methods - strengths, pitfalls and clinical utility for monitoring TgAb-positive patients with differentiated thyroid cancer. Best Pract Res Clin Endocrinol Metab. 2013;27(5):701–12.
213. Feldt-Rasmussen U, Petersen PH, Date J, Madsen CM. Sequential changes in serum thyroglobulin (Tg) and its autoantibodies (TgAb) following subtotal thyroidectomy of patients with preoperatively detectable TgAb. Clin Endocrinol. 1980;12:29–38.
214. Fleck RA, Rapaport SI, Rao LV. Anti-prothrombin antibodies and the lupus anticoagulant. Blood. 1988;72(2):512–9.
215. van der Laken CJ, Voskuyl AE, Roos JC, Stigter van Walsum M, de Groot ER, Wolbink G, et al. Imaging and serum analysis of immune complex formation of radiolabelled infliximab and anti-infliximab in responders and non-responders to therapy for rheumatoid arthritis. Ann Rheum Dis. 2007;66(2):253–6.
216. Richards DB, Cookson LM, Berges AC, Barton SV, Lane T, Ritter JM, et al. Therapeutic clearance of amyloid by antibodies to serum amyloid P component. N Engl J Med. 2015;373(12):1106–14.
217. Latrofa F, Ricci D, Sisti E, Piaggi P, Nencetti C, Marino M, et al. Significance of low levels of thyroglobulin autoantibodies associated with undetectable thyroglobulin after thyroidectomy for differentiated thyroid carcinoma. Thyroid. 2016;26(6):798–806.
218. Pellegriti G, Frasca F, Regalbuto C, Squatrito S, Vigneri R. Worldwide increasing incidence of thyroid cancer: update on epidemiology and risk factors. J Cancer Epidemiol. 2013;2013:965212.
219. Ahn HS, Kim HJ, Welch HG. Korea's thyroid-cancer "epidemic"--screening and overdiagnosis. N Engl J Med. 2014;371(19):1765–7.
220. Oda H, Miyauchi A, Ito Y, Yoshioka K, Nakayama A, Sasai H, et al. Incidences of unfavorable events in the management of low-risk papillary microcarcinoma of the thyroid by active surveillance versus immediate surgery. Thyroid. 2016;26(1):150–5.
221. Davies L, Welch HG. Increasing incidence of thyroid cancer in the United States, 1973-2002. JAMA. 2006;295:2164–7.
222. Zhu C, Zheng T, Kilfoy BA, Han X, Ma S, Ba Y, et al. A birth cohort analysis of the incidence of papillary thyroid cancer in the United States, 1973–2004. Thyroid. 2009;19:1061–6.
223. Udelsman R, Zhang Y. The epidemic of thyroid cancer in the United States: the role of endocrinologists and ultrasounds. Thyroid. 2014;24(3):472–9.
224. Vaccarella S, Franceschi S, Bray F, Wild CP, Plummer M, Dal Maso L. Worldwide thyroid-cancer epidemic? The increasing impact of overdiagnosis. N Engl J Med. 2016;375(7):614–7.
225. Hundahl SA, Cady B, Cunningham MP, Mazzaferri E, McKee RF, Rosai J, et al. Initial results from a prospective cohort study of 5583 cases of thyroid carcinoma treated in the United States during 1996. U.S. and German Thyroid Cancer Study Group. An American College of Surgeons Commission on cancer patient care evaluation study. Cancer. 2000;89(1):202–17.
226. Mazzaferri EL, Kloos RT. Current approaches to primary therapy for papillary and follicular thyroid cancer. J Clin Endocrinol Metab. 2001;86:1447–63.
227. Hay ID, Thompson GB, Grant CS, Bergstralh EJ, Dvorak CE, Gorman CA, et al. Papillary thyroid carcinoma managed at the Mayo Clinic during six decades (1940-1999): temporal trends in initial therapy and long-term outcome in 2444 consecutively treated patients. World J Surg. 2002;26:879–85.
228. Pitoia F, Bueno F, Urciuoli C, Abelleira E, Cross G, Tuttle RM. Outcomes of patients with differentiated thyroid cancer risk-stratified according to the american thyroid association and latin american thyroid society risk of recurrence classification systems. Thyroid. 2013;23:1401–7.
229. Tuttle RM, Leboeuf R. Follow up approaches in thyroid cancer: a risk adapted paradigm. Endocrinol Metab Clin N Am. 2008;37:419–35.
230. Pitoia F, Ward L, Wohllk N, Friguglietti C, Tomimori E, Gauna A, et al. Recommendations of the Latin American Thyroid Society on diagnosis and management of differentiated thyroid cancer. Arq Bras Endocrinol Metabol. 2009;53(7):884.
231. Ashcraft MW, Van Herle AJ. The comparative value of serum thyroglobulin measurements and iodine 131 total body scans in the follow-up of patients with treated differentiated thyroid cancer. Am J Med. 1981;71:806–14.
232. Pineda JD, Lee T, Ain K, Reynolds JC, Robbins J. Iodine-131 therapy for thyroid cancer patients with elevated thyroglobulin and negative diagnostic scan. J Clin Endocrinol Metab. 1995;80:1488–92.
233. Baudin E, Do Cao C, Cailleux AF, Leboulleux S, Travagli JP, Schlumberger M. Positive predictive value of serum thyroglobulin levels, measured during the first year of follow-up after thyroid hormone withdrawal, in thyroid cancer patients. J Clin Endocrinol Metab. 2003;88:1107–11.
234. Smallridge RC, Diehl N, Bernet V. Practice trends in patients with persistent detectable thyroglobulin and negative diagnostic radioiodine whole body scans: a survey of American Thyroid Association members. Thyroid. 2014;24(10):1501–7.
235. Lamartina L, Durante C, Filetti S, Cooper DS. Low-risk differentiated thyroid cancer and radioiodine remnant ablation: a systematic review of the literature. J Clin Endocrinol Metab. 2015;100(5):1748–61.
236. Pacini F, Agate L, Elisei R, Capezzone M, Ceccarelli C, Lippi F, et al. Outcome of differentiated thyroid cancer with detectable serum Tg and negative diagnostic (131)I whole body scan: comparison of patients treated with high (131)I activities versus untreated patients. J Clin Endocrinol Metab. 2001;86:4092–7.

237. Schaap J, Eustatia-Rutten CF, Stokkel M, Links TP, Diamant M, van der Velde EA, et al. Does radioiodine therapy have disadvantageous effects in non-iodine accumulating differentiated thyroid carcinoma. Clin Endocrinol. 2002;57:117–24.
238. Valadão MM, Rosário PW, Borges MA, Costa GB, Rezende LL, Padrão EL, et al. Positive predictive value of detectable stimulated tg during the first year after therapy of thyroid cancer and the value of comparison with Tg-ablation and Tg measured after 24 months. Thyroid. 2006;16:1145–9.
239. Rosario P, Borges M, Reis J, Alves MF. Effect of suppressive therapy with levothyroxine on the reduction of serum thyroglobulin after total thyroidectomy. Thyroid. 2006;16:199–200.
240. Huang SH, Wang PW, Huang YE, Chou FF, Liu RT, Tung SC, et al. Sequential follow-up of serum thyroglobulin and whole body scan in thyroid cancer patients without initial metastasis. Thyroid. 2006;16:1273–8.
241. Giovanella L, Ceriani L, Suriano S, Ghelfo A, Maffioli M. Thyroglobulin measurement before rhTSH-aided (131)I ablation in detecting metastases from differentiated thyroid carcinoma. Clin Endocrinol. 2008;68:659–63.
242. Miyauchi A, Kudo T, Miya A, Kobayashi K, Ito Y, Takamura Y, et al. Prognostic impact of serum thyroglobulin doubling-time under thyrotropin suppression in patients with papillary thyroid carcinoma who underwent total thyroidectomy. Thyroid. 2011;21(7):707–16.
243. Gibelli B, Tredici P, De Cicco C, Bodei L, Sandri MT, Renne G, et al. Preoperative determination of serum thyroglobulin to identify patients with differentiated thyroid cancer who may present recurrence without increased thyroglobulin. Acta Otorhinolaryngol Ital. 2005;25:94–9.
244. Giovanella L, Ceriani L, Ghelfo A, Maffioli M, Keller F. Preoperative undetectable serum thyroglobulin in differentiated thyroid carcinoma: incidence, causes and management strategy. Clin Endocrinol. 2007;67:547–51.
245. Durante C, Puxeddu E, Ferretti E, Morisi R, Moretti S, Bruno R, et al. BRAF mutations in papillary thyroid carcinomas inhibit genes involved in iodine metabolism. J Clin Endocrinol Metab. 2007;92:2840–3.
246. Lazar V, Bidart JM, Caillou B, Mahe C, Lacroix L, Filetti S, et al. Expression of the Na+/I- symporter gene in human thyroid tumors: a comparison study with other thyroid-specific genes. J Clin Endocrinol Metab. 1999;84:3228–34.
247. Gardner DF, Rothman J, Utiger RD. Serum thyroglobulin in normal subjects and patients with hyperthyroidism due to Graves' disease: effects of T3, iodide, 131I and antithyroid drugs. Clin Endocrinol. 1979;11:585–94.
248. Padovani RP, Robenshtok E, Brokhin M, Tuttle RM. Even without additional therapy, serum thyroglobulin concentrations often decline for years after total thyroidectomy and radioactive remnant ablation in patients with differentiated thyroid cancer. Thyroid. 2012;22(8):778–83.
249. Durante C, Montesano T, Attard M, Torlontano M, Monzani F, Costante G, et al. Long-term surveillance of papillary thyroid cancer patients who do not undergo postoperative radioiodine remnant ablation: is there a role for serum thyroglobulin measurement? J Clin Endocrinol Metab. 2012;97:2748–53.
250. Hjiyiannakis P, Mundy J, Harmer C. Thyroglobulin antibodies in differentiated thyroid cancer. Clin Oncol. 1999;11:240–4.
251. Ronga G, Filesi M, Ventroni G, Vestri AR, Signore A. Value of the first serum thyroglobulin level after total thyroidectomy for the diagnosis of metastases from differentiated thyroid carcinoma. Eur J Nucl Med. 1999;26:1448–52.
252. Lima N, Cavaliere E, Tomimori E, Knobel M, Medeieros-Neto G. Prognostic value of serial serum thyroglobulin determinations after total thyroidectomy for differentiated thyroid cancer. J Endocrinol Investig. 2002;25:110–5.
253. Lin JD, Huang MJ, Hsu BR, Chao TC, Hsueh C, Liu FH, et al. Significance of postoperative serum thyroglobulin levels in patients with papillary and follicular thyroid carcinomas. J Surg Oncol. 2002;80:45–51.
254. Hall FT, Beasley NJ, Eski SJ, Witterick IJ, Walfish PG, Freeman JL. Predictive value of serum thyroglobulin after surgery for thyroid carcinoma. Laryngoscope. 2003;113:77–81.
255. Toubeau M, Touzery C, Arveux P, Chaplain G, Vaillant G, Berriolo A, et al. Predictive value for disease progression of serum thyroglobulin levels measured in the postoperative period and after (131) I ablation therapy in patients with differentiated thyroid cancer. J Nucl Med. 2004;45:988–94.
256. Kim TY, Kim WB, Kim ES, Ryu JS, Yeo JS, Kim SC, et al. Serum thyroglobulin levels at the time of 131I remnant ablation just after thyroidectomy are useful for early prediction of clinical recurrence in low-risk patients with differentiated thyroid carcinoma. J Clin Endocrinol Metab. 2005;90:1440–5.
257. Makarewicz J, Adamczewski Z, Knapska-Kucharska M, Lewiński A. Evaluation of the diagnostic value of the first thyroglobulin determination in detecting metastases after differentiated thyroid carcinoma surgery. Exp Clin Endocrinol Diabetes. 2006;114:485–9.
258. Heemstra KA, Liu YY, Stokkel M, Kievit J, Corssmit E, Pereira AM, et al. Serum thyroglobulin concentrations predict disease-free remission and death in differentiated thyroid carcinoma. Clin Endocrinol. 2007;66:58–64.
259. Karatzas T, Vasileiadis I, Zapanti E, Charitoudis G, Karakostas E, Boutzios G. Thyroglobulin antibodies as a potential predictive marker of papillary thyroid carcinoma in patients with indeterminate cytology. Am J Surg. 2016;212:946–52.
260. Shih ML, Lee JA, Hsieh CB, Yu JC, Liu HD, Kebebew E, et al. Thyroidectomy for Hashimoto's

thyroiditis: complications and associated cance. Thyroid. 2008;18:729–34.
261. Tomoda C, Miyauchi A. Undetectable serum thyroglobulin levels in patients with medullary thyroid carcinoma after total thyroidectomy without radioiodine ablation. Thyroid. 2012;22(7):680–2.
262. Angell TE, Spencer CA, Rubino BD, Nicoloff JT, LoPresti JS. In search of an unstimulated thyroglobulin baseline value in low-risk papillary thyroid carcinoma patients not receiving radioactive iodine ablation. Thyroid. 2014;24:1127–33.
263. Spencer CA, Lopresti JS. Measuring thyroglobulin and thyroglobulin autoantibody in patients with differentiated thyroid cancer. Nat Clin Pract Endocrinol Metab. 2008;4(4):223–33.
264. Giovanella L, Imperiali M, Ferrari A, Palumbo A, Furlani L, Graziani MS, et al. Serum thyroglobulin reference values according to NACB criteria in healthy subjects with normal thyroid ultrasound. Clin Chem Lab Med. 2012;50(5):891–3.
265. Spencer CA, LoPresti JS, Fatemi S, Nicoloff JT. Detection of residual and recurrent differentiated thyroid carcinoma by serum Thyroglobulin measurement. Thyroid. 1999;9:435–41.
266. Pacini F, Molinaro E, Castagna MG, Agate L, Elisei R, Ceccarelli C, et al. Recombinant human thyrotropin-stimulated serum thyroglobulin combined with neck ultrasonography has the highest sensitivity in monitoring differentiated thyroid carcinoma. J Clin Endocrinol Metab. 2003;88:3668–73.
267. Mazzaferri EL, Robbins RJ, Spencer CA, Braverman LE, Pacini F, Wartofsky L, et al. A consensus report of the role of serum thyroglobulin as a monitoring method for low-risk patients with papillary thyroid carcinoma. J Clin Endocrinol Metab. 2003;88(4):1433–41.
268. Mazzaferri EL, Kloos RT. Is diagnostic iodine-131 scanning with recombinant human TSH useful in the follow-up of differentiated thyroid cancer after thyroid ablation? J Clin Endocrinol Metab. 2002;87:1486–9.
269. Bachelot A, Cailleux AF, Klain M, Baudin E, Ricard M, Bellon N, et al. Relationship between tumor burden and serum thyroglobulin level in patients with papillary and follicular thyroid carcinoma. Thyroid. 2002;12:707–11.
270. Vitale G, Lupoli GA, Ciccarelli A, Lucariello A, Fittipaldi MR, Fonderico F, et al. Influence of body surface area on serum peak thyrotropin (TSH) levels after recombinant human TSH administration. J Clin Endocrinol Metab. 2003;88:1319–22.
271. Montesano T, Durante C, Attard M, Crocetti U, Meringolo D, Bruno R, et al. Age influences TSH serum levels after withdrawal of l-thyroxine or rhTSH stimulation in patients affected by differentiated thyroid cancer. Biomed Pharmacother. 2007;61:468–71.
272. Braverman L, Kloos RT, Law B Jr, Kipnes M, Dionne M, Magner J. Evaluation of various doses of recombinant human thyrotropin in patients with multinodular goiters. Endocr Pract. 2008;14:832–9.
273. Over R, Nsouli-Maktabi H, Burman KD, Jonklaas J. Age modifies the response to recombinant human thyrotropin. Thyroid. 2010;20:1377–84.
274. Schlumberger M, Charbord P, Fragu P, Lumbroso J, Parmentier C, Tubiana M. Circulating thyrotropin and thyroid hormones in patients with metastases of differentiated thyroid carcinoma: relationship to serum thyrotropin levels. J Clin Endocrinol Metab. 1980;51:513–9.
275. Robbins RJ, Srivastava S, Shaha A, Ghossein R, Larson SM, Fleisher M, et al. Factors influencing the basal and recombinant human thyrotropin-stimulated serum thyroglobulin in patients with metastatic thyroid carcinoma. J Clin Endocrinol Metab. 2004;89:6010–6.
276. Nakabashi CC, Kasamatsu TS, Crispim F, Yamazaki CA, Camacho CP, Andreoni DM, et al. Basal serum thyroglobulin measured by a second-generation assay is equivalent to stimulated thyroglobulin in identifying metastases in patients with differentiated thyroid cancer with low or intermediate risk of recurrence. Eur Thyroid J. 2014;3(1):43–50.
277. Groen AH, Klein Hesselink MS, Plukker JT, Sluiter WJ, van der Horst-Schrivers AN, Brouwers AH, et al. Additional value of a high sensitive thyroglobulin assay in the follow-up of patients with differentiated thyroid carcinoma. Clin Endocrinol. 2016;86(3):419–24.
278. Heilo A, Sigstad E, Fagerlid KH, Håskjold OI, Grøholt KK, Berner A, et al. Efficacy of ultrasound-guided percutaneous ethanol injection treatment in patients with a limited number of metastatic cervical lymph nodes from papillary thyroid carcinoma. J Clin Endocrinol Metab. 2011;96:2750–5.
279. Hay ID, Lee RA, Davidge-Pitts C, Reading CC, Charboneau JW. Long-term outcome of ultrasound-guided percutaneous ethanol ablation of selected "recurrent" neck nodal metastases in 25 patients with TNM stages III or IVA papillary thyroid carcinoma previously treated by surgery and 131I therapy. Surgery. 2013;154(6):1448–54. discussion 54-5
280. Yim JH, Kim EY, Bae Kim W, Kim WG, Kim TY, Ryu JS, et al. Long-term consequence of elevated thyroglobulin in differentiated thyroid cancer. Thyroid. 2013;23(1):58–63.
281. Pacini F, Sabra MM, Tuttle RM. Clinical relevance of thyroglobulin doubling time in the management of patients with differentiated thyroid cancer. Thyroid. 2011;21:691–2.
282. Giovanella L, Trimboli P, Verburg FA, Treglia G, Piccardo A, Foppiani L, et al. Thyroglobulin levels and thyroglobulin doubling time independently predict a positive 18F-FDG PET/CT scan in patients with biochemical recurrence of differentiated thyroid carcinoma. Eur J Nucl Med Mol Imaging. 2013;40:874–80.
283. Miyauchi A, Kudo T, Kihara M, Higashiyama T, Ito Y, Kobayashi K, et al. Relationship of biochemically persistent disease and thyroglobulin-doubling time to age at surgery in patients with papillary thyroid carcinoma. Endocr J. 2013;60(4):415–21.

284. Elisei R, Agate L, Viola D, Matrone A, Biagini A, Molinaro E. How to manage patients with differentiated thyroid cancer and a rising serum thyroglobulin level. Endocrinol Metab Clin N Am. 2014;43(2):331–44.
285. Kelders A, Kennes LN, Krohn T, Behrendt FF, Mottaghy FM, Verburg FA. Relationship between positive thyroglobulin doubling time and 18F-FDG PET/CT-positive, 131I-negative lesions. Nucl Med Commun. 2014;34:176–81.
286. Rossing RM, Jentzen W, Nagarajah J, Bockisch A, Gorges R. Serum thyroglobulin doubling time in progressive thyroid cancer. Thyroid. 2016;26(12):1712–8.
287. Pacini F, Pinchera A. Serum and tissue thyroglobulin measurement: clinical applications in thyroid disease. Biochimie. 1999;81:463–7.
288. Rotman-Pikielny P, Reynolds JC, Barker WC, Yen PM, Skarulis MC, Sarlis NJ. Recombinant human thyrotropin for the diagnosis and treatment of a highly functional metastatic struma ovarii. J Clin Endocrinol Metab. 2000;85:237–44.
289. Russo M, Marturano I, Masucci R, Caruso M, Fornito MC, Tumino D, et al. Metastatic malignant struma ovarii with coexistence of Hashimoto's thyroiditis. Endocrinol Diabetes Metabol Case Rep. 2016;2016:160030.
290. Trimboli P, D'Aurizio F, Tozzoli R, Giovanella L. Measurement of thyroglobulin, calcitonin, and PTH in FNA washout fluids. Clin Chem Lab Med. 2016;55:914–25.
291. Pacini F, Fugazzola L, Lippi F, Ceccarelli C, Centoni R, Miccoli P, et al. Detection of thyroglobulin in fine needle aspirates of nonthyroidal neck masses: a clue to the diagnosis of metastatic differentiated thyroid cancer. J Clin Endocrinol Metab. 1992;74:1401–4.
292. Uruno T, Miyauchi A, Shimizu K, Tomoda C, Takamura Y, Ito Y, et al. Usefulness of thyroglobulin measurement in fine-needle aspiration biopsy specimens for diagnosing cervical lymph node metastasis in patients with papillary thyroid cancer. World J Surg. 2005;29:483–5.
293. Boi F, Baghino G, Atzeni F, Lai ML, Faa G, Mariotti S. The diagnostic value for differentiated thyroid carcinoma metastases of thyroglobulin (Tg) measurement in washout fluid from fine-needle aspiration biopsy of neck lymph nodes is maintained in the presence of circulating anti-Tg antibodies. J Clin Endocrinol Metab. 2006;91:1364–9.
294. Rosario PW, de Faria S, Bicalho L, Alves MF, Borges MA, Purisch S, et al. Ultrasonographic differentiation between metastatic and benign lymph nodes in patients with papillary thyroid carcinoma. J Ultrasound Med. 2005;24:1385–9.
295. Snozek CL, Chambers EP, Reading CC, Sebo TJ, Sistrunk JW, Singh RJ, et al. Serum thyroglobulin, high-resolution ultrasound, and lymph node thyroglobulin in diagnosis of differentiated thyroid carcinoma nodal metastases. J Clin Endocrinol Metab. 2007;92:4278–81.
296. Bruno R, Giannasio P, Chiarella R, Capula C, Russo D, Filetti S, et al. Identification of a neck lump as a lymph node metastasis from an occult contralateral papillary microcarcinoma of the thyroid: key role of thyroglobulin assay in the fine-needle aspirate. Thyroid. 2009;19:531–3.
297. Jeon SJ, Kim E, Park JS, Son KR, Baek JH, Kim YS, et al. Diagnostic benefit of thyroglobulin measurement in fine-needle aspiration for diagnosing metastatic cervical lymph nodes from papillary thyroid cancer: correlations with US features. Korean J Radiol. 2009;10:106–11.
298. Cunha N, Rodrigues F, Curado F, Ilhéu O, Cruz C, Naidenov P, et al. Thyroglobulin detection in fine-needle aspirates of cervical lymph nodes: a technique for the diagnosis of metastatic differentiated thyroid cancer. Eur J Endocrinol. 2007;157:101–7.
299. Suh YJ, Son EJ, Moon HJ, Kim EK, Han KH, Kwak JY. Utility of thyroglobulin measurements in fine-needle aspirates of space occupying lesions in the thyroid bed after thyroid cancer operations. Thyroid. 2012;23(3):280–8.
300. Cappelli C, Pirola I, De Martino E, Gandossi E, Cimino E, Samoni F, et al. Thyroglobulin measurement in fine-needle aspiration biopsy of metastatic lymph nodes after rhTSH stimulation. Head Neck. 2013;35:E21–3.
301. Grani G, Fumarola A. Thyroglobulin in lymph node fine-needle aspiration washout: a systematic review and meta-analysis of diagnostic accuracy. J Clin Endocrinol Metab. 2014;99(6):1970–82.
302. Torres MR, Nóbrega Neto SH, Rosas RJ, Martins AL, Ramos AL, da Cruz TR. Thyroglobulin in the washout fluid of lymph-node biopsy: what is its role in the follow-up of differentiated thyroid carcinoma? Thyroid. 2014;24:7–18.
303. Chung J, Kim EK, Lim H, Son EJ, Yoon JH, Youk JH, et al. Optimal indication of thyroglobulin measurement in fine-needle aspiration for detecting lateral metastatic lymph nodes in patients with papillary thyroid carcinoma. Head Neck. 2014;36(6):795–801.
304. Shi JH, Xu YY, Pan QZ, Sui GQ, Zhou JP, Wang H. The value of combined application of ultrasound-guided fine needle aspiration cytology and thyroglobulin measurement for the diagnosis of cervical lymph node metastases from thyroid cancer. Pak J Med Sci. 2015;31(5):1152–5.
305. Tang S, Buck A, Jones C, Sara Jiang X. The utility of thyroglobulin washout studies in predicting cervical lymph node metastases: one academic medical center's experience. Diagn Cytopathol. 2016;44:964–8.
306. Jeon MJ, Kim WG, Jang EK, Choi YM, Lee YM, Sung TY, et al. Thyroglobulin level in fine-needle aspirates for preoperative diagnosis of cervical lymph node metastasis in patients with papillary thyroid carcinoma: two different cutoff values according to serum thyroglobulin level. Thyroid. 2015;25(4):410–6.
307. Pak K, Suh S, Hong H, Cheon GJ, Hahn SK, Kang KW, et al. Diagnostic values of thyroglobulin measurement in fine-needle aspiration of lymph

nodes in patients with thyroid cancer. Endocrine. 2015;49(1):70–7.
308. Zanella AB, Meyer EL, Balzan L, Silva AC, Camargo J, Migliavacca A, et al. Thyroglobulin measurements in washout of fine needle aspirates in cervical lymph nodes for detection of papillary thyroid cancer metastases. Arq Bras Endocrinol Metabol. 2010;54(6):550–4.
309. Baskin HJ. Detection of recurrent papillary thyroid carcinoma by thyroglobulin assessment in the needle washout after fine-needle aspiration of suspicious lymph nodes. Thyroid. 2004;14(11):959–63.
310. Shin HJ, Lee HS, Kim EK, Moon HJ, Lee JH, Kwak JY. A study on serum antithyroglobulin antibodies interference in thyroglobulin measurement in fine-needle aspiration for diagnosing lymph node metastasis in postoperative patients. PLoS One. 2015;10(6):e0131096.
311. Boi F, Maurelli I, Pinna G, Atzeni F, Piga M, Lai ML, et al. Calcitonin measurement in wash-out fluid from fine needle aspiration of neck masses in patients with primary and metastatic medullary thyroid carcinoma. J Clin Endocrinol Metab. 2007;92:2115–8.
312. Abraham D, Gault PM, Hunt J, Bentz J. Calcitonin estimation in neck lymph node fine-needle aspirate fluid prevents misinterpretation of cytology in patients with metastatic medullary thyroid cancer. Thyroid. 2009;19:1015–6.
313. Massaro F, Dolcino M, Degrandi R, Ferone D, Mussap M, Minuto F, et al. Calcitonin assay in wash-out fluid after fine-needle aspiration biopsy in patients with a thyroid nodule and borderline value of the hormone. J Endocrinol Investig. 2009;32:308–12.
314. Sapin R, d'Herbomez M, Gasser F, Meyer L, Schlienger JL. Increased sensitivity of a new assay for anti-thyroglobulin antibody detection in patients with autoimmune thyroid disease. Clin Biochem. 2003;36:611–6.
315. Donegan D, McIver B, Algeciras-Schimnich A. Clinical consequences of a change in anti-thyroglobulin antibody assays during the follow-up of patients with differentiated thyroid cancer. Endocr Pract. 2014;20:1032–6.
316. Gianoukakis AG. Thyroglobulin antibody status and differentiated thyroid cancer: what does it mean for prognosis and surveillance? Curr Opin Oncol. 2015;27(1):26–32.
317. Lupoli GA, Okosieme OE, Evans C, Clark PM, Pickett AJ, Premawardhana LD, et al. Prognostic significance of thyroglobulin antibody epitopes in differentiated thyroid cancer. J Clin Endocrinol Metab. 2015;100(1):100–8.
318. Spencer CA. New insights for using serum thyroglobulin (Tg) measurement for managing patients with differentiated thyroid carcinomas. Thyroid Int. 2003;4:1–14.
319. Nascimento C, Borget I, Troalen F, Al Ghuzlan A, Deandreis D, Hartl D, et al. Ultrasensitive serum thyroglobulin measurement is useful for the follow-up of patients treated with total thyroidectomy without radioactive iodine ablation. Eur J Endocrinol. 2013;169(5):689–93.
320. Yamada O, Miyauchi A, Ito Y, Nakayama A, Yabuta T, Masuoka H, et al. Changes in serum thyroglobulin antibody levels as a dynamic prognostic factor for early-phase recurrence of thyroglobulin antibody-positive papillary thyroid carcinoma after total thyroidectomy. Endocr J. 2014;61(10):961–5.
321. Tsushima Y, Miyauchi A, Ito Y, Kudo T, Masuoka H, Yabuta T, et al. Prognostic significance of changes in serum thyroglobulin antibody levels of pre- and post-total thyroidectomy in thyroglobulin antibody-positive papillary thyroid carcinoma patients. Endocr J. 2013;60:871–6.
322. Tumino S, Belfiore A. Appearance of antithyroglobulin antibodies as the sole sign of metastatic lymph nodes in a patient operated on for papillary thyroid cancer: a case report. Thyroid. 2000;10:431–3.
323. Slifka MK, Antia R, Whitmire JK, Ahmed R. Humoral immunity due to long-lived plasma cells. Immunity. 1998;8:363–72.
324. Uller RP, Van Herle AJ. Effect of therapy on serum thyroglobulin levels in patients with Graves' disease. J Clin Endocrinol Metab. 1978;46:747–55.
325. Feldt-Rasmussen U, Blichert-Toft M, Christiansen C, Date J. Serum thyroglobulin and its autoantibody following subtotal thyroid resection of Graves' disease. Eur J Clin Investig. 1982;12:203–8.
326. Benvenga S, Bartolone L, Squadrito S, Trimarchi F. Thyroid hormone autoantibodies elicited by diagnostic fine needle biopsy. J Clin Endocrinol Metab. 1997;82:4217–23.
327. Polyzos SA, Anastasilakis AD. Alterations in serum thyroid-related constituents after thyroid fine-needle biopsy: a systematic review. Thyroid. 2010;20:265–71.
328. Izumi M, Larsen PR. Correlation of sequential changes in serum thyroglobulin, triiodothyronine, and thyroxine in patients with Graves' disease and subacute thyroiditis. Metabolism. 1978;27:449–60.
329. Feldt-Rasmussen U, Bech K, Date J, Hyltoft Pedersen P, Johansen K, Nistrup Madsen S. Thyroid stimulating antibodies, thyroglobulin antibodies and serum proteins during treatment of Graves' disease with radioiodine or propylthiouracil. Allergy. 1982;37:161–7.
330. Feldt-Rasmussen U, Bech K, Date J, Petersen PH, Johansen K. A prospective study of the differential changes in serum thyroglobulin and its autoantibodies during propylthiouracil or radioiodine therapy of patients with Graves' disease. Acta Endocrinol. 1982;99:379–85.
331. Stevic I, Dembinski TC, Pathak KA, Leslie WD. Transient early increase in thyroglobulin levels post-radioiodine ablation in patients with differentiated thyroid cancer. Clin Biochem. 2015;48(10-11):658–61.

Management of Post-operative Hypocalcemia

16

Claudio Marcocci

Introduction

Inadequate production of PTH by parathyroid glands is responsible for the occurrence of post-operative (PO) hypocalcemia (HypoCa) (PO-HypoCa) following bilateral thyroid surgery, and, particularly repeated neck surgery [1, 2]. Lobectomy only very rarely may be followed by PO-HypoCa.

Hypocalcemia is defined as ionized serum calcium (Ca) level below the lower limit of normal range. Ionized Ca (Ca^{2+}) measurement is not always easily available in clinical practice. Circulating Ca is present in three forms: ionized (50%), protein-bound (mostly to albumin, about 50%) and complexed to anions (less than 1%). An acceptable indirect estimation of the Ca^{2+} can be obtained by measuring albumin-corrected serum Ca = measured total Ca × [0.8 × (4.0-measured serum albumin, in g/dL)].

PO-HypoCa can be transient, protracted or permanent. Transient PO-HypoCa is usually caused by reversible parathyroid ischemia and resolves within a few weeks, but in some cases it may last longer (protracted PO-HypoCa). Permanent/chronic PO-HypoCa is due to an irreversible parathyroid damage (ischemia, electric scalpel damage and, rarely, presence of parathyroid gland in the pathologic specimen) and persists 6 months after surgery [3, 4].

The rate of PO-HypoCa largely depends upon the experience of the surgeon. Although still debated, an endocrine thyroid surgeon is considered "experienced" when performing one hundred thyroidectomy per year or more [4]. Beside surgical experience, the rate of PO-HypoCa also depends upon the extent of thyroid surgery and the underlying thyroid disorder, the risk being greater in patients undergoing total thyroidectomy and bilateral central lymph node dissection or repeated thyroidectomy [3, 5–7]. Other favoring factors include low 25-hydroxyvitanin D [25(OD)D] levels and hypomagnesemia [1, 2].

The clinical manifestations of PO-HypoCa are strictly related to the speed of onset and the severity of hypocalcemia and may range from asymptomatic cases, when hypocalcemia is mild, to a severe-life threating condition that requires hospital admission and intensive treatment. Symptomatic PO-HypoCa occurs in 30–60% of patients undergoing total thyroidectomy [2, 8].

Post-operative Hypocalcemia

Thyroid surgery is increasingly performed worldwide either with short-term in-hospital admission or on an outpatient basis with perioperative observation. Both strategies have been

C. Marcocci
Department of Clinical and Experimental Medicine, University of Pisa, Endocrine Unit 2, University Hospital of Pisa, Pisa, Italy
e-mail: claudio.marcocci@med.unipi.it

U. K. Mallick et al. (eds.), *Practical Management of Thyroid Cancer*,
https://doi.org/10.1007/978-3-319-91725-2_16

increasingly used following the implementation of minimally invasive techniques and the use of local anesthesia [4, 9, 10]. Prevention and prediction of PO-HypoCa are therefore of utmost importance, since it may delay the discharge of the patient from the hospital and cause admission to the hospital of patients treated on an outpatient basis [9]. Symptoms of hypocalcemia, when occur, usually appear on the first post-operative day, but in some cases hypocalcemia may become clinically manifest even after 3–4 days [11].

Prevention

The best way to prevent PO-HypoCa is to refer all patients with thyroid cancer to experienced endocrine surgeons, and, during thyroidectomy, to identify all parathyroid glands and preserve their blood supply. The risk of permanent PO-HypoCa is closely related to the number of preserved functioning parathyroid glands at surgery [3, 12]. In addition other variables can be evaluated preoperatively and appropriately corrected to prevent or limit PO-HypoCa. Vitamin D status should be assessed by measurement of serum 25(OH)D levels. Vitamin D deficiency, if present, should be corrected before surgery, since it may favor transient PO-HypoCa [13]. Serum magnesium should also be measured since magnesium deficiency impairs the secretion of PTH and its action in target tissues and, therefore, may worsen PO-HypoCa [14, 15]. In patients with high risk of PO-HypoCa perioperative administration of calcitriol has been shown to decrease the incidence of post-operative hypocalcemia and facilitate early hospital discharge after thyroidectomy [16, 17]. In some surgical setting prophylactic treatment with calcium supplements and activated vitamin D is advised to all patients undergoing bilateral thyroidectomy.

It is controversial whether parathyroid gland autotransplantation, which could be considered if there is a high likelihood of permanent PO-HypoCa, may help to preserve parathyroid function. Inadvertently removed parathyroid glands can effectively be grafted intraoperatively with almost complete avoidance of PO-HypoCa [18, 19]. The advantage of transplanting not completely devascularized glands is questionable, since their function is only transiently impaired and may recover better if left *in situ* than if autrotransplanted [3, 20, 21].

Prediction

Several attempts have been made to identify whether perioperative measurement of calcium, PTH either separately or together could predict PO-HypoCa.

As mentioned before hypocalcemia usually presents in the first postoperative day, and therefore measurement of serum calcium on the day after surgery might be a reliable method to predict PO-HypoCa. Indeed, in a prospective study, measurement of Ca^{++} 16 h after thyroidectomy was shown to be a reliable predictor of PO-HypoCa [22]. Moreover, in a retrospective study a rise in serum calcium in samples collected 12 vs 6 h after surgery or a value of serum calcium ≥8 mg/dL predicted normocalcemia at 24 h [23]. Another study has shown that combination of serum calcium levels ≤1.9 mmol/L on the second postoperative day, together with PTH levels ≤15 pg/mL on the first day, had a sensitivity of 96.3% and a specificity of 96.1% for predicting PO-HypoCa, with a PPV of 86.0% and a NPV of 99.0% [24]. However, it should be kept in mind that in a minority of patients hypocalcemia may occur 2–3 days after surgery, and these cases cannot be identified by calcium monitoring in the first 24 h after surgery.

Because of its short half-life, changes in circulating PTH precede changes in serum calcium by hours. Several studies with blood sampling at different times (time of surgery or during the first postoperative day), using different cut-off values of serum PTH, have been performed (see for review [1, 25, 26]). PTH values <10 or 15 pg/mL at 1–6 h after thyroidectomy could predict post-operative hypocalcemia with high sensitivity (92.3–100%) and specificity (72–99%). The high predictive value of serum PTH in the perioperative hours is particularly attracting in the outpatient setting to identify patients that can be discharge safely on the same day of surgery, but also for in-hospital patients to early start appropriate therapy to prevent symptomatic hypocalcemia [21, 27].

Management

The aim of treatment is to control symptoms of hypocalcemia while avoiding side effects and complications. Main treatment options include calcium [oral (dietary or supplements) or intravenous], activated vitamin D (Table 16.1), magnesium, and where available recombinant human $PTH_{1\text{-}84}$. Thiazide diuretics may help to manage hypercalciuria and low phosphate diet and phosphate binders to control hyperphospatemia.

Mild Hypocalcemia

Mild hypocalcemia [corrected calcium ≥7.0 mg/dL (1.75 mmol/L)] is usually, but not necessarily, asymptomatic and cannot be detected unless serum calcium is routinely measured after thyroidectomy. Signs related to neuromuscular irritability (Chvostek and Trousseau signs) may unveil a latent hypocalcemia at physical examination [28]. Oral calcium supplement (usually 1–3 g/daily) alone or combined with active vitamin D metabolites (0.5–1.0 μg calcitriol [1,25$(OH)_2$D] or equivalent doses (1.0–2.0 μg) of alfacalcidiol [1αOHD]) should be considered, particularly in symptomatic patients and in those who have to travel a long journey to get back home.

Moderate to Severe Hypocalcemia

Moderate to severe hypocalcemia (corrected calcium <7.0 mg/dL) is usually symptomatic, even though there is no strict relationship between severity of symptoms and the degree of hypocalcemia. Classical manifestations include paresthesias, carpopedal spasm, tetany, seizures, positive Chvostek's and Trousseau's signs, and prolongation of the QT interval at ECG. The severity of symptoms and the level of corrected serum calcium should guide the treatment [2, 8, 28–30].

Severe hypocalcemia usually requires hospital admission and urgent treatment with intravenous (iv) calcium, until an oral regiment can be started (Fig. 16.1). Calcium gluconate should be preferred, since it is less likely to cause tissue necrosis in the case of extravasation in the adjacent subcutaneous space. One to two ampules of 10% calcium gluconate (one ampule contains 93 mg elemental calcium) diluted in 50–100 mL of 5%dextrose should be infused over a period of 10–20 min. The infusion should not be given more rapidly because of the risk of cardiac complications. ECG monitoring is advised during calcium infusion, particularly in patients taking digoxin, because of the risk of arrhythmias. Calcium infusion will promptly raise the concentration of serum calcium, but its effect is transient and will last no more than 2–4 h. Therefore, a continuous infusion of calcium at a lower rate should follow the initial bolus. A solution containing 1 mg/mL elemental calcium can be prepared by adding 11 ampules of 10% calcium gluconate to 5% dextrose or saline to provide a final volume of 1 l. The solution should be admin-

Table 16.1 Vitamin D and its activeted forms in the management of chronic hypocalcemia[a]

Medication	Typical daily dose	Time to onset of action	Time to offset of action
Calcitriol [1,25$(OH)_2$D]	0.25–2.0 μg once or twice	1–2 days	2–3 days
Alfacalcidiol[b] [1α(OH)D]	0.5–4 μg once	1–2 days	5–7 days
Dihydrotachysterol[b]	0.3–1.0 mg once	4–7 days	7–21 days
Vitamin D_2 (ergocalciferol) or vitamin D_3 (cholecalciferol)[c]	25,000–200,000 IU	10–14 days	14–75 days

[a]Derived from Shoback [1]
[b]This compound is rapidly activated in the liver to 25(OH) dihydrotachysterol
[c]These compound could be used in a setting where activated vitamin D is not available and/or too expensive

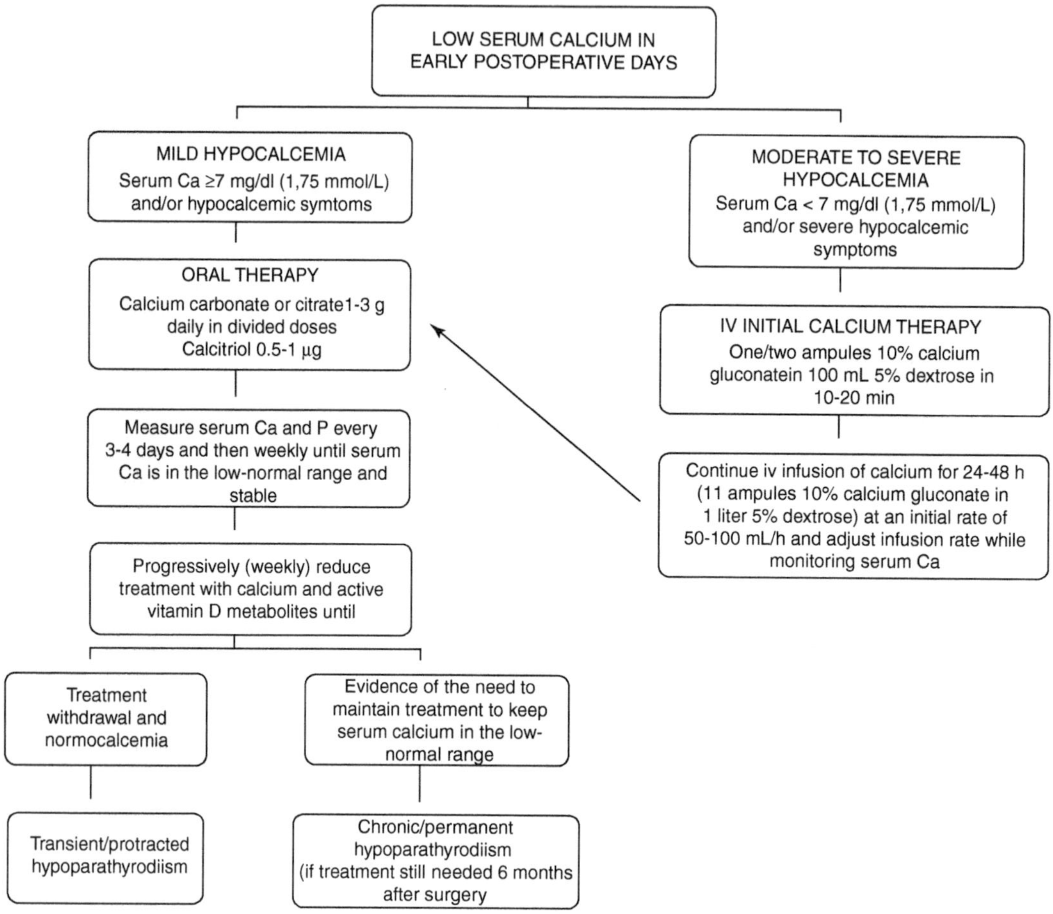

Fig. 16.1 Management of post-operative hypocalcemia. Oral therapy should be the initial management in patients with mild hypocalcemia and/or hypocalcemic symptoms. Conversely, intravenous calcium should be the initial therapy in patients with moderate to severe hypocalcemia and/or the presence of severe hypocalcemia symptoms. In this setting oral therapy with calcium and vitamin D metabolites should be started as soon as practical

istered at an initial rate of 50–100 mL/h and the rate adjusted according to corrected serum calcium level. Serum calcium should be measured at frequent intervals (every 1–2 h initially and every 4–6 h afterwards) and maintained at the lower limit of the normal range, while the patient is asymptomatic. Calcium infusion for 8–10 h using the above protocol will raise serum calcium by approximately 2 mg/dL.

Oral administration of activated vitamin D and calcium should be stared as soon as practical. The use of activated vitamin D (calcitriol or alfacalcidiol) is preferred because of the potency and rapid onset of action and the impaired renal conversion of vitamin D to 1α-hydroxylated metabolites (Table 16.1). Calcitriol is typically initiated at an initial dose of 0.5–1.0 µg twice daily; oral calcium (1–3 g daily in divided doses) is also added.

The possible coexistence of hypomagnesemia should also be considered in patients with acute PO-HypoCa. As mentioned before, hypomagnesemia inhibits PTH secretion and causes a reversible resistance to the action of PTH. If magnesium concentration is low, iv magnesium sulfate should be administered (initial dose 2 g as a 10% solution over 10–20 min, followed by 1 g/h in 100 mL). The intramuscolar route is generally avoided because of pain, high volume of solution, and the risk of sterile abscess. In severely symptomatic patients oral magnesium administration should follow the initial iv calcium bolus.

Recurrence of symptoms of hypocalcemia may indicate the need to increase the rate of calcium infusion. The infusion should be continued until an effective regimen of oral calcium and activated vitamin D is reached (up to 24–48 h or longer) and subsequently slowly tapered.

There is a limited experience on the use of PTH molecules in PO-HypoCa. A small pilot study has shown potential benefits of recombinant human $PTH_{1\text{-}34}$ (teriparatide, 20 μg twice daily) added to calcium and calcitriol therapy, including rapid recovery of hypocalcemic symptoms and shorter duration of hospitalization [31].

Chronic Post-operative Hypocalcemia

Chronic PO-HypoCa is defined by the finding of persistence of hypocalcemia 6 months after thyroid surgery. Persistence of parathyroid insufficiency in patients who required treatment in the immediate postoperative period can be assessed, once attained a stable correction of hypocalcemia, by monitoring serum calcium while progressively (weekly) reducing the treatment with calcium and activated vitamin D. Chronic PO-HypoCa is the most common form of hypoparathyroidism (HypoPT).

The rate of PO-HypoCa ranges between 6.9 to 46%. A large prospective study has shown that about 60–70% of patients recover normal parathyroid function within 4–6 weeks after thyroidectomy (transient PO-HypoCa); the remaining will require continued treatment for additional time (protracted PO-HypoCa), and about 15–20% of them will develop permanent/chronic PO-HypoCa. Thus, the rate of chronic PO-HypoCa ranged between 0.3 and 3.7%, data which are in agreement with those reported by a recent review and meta-analysis [21].

Patients with chronic PO-HypoCa complain of fatigue, tingling fingers and feet, cramping in the hands and feet, "brain fog", numbness around the mouth, muscle cramps and other symptoms, resulting in a lower quality of life (QoL). Because of permanent HypoPT and the inability to reabsorb filtered calcium at the tubular level, patients are prone to develop hypercalciuria, kidney stones, nephrocalcinosis and decreased renal function.

Goals of Management

The goal of therapy of patients with chronic PO-HypoCa is to maintain serum calcium in the low-normal range, control hypocalcemic symptoms, avoid long-term complications and improve the QoL (Table 16.2). Individualized management is necessary and strongly recommended to optimize patient care. Guidelines for the management of chronic PO-HypoCa have only recently developer by the European Society of Endocrinology (ESE) [32], the American Association of Clinical Endocrinologists and the American College of Endocrinology [33], and a panel of international experts [29].

No data are available to define the optimal serum calcium levels during management of chronic PO-HypoCa. According to the ESE guidelines the target serum calcium concentration should be within the lower half of normal range [8.4–9.2 mg/dL (2.1–2.3 mmol/L)], or even slightly below the lower limit, while the patient has no symptoms or signs of hypocalcemia. Maintenance of serum calcium at this target values may help to decrease calcium excretion and avoid the risk of hypercalciuria [34]. Some patients may need higher serum calcium levels to be asymptomatic.

Table 16.2 Goal of therapy of chronic post-operative hypocalcemia

• Improve/eliminate symptoms of hypocalcemia
• Improve the quality of life
• Maintain fasting serum calcium slightly below or at the lower limit of normal range
• Avoid or reduce hypercalciuria
• Maintain serum phosphate in the normal range or slightly above
• Maintain the calcium-phosphate product below 55 mg^2/dl^2 (4.4 $mmol^2/l^2$) to avoid ectopic calcification
• Assure an adequate vitamin D status

Hypercalciuria is a common feature of chronic PO-HypoCa because of the lack of PTH-dependent renal tubular reabsorption of calcium. Hypercalciuria is a risk factor for kidney stones in the general population. Patients with chronic PO-HypoCa have an increased risk of nephrolithiasis, but no data exist to prove whether there is an association with the degree of hypercalciuria [35, 36]. Since it is likely that even in these patients hypercalciuria may increase the risk of nephrolithiasis, 24-h urinary calcium excretion should be maintained in the sex-specific range: <250 mg (6.25 mmol) in women or <300 mg (7.5 mmol) in men or <4 mg (0.1 mmol)/kg body weight in both sexes.

Serum phosphate may be relatively high in patients with PO-HypoCa, because of the lack of the phosphaturic effect of PTH and the increased intestinal phosphate absorption caused by vitamin D treatment [2, 8, 37]. The calcium-phosphate product may be higher than normal and may be responsible of extra-skeletal calcifications, particularly nephrocalcinosis. Thus serum phosphate should be maintained in the normal range, or slightly above, and the calcium-phosphate product below 55 mg^2/dL^2 (4.4 $mmol^2/L^2$) [38].

Magnesium has an important role in the control of PTH secretion and action. Low serum levels of magnesium may reduce the residual function of the parathyroid [39], and cause symptoms similar to those of hypocalcemia. Therefore, serum magnesium should be maintained in the normal range.

A low vitamin D status, as evaluated by measurement of serum 25(OH)D levels, is rather common in the general population, as well as in patients with chronic PO-HypoCa and severe vitamin D deficiency may be associated with muscle dysfunction, a common complain of patients with chronic PO-HypoCa [40]. Administration of activated vitamin D does not influence serum 25(OH) D levels, and therefore, vitamin D supplementation should be considered in patients with hypovitaminosis D, aiming to attain a serum level of 25(OH)D >20 ng/mL (50 nmol/L), and, according to the guidelines of the Endocrine Society, preferably >30 ng/mL (75 nml/L) [41].

Treatment should be personalized to possibly reach the above biochemical targets and, at the same time, a reasonably good overall well-being and QoL. However, since there is no evidence that reaching these goals guarantees long-term benefits to the patients, therapeutic effort with an immediate negative effect on well-being and QoL should be avoided [32].

Conventional Therapy

Once the diagnosis of chronic PO-HypoCa has been confirmed, conventional therapy consists of the administration of oral calcium and activated vitamin D.

Calcium

An adequate calcium intake from dietary sources (mainly dairy products) is advisable, but calcium supplements are often needed to reach the commonly used total daily amount of 1–3 g (sometimes a higher amount may be necessary).

Calcium carbonate (40% elemental calcium: 1 g calcium carbonate contains 600 mg elemental calcium) and calcium citrate (21% elemental calcium: 1 g calcium citrate contains 210 mg elemental calcium) are the most commonly used form of calcium supplementation. Calcium carbonate is preferable because it is more cost-effective and fewer pills per day are needed [42]. Calcium carbonate requires an acidic gastric environment to be absorbed and should be taken with meals. Thus, its bioavailability is reduced in patients with atrophic gastritis or taking proton pump inhibitors. In these circumstances, calcium citrate, which is well absorbed independent of meal and acid environments, should be preferred, where available. Calcium citrate might also be a preferred option for patients who complain of gastrointestinal side effects using calcium carbonate or who prefer to take calcium supplements outside mealtimes [43]. Other forms of calcium (glucobionate, gluconate and lactate, containing lower amount of elemental calcium (6.6, 9, and 13%, respectively)) are not practical oral supplements [29, 30, 43].

The daily amount of calcium supplementation varies among patients. A daily amount of 1–3 g is most commonly used. Since the absorptive gastric capacity is likely saturated with an intake of about 500 mg of calcium in a single ingestion, the use of a higher amount in a single dose should be possibly avoided [43]. A high intake of calcium may lower the dose of vitamin D needed to maintain the optimized serum calcium concentration. On the other hand, by binding to phosphate oral calcium may decrease phosphate absorption and help to lower serum phosphate concentration [44].

Calcium carbonate and calcium citrate interfere with levothyroxine absorption [45]; therefore patients should be advised to take levothyroxine well apart from calcium supplements.

Vitamin D and Its Activated Forms

Activated vitamin D metabolites stimulates intestinal calcium and phosphate absorption and bone remodeling. PTH stimulates renal 1α-hydroxylation of 25(OH)D and the formation of calcitriol. Patients with chronic PO-HypoCa, because of the lack of PTH, have impaired activation of vitamin D.

Prior to the availability of synthetic activated vitamin D, supraphysiological doses of either cholecalciferol (vitamin D_3) or ergocalciferol (vitamin D_2) were used in the management of patients with chronic PO-HypoCa. High doses (25,000 200,000 IU daily) were needed to maintain normocalcemia. Nowadays, activated vitamin D is most commonly used because of the rapid onset and offset of action (Table 16.1). Either calcitriol or alfacalcidiol can be used. They have similar time of onset (1–2 days), but alfacalcidiol has a longer time of offset (5–7 vs 2–3 days). Calcitriol is almost twice as potent as compared to alfacalcidiol in term of the calcemic effect. The initial daily dose needs to be titrated in order to individualize the dosage to keep serum calcium within the target range. The daily dose of calcitriol ranges between 0.25 and 2.0 μg, equal to 0.5–4 μg of alfacalcidiol.

In some countries another activated vitamin D compound, dihydrotachysterol, may also still used. The time to onset and offset of action are 4–7 days and 7–21 days, respectively [46, 47]. Severe hypercalcemia has been reported in a few cases [47].

Where activated vitamin D is not available or to expensive large doses of parent vitamin D can still be used in the management of chronic PO/HypoCa. The half-life of parent vitamin D ranges between 2 and 3 weeks. Particular attention should be paid to the risk of vitamin D toxicity. Serum levels of 25(OH)D should be within the normal range. As in other metabolic bone diseases, levels above 30 ng/mL (75 nmol/L) could be appropriate [41].

As mentioned before, vitamin D deficient patients should be supplemented with vitamin D_2 or D_3 since active vitamin D analogs does not correct hypovitaminosis D.

Optimization of Therapy

Once the target level of serum calcium is reached and the patient is free of symptoms of hypocalcemia, optimization of secondary targets should be considered.

If hypercalciuria is present, it is reasonable to attempt normalizing 24 h urinary calcium excretion, even though no data are available on whether increased urinary calcium excretion in this clinical setting is associated with renal complications. In normal subjects urinary calcium excretion is dependent upon sodium and calcium intake [48]. Therefore, sodium intake should be reduced and, if patients are given large amounts of calcium supplements, the daily dose of activated vitamin D can be increased while decreasing calcium supplements. If the above measures are not sufficient, a thiazide diuretic, that decreases renal calcium excretion, may be considered. The consequent calcium-spearing effect may allow a reduction in the daily calcium supplements. The combination of thiazide with amiloride may further lower urinary calcium excretion and decrease the risk of hypokalemia. In addition, amiloride may reduce urinary magnesium losses [49]. The administration of a thiazide diuretic should be associated with a low-sodium diet. The effect of thiazides is dose-dependent and relatively high doses (50 mg hydrochlorothiazide or 5 mg bendroflumethaizide, twice daily) are required to lower urinary calcium excretion. Chlortalidone and indapamide, thiazide-like diuretics, can also be used and given once daily, because their action lasts longer.

Activated vitamin D stimulates intestinal absorption of phosphate, which may cause hyperphosphatemia and increase the calcium-phosphate product. If hyperphosphatemia is present the intake of phosphate-rich foods should be reduced. In addition, as calcium binds phosphate, increasing the daily dose of calcium supplements may lower the intestinal absorption of phosphate and, at the same time, the requirements of the daily dose of activated vitamin D. If this strategy is adopted, it is advised to measure 24 h-urinary calcium to ensure that it is not abnormally elevated. Finally, phosphate binders can also be considered in troublesome cases.

If serum levels of magnesium are low, magnesium supplements or amiloride may be considered [50]. In chronic hypomagnesemia, a magnesium infusion test (0.5 mmol/kg body weight in 500 mL saline over 6 hours) may be of help in demonstrating intracellular magnesium depletion (24-h urinary magnesium excretion <50% of the infused amount), and, at the same time, treat magnesium deficiency [51].

Monitoring

In patients with PO-HypoCa weekly measurement of serum calcium and phosphate should be performed after surgery until a stable regimen of oral calcium and activated vitamin D supplementation is established. Subsequently, the supplement doses should be gradually tapered while serum calcium and phosphorus are monitored and treatment eventually withdraw if normocalcemia is maintained.

Lifelong monitoring is needed in patients with chronic PO-HypoCa. No study has evaluated how to best monitor these patients. Individualized management is necessary and strongly recommended to optimize patient care. As mentioned before, the target serum calcium concentration is within the low-normal range, with no symptoms of hypocalcemia. However some patients need to have higher serum calcium levels to be symptom-free. A baseline renal imaging has been recommended [52]. The recently published ESE guidelines suggest measuring every 3–6 months biochemical parameters (ionized or albumin-corrected total calcium, magnesium, creatinine (eGFR) and 24-h urinary calcium) and performing renal imaging when patients have symptoms of nephrolithiasis or increasing serum levels of creatinine [32] (Fig. 16.2). When changing the daily dose of calcium or activated vitamin D or introducing a new drug biochemical monitoring should be performed weekly or every other week. Patients should be educated to recognize symptoms of hypo- or hypercalcemia and complications associated with long-term conventional therapy [35, 53]. It is important to note that serum calcium may fluctuate once the therapeutic regimen has been stabilized and may become unstable in several conditions. Indeed, several drugs and conditions may interfere with calcium homeostasis (Table 16.3) and, therefore, patients should be periodically asked whether they are taking new drugs or experiencing gastrointestinal disorders or immobilization.

Long-term Outcomes and Complications

Conventional therapy does not fully restore calcium homeostasis and recent studies have shown that patients do not recover a complete well-being and suffer of several complications. Low QoL, including "bran fog", fatigue, muscle weakness, neuropsychological complaints, have been reported [54–57]. The use of large amount of calcium and activated vitamin D is associated with insidious complications that may become manifest after decades. A chart review study of a large cohort of patients with hypoparathyroidism has shown an increased risk hypercalciuria, nephrocalcinosis, nephrolithiasis and reduction of glomerular filtration rate, which was severe enough to require kidney transplantation in two cases [35]. Moreover, a large cohort study performed in Denmark has also shown an increased risk of renal comorbidieties, neuropsychiatric complications, infections, and seizures [36] (Table 16.4). Bone mineral content is increased in patients with chronic PO-HypoCa, but cancellous bone microarchitecture is abnormal [58].

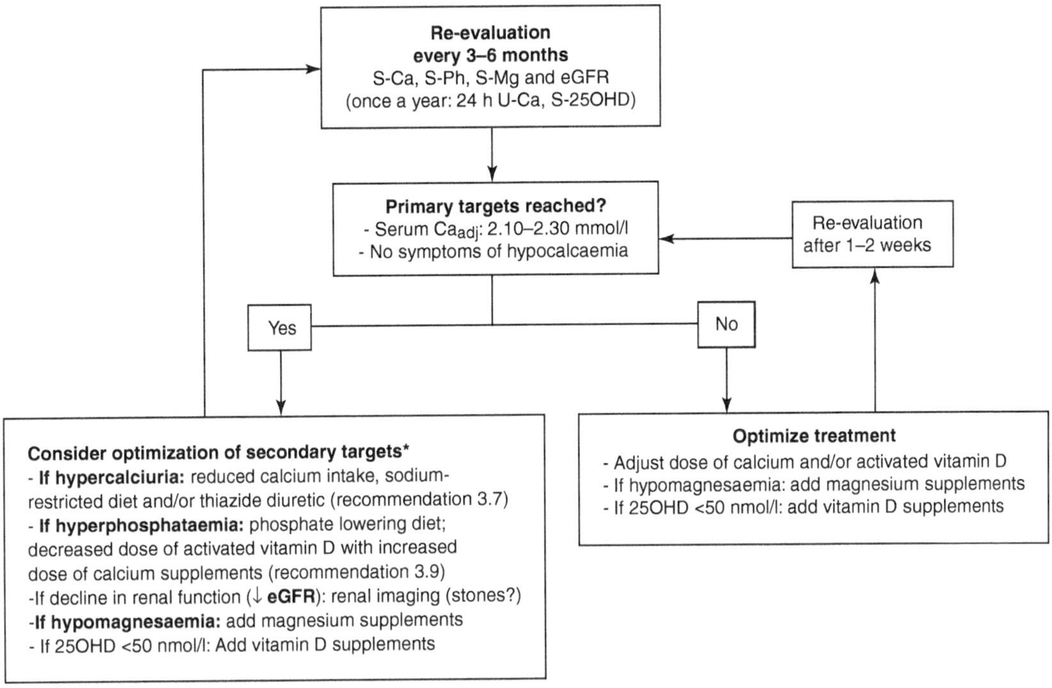

Fig. 16.2 Treatment and monitoring of chronic post-operative hypoparathyroidism. When the primary target has not been reached, the dose of calcium and vitamin D should be adjusted, hypomagnesemia, if present corrected, and vitamin D supplementation considered when needed. When the primary target is reached optimization of therapy is based upon interventions aimed to eventually correct hypercalciuria, hyperphosphatemia, hypomagnesemia and a low vitamin D status. Patients should be re-evaluated every 3–6 month for the risk of chronic complications. (Asterisk) when the dose of oral calcium or active vitamin D is modified serum calcium should be checked after 1–2 weeks (from Bollerslew et al. [32], with permission)

Parathyroid Hormone

Until recently, HypoPT was the only major hormonal insufficiency state not treated with the missing hormone. Almost 90 years ago Fuller Albrigth showed that bovine parathyroid extracts were able abolish symptoms of hypocalcemia, but this therapeutic approach was no further developed because of the occurrence of neutralizing antibodies. Over the last two decades the development of the recombinant human N-terminal, active part of PTH (rhPTH$_{1-34}$, teriparatide) and the full-length recombinant human 1–84 molecule (rhPTH$_{1-84}$) has promoted several studies, which have unshared a new era in the management of this disease. In January 2015 the Food and Drug Administration has approved the use of rhPTH$_{1-84}$ for the management of patients with HypoPT [59] and the European Medical Agency (EMA) has granted a conditional marketing authorisation in the European Union [60].

rhPTH$_{1-34}$

In the studies by Winer et al. subcutaneous injections of rh PTH$_{1-34}$ twice daily were shown to restore normocalcemia and normalize urinary calcium excretion in adults and children, and to be superior when compared to conventional therapy [61, 62]. In most recent studies the administration of rhPTH$_{1-34}$ using a pump delivery system was shown to be superior to the twice-daily injections, in maintaining stable serum calcium levels and avoiding the transient rise in serum calcium that follows the injection [63, 64]. Moreover, urinary calcium was markedly reduced and markers of bone turnover normalized The therapeutic use of rhPTH1-34 in the management of HypoPT has not been further developed.

rh PTH$_{1-84}$

The rational of using the full-length rhPTH$_{1-84}$ is that the native hormone and that the C-terminal part of the molecule may affect additional, yet not well characterized, signaling pathways [65].

Table 16.3 Drug therapy and diseases that may interfere with calcium homeostasis and necessitate changes in therapy and monitoring in patients with chronic post-operative hypocalcemia

Drug/disease	Mechanism	Possible adverse effects in hypoparathyroidism	Action
Loop diuretics	Increased urinary calcium losses	May aggravate hypercalciuria and lower serum calcium levels	Avoid if possible
Thiazide diuretics	Decreased urinary calcium losses	May increase serum calcium levels	May be used in selected patient
Systemic glucocorticoids	Decreased intestinal calcium absorption and increased urinary calcium losses	May cause hypocalcemia	Avoid if possible
Antiresorptive drugs	Decreased bone turnover	May cause hypocalcemia	Rarely needed, as hypoparathyroidism is a state of (very) low bone turnover
Proton pump inhibitors	May cause hypomagnesemia	May lower serum calcium levels and cause symptoms similar to hypocalcemia	Avoid if possible—otherwise magnesium supplements as needed
Chemotherapy: Cisplatin, 5-Fluorouracil, Leucovorin	May cause hypomagnesemia	May lower serum calcium levels and cause symptoms similar to hypocalcemia	Magnesium supplements, as needed
Cardiac glycosides (e.g., digoxin)	Hypercalcemia may predispose to digoxin toxicity Hypocalcemia may reduce the efficacy of digoxin	Arrhythmias	Avoid if possible. If needed, close monitoring by a cardiologist
Diarrhea/gastrointestinal disease	May reduce intestinal absorption of calcium and vitamin D	May cause hypocalcemia	Close monitoring of serum calcium levels with dose adjustments as needed
Changes in (correction of) acid-base balance[a]	The affinity of calcium binding to albumin is pH-dependent (acidosis decreases and alkalosis increased the affinity)	Correction of metabolic acidosis may cause hypocalcemia Correction of metabolic alkalosis may cause hypercalcemia	
Immobilization	Increased bone resorption. In healthy individuals, PTH and 1,25-dihydroxyvitamin D levels are suppressed	May cause hypercalcemia	

[a]Changes in the free (ionized) fraction of serum calcium (Ca^{2+}) cannot be monitored by measuring total calcium levels. Many laboratories report serum Ca^{2+} levels adjusted to a neutral pH value (pH 7.4), which does not reflect the actual serum Ca^{2+} level in a patient with disturbances in acid-base balance. If so, patients may have symptoms despite (apparently) normal calcium levels and Ca^{2+} levels at actual pH should be requested (from Bollerslew et al. [32], with permission, with minor modifications)

Following initial studies, which showed that daily or alternate daily subcutaneous injection of $rhPTH_{1\text{-}84}$ could maintain serum calcium while reducing the need for oral calcium and activated vitamin D supplementation [66, 67], the efficacy and safety of this molecule in the management of chronic HypoPT has been evaluated in Denmark and USA [68, 69].

In 2013 a phase III multicenter, placebo-controlled, double-blind trial (REPLACE) was reported [70]. This study enrolled 134 patients with HypoPT chronically treated with oral

Table 16.4 Comorbidities occurring with an increased prevalence in patients with PO-HypoCa[a]

Organ system	Typical daily dose
Renal	Renal stones
	Nephrocalcinosis
	Impaired renal function
Immunological	Infections
Neuropsychiatric	Neuropsychiatric diseases
	Seizures
	Impaired quality of life
Musculoskeletal	Muscle stiffness/pain

[a]From Bollerslew et al. [32], with permission, with minor modifications)

calcium and activated vitamin D supplements. After a run-in period, in which treatment was adjusted to obtain a stable albumin-corrected serum calcium, patients were randomized (2:1) to receive subcutaneous injections of $rhPTH_{1\text{-}84}$ (50 μg daily) or placebo. Treatment with calcium and activated vitamin D was eventually reduced or even withdrawn, while during the first 5 weeks, the daily dose of $rhPTH_{1\text{-}84}$ could be titrated to 75 or 100 μg. The primary endpoint of the study was the proportion of patients who, at week 24, achieved a 50% or greater reduction of the daily dose of oral calcium and activated vitamin D, while maintaining a serum calcium concentration within the normal range [70]. In the majority (52%) of patients the daily dose of $rhPTH_{1\text{-}84}$ was 100 μg. About half the patients (48; 53%) assigned to $rhPTH_{1\text{-}84}$ met the primary endpoint while this occurred only in one (2%) of those assigned to placebo. Activated vitamin D supplements could be eliminated, while the daily dose of calcium was not greater than 500 mg, in 43% of patients given $rhPTH_{1\text{-}84}$ compared to 5% of those receiving placebo. The rate of adverse events, mostly symptoms related to hypocalcemia, was similar in the two groups. These advantaged of $rhPTH_{1\text{-}84}$ therapy was confirmed in a long term continuous therapy up to 6 years [68]. In addition treatment with $rhPTH_{1\text{-}84}$ increased the bone remodeling rate and improved trabecular bone architecture [71, 72]. Contradictory results have been reported on the effects of $rhPTH_{1\text{-}84}$ therapy on QoL, which is reduced in patients with chronic hypoPT [55, 57]. In a short-term study (6 months) no beneficial effects were shown [57], whereas improvement was demonstrated in a long-term study up to 5 years [55].

The official recommendation is to consider of $rhPTH_{1\text{-}84}$ therapy *"only in patients who cannot be well-controlled on calcium and active forms of vitamin D and for whom the potential benefits are considered to outweigh the potential risk"* [59]. $rhPTH_{1\text{-}84}$ therapy should be started with the subcutaneous administration in the thigh of 50 ug once daily and, at the time, the daily dose of activated vitamin D should be decreased by 50% if serum calcium is above 7.5 mg/dL [59]. Serum calcium should be checked every 3–7 days and the daily dose of $rhPTH_{1\text{-}84}$ titrated every four weeks with the goal of discontinuing active vitamin D therapy and reducing the daily calcium supplements at 500 mg, while the serum calcium be maintained in the low-normal range. Once a stable regimen of therapy has been obtained serum calcium should be monitored every 3–6 months. Hypercalcemia has been reported in some cases [59, 73], but a careful adjustment of the daily dose may decrease this risk. A "black box" in the official recommendation highlights the potential risk of osteosarcoma because of the data showing that both $rhPTH_{1\text{-}34}$ and $rhPTH_{1\text{-}84}$ can cause osterosarcoma in the rats [74, 75]. However, current evidences do not indicate that human subjects treated with either PTH molecules are at increased risk of osteosarcoma [76]. Finally, the *"safety and efficacy in pediatric patients have not been established"*.

The recommendation for the use of $rhPTH_{1\text{-}84}$ leaves wide room to define the patient with HypoPT who is not "well-controlled" with conventional therapy. The Guidelines recently elaborated by a panel of international experts provide a guidance to be followed for considering $rhPTH_{1\text{-}84}$ therapy, where available, in any patient with chronic HypoPT, except patients with autosomal dominant hypocalcemia, a condition due to autosomal dominant mutations of the calcium-sensing receptor [29, 77].

Pregnancy and Lactation

There are limited data to inform treatment strategies in chronic HypoPT in pregnancy and lactation. The ESE Guidelines suggest the use of oral calcium and activated vitamin D as in non-pregnant women and frequent monitoring (every 2–3 weeks) of serum calcium, possibly ionized calcium [32]. A large series including 12 pregnant women reported an overall safety of oral calcium and calcitriol [78]. No studies have addressed the use of $rhPTH_{1\text{-}84}$ therapy in pregnant women and therefore should be used *"only if the potential benefit justifies the potential risk to the fetus"*.

References

1. Marcocci C, Cianferotti L. Postoperative complications-the parathyroids. In: Miccoli P, Davies T, Minuto M, Seybt M, editors. Thyroid surgery preventing and managing complications. 2nd ed. Oxford: Wiley-Blackwell; 2013. p. 227–36.
2. Shoback D. Clinical practice. Hypoparathyroidism. N Engl J Med. 2008;359(4):391–403.
3. Lorente-Poch L, Sancho JJ, Ruiz S, Sitges-Serra A. Importance of in situ preservation of parathyroid glands during total thyroidectomy. Br J Surg. 2015;102(4):359–67.
4. Miccoli P, CE A. Surgical hypoparathyroidism. In: Bilezikian J, editor. The parathyroids basic and clinical concepts. 3rd ed. London: Academic; 2015. p. 737–44.
5. Chen Y, Masiakos PT, Gaz RD, Hodin RA, Parangi S, Randolph GW, et al. Pediatric thyroidectomy in a high volume thyroid surgery center: risk factors for postoperative hypocalcemia. J Pediatr Surg. 2015;50(8):1316–9.
6. Paek SH, Lee YM, Min SY, Kim SW, Chung KW, Youn YK. Risk factors of hypoparathyroidism following total thyroidectomy for thyroid cancer. World J Surg. 2013;37(1):94–101.
7. Puzziello A, Rosato L, Innaro N, Orlando G, Avenia N, Perigli G, et al. Hypocalcemia following thyroid surgery: incidence and risk factors. A longitudinal multicenter study comprising 2,631 patients. Endocrine. 2014;47(2):537–42.
8. Bilezikian JP, Khan A, Potts JT Jr, Brandi ML, Clarke BL, Shoback D, et al. Hypoparathyroidism in the adult: epidemiology, diagnosis, pathophysiology, target-organ involvement, treatment, and challenges for future research. J Bone Miner Res. 2011;26(10):2317–37.
9. Snyder SK, Hamid KS, Roberson CR, Rai SS, Bossen AC, Luh JH, et al. Outpatient thyroidectomy is safe and reasonable: experience with more than 1,000 planned outpatient procedures. J Am Coll Surg. 2010;210(5):575–82.
10. Terris DJ, Snyder S, Carneiro-Pla D, Inabnet WB, Kandil E, Orloff L, et al. American Thyroid Association statement on outpatient thyroidectomy. Thyroid. 2013;23(10):1193–202.
11. Hermann M, Ott J, Promberger R, Kober F, Karik M, Freissmuth M. Kinetics of serum parathyroid hormone during and after thyroid surgery. Br J Surg. 2008;95(12):1480–7.
12. Thomusch O, Machens A, Sekulla C, Ukkat J, Brauckhoff M, Dralle H. The impact of surgical technique on postoperative hypoparathyroidism in bilateral thyroid surgery: a multivariate analysis of 5846 consecutive patients. Surgery. 2003;133(2):180–5.
13. Griffin TP, Murphy MS, Sheahan P. Vitamin D and risk of postoperative hypocalcemia after total thyroidectomy. JAMA Otolaryngol Head Neck Surg. 2014;140(4):346–51.
14. Kannan S, Mahadevan S, Velayutham P, Bharath R, Kumaravel V, Muthukumaran J, et al. Estimation of magnesium in patients with functional hypoparathyroidism. Ind J Endocrinol Metabol. 2014;18(6):821–5.
15. Wilson RB, Erskine C, Crowe PJ. Hypomagnesemia and hypocalcemia after thyroidectomy: prospective study. World J Surg. 2000;24(6):722–6.
16. Sanabria A, Dominguez LC, Vega V, Osorio C, Duarte D. Routine postoperative administration of vitamin D and calcium after total thyroidectomy: a meta-analysis. Int J Surg. 2011;9(1):46–51.
17. Tartaglia F, Giuliani A, Sgueglia M, Biancari F, Juvonen T, Campana FP. Randomized study on oral administration of calcitriol to prevent symptomatic hypocalcemia after total thyroidectomy. Am J Surg. 2005;190(3):424–9.
18. Lo CY, Lam KY. Parathyroid autotransplantation during thyroidectomy: is frozen section necessary? Arch Surg. 1999;134(3):258–60.
19. Olson JA Jr, DeBenedetti MK, Baumann DS, Wells SA Jr. Parathyroid autotransplantation during thyroidectomy. Results of long-term follow-up. Ann Surg. 1996;223(5):472–8. discussion 8–80
20. Promberger R, Ott J, Kober F, Mikola B, Karik M, Freissmuth M, et al. Intra- and postoperative parathyroid hormone-kinetics do not advocate for autotransplantation of discolored parathyroid glands during thyroidectomy. Thyroid. 2010;20(12):1371–5.
21. Edafe O, Antakia R, Laskar N, Uttley L, Balasubramanian SP. Systematic review and meta-analysis of predictors of post-thyroidectomy hypocalcaemia. Br J Surg. 2014;101(4):307–20.
22. Bentrem DJ, Rademaker A, Angelos P. Evaluation of serum calcium levels in predicting hypoparathyroidism after total/near-total thyroidectomy or parathyroidectomy. Am Surg. 2001;67(3):249–51. discussion 51–2
23. Nahas ZS, Farrag TY, Lin FR, Belin RM, Tufano RP. A safe and cost-effective short hospital stay protocol to identify patients at low risk for the development of significant hypocalcemia after total thyroidectomy. Laryngoscope. 2006;116(6):906–10.

24. Asari R, Passler C, Kaczirek K, Scheuba C, Niederle B. Hypoparathyroidism after total thyroidectomy: a prospective study. Arch Surg. 2008;143(2):132–7. discussion 8
25. Lee DR, Hinson AM, Siegel ER, Steelman SC, Bodenner DL, Stack BC Jr. Comparison of intraoperative versus postoperative parathyroid hormone levels to predict hypocalcemia earlier after total thyroidectomy. Otolaryngol Head Neck Surg. 2015;153(3):343–9.
26. Grodski S, Serpell J. Evidence for the role of perioperative PTH measurement after total thyroidectomy as a predictor of hypocalcemia. World J Surg. 2008;32(7):1367–73.
27. Raffaelli M, De Crea C, Carrozza C, D'Amato G, Zuppi C, Bellantone R, et al. Combining early postoperative parathyroid hormone and serum calcium levels allows for an efficacious selective post-thyroidectomy supplementation treatment. World J Surg. 2012;36(6):1307–13.
28. Cooper MS, Gittoes NJ. Diagnosis and management of hypocalcaemia. BMJ. 2008;336(7656):1298–302.
29. Bilezikian JP, Brandi ML, Cusano NE, Mannstadt M, Rejnmark L, Rizzoli R, et al. Management of Hypoparathyroidism: present and future. J Clin Endocrinol Metab. 2016;101(6):2313–24.
30. Walker Harris V, Jan De Beur S. Postoperative hypoparathyroidism: medical and surgical therapeutic options. Thyroid. 2009;19(9):967–73.
31. Shah M, Bancos I, Thompson GB, Richards ML, Kasperbauer JL, Clarke BL, et al. Teriparatide therapy and reduced postoperative hospitalization for postsurgical hypoparathyroidism. JAMA Otolaryngol Head Neck Surg. 2015;141(9):822–7.
32. Bollerslev J, Rejnmark L, Marcocci C, Shoback DM, Sitges-Serra A, van Biesen W, et al. European Society of Endocrinology Clinical Guideline: treatment of chronic hypoparathyroidism in adults. Eur J Endocrinol. 2015;173(2):G1–20.
33. Stack BC Jr, Bimston DN, Bodenner DL, Brett EM, Dralle H, Orloff LA, et al. American association of clinical endocrinologists and American college of endocrinology disease state clinical review: postoperative hypoparathyroidism--definitions and management. Endocr Pract. 2015;21(6):674–85.
34. Rathod A, Bonny O, Guessous I, Suter PM, Conen D, Erne P, et al. Association of urinary calcium excretion with serum calcium and vitamin D levels. Clin J Am Soc Nephrol. 2015;10(3):452–62.
35. Mitchell DM, Regan S, Cooley MR, Lauter KB, Vrla MC, Becker CB, et al. Long-term follow-up of patients with hypoparathyroidism. J Clin Endocrinol Metab. 2012;97(12):4507–14.
36. Underbjerg L, Sikjaer T, Mosekilde L, Rejnmark L. The epidemiology of nonsurgical hypoparathyroidism in Denmark: a nationwide case finding study. J Bone Miner Res. 2015;30(9):1738–44.
37. Khan MI, Waguespack SG, Hu MI. Medical management of postsurgical hypoparathyroidism. Endocr Pract. 2011;17(Suppl 1):18–25.
38. Caudarella R, Vescini F, Buffa A, Francucci CM. Hyperphosphatemia: effects on bone metabolism and cardiovascular risk. J Endocrinol Investig. 2007;30(6 Suppl):29–34.
39. Rodriguez-Ortiz ME, Canalejo A, Herencia C, Martinez-Moreno JM, Peralta-Ramirez A, Perez-Martinez P, et al. Magnesium modulates parathyroid hormone secretion and upregulates parathyroid receptor expression at moderately low calcium concentration. Nephrol Dial Transplant. 2014;29(2):282–9.
40. Autier P, Boniol M, Pizot C, Mullie P. Vitamin D status and ill health: a systematic review. Lancet Diabetes Endocrinol. 2014;2(1):76–89.
41. Holick MF, Binkley NC, Bischoff-Ferrari HA, Gordon CM, Hanley DA, Heaney RP, et al. Evaluation, treatment, and prevention of vitamin D deficiency: an Endocrine Society clinical practice guideline. J Clin Endocrinol Metab. 2011;96(7):1911–30.
42. Heaney RP, Dowell MS, Bierman J, Hale CA, Bendich A. Absorbability and cost effectiveness in calcium supplementation. J Am Coll Nutr. 2001;20(3):239–46.
43. Straub DA. Calcium supplementation in clinical practice: a review of forms, doses, and indications. Nutr Clin Pract. 2007;22(3):286–96.
44. Malberti F. Hyperphosphataemia: treatment options. Drugs. 2013;73(7):673–88.
45. Zamfirescu I, Carlson HE. Absorption of levothyroxine when coadministered with various calcium formulations. Thyroid. 2011;21(5):483–6.
46. Kanis JA, Russell RG. Rate of reversal of hypercalcaemia and hypercalciuria induced by vitamin D and its 1alpha-hydroxylated derivatives. Br Med J. 1977;1(6053):78–81.
47. Quack I, Zwernemann C, Weiner SM, Sellin L, Henning BF, Waldherr R, et al. Dihydrotachysterol therapy for hypoparathyroidism: consequences of inadequate monitoring. Five cases and a review. Exp Clin Endocrinol Diabetes. 2005;113(7):376–80.
48. Porter RH, Cox BG, Heaney D, Hostetter TH, Stinebaugh BJ, Suki WN. Treatment of hypoparathyroid patients with chlorthalidone. N Engl J Med. 1978;298(11):577–81.
49. Murdoch DL, Forrest G, Davies DL, McInnes GT. A comparison of the potassium and magnesium-sparing properties of amiloride and spironolactone in diuretic-treated normal subjects. Br J Clin Pharmacol. 1993;35(4):373–8.
50. Dai LJ, Ritchie G, Kerstan D, Kang HS, Cole DE, Quamme GA. Magnesium transport in the renal distal convoluted tubule. Physiol Rev. 2001;81(1):51–84.
51. Fatemi S, Ryzen E, Flores J, Endres DB, Rude RK. Effect of experimental human magnesium depletion on parathyroid hormone secretion and 1,25-dihydroxyvitamin D metabolism. J Clin Endocrinol Metab. 1991;73(5):1067–72.
52. Boyce AM, Shawker TH, Hill SC, Choyke PL, Hill MC, James R, et al. Ultrasound is superior to computed tomography for assessment of medullary nephrocalcinosis in hypoparathyroidism. J Clin Endocrinol Metab. 2013;98(3):989–94.

53. Underbjerg L, Sikjaer T, Mosekilde L, Rejnmark L. Cardiovascular and renal complications to postsurgical hypoparathyroidism: a Danish nationwide controlled historic follow-up study. J Bone Miner Res. 2013;28(11):2277–85.
54. Arlt W, Fremerey C, Callies F, Reincke M, Schneider P, Timmermann W, et al. Well-being, mood and calcium homeostasis in patients with hypoparathyroidism receiving standard treatment with calcium and vitamin D. Eur J Endocrinol. 2002;146(2):215–22.
55. Cusano NE, Rubin MR, McMahon DJ, Irani D, Anderson L, Levy E, et al. PTH(1-84) is associated with improved quality of life in hypoparathyroidism through 5 years of therapy. J Clin Endocrinol Metab. 2014;99(10):3694–9.
56. Hadker N, Egan J, Sanders J, Lagast H, Clarke BL. Understanding the burden of illness associated with hypoparathyroidism reported among patients in the PARADOX study. Endocr Pract. 2014;20(7):671–9.
57. Sikjaer T, Rolighed L, Hess A, Fuglsang-Frederiksen A, Mosekilde L, Rejnmark L. Effects of PTH(1-84) therapy on muscle function and quality of life in hypoparathyroidism: results from a randomized controlled trial. Osteoporos Int. 2014;25(6):1717–26.
58. Shoback DM, Bilezikian JP, Costa AG, Dempster D, Dralle H, Khan AA, et al. Presentation of hypoparathyroidism: etiologies and clinical features. J Clin Endocrinol Metab. 2016;101(6):2300–12.
59. NATPARA [package insert]. Shire-NPS Pharmaceuticals, Inc. 2015. Available from: http://www.fda.gov/Drugs/.
60. European Medicines Agency (EMA). First hormone replacement therapy for parathyroid disorder. London; 2017.
61. Winer KK, Ko CW, Reynolds JC, Dowdy K, Keil M, Peterson D, et al. Long-term treatment of hypoparathyroidism: a randomized controlled study comparing parathyroid hormone-(1-34) versus calcitriol and calcium. J Clin Endocrinol Metab. 2003;88(9):4214–20.
62. Winer KK, Yanovski JA, Sarani B, Cutler GB Jr. A randomized, cross-over trial of once-daily versus twice-daily parathyroid hormone 1-34 in treatment of hypoparathyroidism. J Clin Endocrinol Metab. 1998;83(10):3480–6.
63. Winer KK, Fulton KA, Albert PS, Cutler GB Jr. Effects of pump versus twice-daily injection delivery of synthetic parathyroid hormone 1-34 in children with severe congenital hypoparathyroidism. J Pediatr. 2014;165(3):556–63.e1.
64. Winer KK, Zhang B, Shrader JA, Peterson D, Smith M, Albert PS, et al. Synthetic human parathyroid hormone 1-34 replacement therapy: a randomized crossover trial comparing pump versus injections in the treatment of chronic hypoparathyroidism. J Clin Endocrinol Metab. 2012;97(2):391–9.
65. Cupp ME, Nayak SK, Adem AS, Thomsen WJ. Parathyroid hormone (PTH) and PTH-related peptide domains contributing to activation of different PTH receptor-mediated signaling pathways. J Pharmacol Exp Ther. 2013;345(3):404–18.
66. Rubin MR, Sliney J Jr, McMahon DJ, Silverberg SJ, Bilezikian JP. Therapy of hypoparathyroidism with intact parathyroid hormone. Osteoporos Int. 2010;21(11):1927–34.
67. Sikjaer T, Rejnmark L, Rolighed L, Heickendorff L, Mosekilde L, Hypoparathyroid Study G. The effect of adding PTH(1-84) to conventional treatment of hypoparathyroidism: a randomized, placebo-controlled study. J Bone Miner Res. 2011;26(10):2358–70.
68. Rubin MR, Cusano NE, Fan WW, Delgado Y, Zhang C, Costa AG, et al. Therapy of hypoparathyroidism with PTH(1-84): a prospective six year investigation of efficacy and safety. J Clin Endocrinol Metab. 2016;101(7):2742–50.
69. Sikjaer T, Amstrup AK, Rolighed L, Kjaer SG, Mosekilde L, Rejnmark L. PTH(1-84) replacement therapy in hypoparathyroidism: a randomized controlled trial on pharmacokinetic and dynamic effects after 6 months of treatment. J Bone Miner Res. 2013;28(10):2232–43.
70. Mannstadt M, Clarke BL, Vokes T, Brandi ML, Ranganath L, Fraser WD, et al. Efficacy and safety of recombinant human parathyroid hormone (1-84) in hypoparathyroidism (REPLACE): a double-blind, placebo-controlled, randomised, phase 3 study. Lancet Diabetes Endocrinol. 2013;1(4):275–83.
71. Cipriani C, Abraham A, Silva BC, Cusano NE, Rubin MR, McMahon DJ, et al. Skeletal changes after restoration of the euparathyroid state in patients with hypoparathyroidism and primary hyperparathyroidism. Endocrine. 2017;55(2):591–8.
72. Silva BC, Rubin MR, Cusano NE, Bilezikian JP. Bone imaging in hypoparathyroidism. Osteoporos Int. 2017;28(2):463–71.
73. Cusano NE, Rubin MR, McMahon DJ, Zhang C, Ives R, Tulley A, et al. Therapy of hypoparathyroidism with PTH(1-84): a prospective four-year investigation of efficacy and safety. J Clin Endocrinol Metab. 2013;98(1):137–44.
74. Jolette J, Wilker CE, Smith SY, Doyle N, Hardisty JF, Metcalfe AJ, et al. Defining a noncarcinogenic dose of recombinant human parathyroid hormone 1-84 in a 2-year study in Fischer 344 rats. Toxicol Pathol. 2006;34(7):929–40.
75. Vahle JL, Sato M, Long GG, Young JK, Francis PC, Engelhardt JA, et al. Skeletal changes in rats given daily subcutaneous injections of recombinant human parathyroid hormone (1-34) for 2 years and relevance to human safety. Toxicol Pathol. 2002;30(3):312–21.
76. Cipriani C, Irani D, Bilezikian JP. Safety of osteoanabolic therapy: a decade of experience. J Bone Miner Res. 2012;27(12):2419–28.
77. Brandi ML, Bilezikian JP, Shoback D, Bouillon R, Clarke BL, Thakker RV, et al. Management of Hypoparathyroidism: summary statement and guidelines. J Clin Endocrinol Metab. 2016;101(6):2273–83.
78. Callies F, Arlt W, Scholz HJ, Reincke M, Allolio B. Management of hypoparathyroidism during pregnancy--report of twelve cases. Eur J Endocrinol. 1998;139(3):284–9.

17 Radioiodine Refractory Thyroid Cancer

Amandine Berdelou, Sophie Leboulleux, and Martin Schlumberger

Introduction

Radioiodine refractory thyroid cancer is uncommon, with an estimated incidence of 4 to 5 cases per million population [1, 2]. It occurs more frequently in older patients, in those with poorly differentiated thyroid cancer, in those with large metastases, and in those with high FDG uptake on PET scan [3–6].

In the absence of effective treatment modalities, patients with advanced refractory disease have a median survival rate of 3–6 years and a 10 year survival rate of only 10% [3]. In recent years, major therapeutic progresses have been achieved.

In accordance with the American Thyroid Association guidelines [7], we propose a definition for refractory thyroid cancer, and the criteria to be used in those patients for considering a treatment with kinase inhibitors. Then, data obtained in these patients during treatment with kinase inhibitors are reviewed.

Definition of Refractory Thyroid Cancer

Radioiodine (RAI) treatment is the first line systemic treatment in patients with advanced disease. Efficacy of ^{131}I treatment is assessed by functional parameters (serum Thyroglobulin (Tg) level and quantitative ^{131}I uptake in metastases on post-therapy whole body scan (WBS)) and by tumor volume on anatomical imaging with CT scan and MRI. Favorable responses are characterized by parallel decreases in tumor volume and in functional parameters. In contrast, a decrease in ^{131}I uptake without a parallel decrease in tumor volume denotes the destruction of differentiated cells with high uptake and the persistence of less differentiated cells that are likely to progress. Indeed, the practitioner should ascertain that decreased RAI uptake is not due to iodine contamination or to insufficient TSH stimulation.

A cure is frequently achieved with RAI treatments in young patients with small metastases from well-differentiated thyroid cancer who have high RAI uptake in neoplastic foci. These patients represent about one third of all patients with an advanced disease. In the other two thirds, partial response and long-term stabilization may be obtained, but cure is rarely achieved [3]. In these patients with advanced disease, it is important to recognize when RAI treatment is no longer beneficial in order to avoid unnecessary treatments. At that point, the disease is considered RAI-refractory and alternative local or systemic therapies may be considered. The likelihood of obtaining a complete response is reduced when 18F-FDG uptake on PET scan is high in the tumor foci [4–6]. However, the decision to abandon RAI

A. Berdelou · S. Leboulleux · M. Schlumberger (✉)
Gustave Roussy, Villejuif, France
e-mail: martin.schlumberger@gustaveroussy.fr

U. K. Mallick et al. (eds.), *Practical Management of Thyroid Cancer*,
https://doi.org/10.1007/978-3-319-91725-2_17

therapy should not be based only on the presence or intensity of 18F-FDG uptake.

Most patients with RAI-refractory DTC fall into four categories [2, 7]: *(a) Patients with metastatic disease that does not take-up ^{131}I at the time of the first ^{131}I treatment.* For these patients, treatment with ^{131}I does not provide any benefit. This group includes patients with structurally evident disease with no ^{131}I uptake on a diagnostic WBS, because in such patients ^{131}I uptake when present on post-therapy WBS will not deliver sufficiently high radiation doses to induce benefit [8]. *(b) Patients whose tumors lose the ability to take-up ^{131}I after previous evidence of uptake.* This is frequently observed in patients with large metastases and is due to the eradication by ^{131}I treatment of differentiated cells able to take-up ^{131}I but not of less differentiated cells that do not take-up ^{131}I and that are likely to progress. *(c) Patients with ^{131}I uptake retained in some lesions but not in others.* This is frequently shown by ^{124}I studies on PET scan in patients with multiple large metastases [9] and by comparing results of ^{131}I WBS with other imaging modalities (FDG-PET or CT scans). In such patients, progression is likely to occur in metastases without ^{131}I uptake (with usually presence of high FDG uptake) and ^{131}I treatment will not be beneficial [4–6] *(d) Patients with metastatic disease that progresses despite significant uptake of ^{131}I in all metastases and adequate ^{131}I treatment.* It has been shown that if progression occurs following a course of adequate radioiodine treatment, subsequent ^{131}I treatment will be ineffective [10]. Also, the administration of large ^{131}I activities based on blood dosimetry does not improve the efficacy of ^{131}I as compared to standard activities of 3.7 GBq [11].

The situation for patients with persistent visible ^{131}I uptake in all lesions who are not cured despite several treatment courses but whose disease does not progress according to cross section imaging is less clear (particularly after receiving more than 22 GBq-600 mCi of ^{131}I). For these patients, further ^{131}I treatment may prolong tumor response but the probability of obtaining a cure is low [3] and side effects may significantly increase, including the risk of secondary cancers and leukemias [12]. The decision to continue ^{131}I treatment in such patients is generally based on their response to previous treatment courses, persistence of a significant level of ^{131}I uptake on the previous post-therapy WBS, low FDG uptake in tumor foci, and absence of side effects. If these patients are not re-treated with ^{131}I, they are followed-up as detailed below. Also, patients may achieve dissociated response with a tumor response in most lesions but with one or a few lesions that do not respond or even progress. Progressive lesions may require focal treatments and the decision to continue ^{131}I treatment is then based on a case by case decision.

Finally, thyroidectomy is not feasible in some patients with advanced disease and ^{131}I treatment is usually not administered. In these patients, ^{131}I uptake status cannot be assessed and they are managed as RAI-refractory patients.

Focal Treatment Modalities

Therapy of Local and Regional Recurrences

Surgery is the main treatment for neck and mediastinum recurrences, and its indication should take into account the size and extent of the recurrence and of distant metastases. When the surgical resection of the tumor is not feasible or has been incomplete, external radiation therapy to the neck and mediastinum may be indicated for local tumor control, in particular in the absence of known distant metastases [13, 14].

Surgery and external radiation therapy to the neck may also be indicated in patients with tumor invading the aerodigestive structures, and may be necessary before initiating a treatment with kinase inhibitors to avoid fatal bleeding [15–17]. DTC invading the central airway may be amenable to laser or photodynamic therapy or airway stenting.

Focal Treatment for Distant Metastases

Focal treatment modalities are performed in patients with local symptoms or at high risk of local complication, preferably before initiation of systemic treatment, and may permit to postpone systemic treatment [7]. Surgery may be indicated on bone metastases in patients with orthopedic or neurological complications or at high risk of such complications and in case of a single or a few metastases located in bone, brain, lungs or liver. External radiation therapy can induce rapid relief of bone pain and slower recalcification of bone lesions [18]. For brain metastases not amenable to surgery or as first line treatment, stereotactic irradiation is preferred to whole brain irradiation, whenever possible because the life expectancy of metastatic DTC may be long and this modality yields fewer neurological complications [19]. Finally, percutaneous thermal ablation (radiofrequency or cryo-ablation) for bone (eventually combined with cement injection), lung or liver metastases is becoming the preferred focal treatment modality for a number of metastatic patients [20, 21]. It is less aggressive than surgical resection, proved to be locally efficient and can be combined with other focal treatment modalities.

Bone Directed Therapies

Two thirds of patients with bone metastases from DTC develop skeletal-related events within a year following the diagnosis of bone metastases [22]. Focal treatment modalities are used in patients with threatening and/or symptomatic bone lesions before initiation of systemic treatment. Unfortunately, bone progression commonly occurs during kinase inhibitor therapy despite maintained benefit with respect to other metastases, and bone-directed therapy should be considered in patients with multiple progressing and/or symptomatic bone metastases even if kinase inhibitor therapy is intended or ongoing. In other solid tumors, bisphosphonates (especially IV infusion of zoledronic acid every 3 months) and the RANK-ligand-directed agent (monthly sub-cutaneous injection of denosumab) have been shown to delay time to occurrence of skeletal-related events and to improve symptoms with similar efficacy [23, 24]. Two small studies have indicated potential benefit from bisphosphonates in DTC bone metastases [25, 26]. Risks are similar with both types of medicine and include hypocalcemia, prompting the concomitant use of supplemental calcium and vitamin D therapy, and non-healing oral lesions and jaw osteonecrosis indicating dental/oral surgical evaluation prior to their initiation [23]. The optimal duration of bone directed therapies remains unknown. The risk of jaw osteonecrosis increases after two years of treatment and the risk/benefit balance should then be reevaluated.

Systemic Treatment

Initiation of Systemic Treatment

Once ^{131}I treatment is abandoned, levothyroxine treatment is used to maintain serum TSH at a low or undetectable level (Table 17.1). Refractory thyroid cancers encompass a heterogeneous group of patients with regards to progression rate and life expectancy. Indeed, more aggressive tumors are poorly differentiated, occur in older patients, have no initial RAI uptake but a high FDG uptake, and usually large metastases. In contrast, young patients with small lung metastases from a well differentiated thyroid carcinoma can be asymptomatically stable for long periods of time [3, 7, 27]. However, there are exceptions and the rate of progression should be documented by imaging in each patient.

Surveillance includes a FDG-PET scan or a CT scan of the neck, chest, abdomen and pelvis with contrast, at an interval of usually 3–6 months that is dictated by the pace of prior disease pro-

Table 17.1 Treatment modalities in patients with refractory thyroid cancer

• L-T4 treatment: serum TSH <0.5 mU/L
• Focal treatments when needed
• Imaging follow-up every 4–6 months
– Stable disease: follow-up
– Progression (>20% (RECIST) in 6–12 months and significant tumor burden: systemic treatment
Inclusion in a trial
Chemotherapy: low efficacy, significant toxicity
Targeted therapy as first line

gression and by the rate of serum Tg increase [2, 7, 28]. In the absence of documented progression, follow-up with anatomical imaging is maintained every 6–12 months on levothyroxine suppressive treatment but without any other treatment, because the benefits of novel therapies may be largely outweighed by drug toxicities.

The decision to initiate systemic treatment in patients with refractory disease is based on several parameters, including tumor burden, disease progression, symptoms or high risk of local complications, age and general condition of the patient, and absence of contraindications [2]. Treatment should be initiated preferably before the occurrence of an invasion of the aero-digestive tract or of an encasement of large vessels that increases the risk of severe bleeding during treatment [15–17].

Progression rate can be evaluated by the doubling time of serum Tg [28] but should always be confirmed by imaging using Response Evaluation Criteria in Solid Tumors (RECIST) [29]. Indeed, patients with multiple lesions >1–2 cm and with RECIST progression within less than 12 months are considered for systemic treatment. In the SELECT trial, median PFS in the placebo group and benefits of lenvatinib treatment were similar whatever the criteria used for the definition of refractory disease, but all patients had documented progression before inclusion in the trial [30].

On the contrary, patients with few and/or small metastatic lesions <1 cm, and those with no evidence of progression in less than 12 months are considered for follow-up without systemic treatment [1, 2, 7]. Some patients with large tumor burden and lacking ^{131}I uptake and for whom there is no data on progression, may be considered for systemic treatment based on high uptake of FDG on PET scanning, on aggressive primary tumor histology [4–6], or when there is a short-term risk of local complications.

Cytotoxic Chemotherapy

Cytotoxic chemotherapies provided low response rates (from 0 to 22% with the most frequently used agent, doxorubicin at a dose of 60 mg/m^2 every 3–4 weeks) and toxicity was high [31]. Combination doxorubicin-cisplatin yielded similar low response rates to that of doxorubicin alone, but major toxicity was the added drawback. Very few trials have been reported on only limited series of patients with other cytotoxic agents. Paclitaxel appeared effective in a limited series of patients and the combination of gemcitabine and oxaliplatin appeared to be effective in some isolated patients [32, 33].

Treatment with interferon-α or interleukin-2, either alone or in combination with doxorubicin, or with somatostatin analogs failed to yield any tumor response. In some in vitro studies, retinoic acid analogs decreased the tumor growth rate and increased the expression of the sodium-iodine symporter. However, in clinical trials only minimal tumor effect and a small increase in ^{131}I uptake were observed in only few patients [34].

Molecular-targeted Therapy

Rationale

In most DTC patients, an initiating carcinogenic event is found and molecular targeted therapy can be given with a scientific rationale [1, 35–37]. Gene rearrangements (*RET-PTC* and *NTRK*) or point mutations of the *RAS* and *BRAF* genes are found in the majority of papillary thyroid cancers, resulting in the activation of the MAP kinase pathway. *RAS* mutations are found in 40% of follicular carcinomas and in 25% of poorly differentiated thyroid cancers. The PI3K-AKT pathway is frequently activated in follicular and poorly differentiated carcinomas [38–40]. Angiogenesis is activated in thyroid cancers, with an overproduction of VEGF by cancer cells and an overexpression of VEGF receptors by cancer and endothelial cells [41, 42]. Furthermore, other pathways such as the FGFR and PDGFR pathways may also be activated [43, 44].

Up to now, most kinase inhibitors that have been used in refractory thyroid cancers are antiangiogenic drugs and some also target kinases in the MAP kinase pathway (Table 17.2). The relative role of the inhibition of each target or of their combined inhibition on tumor response is currently unknown.

Results of Clinical Trials with Anti-angiogenic Drugs

In phase 2 trials with these agents, partial responses were observed in 0–59% of patients and long-term stable disease in at least another third (Table 17.2). Comparison of the outcomes among these compounds is at the present time not possible, but the response rates recently reported (around 50% or even higher) with pazopanib [45], lenvatinib [30, 46] and cabozantinib [47] seem higher than in previous reports with axitinib [48, 49], motesanib [50], sorafenib [51–56], sunitinib [57, 58], and vandetanib [59, 60]. It also appears that most drugs are more effective on metastases located in lymph nodes, liver and lungs than in bones.

Even more importantly, is the benefit observed in progression free survival (PFS) with these agents when compared with placebo, firstly in one randomized phase 2 trial (vandetanib vs placebo) and then in two phase 3 trials (sorafenib vs placebo and lenvatinib vs placebo). The lack of demonstrated improvement in overall survival versus placebo might have been related to the crossover design of these randomized studies.

The ZACTHYF trial was a multicentre, randomized phase 2 study with vandetanib (300 mg/day) vs placebo on 145 patients with RAI-refractory locally advanced or metastatic DTC that had progressed within the past 14 months. Vandetanib significantly prolonged PFS compared with placebo (hazard ratio: 0.63, $p = 0.008$; median: 11.1 vs 5.9 months), with a partial response rate of 8% [59]. The VERIFY phase 3 trial (vandetanib 300 mg vs placebo) then performed on 228 patients showed a non significant prolongation of PFS (HR: 0.75; $P = 0.080$; median: 10.0 vs 5.7 months), with a partial response rate of 5% [60].

Table 17.2 Tyrosine kinase inhibitors used in patients with RAI refractory differentiated thyroid cancer

	VEGFR	Other targets	n	PR (%)	SD >6 months (%)
Axitinib Cohen [48] Locati [49]	+	RET, PDGFR, KIT	45 45	31 38	38 29
Cabozantinib Cabanillas [47]	+	RET, C-MET	15	53	40
Lenvatinib Cabanillas [46] Schlumberger (Phase III vs placebo) [30]	+	RET, FGFR, PDGFR,C-KIT	58 392	59 65	36 Median PFS 18.3 vs 3.6 months
Motesanib Sherman [50]	+	PDGFR, KIT, RET	93	14	33
Pazopanib Bible [45]	+	PDGFR, KIT	37	49	
Sorafenib Kloos [55] Gupta [53] Hoftijzer [54] Ahmed [51] Capdevila [52] Brose (Phase III vs placebo) [56]	+	RET, RAF, PDGFR, KIT	58 25 32 19 16 417	5 23 25 18 19 12	58 53 36 79 50 Median PFS 10.8 vs 5.8 months
Sunitinib Atallah [58] Carr [57]	+	RET, PDGFR, KIT	57 29	35 28	68 46
Vandetanib Leboulleux (Phase II vs placebo) [59] Bastholt (Phase III vs placebo) [60]	+	RET, EGFR	145 228	8 5	Median PFS: 11.1 vs 5.9 months Median PFS : 10.0 vs 5.7

The DECISION trial was a multicenter, randomized (1:1) phase 3 study of sorafenib (400 mg twice-daily) vs placebo in 417 patients with RAI-refractory locally advanced or metastatic DTC that had progressed within the past 14 months [56]. The mean daily study sorafenib dose was 651 mg. Sorafenib treatment significantly improved PFS compared with placebo (HR: 0.587; 95%CI 0.454–0.758; $p < 0.0001$; median 10.8 versus 5.8 months) and the partial response rate was 12%. The improvement in PFS was seen in all clinical and biomarker subgroups. Median thyroglobulin levels rose in the placebo group and decreased and then paralleled progression in the sorafenib-treated group. The safety profile of sorafenib was as expected, with most adverse events being grade 1 and 2. The most common treatment-emergent adverse events in the sorafenib arm were dermatological- hand-foot skin reaction (76%), alopecia (67%) and rash/desquamation (50%)– but also included diarrhea (68%), fatigue (49%), weight loss (46%), and hypertension (40%). Serious AEs occurred in more than 30% of patients, the most frequent being secondary malignancy (4.3%), dyspnea (3.4%), and pleural effusion (2.9%). Toxicities led to dose reduction in 64% of patients and to drug withdrawal in 19%.

The SELECT trial was a multicenter, randomized (2:1) phase 3 study of lenvatinib (24 mg/day) vs placebo in 392 patients with RAI-refractory locally advanced or metastatic DTC that had progressed within the past 13 months, as confirmed by independent radiological review [30]. The mean daily study lenvatinib dose was 16.8 mg, with a median time to first dose reduction of 3 months. Lenvatinib treatment significantly improved PFS compared with placebo (HR: 0.21; 99% CI: 0.14–0.31, $P < 0.001$; median PFS: 18.3 vs 3.6 months). At year 2, progression events occurred in 86% of those in the placebo arm and only in 41% of subjects in the treatment arm. The objective response rate was 65% with complete responses in 2%, with a median time to objective response of 2 months. Similar benefits were observed in the 20% of patients who had received prior VEGF-targeted therapy. The improvement in PFS was seen in all clinical and biomarker subgroups. Treatment-related adverse events were reported in all patients in the lenvatinib group. Most often these were hypertension (68%), fatigue (64%), diarrhea (59%), and decreased appetite (50%). Proteinuria occurred in 32%. The most frequent grade 3 or higher treatment-related AEs were hypertension (42%), proteinuria (10%), arterial and venous thromboembolic events (2.7% and 3.8%, respectively), acute renal failure (1.9%), QTc prolongation (1.5%), and hepatic failure (0.4%). Toxicities led to dose reduction in 68% of the patients and to drug withdrawal in 14% of patients. In the active treatment arm, there were 20 fatalities compared with 6 in the placebo arm. Investigators attributed 6 fatalities (2%) directly to the use of lenvatinib. One person died from a pulmonary embolism, 1 died due to hemorrhagic stroke, and the other 4 patients died due to general health deterioration.

Metabolic consequences of kinase inhibitor treatment are relevant in DTC patients. The increased need of levothyroxine is frequent and serum TSH should be measured at each control. In athyreotic subjects with advanced DTC treated with sorafenib, this was attributed to an increased activity of type 3 deiodinase that converts T4 in inactive rT3 [61], and to a decrease in clearance of rhTSH [62]. An increased need in calcium and vitamin D analog may occur particularly in patients already treated for post-operative hypoparathyroidism, and ionized calcium should be measured at each control during treatment, and also when kinase inhibitor treatment is withdrawn, then to avoid severe hypercalcemia.

Aero-digestive fistula formation and bleeding have been reported in patients with tumor involvement of the aero-digestive tract that may require intervention before initiating any treatment with kinase inhibitors [15, 17]. In a retrospective analysis, there were 3 predictive factors of bleeding: aero-digestive tumor invasion, poorly differentiated histotype and history of previous neck irradiation [16]. Furthermore, cholecystitis, active peptic ulcer, inflammatory bowel disease may increase the risk of gastrointestinal bleeding or fistula.

Toxicities of these kinase inhibitors included fatigue, diarrhea, hypertension and skin toxicities, that induced a decrease in the quality of life, but there was no unexpected toxicity. Toxicities led to dose reduction in 11–73% of patients and to drug withdrawal in 7–25%. This suggests that these treatments should be initiated only in patients with significant tumor burden and with documented progressive disease. Also, prevention of adverse events whenever possible, education of patients and of care providers, assessment of adverse events using standardized guidelines [63] and their early management are mandatory and represent the best way to improve patient's compliance. This also suggests that these patients should be managed by experienced teams.

In conclusion, despite the absence of direct comparison, lenvatinib seems more effective with an almost 15 month improvement in median PFS compared with placebo and a response rate as high as 65%, with a few complete responses. These data are even more meaningful when considering that the SELECT trial enrolled patients with more advanced and more aggressive disease (as shown by a shorter median PFS in the placebo arm), some of whom had been previously treated with a TKI. However, efficacy and toxicity of lenvatinib have still to be evaluated in real life, outside the frame of a controlled trial and this will also permit to refine its indications. Also, trials are necessary to determine optimal initial dosages.

Predictive Factors of Drug Efficacy

In both the DECISION and SELECT trials, benefits of sorafenib or lenvatinib were observed in patients with mutated or wild type RAS or BRAF status, and this status cannot be used to predict response to treatment [30, 56].

Basal levels of some cytokines or angiogenic factors or changes in their serum level at 1–2 weeks have been associated with tumor response [64, 65]. These studies have shown the promise of using biomarkers in predicting drug efficacy, which needs to be refined before they can be used in clinical practice.

Comparison of FDG uptake on PET/CT at 1–2 weeks with baseline FDG uptake has produced inconsistent results and the interest of repeated FDG-PET/CT in the management of DTC patients during treatment with these new drugs is still unclear. During treatment with sunitinib, a decrease in FDG uptake was associated with subsequent tumor response, and an increase with subsequent tumor progression [57].

Other Medications

Mutation screening is performed on a routine basis in these patients, because the presence of a driver mutation may lead to use a specific inhibitor. However, larger series of patients are needed for defining the clinical utility of this approach. Also, many data have been obtained on thyroid tumor tissues that were resected long before treatment and analysis of the metastatic tumor tissue at the time of treatment would probably be more informative. In one study, the BRAF or RAS mutations found in the primary tumor were also present in the metastases, and additional mutations (PIK3CA or AKT1) were found in some metastatic tissues [38].

The presence of *BRAF* mutation was an inclusion criteria in two phase 2 trials with a BRAF inhibitor, vemurafenib or dabrafenib. In the phase 2 trial of vemurafenib in 26 PTC patients, 10 (39%) achieved a partial response [66] and in a retrospective study on 15 patients the partial response rate was 47% [67]. In 14 patients with a metastatic thyroid cancer included in a phase 1 trial of dabrafenib, 4 partial responses were observed [68].

Mutation in ALK (Anaplastic Lymphoma Kinase) gene has been reported in few DTC patients and may be used as a target for an ALK inhibitor [69].

Other pathways, such as the PI3K-AKT pathway [39, 40] are activated in some follicular and poorly differentiated carcinomas and trials with inhibitors of this pathway are ongoing, used either alone or in combination with an anti-angiogenic drug or an inhibitor of the MAP kinase pathway.

Another potential way of treating these patients is to restore the ability of radioiodine uptake in tumor cells, and then to treat with radioiodine following a preparation with rhTSH stimulation. The use of retinoic acid analogs or of sorafenib did not produce significant increase in uptake [34, 54]. However, in a pilot study on 20 patients with metastatic differentiated thyroid carcinomas with no significant radioiodine uptake, lesional dosimetry with ^{124}I PET imaging was performed after rhTSH stimulation before and then after 4 weeks of treatment with a MEK inhibitor, selumetinib. Twelve patients demonstrated increased tumoral ^{124}I uptake, and 8 of these 12 patients achieved sufficient iodine uptake after selumetinib to warrant treatment with ^{131}I: 5 achieved a RECIST partial responses and the other 3 had a stable disease. Of the 20 patients, 9 patients had tumors with the V600E *BRAF* mutation, 5 patients had tumors with *NRAS* mutations at codon 61, 3 patients had tumors with *RET/PTC* rearrangements, and the remaining 3 patients were wild-type for these alterations. Interestingly, of the 8 patients with a major increased ^{124}I uptake, 5 were found to have *NRAS* mutations, one a *BRAF* mutation, one a *RET/PTC* rearrangement and one patient was wild-type [70]. In another study on 10 patients with advanced papillary thyroid cancer with a BRAF mutation, and who had no ^{131}I uptake in tumor foci, treatment with dabrafenib for 25 days induced uptake in 6, who were then treated with ^{131}I and 2 had partial responses [71]. This approach may be relevant in patients at high risk of recurrence in a post-operative adjuvant setting and also in patients with small metastases with a slow progression rate and with a baseline radioiodine uptake that is absent or too low to allow significant radiation doses to be delivered.

Immunological intervention may use two directions. One is guided by the increased number of Tumor Associated Macrophages (TAMs) in aggressive tumors [72, 73]. It has recently been reported in BRAF transgenic mice that depletion of TAM through inhibition of the Colony Stimulating Factor 1 (CSF1) pathway that attracts TAMs into the tumor impairs tumor progression [74]. Another one is tumor evasion from immunosurveillance. This can occur through a variety of mechanisms, such as through the abnormal expression of an inhibitor of T-cell function, CTLA-4, PD-1 or PD-L1. Blockade with monoclonal antibodies directed at these immune checkpoints has emerged as a successful treatment approach for patients with advanced melanoma and other cancer types [75]. Interestingly, BRAF mutated papillary thyroid cancer have a higher expression of CTLA-4 and PD-L1 compared to BRAF wild type tumors [76]. There is no available data on treatment with these antibodies in refractory DTC, but immunotherapies either alone or in combination with TKI represent a future avenue of research in these patients.

Clinical Practice and Future Developments

At the present time, the kinase inhibitors sorafenib and lenvatinib are the only drugs to be approved by EMA and FDA for patients with radioiodine-refractory DTC with significant tumor burden and in whom progression has been documented. In countries where labelled drugs are available, the choice of the first drug is based on efficacy, tolerance and clinical presentation of the patient. Consideration to participation in clinical trials should be given to all patients, even in countries where a drug is currently approved [77]. For selected patients with progressive refractory disease in whom a treatment with an approved medication must be withdrawn and who are not suitable candidates for clinical trials, several expensive drugs, such as sunitinib, pazopanib or cabozantinib which are commercially available because they are approved for other malignancies have entered into clinical use.

Before initiation of systemic treatment, a comprehensive review is necessary to ascertain the patient's suitability for therapy [7, 63]. An initial evaluation includes assessment of the patient's performance status. Little is known about the tolerability of TKIs in patients with a poor performance status (*e.g.*, ECOG 2 or more) because all trials with TKIs have excluded these patients. Cardiovascular history, poor blood pressure control, and hematological, renal, and hepatic abnormalities may contraindicate any TKI treatment or may indicate treatment initiation at a lower dosage (Tables 17.3 and 17.4).

Tumor responses were observed in only a fraction of patients and most were partial and

Table 17.3 Comorbidities discouraging the use of TKIs

Uncontrolled high blood pressure
Recent cardiovascular event
Prolonged QTc interval and history of significant arrhythmia
Poor general condition (ECOG >2) and short life expectancy
Cachexia, poor nutrition, sarcopenia
Active or recent gastrointestinal disease: cholecystitis, diverticulitis, inflammatory bowel disease, recent bowel resection
Liver disease Renal impairment: creatinine clearance <60 ml/mn; proteinuria>1 g/24 h
Recent bleeding (ulcer, esotracheal tumor involvement), coagulopathy or anticoagulant treatment
Recent tracheal radiation therapy
Untreated brain metastases (controversial)

transient. The duration of treatment is not yet validated and, for this reason, treatment is usually given as long as toxicities remain manageable and there is no evidence of tumor progression. One unresolved question is when treatment should be stopped in patients with progression in a single or in a few metastases which can benefit from focal treatments when a tumor response is observed in the other lesions? This is frequently the case of patients with bone metastases. Another unresolved question is until when should treatment be maintained in patients who responded and then slowly progressed? It appeared that progression rate does not change when treatment is maintained, as shown by studying secondary PFS in the DECISION trial [78]. However, accelerated disease progression has been reported after discontinuation of treatment, indicating that patients with progressive disease should not remain untreated for long periods of time [79]. This can be achieved by either maintaining treatment when there is still some clinical benefits, or using another medication when this is available; indeed, PFS with a second line treatment was similar to the PFS observed with a first line treatment [80, 81]. However, benefits of further treatment lines with other anti-angiogenic drugs are questionable, and this may indicate that future studies should test cross-resistance between drugs and alternatively drugs targeted at other abnormalities that are present in the tumor tissue should

Table 17.4 Frequent toxicities observed during treatment with TKIs

HTA Control blood pressure before treatment initiation to less than 120/80 Frequent blood pressure self-monitoring, in particular during the first 8 weeks of treatment Treat any high blood pressure (calcium channel blockers may be the most effective)
Cardiotoxicity Pre-therapy: ECG. Echocardiogram is recommended in any patient with cardiac history (hypertension, symptoms consistent with congestive heart failure or coronary artery disease)
QTc prolongation Do not initiate treatment if >480 ms Serial monitor of ECG and electrolytes Correct any electrolyte abnormality and avoid drugs known to prolong QTc Discontinue treatment if QTc ≥500 ms
Fatigue and loss of weight Increase or at least maintain physical activity; fractionated meals; take pills in the evening Monitor other causes (anemia, depression, electrolyte disturbance, hypothyroidism)
Diarrhea Loperamide and/or codeine and/or clay Dietary changes (eat low-fiber foods; avoid high-fat or spicy foods, alcohol, and caffeinated or carbonated drinks; hydration)
Dermatological *Rash*: Use perfume-free soaps and wear loose, natural-fabric clothing; avoid hot or cold water; topical corticosteroids or antihistamines *Hand-foot syndrome*: Prevention: local care of feet and hands, urea cream 10% on hands and feet. Use cotton socks and comfortable shoes, avoid traumatisms and avoid hot/cold water. Treatment: thick urea-based cream (30%), topical lidocaine if painful *Alopecia*: Inform the patient that it is temporary, usually recovering after the treatment, and does not require any treatment *Photosensitivity*: avoid sun exposure, cover the skin with clothes, use sunscreen creams *Mucositis*: mouth wash with lidocaine + sucralfate, salt and sodium bicarbonate, chlorhexidine
Proteinuria If ≥3 g/24 h: withhold treatment Resume at reduced dose when proteinuria is <1 g/24 h *Hepatotoxicity*: Increase of alanine serum transferase, alkaline phosphatase and bilirubin by three- to fivefold should lead to dose reduction or treatment discontinuation *Hypothyroidism*: Monitor TSH levels monthly and adjust levothyroxine dosage *Hypocalcemia*: Monitor blood calcium levels at least monthly and replace calcium + vitamin D as necessary *Hematological toxicities*: neutropenia, lymphopenia, thrombopenia *Pancreatitis*: increase of serum amylase

be used. Combination or sequential treatments may also be studied.

In conclusion, despite the many advances achieved in recent years, there are still many questions to be answered, such as which drug should be used as first line treatment, what is the mechanism of resistance in case of progression (pharmacodynamics or intra-tumor mechanism), for how long treatment should be maintained, interest of combination therapy, interest of other drugs, and many others. Thus, there is a need for trials and recent experience performed in the frame of clinical networks have shown that inclusion of the expected number of thyroid cancer patients to reach statistically significant conclusions is possible in a limited period of time.

References

1. Xing MM, Haugen B, Schlumberger M. Progress in molecular-based management of differentiated thyroid cancer. Lancet. 2013;381:1058–69.
2. Schlumberger M, Brose M, Elisei R, et al. Definition and management of radioactive iodine-refractory differentiated thyroid cancer: recommendations by an international expert panel. Lancet Diabetes Endocrinol. 2014;2:356–8.
3. Durante C, Haddy N, Baudin E, et al. Long-term outcome of 444 patients with distant metastases from papillary and follicular thyroid carcinoma: benefits and limits of radioiodine therapy. J Clin Endocrinol Metab. 2006;91:2892–9.
4. Rivera M, Ghossein RA, Schoder H, Gomez D, Larson SM, Tuttle RM. Histopathologic characterization of radioactive iodine-refractory fluorodeoxyglucose-positron emission tomography-positive thyroid carcinoma. Cancer. 2008;113:48–56.
5. Robbins RJ, Wan Q, Grewal RK, et al. Real-time prognosis for metastatic thyroid carcinoma based on 2-[18F]fluoro-2-deoxy-D-glucose-positron emission tomography scanning. J Clin Endocrinol Metab. 2006;91:498–505.
6. Deandreis D, Al Ghuzlan A, Leboulleux S, et al. Do histological, immunohistochemical and metabolic (radioiodine and fluorodeoxyglucose uptake) patterns of metastatic thyroid cancer correlate with patient outcome? Endocr Relat Cancer. 2011;18:159–69.
7. Haugen BR, Alexander EK, Bible KC, et al. 2015 American Thyroid Association Management Guidelines for adult Patients with Thyroid Nodules and Differentiated Thyroid Cancer. Thyroid. 2016;26:1–133.
8. Sabra MM, Grewal RK, Tala H, Larson SM, Tuttle RM. Clinical outcomes following empiric radioiodine therapy in patients with structurally identifiable metastatic follicular cell-derived thyroid carcinoma with negative diagnostic but positive post-therapy 131I whole-body scans. Thyroid. 2012;22:877–83.
9. Sgouros G, Kolbert KS, Sheikh A, et al. Patient-specific dosimetry for 131I thyroid cancer therapy using 124I PET and 3-dimensional-internal dosimetry (3D-ID) software. J Nucl Med. 2004;45:1366–72.
10. Vaisman F, Tala H, Grewal R, Tuttle RM. In differentiated thyroid cancer, an incomplete structural response to therapy is associated with significantly worse clinical outcomes than only an incomplete thyroglobulin response. Thyroid. 2011;21:1317–22.
11. Deandreis D, Rubino C, Tala H, et al. Comparison of empiric versus whole body/blood clearance dosimetry-based approach to radioactive iodine treatment in patients with metastases from differentiated thyroid cancer. J Nucl Med. 2017;58(5):717–22.
12. Rubino C, De Vathaire F, Dottorini ME, et al. Second primary malignancies in thyroid cancer patients. Br J Cancer. 2003;89:1638–44.
13. Tufano RP, Clayman G, Heller KS, et al. Management of recurrent/persistent nodal disease in patients with differentiated thyroid cancer: a critical review of the risks and benefits of surgical intervention versus active surveillance. Thyroid. 2015;25:15–27.
14. Romesser PB, Sherman EJ, Shaha AR, et al. External beam radiotherapy with or without concurrent chemotherapy in advanced or recurrent non-anaplastic nonmedullary thyroid cancer. J Surg Oncol. 2014; 110:375–82.
15. Licitra L, Locati L. Antiangiogenetic TKIs and advanced RAI-resistant thyroid cancer: time for treatment strategy rethinking? Thyroid. 2014;24:1815.
16. Lamartina L, Ippolito S, Danis M, et al. Antiangiogenic tyrosine kinase inhibitors: occurrence and risk factors of hemoptysis in refractory thyroid cancer. J Clin Endocrinol Metab. 2016;101:2733–41.
17. Blevins DP, Dadu R, Hu M, et al. Aerodigestive fistula formation as a rare side effect of antiangiogenic tyrosine kinase inhibitor therapy for thyroid cancer. Thyroid. 2014;24:918–22.
18. Tubiana M, Haddad E, Schlumberger M, Hill C, Rougier P, Sarrazin D. External radiotherapy in thyroid cancers. Cancer. 1985;55:2062–71.
19. Lo SS, Fakiris AJ, Chang EL, et al. Stereotactic body radiation therapy: a novel treatment modality. Nat Rev Clin Oncol. 2010;7:44–54.
20. Deandreis D, Leboulleux S, Dromain C. Role of FDG PET/CT and chest CT in the follow-up of lung lesions treated with radiofrequency ablation. Radiology. 2011;258:270–6.
21. Quan GM, Pointillart V, Palussiere J, Bonichon E. Multidisciplinary treatment and survival of patients with vertebral metastases from thyroid carcinoma. Thyroid. 2012;22:125–30.
22. Farooki A, Leung V, Tala H, Tuttle RM. Skeletal-related events due to bone metastases from differentiated thyroid cancer. J Clin Endocrinol Metab. 2012;97:2433–9.
23. Coleman R, Gnant M, Morgan G, Clezardin P. Effects of bone-targeted agents on cancer progression and mortality. J Natl Cancer Inst. 2012;104:1059–67.

24. Wardley A, Davidson N, Barrett-Lee P, et al. Zoledronic acid significantly improves pain scores and quality of life in breast cancer patients with bone metastases: a randomised, crossover study of community vs hospital bisphosphonate administration. Br J Cancer. 2005;92:1869–76.
25. Vitale G, Fonderico F, Martignetti A, et al. Pamidronate improves the quality of life and induces clinical remission of bone metastases in patients with thyroid cancer. Br J Cancer. 2001;84:1586–90.
26. Orita Y, Sugitani I, Toda K, Manabe J, Fujimoto Y. Zoledronic acid in the treatment of bone metastases from differentiated thyroid carcinoma. Thyroid. 2011;21:31–5.
27. Kwong N, Marqusee E, Gordon MS, et al. Long-term, treatment-free survival in select patients with distant metastatic papillary thyroid cancer. Endocr Connect. 2014;3:207–14.
28. Miyauchi A, Kudo T, Miya A, et al. Prognostic impact of serum thyroglobulin doubling-time under thyrotropin suppression in patients with papillary thyroid carcinoma who underwent total thyroidectomy. Thyroid. 2011;21:707–16.
29. Eisenhauer EA, Therasse P, Bogaerts J, et al. New response evaluation criteria in solid tumours: revised RECIST guideline (version 1.1). Eur J Cancer. 2009;45:228–47.
30. Schlumberger M, Tahara M, Wirth LJ, et al. Lenvatinib versus placebo in radioiodine-refractory thyroid cancer. N Engl J Med. 2015;372:621–30.
31. Sherman SI. Cytotoxic chemotherapy for differentiated thyroid carcinoma. Clin Oncol (R Coll Radiol). 2010;22:464–8.
32. Crouzeix G, Michels JJ, Sevin E, Aide N, Vaur D, Bardet S. Unusual short-term complete response to two regimens of cytotoxic chemotherapy in a patient with poorly differentiated thyroid carcinoma. J Clin Endocrinol Metab. 2012;97:3046–50.
33. Spano JP, Vano Y, Vignot S, et al. GEMOX regimen in the treatment of metastatic differentiated refractory thyroid carcinoma. Med Oncol. 2012;29:1421–8.
34. Grüning T, Tiepolt C, Zöphel K, Bredow J, Kropp J, Franke WG. Retinoic acid for redifferentiation of thyroid cancer-does it hold its promise? Eur J Endocrinol. 2003;148:395–402.
35. Phay JE, Ringel MD. Metastatic mechanisms in follicular cell-derived thyroid cancer. Endocr Relat Cancer. 2013;20:R307–19.
36. Cancer Genome Atlas Research Network. Integrated genomic characterization of papillary thyroid carcinoma. Cancer Genome Atlas Research Network. Cell. 2014;159:676–90.
37. Fagin JA, Wells SA Jr. Biologic and clinical perspectives on thyroid cancer. N Engl J Med. 2016;375:1054–67.
38. Ricarte-Filho JC, Ryder M, Chitale DA, et al. Mutational profile of advanced primary and metastatic radioactive iodine-refractory thyroid cancers reveals distinct pathogenetic roles for BRAF, PIK3CA, and AKT1. Cancer Res. 2009;69:4885–93.
39. Ringel MD, Hayre N, Saito J, et al. Overexpression and overactivation of Akt in thyroid carcinoma. Cancer Res. 2001;61:6105–11.
40. Xing M. Genetic alterations in the phosphatidylinositol-3 kinase/Akt pathway in thyroid cancer. Thyroid. 2010;20:697–706.
41. Bunone G, Vigneri P, Mariani L, et al. Expression of angiogenesis stimulators and inhibitors in human thyroid tumors and correlation with clinical pathological features. Am J Pathol. 1999;155:1967–76.
42. Klein M, Vignaud JM, Hennequin V, et al. Increased expression of the vascular endothelial growth factor is a pejorative prognosis marker in papillary thyroid carcinoma. J Clin Endocrinol Metab. 2001;86:656–8.
43. Guo M, Liu W, Serra S, Asa SL, Ezzat S. FGFR2 isoforms support epithelial-stromal interactions in thyroid cancer progression. Cancer Res. 2012;72:2017–27.
44. St Bernard R, Zheng L, Liu W, Winer D, Asa SL, Ezzat S. Fibroblast growth factor receptors as molecular targets in thyroid carcinoma. Endocrinology. 2005;146:1145–53.
45. Bible KC, Suman VJ, Molina JR, et al. Efficacy of pazopanib in progressive, radioiodine-refractory, metastatic differentiated thyroid cancers: results of a phase 2 consortium study. Lancet Oncol. 2010;11:962–72.
46. Cabanillas ME, Schlumberger M, Jarzab B, et al. A phase 2 trial of lenvatinib (E7080) in advanced, progressive, radioiodine-refractory, differentiated thyroid cancer: A clinical outcomes and biomarker assessment. Cancer. 2015;121:2749–56.
47. Cabanillas M, Brose M, Holland J, Ferguson KC, Sherman SI. A phase I study of cabozantinib (XL184) in patients with differentiated thyroid cancer. Thyroid. 2014;24:1508–14.
48. Cohen EE, Rosen LS, Vokes EE, et al. Axitinib is an active treatment for all histologic subtypes of advanced thyroid cancer: results from a phase II study. J Clin Oncol. 2008;26:4708–13.
49. Locati LD, Licitra L, Agate L, et al. Treatment of advanced thyroid cancer with axitinib: Phase 2 study with pharmacokinetic/pharmacodynamic and quality-of-life assessments. Cancer. 2014;120:2694–703.
50. Sherman SI, Wirth LJ, Droz JP, et al. Motesanib diphosphate in progressive differentiated thyroid cancer. N Engl J Med. 2008;359:31–42.
51. Ahmed M, Barbachano Y, Riddell A, et al. Analysis of the efficacy and toxicity of sorafenib in thyroid cancer: a phase II study in a UK based population. Eur J Endocrinol. 2011;165:315–22.
52. Capdevila J, Iglesias L, Halperin I, et al. Sorafenib in metastatic thyroid cancer. Endocr Relat Cancer. 2012;19:209–16.
53. Gupta-Abramson V, Troxel AB, Nellore A, et al. Phase II trial of sorafenib in advanced thyroid cancer. J Clin Oncol. 2008;26:4714–9.
54. Hoftijzer H, Heemstra KA, Morreau H, et al. Beneficial effects of sorafenib on tumor progression, but not on radioiodine uptake, in patients with differentiated thyroid carcinoma. Eur J Endocrinol. 2009;161:923–31.

55. Kloos RT, Ringel MD, Knopp MV, et al. Phase II trial of sorafenib in metastatic thyroid cancer. J Clin Oncol. 2009;27:1675–84.
56. Brose MS, Nutting CM, Jarzab B, et al. A randomized trial of sorafenib for 131I-refractory differentiated thyroid cancer. Lancet. 2014;384:319–28.
57. Carr LL, Mankoff DA, Goulart BH, et al. Phase II study of daily sunitinib in FDG-PET-positive, iodine-refractory differentiated thyroid cancer and metastatic medullary carcinoma of the thyroid with functional imaging correlation. Clin Cancer Res. 2010;16:5260–8.
58. Atallah V, Hocquelet A, Do Cao C, et al. Activity and safety of sunitinib in patients with advanced radioiodine refractory thyroid carcinoma : a retrospectuve analysis of 57 patients. Thyroid. 2016;26:1085–92.
59. Leboulleux S, Bastholt L, Krause T, et al. Vandetanib in locally advanced or metastatic differentiated thyroid cancer: a randomised, double-blind, phase 2 trial. Lancet Oncol. 2012;13:897–905.
60. Bastholt L, Schlumberger MJ, Fagin JA et al. Vandetanib in patients with locally advanced or metastatic differentiated thyroid cancer who are refractory or unsuitable for radioiodine therapy: a phase III study (VERIFY). Abstract; 2016 ETA meeting, Copenhagen. 2016.
61. Abdulrahman RM, Verloop H, Hoftijzer H, et al. Sorafenib-induced hypothyroidism is associated with increased type 3 deiodination. J Clin Endocrinol Metab. 2010;95:3758–62.
62. Verloop H, Smit JW, Dekkers OM. Sorafenib therapy decreases the clearance of thyrotropin. Eur J Endocrinol. 2013;168:163–7.
63. Carhill AA, Cabanillas ME, Jimenez C, et al. The noninvestigational use of tyrosine kinase inhibitors in thyroid cancer: establishing a standard for patient safety and monitoring. J Clin Endocrinol Metab. 2013;98:31–42.
64. Bass MB, Sherman SI, Schlumberger MJ, et al. Biomarkers as predictors of response to treatment with motesanib in patients with progressive advanced thyroid cancer. J Clin Endocrinol Metab. 2010;95:5018–27.
65. Tahara M, Schlumberger M, Elisei R et al. Pharmacodynamic biomarkers of outcomes in the phase 3 study of lenvatinib in 131I-refractory differentiated thyroid cancer (SELECT). Abstract 6014. ASCO 2016. 2016.
66. Brose MS, Cabanillas ME, Cohen EE, et al. Vemurafenib in patients with BRAF(V600E)-positive metastatic or unresectable papillary thyroid cancer refractory to radioactive iodine: a non-randomised, multicentre, open-label, phase 2 trial. Lancet Oncol. 2016;17:1272–82.
67. Dadu R, Shah K, Busaidy NL, et al. Efficacy and tolerability of vemurafenib in patients with BRAFV600E-positive papillary thyroid cancer: M.D. anderson cancer center off label experience. J Clin Endocrinol Metab. 2015;100:77–81.
68. Falchook GS, Millward M, Hong DS, et al. BRAF inhibitor dabrafenib in patients with metastatic-BRAF-mutant thyroid cancer. Thyroid. 2015;25:71–7.
69. Hamatani K, Mukai M, Takahashi K, Hayashi Y, Nakachi K, Kusunoki Y. Rearranged anaplastic lymphoma kinase (ALK) gene in adult-onset papillary thyroid cancer amongst atomic bomb survivors. Thyroid. 2012;22:1153–9.
70. Ho AL, Grewal RK, Leboeuf R, Sherman EJ, et al. Selumetinib-enhanced radioiodine uptake in advanced thyroid cancer. N Engl J Med. 2013;368:623–32.
71. Rothenberg SM, McFadden DG, Palmer EL, Daniels GH, Wirth LJ. Redifferentiation of iodine-refractory BRAF V600E-mutant metastatic papillary thyroid cancer with dabrafenib. Clin Cancer Res. 2015;21:1028–35.
72. Ryder M, Ghossein RA, Ricarte-Filho JC, Knauf JA, Fagin JA. Increased density of tumor-associated macrophages is associated with decreased survival in advanced thyroid cancer. Endocr Relat Cancer. 2008;15:1069–74.
73. Caillou B, Talbot M, Weyemi U, et al. Tumor-associated macrophages (TAMs) form an interconnected cellular supportive network in anaplastic thyroid carcinoma. PLoS One. 2011;6:e22567.
74. Ryder M, Gild M, Hohl TM, et al. Genetic and pharmacological targeting of CSF-1/CSF-1R inhibits tumor-associated macrophages and impairs BRAF-induced thyroid cancer progression. PLoS One. 2013;8(1):e54302.
75. Ott PA, Hodi FS, Robert C. CTLA-4 and PD-1/PD-L1 blockade: new immunotherapeutic modalities with durable clinical benefit in melanoma patients. Clin Cancer Res. 2013;19:5300–9.
76. Angell TE, Lechner MG, Jang JK, Correa AJ, LoPresti JS, Epstein AL. BRAF V600E in papillary thyroid carcinoma is associated with increased programmed death ligand 1 expression and suppressive immune cell infiltration. Thyroid. 2014;24:1385–93.
77. Tsimberidou AM, Vaklavas C, Wen S, et al. Phase I clinical trials in 56 patients with thyroid cancer: the M. D. Anderson Cancer Center experience. J Clin Endocrinol Metab. 2009;94:4423–32.
78. Schlumberger M, Nutting C, Jarzab B et al. Exploratory analysis of outcomes for patients with locally advanced or metastatic radioactive iodine-refractory differentiated thyroid cancer (RAI-rDTC) receiving open-label sorafenib post-progression on the phase III DECISION trial. Abstract, ETA 2014, Santiago di Compostella. 2014.
79. Yun KJ, Kim W, Kim EH, et al. Accelerated disease progression after discontinuation of sorafenib in a patient with metastatic papillary thyroid cancer. Endocrinol Metab. 2014;29:388–93.
80. Dadu R, Devine C, Hernandez M, et al. Role of salvage targeted therapy in differentiated thyroid cancer patients who failed first-line sorafenib. J Clin Endocrinol Metab. 2014;99:2086–94.
81. Massicotte MH, Brassard M, Claude-Desroches M, et al. Tyrosine kinase inhibitor treatments in patients with metastatic thyroid carcinomas: a retrospective study of the TUTHYREF network. Eur J Endocrinol. 2014;170:575–82.

Part VI

Medullary Thyroid Carcinoma and Familial Non Medullary Thyroid Cancer

18 Practical Management of Thyroid Cancer: A Multidisciplinary Approach-Medullary Thyroid Cancer

Anna I. Kaleva, Ashok R. Shaha, and Iain J. Nixon

Introduction

Medullary thyroid cancer (MTC) is one of the less common histological types of thyroid malignancy, only accounting for 1–2% of thyroid cancers [1]. It was first recognised as an entity in 1906 by Jaquet and subsequently described in more definitive detail by Hazard and Crile [2]. In practical terms its biology differs from the more common papillary cancer and as such, requires a different therapeutic approach. This chapter describes the current understanding of the biology of this thyroid cancer type and practical considerations useful for the multi-disciplinary care of these patients.

The Patient Population and Cancer Genetics

MTC can occur either sporadically (75% of cases) or be inherited by patients with multiple endocrine neoplasia type 2 (MEN2) or familial medullary thyroid cancer (FMTC) (25% of cases). The most commonly associated genetic mutation with this condition is in the RET proto-oncogene located on chromosome 10. It is responsible for a transmembrane receptor of the tyrosine kinase family. The majority of patients who present with MTC in the setting of MEN2 and FMTC have mutations in this gene, as well as more than 50% of patients with sporadic disease [3–8]. Increased understanding of the different RET mutations and their associated disease phenotypes has led to the ability to risk stratify disease - mutations known to date have been classified as either moderate, high or highest risk in the recent ATA guidelines (Table 18.1). An algorithm outlining an approach to the management of patients with such mutations is outlined in Fig. 18.1. If a new MTC is diagnosed, good practice dictates that investigation for other features of MEN is performed, in particular to assess for the presence of phaeochromocytoma and hyperparathyroidism [1, 9]. Furthermore, if no RET mutation is identified or there is a mismatch between the genotype and phenotype present, the ATA guidelines recommend more detailed genetic sequencing of the coding region. An additional consideration during initial management of these patients is the potential for inheritance and the effect this may have on both the index patient and their affected offspring. Current guidelines recommend testing first-degree relatives of patients harbouring disease which shows a phenotype suggestive of either FMTC or

A. I. Kaleva (✉)
Ipswich Hospital NHS Trust, Ipswich, UK

A. R. Shaha
Memorial Sloan Kettering Cancer Center, New York, NY, USA

I. J. Nixon
NHS Lothian, Edinburgh, UK

U. K. Mallick et al. (eds.), *Practical Management of Thyroid Cancer*,
https://doi.org/10.1007/978-3-319-91725-2_18

MEN2. Hence, in the multi-disciplinary team a consideration of the psychological burden of this diagnosis on both the patient and their relatives must be considered, and families counselled appropriately. With respect to the children of index patients, screening may be performed as soon as the initial case is diagnosed. If an infant is identified as being at risk of inherited MTC, an understanding of the genotype-phenotype and the risk of developing aggressive MTC is summarised in the American Thyroid Association Guidelines on medullary thyroid cancer [10]. These classify patients in categories A-D with families at lower risk, (class A) children requiring investigation within the first 5 years of life and appropriate management thereafter. In contrast, those children from families at highest risk (class D) should be screened as soon as possible after birth, and scheduled for surgery within the first year of life if the mutation is confirmed. Clearly, the process of counselling in relation to familial screening, interpretation of results and discussion of the approach to subsequent therapy should be coordinated by an experienced team with the help of the geneticist. Difficulties can arise if a parent does not want to inform their children of a potentially malignant thyroid lesion. The ATA guidelines state that clinicians in these situations may need to seek further advice and guidance from previous cases.

Table 18.1 RET protooncogene mutations recognised to date, their genetic location and estimated risk (adapted from the ATA guidelines)

Mutation	Exon	Level of risk as per ATA guidelines
G533C	8	Moderate
C609F/G/R/S/Y	10	Moderate
C611F/G/S/Y/W	10	Moderate
C618F/R/S	10	Moderate
C620F/R/S	10	Moderate
C630R/Y	11	Moderate
D631Y	11	Moderate
C634F/G/R/S/W/Y	11	High
K666E	11	Moderate
E768D	13	Moderate
L790F	13	Moderate
V804L	14	Moderate
V804M	14	Moderate
A883F	15	High
S891A	15	Moderate
R912P	16	Moderate
M918T	16	Highest

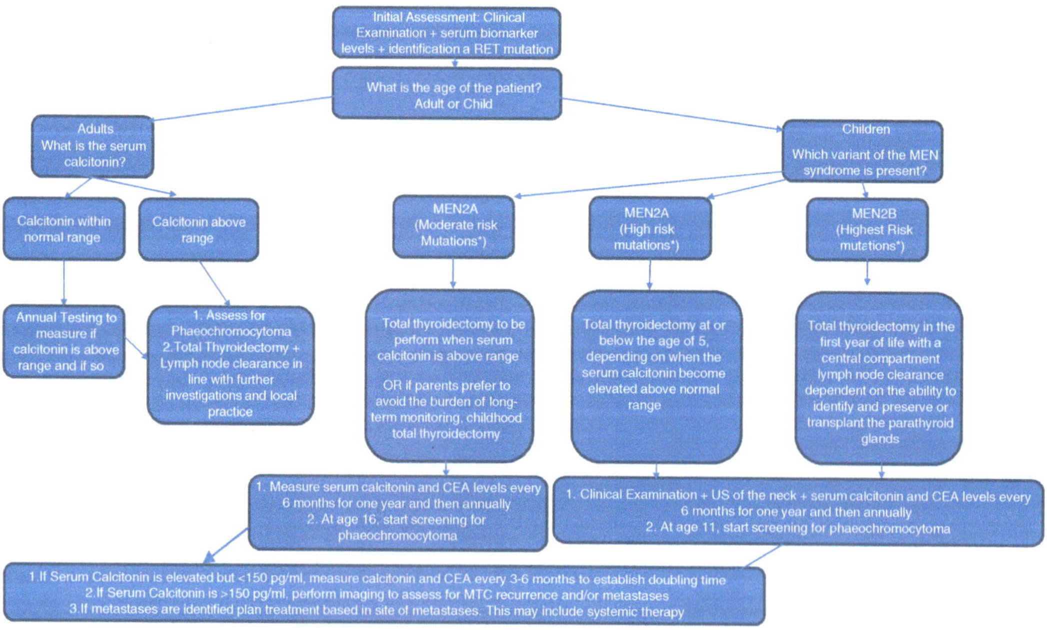

Fig. 18.1 Algorithm for management of patients once a RET protooncogene mutation has been identified

Investigations

Most patients will present with a thyroid nodule and the evaluation of this nodule should include clinical history, physical examination, ultrasound and fine needle aspiration and cytology (FNAC) [1]. Clearly a family history is critical, as is any suggestion of voice change, or dysphagia which may suggest invasive local disease. Clinical examination should include both palpation of the neck and assessment of vocal cord mobility.

A number of ultrasound features have been recognised to suggest malignancy including microcalcifications, cystic aspect, peripheral vascularity, hyperechogenicity and rounded shape [11]. Fine needle aspiration cytology of such nodules will often reveal trabecular, insular, glandular and amyloid-rich cellular arrangement and morphologic features [12].

In terms of cytology, MTC cells may be plasmacytoid, spindle-shaped or epitheliod and tend to not be very cohesive. However, these features are not very specific for MTC and for example an epitheliod MTC can be mistaken for a follicular lesion. The most significant findings suggestive of MTC are a dispersed cell pattern of polygonal or triangular cells, azurophilic cytoplasmic granules, eccentrically placed nuclei with coarse granular chromatin and amyloid [13]. Furthermore, unlike RET mutations, these light microscopy features do not correlate well to specific patterns of cancer behaviour [14]. Therefore, additional testing such as immunolocalisation of calcitonin and confirmation of the absence of thyroglobulin staining is often necessary to reduce the risk of false positive results. If these results are suggestive of MTC then the biochemical tests including serum calcitonin and CEA should be performed before commencing any treatment. In particular, in patients with inconclusive FNAC results, biochemical testing is strongly recommended [1]. These help both in accurate diagnosis and as prognostic markers.

Unlike thyroid tumours of follicular origin, MTC originates from parafollicular C-cells which do not concentrate iodine but do produce tumour markers including calcitonin and carcioembryogenic antigen (CEA). The parafollicular C-cells are located in the upper poles of the thyroid gland and hence MTC nodules are often found in this location.

Baseline levels of serum calcitonin and CEA baseline levels, and doubling times during follow up in particular do correlate with prognosis. In cases with markedly elevated calcitonin levels, rates of lateral neck involvement are high, and in the recent ATA guidelines recommendations, a serum calcitonin of >200 pg/mL should prompt consideration of lateral neck node surgery in the elective setting. However, the routine clinical benefit of testing FNAC samples for calcitonin is as yet not clearly defined, in particular when weighed against the cost of testing. Furthermore, calcitonin results need to be interpreted in the context of a patient's current clinical status e.g. a septic patient or one with renal failure may have raised levels of procalcitonin which in some assays will give a positive result for calcitonin. Interestingly, a high procalcitonin to calcitonin ratio has been shown to correlate with shorter disease-free survival [15, 16]. However, in practice few centres test for procalcitonin routinely, and the cost involved. Also, when testing calcitonin levels in children, it is important to be aware that for the under 3 years old patients it can be elevated independently of MTC and this is even more significant for infants under 6 months of age [1]. It is important to bear in mind that CEA is also not specific marker for MTC and hence it is tested for alongside calcitonin. False positive CEA results are a risk as they can occur in tobacco smokers and patients with gastrointestinal inflammatory conditions.

Ultrasound of the thyroid and the neck are routinely performed in evaluation of a suspected thyroid nodule. Once the diagnosis of MTC is suggested, additional investigations should include a contrast CT scan of the neck and chest. In those with extensive neck disease, or significantly elevated tumour markers, further investigations such as an MRI of the liver and an axial MRI as well as bone scintigraphy. At present, there is no evidence to support the use of PET-CT.

Treatment

Once a diagnosis of MTC is made, the approach to management will depend on clinical findings, imaging studies and assessment of tumour markers [1]. In terms of management of the primary lesion, total thyroidectomy is recommended. This removes all at-risk C-cells in both thyroid lobes. Although wide surgical margins can rarely be achieved in thyroid surgery, an attempt should be made to completely eradicate all disease from the thyroid bed with the initial surgical procedure. When advanced disease is suspected based upon either examination or imaging studies, a careful balance between operative morbidity and disease outcome must be made. Invasion of local structures including the recurrent laryngeal nerve, trachea, larynx and oesophagus can all be managed with adequate planned surgical excision with reconstruction as appropriate. However, if this is in the setting of widespread disseminated disease, such an aggressive approach may not be appropriate.

When nodal disease is identified on preoperative imaging, a compartment orientated therapeutic neck dissection is indicated. Interestingly it doesn't appear to correlate with intra-operative tumour size measurement. Unfortunately, despite nodal involvement being common, it can often go undetected. In studies of prophylactic necks dissection, occult nodal disease has been identified on histological analysis in around 75% of cases [17]. The likelihood of central compartment nodal involvement correlates with the stage of the tumour: 14% of patients with T1 tumours have central node involvement, compared to 86% of patients with T4 tumours. This is also true for lateral node involvement, 11% in T1 patients versus 93% in T4 patients [18]. When disease is limited to the central neck, a bilateral level VI and VII dissection should be performed.

The situation regarding the lateral compartment of the neck is more complex. Lateral neck nodal involvement is common. Some studies have suggested that ipsilateral neck nodes are involved in up to 80% of cases. Contralateral neck nodes are involved in up to half of cases [19]. When disease is identified in the lateral neck, dissection of levels II-V as well as bilateral central neck dissection should be performed. In the absence of imaging detected nodal disease, due to the high rates of occult disease, prophylactic central neck dissection is recommended. However, lateral neck dissection is associated with surgical morbidity [20], and ultrasound assessment is more accurate than in the central neck compartment. In addition, rates of biochemical cure are low in patients who have lateral neck disease at the time of presentation. For these reasons, prophylactic surgery has not been widely recommended. However, work by groups who take a more aggressive stance towards treatment of the lateral neck has shown that in the presence of multiple central lymph node metastases or a particularly high pre-operative calcitonin, rates of occult metastasis to the ipsilateral lateral neck are high. In the hands of high volume, experienced surgeons, lateral neck surgery can be performed with lower levels of morbidity. Such results are unlikely to be achieved in less experienced hands and as such this approach has not been endorsed in international guidelines.

For patients with a calcitonin level is <20 pg/mL, the evidence suggests that they are highly unlikely to have any metastases [21] and prophylactic lymph node clearance may be unjustifiable. Calcitonin levels >50 pg/mL correlate with a significant rate of metastases in the central neck compartment, levels >200 pg/mL correlate with a significant rate of metastases in the lateral neck compartment, and levels >500 pg/mL with metastases in the upper mediastinum [21]. Therefore, when calcitonin levels are significantly elevated and ipsilateral nodes are seen to be involved, contralateral prophylactic lateral neck dissection as a secondary procedure has also been recommended. The groups who argue for prophylactic surgery, have shown that with this aggressive approach to management, high levels of biochemical cure can be achieved. However, such findings should be seen in context. Many patients who present with disease which has spread beyond the central neck will not achieve biochemical cure in the long term, particularly if the contralateral lateral neck is involved. This balance between treatment morbidity and oncological outcome highlights the importance that such cases are referred to expert centres for management.

In terms of non-surgical medical options, there is little evidence to support their use. Unlike follicular cell derived thyroid cancer, iodine is not concentrated in MTC and therefore radioactive iodine is not effective [22]. In addition, external beam radiotherapy or chemotherapy have not demonstrated efficacy in MTC, and therefore in the presence of resectable disease surgery remains the mainstay of treatment [23, 24].

For locally advanced and metastatic MTC, surgery is often still appropriate, however there needs to be an emphasis on minimising any surgical morbidity and complications. This includes strategies to preserve speech and swallowing, such as less aggressive lymph node clearance or even some of the non-surgical options. For certain symptoms these latter options may have less evidence as successful curative recommendations. They may have a role in symptom control due to local tumour morbidity. The precise strategy will vary according to the anatomy of the patient and the tumour and this is another example of where a multi-disciplinary approach, by team members who deal with a high volume of MTC is likely to be highly beneficial [1].

As well as surgical options, there is increasing evidence for targeted therapies. Currently the two FDA and EMA approved drugs include Vandetanib which targets RET, vascular endothelial growth factor receptors (VEGFRs) and Epidermal Growth Factor Receptor (EGFR) signalling and Cabozantinib an inhibitor of Met tyrosine kinase, RET and the VEGFRs [25]. Other targeted therapies include Sorafenib, a multi kinase inhibitor which acts on VEGFRs, platelet-derived growth factor receptors (PDGFRs) and Raf family kinases, Sunitinib, a tyrosine kinase inhibitor which also acts on PDGFRs and VEGFRs which have been used and are undergoing further evaluations in trials. Currently available drugs include Vandetanib which targets RET, vascular endothelial growth factor receptors (VEGFRs) and Epidermal Growth Factor Receptor (EGFR) signalling; Sorafenib, a tyrosine kinase inhibitor which acts on VEGFRs, platelet-derived growth factor receptors (PDGFRs) and Raf family kinases; Sunitinib, another tyrosine kinase inhibitor which also acts on PDGFRs and VEGFRs and Cabozantinib an inhibitor of Met tyrosine kinase, RET and the VEGFRs [25]. Although these treatments have a role in the management of unresectable and progressive disease, they require long term therapy and are associated with significant side effects. Many patients who commence such therapy will require dose reduction or development cardiac or GI symptoms may require cessation of therapy. These will be discussed in more detail in the next chapter.

Prophylactic Thyroid Surgery

In patients with hereditary cancer syndromes prophylactic thyroidectomy is indicated if the genetic mutation causing the malignancy is characterised by complete or near complete penetrance. The timing of surgery will depend on the specific genetic mutation as well as imaging and biochemical studies (Fig. 18.1). In particular detailed DNA analysis of RET mutations as well as basal and/or stimulated calcitonin levels are used to decide on prophylactic surgery. Therefore another factor in the decision making process needs to be the patients' likely compliance with future periodic evaluation. Some parents may opt for thyroidectomy over 6-monthly monitoring for an extended period of time and hence should be offered the choice.

More specifically, MEN2A patients with high risk mutations (ATA-H see Table 18.1) such as codon 634 mutations develop MTC in their early years and hence, should be monitored from age 3 with serial ultrasound examinations and biochemical measurements with a low threshold for early surgery. Most of these children should have thyroidectomy before the age of 5. The precise timing will depend on the findings on ultrasound and blood tests. Mutations considered to convey moderate risk (ATA-MOD see Table 18.1) typically cause MTC later but there is a significant degree of variability in clinical expression within this group. For example, codon C609S mutations have been reported to present with MTC anywhere between 9 and 40 years old. Therefore, for the ATA-MOD group, the ATA guidelines recommend monitoring to start at age 5 [1]. As for the extent of surgery, if the Calcitonin levels are less than 40 pg/mL, the likelihood of lymph node metastases is very low and hence central neck dissection is not recommended.

MEN2B patients in the highest risk category (ATA-HST see Table 18.1) such as RET codon M918T mutations can develop MTC with nodal metastases in the first year of life. Hence, surgery in the first year of life is recommended. However, the precise timing can be difficult to decide as calcitonin levels can be very high regardless of disease state. Neck dissection in these patients carries a very high risk of inadvertent parathyroidectomy and hence is only recommended when the parathyroid glands are identified and preserved intra-operatively. Prompt management in these patients is more difficult in de novo RET mutations and hence clinicians need to have an awareness of the non-endocrine manifestations of MEN2B which may act as the presenting features of the condition, such as ganglioneuromatosis, oral symptoms, ocular manifestations and skeletal abnormalities. Fortunately the cure rate with thyroidectomy in these patients appears to be higher [26].

However, in young children, the morbidity of thyroidectomy is often high, firstly because it is not a commonly performed surgical procedure but also, because differentiating the parathyroid glands from normal tissue is more challenging. Post-operative hypoparathyroidism is more common in paediatric patients than adults. Also, amongst paediatricians there is significant concern regarding insufficient thyroid replacement post-operatively and the potential impact of hypothyroidism on growth and brain development [27]. Therefore, such patients should be considered for referral to high volume centres with significant paediatric endocrine expertise.

Follow-up

TNM staging as described in Tables 18.2 and 18.3 is used for estimating survival in thyroid cancer, however it does not incorporate specific features of MTC such as genetics (Fig. 18.1) and tumour markers which have prognostic significance in MTC. In particular, if all thyroid disease

Table 18.2 TNM staging of thyroid cancer

TNM classification for thyroid cancer	
Primary tumour (T)	
T_x	Primary tumour cannot be assessed
T0	No evidence of primary tumour
T1	Tumour 2 cm or less in greatest dimension, limited to the thyroid
$T1_a$	Tumour 1 cm or less, limited to the thyroid
$T1_b$	Tumour >1 cm, but <2 cm, in greatest dimension and limited to the thyroid
T2	Tumour >2 cm, but <4 cm, in the greatest dimension, limited to the thyroid
T3	Tumour >4 cm in greatest dimension limited to the thyroid, or any tumour with minimal extrathyroid extension (e.g., extension to sternothyroid muscle or perithyroid soft tissues)
$T4_a$	Moderately advanced disease; tumour of any size extending beyond the thyroid capsule to invade subcutaneous soft tissues, larynx, trachea, oesophagus, or recurrent laryngeal nerve
$T4_b$	Very advanced disease; tumour invades prevertebral fascia or encases carotid artery or mediastinal vessels
Regional node involvement (N)	
NX	Regional lymph nodes cannot be assessed
N0	No regional lymph node metastasis
N1	Regional lymph node metastasis
$N1_a$	Metastasis to the central compartments (level VI, pretracheal, paratracheal, and pre-laryngeal/ Delphian lymph nodes)
$N1_b$	Metastasis to unilateral, bilateral, or contralateral compartment cervical (levels I, II, III, IV, or V) or retropharyngeal or superior mediastinal lymph nodes (level VII)
Distant metastases (M)	
M0	No distant metastasis
M1	Distant metastasis

Table 18.3 The American Joint Committee Classification on cancer staging

American Joint Committee on Cancer Staging	
Stage I	T1, N0, M0
Stage II	T2, N0, M0 T3, N0, M0
Stage III	T1, N1a, M0 T2, N1a, M0 T3, N1a, M0
Stage IVA	T4a, N0, M0 T4a, N1a,M0 T1, N1b, M0 T2, N1b, M0 T3, N1b, M0 T4a, N1b, M0
Stage IVB	T4b, any N, M0
Stage IVC	Any T, any N, M1

is eradicated, then calcitonin is undetectable. The literature suggests that the optimum time to measure calcitonin and expect it to be at its nadir is 3 months post-operatively. If undetectable at this time, levels should be measured every 6 months for one year, and then annually thereafter.

An increase in calcitonin post-operatively indicates tumour recurrence [28]. Although the presence of a rising calcitonin confirms recurrent disease, calcitonin doubling time has been shown to be useful as a prognostic tool. One study showed that in those with a calcitonin doubling time less than 6 months, 5 year survival is 25% and 10 year survival is 8%. In contrast, if the doubling time is between 6 months and 24 months, 5 year survival is 97% and the 10 year survival is 37% [29]. Once recurrent disease is suspected, imaging will be required in the form of ultrasound and CT scans to identify structural disease [30, 31]. The absolute level of calcitonin is useful to target investigations. If levels are raised but remain below 150 pg/mL, this suggests that persistent or recurrent disease will be limited to the lymph nodes of the neck [1, 32]. If levels exceed 150 pg/ml, disseminated disease should be suspected and clinicians should consider additional imaging of the chest, liver and bones. In such cases PET scanning may also be considered. For those patients with recurrent disease, clinical decision making is challenging. Although disease cure at this stage is unlikely, surgery may be indicated to minimize complications and maintain speech and swallowing. Clearly factors such as structural disease trajectory and calcitonin doubling times will be taken in to consideration when planning treatment of such complex cases [1].

Conclusion

Medullary thyroid cancer is rare. Unlike other thyroid cancers, MTC more commonly presents with advanced local disease and nodal metastases to the neck making this condition challenging to cure. Careful pre-operative assessment includes an accurate clinical and family history, thorough examination, comprehensive imaging with targeted biopsies and biochemical assessment of tumour markers. The information provided allows disease management teams to tailor the treatment approach to the individual patients. However, genetic testing should also be performed to identify those family members at risk of inherited disease and guide further investigation and treatment thereafter.

Following identification of disease, the mainstay of treatment is surgical. Although those with limited disease can be cured with appropriate surgical intervention, a significant number of patients will either present with advanced disease or recur during follow up. Progress in the development of targeted therapies now offers treatment options to even those with the most advanced disease.

As in all of medicine, clinicians involved in the management of MTC should balance the morbidity of treatment against the likelihood of cure. Such balance is best managed in high volume centres with expertise in managing complex cases which require input from a wide multi-disciplinary team. Consideration of clinical, radiological, biochemical, genetic, surgical and endocrine factors combined will allow disease management teams to optimise the oncological outcome for patients and families with medullary thyroid cancer.

References

1. Wells SA Jr, Asa SL, Dralle H, Elisei R, Evans DB, Gagel RF, et al. Revised American Thyroid Association guidelines for the management of medullary thyroid carcinoma. Thyroid. 2015;25(6):567–610.
2. Hazard JB, Hawk WA, Crile G Jr. Medullary (solid) carcinoma of the thyroid; a clinicopathologic entity. J Clin Endocrinol Metab. 1959;19(1):152–61.
3. Donis-Keller H, Dou S, Chi D, Carlson KM, Toshima K, Lairmore TC, et al. Mutations in the RET proto-oncogene are associated with MEN 2A and FMTC. Hum Mol Genet. 1993;2(7):851–6.
4. Mulligan LM, Kwok JB, Healey CS, Elsdon MJ, Eng C, Gardner E, et al. Germ-line mutations of the RET proto-oncogene in multiple endocrine neoplasia type 2A. Nature. 1993;363(6428):458–60.
5. Carlson KM, Dou S, Chi D, Scavarda N, Toshima K, Jackson CE, et al. Single missense mutation in the tyrosine kinase catalytic domain of the RET protooncogene is associated with multiple endocrine neoplasia type 2B. Proc Natl Acad Sci U S A. 1994;91(4):1579–83.
6. Hofstra RM, Landsvater RM, Ceccherini I, Stulp RP, Stelwagen T, Luo Y, et al. A mutation in the RET proto-oncogene associated with multiple endocrine

neoplasia type 2B and sporadic medullary thyroid carcinoma. Nature. 1994;367(6461):375–6.
7. Eng C, Smith DP, Mulligan LM, Nagai MA, Healey CS, Ponder MA, et al. Point mutation within the tyrosine kinase domain of the RET proto-oncogene in multiple endocrine neoplasia type 2B and related sporadic tumours. Hum Mol Genet. 1994;3(2):237–41.
8. Marsh DJ, McDowall D, Hyland VJ, Andrew SD, Schnitzler M, Gaskin EL, et al. The identification of false positive responses to the pentagastrin stimulation test in RET mutation negative members of MEN 2A families. Clin Endocrinol. 1996;44(2):213–20.
9. Brandi ML, Gagel RF, Angeli A, Bilezikian JP, Beck-Peccoz P, Bordi C, et al. Guidelines for diagnosis and therapy of MEN type 1 and type 2. J Clin Endocrinol Metab. 2001;86(12):5658–71.
10. Kloos RT, Eng C, Evans DB, Francis GL, Gagel RF, American Thyroid Association Guidelines Task Force, et al. Medullary thyroid cancer: management guidelines of the American Thyroid Association. Thyroid. 2009;19(6):565–612.
11. Leenhardt L, Erdogan MF, Hegedus L, Mandel SJ, Paschke R, Rago T, et al. 2013 European thyroid association guidelines for cervical ultrasound scan and ultrasound-guided techniques in the postoperative management of patients with thyroid cancer. Eur Thyroid J. 2013;2(3):147–59.
12. Schroder S, Bocker W, Baisch H, Burk CG, Arps H, Meiners I, et al. Prognostic factors in medullary thyroid carcinomas. Survival in relation to age, sex, stage, histology, immunocytochemistry, and DNA content. Cancer. 1988;61(4):806–16.
13. Papaparaskeva K, Nagel H, Droese M. Cytologic diagnosis of medullary carcinoma of the thyroid gland. Diagn Cytopathol. 2000;22(6):351–8.
14. Rios A, Rodriguez JM, Febrero B, Acosta Ortega JM, Torregrosa N, Balsalobre M, et al. Histological and immunohistochemical profile of sporadic and familial medullary thyroid carcinoma. Endocrinol Nutr. 2011;58(10):521–8.
15. Algeciras-Schimnich A, Preissner CM, Theobald JP, Finseth MS, Grebe SK. Procalcitonin: a marker for the diagnosis and follow-up of patients with medullary thyroid carcinoma. J Clin Endocrinol Metab. 2009;94(3):861–8.
16. Walter MA, Meier C, Radimerski T, Iten F, Kranzlin M, Muller-Brand J, et al. Procalcitonin levels predict clinical course and progression-free survival in patients with medullary thyroid cancer. Cancer. 2010;116(1):31–40.
17. Weber T, Schilling T, Frank-Raue K, Colombo-Benkmann M, Hinz U, Ziegler R, et al. Impact of modified radical neck dissection on biochemical cure in medullary thyroid carcinomas. Surgery. 2001;130(6):1044–9.
18. Machens A, Hinze R, Thomusch O, Dralle H. Pattern of nodal metastasis for primary and reoperative thyroid cancer. World J Surg. 2002;26(1):22–8.
19. Moley JF, DeBenedetti MK. Patterns of nodal metastases in palpable medullary thyroid carcinoma: recommendations for extent of node dissection. Ann Surg. 1999;229(6):880–7. discussion 7–8
20. McMullen C, Rocke D, Freeman J. Complications of bilateral neck dissection in thyroid cancer from a single high-volume center. JAMA Otolaryngol Head Neck Surg. 2017;143:376–81.
21. Machens A, Dralle H. Biomarker-based risk stratification for previously untreated medullary thyroid cancer. J Clin Endocrinol Metab. 2010;95(6):2655–63.
22. Brierley J, Tsang R, Simpson WJ, Gospodarowicz M, Sutcliffe S, Panzarella T. Medullary thyroid cancer: analyses of survival and prognostic factors and the role of radiation therapy in local control. Thyroid. 1996;6(4):305–10.
23. Orlandi F, Caraci P, Berruti A, Puligheddu B, Pivano G, Dogliotti L, et al. Chemotherapy with dacarbazine and 5-fluorouracil in advanced medullary thyroid cancer. Ann Oncol. 1994;5(8):763–5.
24. Petursson SR. Metastatic medullary thyroid carcinoma. Complete response to combination chemotherapy with dacarbazine and 5-fluorouracil. Cancer. 1988;62(9):1899–903.
25. Nixon IJ, Shaha AR, Tuttle MR. Targeted therapy in thyroid cancer. Curr Opin Otolaryngol Head Neck Surg. 2013;21(2):130–4.
26. Brauckhoff M, Gimm O, Weiss CL, Ukkat J, Sekulla C, Brauckhoff K, et al. Multiple endocrine neoplasia 2B syndrome due to codon 918 mutation: clinical manifestation and course in early and late onset disease. World J Surg. 2004;28(12):1305–11.
27. Frank-Raue K, Buhr H, Dralle H, Klar E, Senninger N, Weber T, et al. Long-term outcome in 46 gene carriers of hereditary medullary thyroid carcinoma after prophylactic thyroidectomy: impact of individual RET genotype. Eur J Endocrinol. 2006;155(2):229–36.
28. Engelbach M, Gorges R, Forst T, Pfutzner A, Dawood R, Heerdt S, et al. Improved diagnostic methods in the follow-up of medullary thyroid carcinoma by highly specific calcitonin measurements. J Clin Endocrinol Metab. 2000;85(5):1890–4.
29. Barbet J, Campion L, Kraeber-Bodere F, Chatal JF, Group GTES. Prognostic impact of serum calcitonin and carcinoembryonic antigen doubling-times in patients with medullary thyroid carcinoma. J Clin Endocrinol Metab. 2005;90(11):6077–84.
30. Boi F, Maurelli I, Pinna G, Atzeni F, Piga M, Lai ML, et al. Calcitonin measurement in wash-out fluid from fine needle aspiration of neck masses in patients with primary and metastatic medullary thyroid carcinoma. J Clin Endocrinol Metab. 2007;92(6):2115–8.
31. Kudo T, Miyauchi A, Ito Y, Takamura Y, Amino N, Hirokawa M. Diagnosis of medullary thyroid carcinoma by calcitonin measurement in fine-needle aspiration biopsy specimens. Thyroid. 2007;17(7):635–8.
32. Pellegriti G, Leboulleux S, Baudin E, Bellon N, Scollo C, Travagli JP, et al. Long-term outcome of medullary thyroid carcinoma in patients with normal postoperative medical imaging. Br J Cancer. 2003;88(10):1537–42.

19 Medullary Thyroid Cancer: Diagnosis and Non Surgical Management

Rossella Elisei and Antonio Matrone

Introduction

Medullary thyroid carcinoma (MTC) is a neuroendocrine tumor originating from the parafollicular C-cells [1, 2] which are localized in the thyroid with the function to secrete mainly calcitonin (Ct) and other peptides such as chromogranin, serotonin, somatostatin, or calcitonin gene related peptide (CGRP) [3]. They are located adjacent to the thyroid follicles and reside in the connective tissue within the basement membrane, which surrounds the entire thyroid follicle. Until recently, parafollicular C-cells were believed to be derived from neural crest cells but genetic lineage tracing in mice arose the hypothesis of an endoderm origin of mammalian C-cell progenitors [4, 5]. The expression of E-cadherin, which is consistent with an origin different from the neural crest-derived mesenchyme, seems to support this hypothesis [6].

Parafollicular C-cells are normally concentrated in the upper and the middle thirds of the thyroid, but when hyperplastic they can be found predominantly in the middle and lower thirds of the lateral lobes. Exceptionally, some C-cells are present in the isthmic region [7]. The parafollicular C-cells represent only 0.1% of all thyroid cells and, normally, they are not visible at a common Hematoxilin-Eosin tissue stained histology while become detectable if an immunohistochemistry with an anti-Ct antibody is performed. Because of its origin, MTC appears as a separate entity from the other differentiated thyroid carcinomas.

The incidence of MTC is unknown but its prevalence is generally reported as 5–10% in all thyroid malignancies, 0.4–1.4% in all thyroid nodules and less than 1% in thyroids of subjects submitted to autopsy. Nowadays MTC is recognized by the national Health Institute (NIH) as a rare disease [8]. At variance with papillary (PTC) and follicular (FTC) carcinomas, which are 4 times more prevalent in females than in males [9], no difference in sex distribution is reported. The median age at diagnosis is 45–55 years, but a wide range of age at onset is present [10–13].

Up to now, no specific risk factors for the development of MTC have been discovered. Although no environmental factors or ethnical differences have been identified, some associations with pre-existing thyroid diseases and/or other disorders such as hypertension, allergies and gallbladder disease have been reported in a pooled analysis of epidemiological studies [14].

One peculiarity of MTC is that it can arise as a sporadic form, which accounts for 75% of cases, or in the context of familial syndromes, which represent the remaining 25%. When sporadic, it affects

R. Elisei (✉) · A. Matrone
Endocrine Unit, Department of Clinical and Experimental Medicine, University Hospital of Pisa, Pisa, Italy
e-mail: rossella.elisei@med.unipi.it; anto.matrone@virgilio.it

U. K. Mallick et al. (eds.), *Practical Management of Thyroid Cancer*,
https://doi.org/10.1007/978-3-319-91725-2_19

one single person inside the kindred while in the familial cases a dominant mendelian autosomal transmission of the disease can be observed, often associated with other endocrine neoplasia such as pheocromocytoma (PHEO) and/or hyperparathyroidism due to parathyroid hyperplasia or multiple adenomatosis (PTHAd) [15]. These syndromes are called multiple endocrine neoplasia (MEN) and are distinguished into 3 phenotypes according to the combination of endocrine neoplasia and other non endocrine disorders (Table 19.1). Only the hereditary form affects children and, generally, the most aggressive is the syndrome (i.e. MEN IIB) the youngest is the clinically affected child [16–18].

The pathogenesis of MTC has been deeply studied in the last 25 years after the recognition that the activation of the *RET* protoncogene was strongly correlated with the development of the hereditary form of MTC [19–21]. More recently, a very important role of *RET* mutations has been demonstrated also in the sporadic forms since about 50% of them have been found to carry a somatic *RET* mutation which is also related to a greater aggressiveness and a poor outcome of the disease [22]. Up to now, no data are available regarding the possible causes of induction of *RET* mutation.

The clinical behavior of MTC is much less favorable when compared with that of the other well-differentiated thyroid carcinomas even though it is not as unfavourable as that of anaplastic carcinoma [23]. A 10-year survival of about 50% of MTC patients is reported in several series. The stage of the disease at diagnosis is the most important prognostic factor for both the cure and survival of these patients as demonstrated by the evidence that if an early diagnosis is performed, possibly when the neoplastic disease is still intrathyroid, 90% of patients can survive up to 35 years [24, 25].

Table 19.1 Typical clinical manifestations of the three Multiple Endocrine Neoplasia Syndromes

Clinical manifestations[a]	MEN IIA	MEN IIB	FMTC
Medullary thyroid cancer	100%	100%	100%
Pheochromocytoma	60%	45%	No
Parathyroid adenomas	20%	No	No
Cutaneous lichen amyloidosis	20%	No	No
Marfanoid habitus	No	100%	No
Skeletal alterations	No	10%	No
Megacolon	No	40%	No
Mucosal Neurinomas	No	90%	No
Corneal hypertrophy	No	65%	No
Hirschsprung disease	2%	No	No

[a]The prevalence of the different clinical manifestations reported in this table are derived from the data of Pisa registry of MEN II syndromes

Diagnosis of Medullary Thyroid Carcinoma

Clinical Presentation of MTC

The diagnosis of MTC is very much dependent on its clinical presentation. Usually, the most common clinical presentation of a sporadic MTC is a thyroid nodule, either single or belonging to a series of nodules configuring the clinical picture of a multinodular goiter. The association of thyroid nodular disease with a lump in the lateral part(s) of the neck may induce the clinician to suspect a thyroid malignancy but not specifically a MTC. With the exception of the simultaneous presence of diarrhea and/or flushing syndrome, which is however rare and usually related to an advanced metastatic disease with high serum levels of Ct, there are no symptoms or signs that can induce the suspicion of a case of MTC.

At variance, the suspicions of a hereditary MTC can easily originate when a familial history of MTC is present or if the same patient has already been diagnosed with a PHEO or a PTHAd. The presence of mucosal neurinomas of the tongue or conjunctivas in particular if associated to a marfanoid habitus and/or skeletal alterations, should immediately suggest the diagnosis of MEN IIB and induce to the search for an MTC. Similarly, the presence of an interscapular cutaneous itchy lesion, named cutaneous lichen amyloidosis (CLA), is also highly suspicious of MEN IIA since this lesion is almost exclusively found in subjects with this syndrome.

The Diagnostic Work Up in the Sporadic Forms of MTC

As mentioned above, the sporadic MTC appears as a thyroid nodule, single or in the context of a multinodular goiter. Physical examination of the neck does not offer any significant diagnostic elements especially nowadays that the majority of nodules are not palpable and incidentally discovered by neck ultrasound often performed for other purposes [26]. Once the nodule has been discovered a classical work up for thyroid nodular disease is then performed.

Neck Imaging Tools

The MTC ultrasonography usually shows a nodule with an intermediate or high suspicion pattern of malignancy [27] mainly due to the hypoechogenicity, the presence of microcalcifications and a high intranodular vascularization but without any specific or peculiar feature to induce a specific suspicion of MTC. No major differences between the ultrasound pattern of MTC and the other differentiated thyroid carcinoma such as PTC and FTC, have been identified so far [28]. In case of a suspicious thyroid nodule, ultrasound should be extended to the lateral regions of the neck in order to identify suspicious lymph nodes to be submitted to a fine needle aspiration for cytological (FNAC) examination. Thyroid scintiscan, either with 131-I or Tc99, is not commonly indicated but, if performed, MTC appears as a cold nodule similarly to any other thyroid malignancy.

Fine Needle Aspiration Cytology

Fine needle aspiration cytology (FNAC) is performed according to the standard procedure both for the collection of the cytological material, the preparation of the smear and the cytological examination. Standard staining shows the typical MTC "salt and pepper" and "plasmacytoid" appearance of cells. Cells shape varies from oval to round, they can be large polygonal or spindled and are usually isolated. Cytoplasm may be abundant or scanty and usually contains acidophilic granulation visible with specific stains (May-Grunwald-Giemsa). Nuclei, of which there are two or even more, are preferentially round-shaped and eccentrically localized. Amyloid is frequently detectable as clumps of amorphous material, and revealed by Red Congo staining [29, 30]. The immunocytochemistry for Ct and/or chromogranin should be performed if a diagnostic uncertainty is present [31, 32]. Although the cytological pattern of MTC is generally typical, there are several series that show a high percentage of failure in making a presurgical diagnosis by FNAC [33–36]. Recently, this difficulty has been even better demonstrated in a multicentric international study in which the clinical charts of 313 patients, followed in 12 different Institutions located in seven different countries, were evaluated. The authors clearly demonstrated that FNAC was able to make a presurgical diagnosis of MTC only in less than 50% of cases thus negatively impacting on the decision of the surgical treatment extension [37]. Among other explanations, cytological negative results might be due to the fact that MTC could be present in one nodule, in the context of a multinodular goiter, not submitted to FNAC. In this condition, serum Ct measurement is more reliable, since it is elevated even in the presence of microfoci of MTC [34, 38].

Serum Calcitonin

Calcitonin is the most specific and sensitive MTC serum marker, both before and after thyroidectomy [2, 39, 40]. It is a small polypeptide hormone of 32 aminoacids normally produced almost exclusively by C cells. Several studies have demonstrated that routine measurement of serum Ct is the most accurate diagnostic tool for the detection of MTC in patients with thyroid nodules [34–36, 38, 41–43]. In all series the sensitivity of serum Ct was more accurate than that of cytology. Nevertheless, there are still controversial opinions on the role of a routine measurement of basal serum Ct in the work up of thyroid nodules and the new American Thyroid Association guidelines does not suggest in favour or against this procedure leaving the choice to the experience of the physicians on the usefulness of this practice in the management of their patients [44]. However, a good compromise could be the recommendation suggested by the American Association of Clinical Endocrinologists, American College of Endocrinology, and Italian Association of Endocrinologists which indicates to determine serum Ct in thyroid nodules with suspicious ultrasound features or indeterminate cytologic findings [45]. If the routine measurement of serum Ct is not adopted in the clinical work up of thyroid nodules, it could be helpful at least when a surgical treatment is planned for a nodule with an indeterminate cytology or with a malignant cytology no better specified, to plan, in case of elevated values, the right surgical treatment that, at the present, is total thyroidectomy and at least the dissection of the central neck node compartment [44]. This will be also useful to avoid incidental histological diagnosis of MTC which is always followed by the uncertainty to complete or not complete the surgical treatment [46, 47].

The major concerns about the routinely use of serum Ct measurement in thyroid nodules are (a) the cost effectiveness; (b) the low specificity of several assays used to measure serum Ct; (c) the presence of heterophilic antibodies; (d) the association of elevated levels of serum Ct in other diseases than MTC. The problem of the cost effectiveness is not negligible since the prevalence of MTC is rather low and varying form 0.4 to 1.4% among thyroid nodules [10–12, 34]. However, a study performed in USA showed that the cost-effectiveness of the routine measurement of serum Ct in thyroid nodules is comparable to that of the measurement of thyroid stimulating hormone, colonoscopy, and mammography screening [48]. The low specificity of some Ct assays is the real problem since in several studies it has been demonstrated that cases with detectable levels of serum Ct, but less than 50 pg/ml, and submitted to thyroidectomy did not show any MTC at histology [49]. On this regard it is useful to say that the comparison of results obtained by measuring the same sample with different assays has shown a significant analytical inaccuracy and, as a consequence, patient classification was highly dependent on the assay used [50]. Moreover, several of these assays are affected by the presence of heterophilic antibodies in the blood of patients that can interfere in the assay, thus producing false positive results [51]. The interpretation of serum Ct measurement must also take into account of those cases of hypercalcitoninemia not related to MTC. There are several other conditions, both physiological and pathological, in which basal levels of serum Ct may be found to be elevated, and a differential diagnosis is needed [52]. Usually a well collected personal/familial medical history and an accurate physical examination will be of great help in identifying other reasons for the production of Ct such as other malignancies, mainly of neuroendocrine origin or advanced malignancies in which the Ct secretion is related to a paraneoplastic syndrome [53–56]. Very frequently, elevated values of Ct can be found in patients with renal failure [57] and in those with the Zollinger's syndrome [58]. In both cases C-cell hyperplasia was observed in the thyroid of those few patients who have been surgically treated. It is known that C-cell hyperplasia can also be associated with lymphocytic thyroiditis and FTC or, more frequently, PTC microcarcinoma [59, 60] which represent other differential diagnosis to be excluded.

Because of all the aforementioned reasons, elevated basal serum Ct, especially of medium–low level (i.e <100 pg/ml) should not be immediately considered as diagnostic of MTC. These medium-low levels of serum Ct should be further investigated by submitting the patient to a stimulation test with the administration of calcium (Table 19.2) to confirm that the Ct is really secreted by a MTC: a significant increase of serum Ct (usually 3–4 times the basal level) is observed in patients with MTC [61, 62] but not in those with elevated basal serum Ct deriving from other sources or due to artifacts [51, 55, 63]. However, also for the stimulation test and in particular for the significance of the Ct peak after stimulation there are controversial opinions [49, 64] and the final consideration is that each laboratory should identify its own basal and stimulated Ct cut-off with its negative and positive predictive value to be used for diagnostic purposes. Although the routine measurement of serum Ct in all thyroid nod-

Table 19.2 modalities of execution of calcium stimulation test for serum calcitonin

Steps	
(a)	Patient must be weighted
(b)	2.5 mg of Calcium element (or 25 mg of Calcium gluconate) per 1 kg or 2.2 lbs of weight should be taken
(c)	The volume above calculated must be diluted up to 50 ml with standard saline solution
(d)	The i.v. infusion of the 50 ml containing calcium should be rather rapidly administered (in 10 min)
(e)	Blood should be taken before the infusion and 2, 5, 15 and 30 min after the complete infusion of the calcium for calcitonin measurement

ules is still controversial [65, 66], evidence has been provided that this approach allows an early diagnosis and treatment, thus significantly improving the outcome of this potentially lethal disease [67].

Calcitonin Measurement in the Washout of the Needle Used for FNA

If the cytological diagnosis is not defined and the serum Ct is in the grey zone of the assay (i.e. >20 but less than 100 pg/ml) the Ct measurement in the washout of the needle used for the puncture of the suspected thyroid nodule may be crucial [68, 69]. This approach is of particular diagnostic utility to ascertain the nature of neck lymph nodes, especially before thyroidectomy, to plan the surgical approach or the most appropriate therapeutic strategies.

Other Serum Markers

Other than Ct several other peptides are released by the malignant transformed C cells [3]. Among them, the most useful in the management of MTC, especially in the follow up, is the carcino embryonic antigen (CEA) which is usually elevated when the disease is diffuse and distant metastases are present [70, 71]. The serum CEA value is related to the tumoral burden and it is very useful in monitoring the progression of the disease since its level increases when the disease progresses. Serum CEA determination is not part of the work up of thyroid nodule(s) but, if it is incidentally found to be elevated and a thyroid nodule is present, the measurement of serum Ct is indicated [72].

Serum chromogranin may also be elevated in patients with MTC. It is not specific since elevated values have been reported in patients with neither clinical nor biochemical evidence of a primary MTC [73]. Immunohistochemistry for chromogranin more than its serum level is relevant for the diagnosis of MTC especially if the MTC is secreting low amount of Ct.

As in many other neuroendocrine tumors, somatostatin, gastrin releasing peptide, vasoactive intestinal peptide, neuron-specific enolase, calcitonin-gene-related peptide (CGRP) and other neuroendocrine substances may be produced abnormally but none of these peptides are useful for diagnosis [3, 74–76]. Some of these products are responsible of some clinical manifestations such as flushing and diarrhea syndrome [77, 78].

Recently it has been demonstrated a poor prognostic role of carbohydrate antigen 19.9 (CA 19.9) in advanced MTC cases, which seems to be significantly correlated with a short survival once it becomes elevated [79–81]. No MTC diagnostic role for CA 19.9 has been demonstrated so far.

The Histological Diagnosis

Histologically, MTC is pleiomorphic with rounded or spindle cells characteristically organized in nested patterns. Mitosis are rather rare, nuclei are uniform and secretory granules are dispersed in the eosinophilic cytoplasm. Amyloid substance is frequently present (60–80%) between tumoral cells [82]. Whenever a doubt is present and a differential diagnosis from anaplastic, Hurthle cell or insular carcinoma is needed, especially if pseudopapillary elements or giants cells are present, the immunohistochemistry for Ct and chromogranin can easily solve the problem since its positivity is diagnostic of MTC [83].

A mixed form of MTC is also described [84]. It is characterized by the simultaneous presence of parafollicular and follicular cell features, with positive immunohistochemistry for both Ct and thyroglobulin (Tg). On this regard, it is worth noting that the association of MTC and PTC in the same thyroid gland seems to be quite frequent [85, 86]. Molecular studies have shown that genes theoretically specific of the parafollicular C cells (i.e. normal *RET* gene) are expressed in PTC as well as genes theoretically specific of the follicular cells (i.e. Tg, TSH receptor, thyroid transcription factor 1) are indeed expressed also in MTC [5, 87–89]. Despite all these observations, it is still controversial if the mixed MTC is a real separate histological entity, originating from an ancestral stem cell able to differentiate as both follicular and parafollicular cell, or the consequence of the collision of two distinct tumors, MTC and PTC, originating in the same thyroid gland. The oncogene alterations present in the two malignant neoplasm belonging to the same gland have been demonstrated to be different and separate suggesting a separate origin of the two tumors [90].

If the cytology turns out to be negative or indeterminate and serum Ct has not been measured, MTC can be an incidental histological finding. This event is rare but does exist. It causes problems in taking the decision how to proceed particularly if the patient has been submitted to a surgical treatment that is not the recommended one for MTC [44]. On this regard it is worth noting that in a recent multicentric study it has been demonstrated that 5.6% and 17% of sporadic cases are bilateral and multifocal, respectively [46]. This finding suggests that total thyroidectomy should remain the standard of care for initial surgery if the presurgical diagnosis is known. The need to perform a completion thyroidectomy after an incidental histological finding of MTC could be indicated by the basal and/or stimulated levels of serum Ct.

The *RET* Genetic Screening

After 20 years from the discovery that germline *RET* oncogene mutations are responsible of hereditary cases of MTC [19, 21, 91] it is recognised worldwide that *RET* genetic screening must be performed in all patients with MTC, independently from their apparent sporadic origin [92]. The rationale of this screening is lying in the evidence that 5–10% of apparently sporadic MTC cases are found to harbour a germline *RET* mutation being "de novo" or misdiagnosed familial cases [93]. This finding is of great relevance for the early discovery of the other gene carries in the family who are unaware of their condition and sometimes already affected.

Although not yet introduced as a standard of care, *RET* gene analysis would be useful if performed also in the tumoral tissue, either in the fresh or in the paraffin embedded tumoral tissue, of ascertained sporadic cases. There are at least three main reasons to perform this procedure: (a) the discovery of a somatic mutation, that usually occurs in 45% of cases, confirms the sporadic nature of the tumor [94]; (b) the prognostic value of the presence/absence of the somatic mutation [22]; (c) the future possibility for *RET* mutated patients to be treated with drugs specifically aimed at inhibiting the altered *RET* gene [95].

When familial, MTC is one of the components of the Multiple Endocrine Neoplasia type II (MEN II) syndrome, which is an autosomal dominant inherited syndrome with a variable degree of expressivity and an age related penetrance. As shown in Table 19.1, three different hereditary syndromes can be classified according to the involved organs: (a) multiple endocrine neoplasia type IIA (MEN IIA), a syndrome consisting of MTC, PHEO and PTHAd [96]; (b) multiple endocrine neoplasia type IIB (MEN IIB), a syndrome consisting of MTC, PHEO, mucosal neurinomas, ganglioneuromatosis, habitus marfanoid and skeletal alterations [97]; (c) familial medullary thyroid carcinoma (FMTC), which is characterized by the presence of a inheritable MTC with no apparent association with other endocrine neoplasia [98]. After the introduction of the RET genetic screening, the relative prevalence of the FMTC syndrome has been found to be much higher (from 10 to 50% of all MEN syndromes). The increased number of FMTC is mainly due to the high number of apparently sporadic MTC demonstrated to be familial cases by the *RET* mutation analysis [93, 99, 100].

The Work Up for the Identification of the Other Neoplasia of MEN II Syndromes

The evaluation of the thyroid nodule in the hereditary form is performed in the same way as that recommended for sporadic cases, while the hereditary forms require mandatory simultaneous examination of adrenal and parathyroid glands. This research can be guide by the type of *RET* mutation since it is known that there is an important correlation between the genotype and the phenotype (Table 19.3) with some mutations strictly associated to MEN IIA, others with MEN IIB or FMTC.

With the exception of a few examples [101, 102], the development and the diagnosis of PHEO usually follows the development and the diagnosis of MTC. PHEO is usually bilateral but its development can be metachronous with years of latency between the two tumoral mass growth. Symptoms of PHEO are not specific and may be confused with those caused by anxiety. Hypertension is very rare, especially at the beginning of the disease. An elevated value of the daily urinary excretion of epinephrine (or adrenaline) is observed as the first alteration of catecholamine production. Norepinephrine (or noradrenaline) usually increases only later in the course of the disease, thus the earliest biochemical abnormality is an elevated ratio of epinephrine-to-norepinhephrine [103, 104]. As reported in the recent published European guidelines for the management of patients with PHEO [105], the measurement of plasmatic metanephrines, the o–methylated metabolites of catecholamines (both adrenaline and noradrenaline), offer great advantages for an early diagnosis of PHEO over standard measurements of plasmatic catecholamines. Tests for plasmatic metanephrines are more specific and sensitive than those for catecholamines: while normal plasmatic concentrations of metanephrines exclude the diagnosis of pheochromocytoma, normal plasmatic concentrations of catecholamines do not [106, 107]. Once the biochemical suspicious of a PHEO has been arisen, an abdomen ultrasound associated or not with a computerized tomography (CT) and/or magnetic resonance imaging (MRI), may be useful for the localization of the adrenal mass [108, 109]. If there is no demonstrable adrenal mass by CT or MRI scanning, 131-I metaiodobenzylguanidine, a catecholamine analogue actively concentrated by chromaffin tissue, can be used to investigate the presence of an extra-adrenal tumor [110]. Although frequently bilateral, as above mentioned, it is useful to know that PHEO is often asynchronous and several years can separate the appearance of the contra lateral PHEO. For this reason, the unilateral adrenal gland surgical treatment is preferred if the PHEO is present only in one gland. A yearly periodic monitoring of the other adrenal gland is recommended to early identify the second PHEO.

Parathyroid glands may also be involved in MEN IIA. Both adenomas and hyperplasia may be associated with an increase of the parathyroid hormone (PTH) secretion, resulting in hypercalcemia and hypercalciuria in more advanced cases [111]. The earliest serum abnormality detected is a moderately elevated level of serum PTH with normal-high levels of calcemia. In doubtful cases, a calcium infusion test that is unable to suppress the parathyroid hormone secretion will be helpful for the diagnosis [112]. A secondary hyper PTH due to low levels of serum Vitamin D

Table 19.3 Correlation between *RET* mutations and clinical syndromes as described in the ATA 2015 guidelines

Clinical syndrome	*RET* mutation(s)
MEN IIB	M918T (97%) A883F Double mutations
MEN IIA	C634F/G/R/S/W/Y C609F/G/R/S/Y[a] C611F/G/S/Y/W[a] C618F/R/S[a] C620F/R/S[a]
MEN IIA or FMTC	G533C D631Y K666E L790F V804L/M S891A
FMTC	E768D R912P

[a]Mutations regarding these 4 codons can both activate and inhibit the *RET* function, in fact they are called "Janus" mutations and the syndrome can include also the Hirschsprung disease

must be excluded. A neck ultrasound will be useful when a suspicion of parathyroid adenomas is present: the parathyroid adenoma(s) is usually well recognizable as a extrathyroidal mass at the upper and/or lower limit of both thyroid lobes. A dual-phase (early- and delayed-phase) parathyroid scintiscan with ^{99m}Tc Sestamibi can discover parathyroid adenomas not identified with neck ultrasound because too small or because ectopically localized far from thyroid. The dual phase technique is based on the observation that ^{99m}Tc sestamibi washes out more rapidly from the thyroid gland than from hyperfunctioning parathyroid glands [113].

The Genetic Screening for the Identification of Gene Carriers

Once an index case has been confirmed to be hereditary because harbouring a germline *RET* mutation, all first degree relatives should be screened for the presence of the same mutation in their constitutive DNA (i.e. gene carriers). While negative cases can avoid to be re-checked over the years since they are not at risk to develop the MTC, gene carriers must be submitted to a clinical, biochemical (i.e. basal Ct measurement) and neck ultrasound evaluation for the early discovery of the disease. If both of them are negative or normal a calcium stimulation test for Ct is usually recommended [114]. The therapeutic strategies and follow up protocols of gene carriers have been changed over the years. Immediately after the discovery that *RET* mutations were responsible of the hereditary forms the surgical practice of prophylactic thyroidectomy in all children *RET* positive was strongly advocated [115]. Nowadays it is clear that *RET* mutations are different in terms of penetrance and the age of development of MTC can greatly vary from one to the other being the M918T and the non cysteine mutations (i.e. V804M, S891A, L790F, etc) the most and the less transforming and aggressive, respectively. For these reasons the ATA guidelines [44] distinguish the mutations into different classes of risk and the timing of thyroidectomy in gene carriers should take into consideration several factors including the level of risk of the mutation and the basal and stimulated value of serum Ct [44, 92]. The periodical evaluation of serum Ct, both basal and stimulated, may be very useful in identifying the right time to perform an early and safe thyroidectomy [114].

Diagnosis of Persistent or Recurrent Disease

Independently from the sporadic or hereditary nature of the MTC, the first control after surgery should be done 3 months after the surgical treatment, including physical examination, neck ultrasound and measurement of serum FT3, FT4, TSH, Ct and CEA. Measurement of FT3, FT4 and TSH are requested for monitoring the L-tyroxine (L-T4) replacement therapy. Serum Ct is the specific marker to be used for the follow up of MTC patients. CEA measurement is relevant to have a better idea about the tumoral burden and the degree of differentiation of the tumor since, when dedifferentiated, serum Ct can be relatively low and CEA rather elevated.

Due to the prolonged half-lives, if performed too early, measurement of serum Ct may be misleading, especially if a high serum concentration was present pre operatively [116]. If postoperative basal Ct is undetectable, the patient can be considered as cured with a risk of recurrence of about 10% [117]. There are controversial opinions if it could be useful to perform a stimulation test in patients with a postoperative undetectable serum Ct [44]. A study performed in large series of patients with prolonged follow up has shown that only 3.3% of those patients who had one post operative negative stimulation test subsequently become positive [118] thus improving the prognostic value of the measurement of stimulated Ct respect to the basal.

Frequently basal and/or stimulated serum Ct is persistently elevated after initial surgery. Because serum Ct is a very sensitive and specific MTC marker, the finding of detectable serum levels of basal or stimulated Ct is an indication of persistent disease. In patients with persistent disease, serum CEA concentration should be monitored because both high and increasing levels are strongly suggestive of a progressive disease [70, 71]. In the majority of cases, the challenge is to find the source of production of Ct and CEA. About 50% of patients not cured at surgery have no evidence of metastatic disease when studied with the traditional imaging techniques. Several studies demonstrated that when serum Ct is less than 150 pg/ml it is very unlikely to find the origin of the Ct production and thus the metastatic lesions. For this reason the new ATA guidelines suggest to perform imaging procedures only when serum Ct is >150 pg/mL [44]. The only imaging procedure that can be performed when serum Ct is less than 150 pg/ml is the neck ultrasound since the neck is the site with the highest frequency of local recurrence and node metastases. A total body CT scan with contrast medium and a bone scintigraphy are suggested as the most sensitive procedures [119]. MRI is very useful for the detection of small liver metastases which, at CT scan are often interpreted as small angiomas. Other imaging techniques such as Octrescan, 123-metaiodobenzylguanidine (MIBG), and positron emission tomography (PET) may be useful although at present they do not appear to be particularly sensitive, especially in the presence of micrometastases [120–122]. A greater sensitivity of PET can be obtained by using 18F-DOPA which can be complimentary to 18F-FDG standard PET [123, 124] even if both of them are rarely able to find metastatic lesions in patients with detectable but low levels of serum Ct [125]. As far as PET is considered, in the last years new radiopharmaceuticals have been identified and demonstrated to be more specific for MTC such as (68) Ga-labeled somatostatin analogues (Ga68-Dotatoc or Dotatate) [126] but their sensitivity is related to the presence of somatostatin receptors which are usually positive in <50% of MTC. Their use is relevant if a therapy with (177)Lu-labeled or (90)Y-labeled somatostatin analogues would be performed.

The most accurate technique for the localization of occult metastases is probably the measurement of serum Ct after selective venous sampling catheterization: the presence of a gradient in the neck, in the mediastinum or in the supra-hepatic veins suggests the presence of a metastatic disease in the district where the higher levels of serum Ct have been found. However, this method is highly invasive and does not significantly improve the rate of cure and nowadays is very rarely indicated [127–129].

Non Surgical Management

When patients are not cured by the primary surgical treatment, which should include total thyroidectomy and central neck lymphnode dissection, other therapeutic procedures are indicated according to the localization and the number of lesions. In planning a therapeutic strategy it should be taken into account that most distant metastases found during follow up are small at the time of their recognition and that their growth is usually rather slow. These lesions are compatible with a long period of good quality of life. In these cases, an aggressive therapeutic approach may not be indicated, unless an evident rapid progressive disease is demonstrated. Nowadays, there are new drugs, named tyrosine kinase inhibitors (TKI), that have been approved for the treatment of advanced and progressive MTC. Nevertheless, before starting these systemic therapies some considerations must be done regarding the number, the size and the rate of growth of the lesions. Whenever possible a local treatment should be preferred and systemic therapy should be postponed to the evidence of a multimetastatic progressive disease [130].

Local Treatments

(a) *External radiotherapy (ERBT)*: although MTC is not very sensitive to radiation, EBRT may be indicated in some cases. A local inoperable disease or a lymphnodal recurrent disease already treated 2 or 3 times by surgery can be treated with ERBT with the aim to stop the growth or at least to reduce the rate of growth [131]. There are data suggesting an improved local control of the disease with a longer interval between treatment and recurrence of regional or local disease in patients treated with ERBT with respect to those untreated [132, 133]. With the same purpose, but also to reduce the pain, ERBT can be used in some cases of bone metastases. Brain metastases may be also treated with ERBT, with a stereotactic radiosurgery (SRS) and/or a whole brain radiotherapy (WBRT), and a rapid and reliable response may be obtained [134]. Radiation therapy of lung metastases is not indicated for the high risk of radiation fibrosis and respiratory dysfunction.

(b) *Radiofrequency thermoablation (RT)*: this is a procedure based on the use of electromagnetic waves that induce movement and consequently the production of heat that will kill the tumoral cells. This treatment is applicable to local disease but also to bone, liver and lung lesions if technically possible [135–137]. This treatment is of particular utility when the lesion to be treated is the only site of disease or the only one among others that is growing and a surgical treatment cannot be performed.

(c) *Treatment of tracheal infiltration or compression*: when tracheal infiltration is present and an invasion of the tracheal lumen is evident at tracheobroncoscopy, a disobstructive laser treatment can be performed and periodically repeated if necessary. An endotracheal stent may be applied to reduce the risk of suffocation when the trachea is compressed by an adjacent tumoral mass [138].

(d) *Conventional transarterial chemoembolization (cTACE) or radioembolization*: these techniques are commonly used for a palliative treatment of advanced hepatocellular carcinoma but in some advanced cases of liver metastatic disease can be also applied in MTC. These procedures have been demonstrated to be of particular benefit when liver metastases are smaller than 3 cm and the liver involvement is less than 30% [139].

Systemic Therapy

(a) *Chemotherapy*: no clinical advantages have been shown in several small-scale trials published to date in which advanced, metastatic MTC were treated with chemotherapy [140]. Thus, nowadays chemotherapy is not more indicated and should be reserved to those few patients who, for any reasons, cannot be treated with the new targeted therapies. In these cases the reduction of the growth rate and the achievement of a stabilization of the disease represents a satisfactory result, although we are conscious that these effects are not durable or very short. A high dose of doxorubicine (75 mg/m^2 every 3–4 weeks) remains the most effective chemotherapeutic agent with a response rate of 15–20% in terms of stabilization of the disease. The same response rate is obtained when doxorubicin is used alone or in combination with other drugs such as 5-fluorouracile, dacarbazine, streptozocin, cyclo-phosphamide and vincristine [141, 142]. Since major toxic effects are frequently observed and the response is only partial and short lived, chemotherapy should not be used in patients with stable or slowly progressive disease.

(b) *Radionuclide therapy*: MTC is a neuroendocrine tumor and 30–50% of cases express somatostatin receptors as ascertained by octreoscan [120] and nowadays even better by 68Ga-DOTATATE or DOTATOC PET/CT [143]. Over the years, different types of octreotide, from the native to the long-acting analogues, have been explored as potential therapeutic agents. In the majority of cases, a significant reduction in serum Ct has been demonstrated [144]. Unfortunately, no evidence of a parallel reduction of the number and/or the size of tumor lesions has been shown. Inconstant and transient effects in reducing symptoms such as flushing and diarrhea are not sufficient to recommend the administration of somatostatin analogues in metastatic MTC patients. No improvement in the therapeutic effect has been observed when the somatostatin analogues have been combined with α-interferon [144]. The possibility to use (90)Yttrium and/or (177) Lutetium labeled somatostatin analogs seems to be promising although limited to a 30% of somatostatin positive MTC [145, 146].

(c) *Targeted therapies with tyrosine kinase inhibitors*: Current systemic therapeutic options for advanced and progressive MTC are represented by targeted tyrosine kinase inhibitors (TKIs) therapies specifically directed against signal transduction pathways and or genetic alteration of MTC (Table 19.4). Although several TKIs have been tested on advanced and progressive MTC only two drugs, vandetanib and cabozantinib, have been approved by both the Food and Drug Administration (FDA) and the European Medicine Agency (EMA) for the therapy of these patients after the phase III clinical ZETA and EXAM studies [147, 148].

Although with different patterns, both vandetanib and cabozantinb are small molecules able to block multiple tyrosine kinases with different activities that make the difference between the two drugs. Both of them should be started if the progression of the disease, as assessed according to following Response Evaluation Criteria in Solid Tumors (RECIST), has been documented in the last 12/14 months or according to clinical judgment in very advanced cases. The choice of one or the other drug is very much dependent on the availability of the drug since not all countries have both drugs approved and reimbursed. However, in those countries where both of them can be prescribed, the choice must take into consideration the patient clinical features and drug characteristics. According to the results of the phase III studies [147, 148] the effect of cabozantinib seems to be more rapid but with a safety profile more demanding in its management (Table 19.5). Cabozantinb has been tested also in patients who had been previoulsy treated with other TKIs and the results showed that it works in terms of prolongation of the progression free survival thus suggesting that it can be used as second line. This information is unavailable for vandetanib that is apparently more manageable but slower in determining the disease control. Vandetanib, but not cabozantinib, has been tested also in children with a dedicated scheme of administration and the results showed that it is safe and effective also in the control of the childhood MTC [149]. Moreover, there are several reported evidences that the ectopic ACTH secretion and the consequent paraneoplastic Cushing's syndrome, which is frequently present when the disease is multimetastatic and advanced, is reverted and cured by the administration of vandetanib [150–153]. Vandetanib cannot be used in patients who have a prolonged QTc (>450 ms in men and >470 ms in females) while cabozantib has not this limitation. Side effects are similar but the prevalence of each one of them is different according to the drug that is used (Table 19.5). Despite a significant advantage in prolonging the progression free survival time has been demon-

Table 19.4 Tyrosine kinase inhibitors approved for the treatment of advanced MTC and their molecular targets

Drug	VEGFR	cKIT	RET	PDGFR	FGFR	EGFR	BRAF	MEK	mTOR	Others
Vandetanib	+	–	+	–	–	+	–	–	–	RET fusions
Cabozantinib	+	+	+	+	–	–	–	–	–	MET RET fusions

Table 19.5 Adverse events reported in more than 30% of patients at least in one of the two Phase III studies exploring the impact of two tyrosine kinase inhibitors on the prolongation of the progression free survival

Phase III clinical trial	Drug	Tumor	Hypertension (%)	Diarrhoea (%)	Skin rash (%)	Anorexia (%)	Nausea (%)	Weight loss (%)	Fatigue (%)	QTc prolongation (%)
ZETA	Vandetanib	MTC	32	56	45	21	33	10	24	14
EXAM	Cabozantinib	MTC	32	63	19	45	43	47	40	NE[a]

[a]*NE* not evaluated

strated by the use of both drugs, so far, none of them showed an increase of the overall survival.

Both drugs, as all TKI, are cytostatic and not cytotoxic thus they can stop the growth of the cells but they do not kill them and for this reason they must be continued until the evidence of clinical benefit. However, from the results of the two studies is clearly evident that sooner or later a sort of resistance is developed and the clinicians must decide to continue or to stop the drug. Further studies to analyse the possibility to use the two drugs in an alternated modality or combined between them or with other drugs, either working with the same mechanism or by modulating the immune system, will be the challenge of the next future.

Conclusions

MTC is a rare disease whose clinical presentation is similar to that of any other thyroid tumors and the only diagnostic marker is represented by elevated levels of serum Ct. Fine needle aspiration cytology is the only other presurgical diagnostic tool although it fails in obtaining a precise diagnosis of MTC in about half of the cases. Nevertheless, an early presurgical diagnosis is fundamental to obtain a definitive cure with the surgical treatment. Once this cannot be obtained, the disease becomes chronic and, if progressing, it requires further therapies that can be either local treatments, such as radiofrequency ablation and chemoembolization, if the progression is related to one lesion or systemic when a simultaneous progression of several lesions is happening. At the present, the systemic therapy of choice is represented by two tyrosine kinase inhibitors, vandetanib and cabozantinib, that have been approved by both FDA and EMA for the treatment of advanced and progressive MTC. Considering the rarity of the disease, the difficulty of an early diagnosis, the possibility that it can be familial other than sporadic and that the management of the persistent disease can be challenging it is recommended that MTC patients should be followed by a multidisciplinary team in a specialized center.

References

1. Hazard JB, Hawk WA, Crile G Jr. Medullary (solid) carcinoma of the thyroid; a clinicopathologic entity. J Clin Endocrinol Metab. 1959;19:152–61.
2. Melvin KE, Tashjian AH Jr. The syndrome of excessive thyrocalcitonin produced by medullary carcinoma of the thyroid. Proc Natl Acad Sci U S A. 1968;59:1216–22.
3. Pacini F, Basolo F, Elisei R, Fugazzola L, Cola A, Pinchera A. Medullary thyroid cancer. An immunohistochemical and humoral study using six separate antigens. Am J Clin Pathol. 1991;95:300–8.
4. Johansson E, Andersson L, Ornros J, et al. Revising the embryonic origin of thyroid C cells in mice and humans. Development. 2015;142:3519–28.
5. Nilsson M, Williams D. On the origin of cells and derivation of thyroid cancer: C cell story revisited. Eur Thyroid J. 2016;5:79–93.
6. Kameda Y, Nishimaki T, Chisaka O, Iseki S, Sucov HM. Expression of the epithelial marker E-cadherin by thyroid C cells and their precursors during murine development. J Histochem Cytochem. 2007;55:1075–88.
7. Gmunder-Lehner RB, Okamoto E, Hedinger C. Distribution of C cells in the human thyroid gland. Schweiz Med Wochenschr. 1983;113:1385–94.
8. https://rarediseases.info.nih.gov/diseases/7004/thyroid-cancer-medullary.
9. National Cancer Institute - Surveillance, Epidemiology and End Result Program.
10. Bergholm U, Adami HO, Telenius-Berg M, Johansson H, Wilander E. Incidence of sporadic and familial medullary thyroid carcinoma in Sweden 1959 through 1981. A nationwide study in 126 patients. Swedish MCT Study Group. Acta Oncol. 1990;29:9–15.
11. Christensen SB, Ljungberg O, Tibblin S. A clinical epidemiologic study of thyroid carcinoma in Malmo, Sweden. Curr Probl Cancer. 1984;8:1–49.
12. Bondeson L, Ljungberg O. Occult thyroid carcinoma at autopsy in Malmo, Sweden. Cancer. 1981;47:319–23.
13. Bhattacharyya N. A population-based analysis of survival factors in differentiated and medullary thyroid carcinoma. Otolaryngol Head Neck Surg. 2003;128:115–23.
14. Negri E, Ron E, Franceschi S, et al. Risk factors for medullary thyroid carcinoma: a pooled analysis. Cancer Causes Control. 2002;13:365–72.
15. Romei C, Pardi E, Cetani F, Elisei R. Genetic and clinical features of multiple endocrine neoplasia types 1 and 2. J Oncol. 2012;2012:705036.
16. Machens A, Niccoli-Sire P, Hoegel J, et al. Early malignant progression of hereditary medullary thyroid cancer. N Engl J Med. 2003;349:1517–25.
17. Niccoli-Sire P, Murat A, Baudin E, et al. Early or prophylactic thyroidectomy in MEN 2/FMTC gene carriers: results in 71 thyroidectomized patients. The French Calcitonin Tumours Study Group (GETC). Eur J Endocrinol. 1999;141:468–74.

18. Sanso GE, Domene HM, Garcia R, et al. Very early detection of RET proto-oncogene mutation is crucial for preventive thyroidectomy in multiple endocrine neoplasia type 2 children: presence of C-cell malignant disease in asymptomatic carriers. Cancer. 2002;94:323–30.
19. Mulligan LM, Kwok JB, Healey CS, et al. Germline mutations of the RET proto-oncogene in multiple endocrine neoplasia type 2A. Nature. 1993;363:458–60.
20. Mulligan LM, Marsh DJ, Robinson BG, et al. Genotype-phenotype correlation in multiple endocrine neoplasia type 2: report of the International RET Mutation Consortium. J Intern Med. 1995;238:343–6.
21. Donis-Keller H, Dou S, Chi D, et al. Mutations in the RET proto-oncogene are associated with MEN 2A and FMTC. Hum Mol Genet. 1993;2:851–6.
22. Elisei R, Cosci B, Romei C, et al. Prognostic significance of somatic RET oncogene mutations in sporadic medullary thyroid cancer: a 10-year follow-up study. J Clin Endocrinol Metab. 2008;93:682–7.
23. Christensen SB, Ljungberg O. Mortality from thyroid carcinoma in Malmo, Sweden 1960-1977. A clinical and pathologic study of 38 fatal cases. Cancer. 1984;54:1629–34.
24. Gharib H, McConahey WM, Tiegs RD, et al. Medullary thyroid carcinoma: clinicopathologic features and long-term follow-up of 65 patients treated during 1946 through 1970. Mayo Clin Proc. 1992;67:934–40.
25. Kebebew E, Ituarte PH, Siperstein AE, Duh QY, Clark OH. Medullary thyroid carcinoma: clinical characteristics, treatment, prognostic factors, and a comparison of staging systems. Cancer. 2000;88:1139–48.
26. Acar T, Ozbek SS, Acar S. Incidentally discovered thyroid nodules: frequency in an adult population during Doppler ultrasonographic evaluation of cervical vessels. Endocrine. 2014;45:73–8.
27. Valderrabano P, Klippenstein DL, Tourtelot JB, et al. New American thyroid association sonographic patterns for thyroid nodules perform well in medullary thyroid carcinoma: institutional experience, systematic review, and meta-analysis. Thyroid. 2016;26:1093–100.
28. Lee S, Shin JH, Han BK, Ko EY. Medullary thyroid carcinoma: comparison with papillary thyroid carcinoma and application of current sonographic criteria. AJR Am J Roentgenol. 2010;194(4):1090.
29. Soderstrom N, Telenius-Berg M, Akerman M. Diagnosis of medullary carcinoma of the thyroid by fine needle aspiration biopsy. Acta Med Scand. 1975;197:71–6.
30. Mendonca ME, Ramos S, Soares J. Medullary carcinoma of thyroid: a re-evaluation of the cytological criteria of diagnosis. Cytopathology. 1991;2:93–102.
31. Takeichi N, Ito H, Okamoto H, Matsuyama T, Tahara E, Dohi K. The significance of immunochemically staining calcitonin and CEA in fine-needle aspiration biopsy materials from medullary carcinoma of the thyroid. Jpn J Surg. 1989;19:674–8.
32. Papaparaskeva K, Nagel H, Droese M. Cytologic diagnosis of medullary carcinoma of the thyroid gland. Diagn Cytopathol. 2000;22:351–8.
33. Forrest CH, Frost FA, de Boer WB, Spagnolo DV, Whitaker D, Sterrett BF. Medullary carcinoma of the thyroid: accuracy of diagnosis of fine-needle aspiration cytology. Cancer. 1998;84:295–302.
34. Pacini F, Fontanelli M, Fugazzola L, et al. Routine measurement of serum calcitonin in nodular thyroid diseases allows the preoperative diagnosis of unsuspected sporadic medullary thyroid carcinoma. J Clin Endocrinol Metab. 1994;78:826–9.
35. Rieu M, Lame MC, Richard A, et al. Prevalence of sporadic medullary thyroid carcinoma: the importance of routine measurement of serum calcitonin in the diagnostic evaluation of thyroid nodules. Clin Endocrinol. 1995;42:453–60.
36. Niccoli P, Wion-Barbot N, Caron P, et al. Interest of routine measurement of serum calcitonin: study in a large series of thyroidectomized patients. The French Medullary Study Group. J Clin Endocrinol Metab. 1997;82:338–41.
37. Essig GF Jr, Porter K, Schneider D, et al. Fine needle aspiration and medullary thyroid carcinoma: the risk of inadequate preoperative evaluation and initial surgery when relying upon FNAB cytology alone. Endocr Pract. 2013;19:920–7.
38. Vierhapper H, Raber W, Bieglmayer C, Kaserer K, Weinhausl A, Niederle B. Routine measurement of plasma calcitonin in nodular thyroid diseases. J Clin Endocrinol Metab. 1997;82:1589–93.
39. Tashjian AH Jr, Melvin EW. Medullary carcinoma of the thyroid gland. Studies of thyrocalcitonin in plasma and tumor extracts. N Engl J Med. 1968;279:279–83.
40. Dube WJ, Bell GO, Aliapoulios MA. Thyrocalcitonin activity in metastatic medullary thyroid carcinoma. Further evidence for its parafollicular cell origin. Arch Intern Med. 1969;123:423–7.
41. Kaserer K, Scheuba C, Neuhold N, et al. C-cell hyperplasia and medullary thyroid carcinoma in patients routinely screened for serum calcitonin. Am J Surg Pathol. 1998;22:722–8.
42. Ozgen AG, Hamulu F, Bayraktar F, et al. Evaluation of routine basal serum calcitonin measurement for early diagnosis of medullary thyroid carcinoma in seven hundred seventy-three patients with nodular goiter. Thyroid. 1999;9:579–82.
43. Hahm JR, Lee MS, Min YK, et al. Routine measurement of serum calcitonin is useful for early detection of medullary thyroid carcinoma in patients with nodular thyroid diseases. Thyroid. 2001;11:73–80.
44. Wells SA Jr, Asa SL, Dralle H, et al. Revised American Thyroid Association guidelines for the management of medullary thyroid carcinoma. Thyroid. 2015;25:567–610.
45. Gharib H, Papini E, Garber JR, et al. American Association of Clinical Endocrinologists, American College of Endocrinology, and Associazione Medici Endocrinologi Medical Guidelines for Clinical

Practice for the diagnosis and management of thyroid nodules--2016 update. Endocr Pract. 2016;22:622–39.
46. Essig GF Jr, Porter K, Schneider D, et al. Multifocality in sporadic medullary thyroid carcinoma: an international multicenter study. Thyroid. 2016;26:1563–72.
47. Ahmed SR, Ball DW. Incidentally discovered medullary thyroid cancer: diagnostic strategies and treatment. J Clin Endocrinol Metab. 2011;96:1237–45.
48. Cheung K, Roman SA, Wang TS, Walker HD, Sosa JA. Calcitonin measurement in the evaluation of thyroid nodules in the United States: a cost-effectiveness and decision analysis. J Clin Endocrinol Metab. 2008;93(6):2173–80.
49. Costante G, Meringolo D, Durante C, et al. Predictive value of serum calcitonin levels for preoperative diagnosis of medullary thyroid carcinoma in a cohort of 5817 consecutive patients with thyroid nodules. J Clin Endocrinol Metab. 2007;92:450–5.
50. Martinetti A, Seregni E, Ferrari L, et al. Evaluation of circulating calcitonin: analytical aspects. Tumori. 2003;89:566–8.
51. Tommasi M, Brocchi A, Cappellini A, Raspanti S, Mannelli M. False serum calcitonin high levels using a non-competitive two-site IRMA. J Endocrinol Investig. 2001;24:356–60.
52. Elisei R. Routine serum calcitonin measurement in the evaluation of thyroid nodules. Best Pract Res Clin Endocrinol Metab. 2008;22:941–53.
53. Tsolakis AV, Portela-Gomes GM, Stridsberg M, et al. Malignant gastric ghrelinoma with hyperghrelinemia. J Clin Endocrinol Metab. 2004;89:3739–44.
54. Mullerpatan PM, Joshi SR, Shah RC, et al. Calcitonin-secreting tumor of the pancreas. Dig Surg. 2004;21(4):321.
55. Samaan NA, Castillo S, Schultz PN, Khalil KG, Johnston DA. Serum calcitonin after pentagastrin stimulation in patients with bronchogenic and breast cancer compared to that in patients with medullary thyroid carcinoma. J Clin Endocrinol Metab. 1980;51:237–41.
56. Monsieur I, Meysman M, Noppen M, et al. Non-small-cell lung cancer with multiple paraneoplastic syndromes. Eur Respir J. 1995;8:1231–4.
57. Akan B, Bohmig G, Sunder-Plassmann G, Borchhardt KA. Prevalence of hypercalcitoninemia in patients on maintenance dialysis referred to kidney transplantation. Clin Nephrol. 2009;71:538–42.
58. Lamers CB, Hackeng WH, Thien T, van Tongeren JH. Serum concentrations of immunoreactive calcitonin in patients with hypergastrinaemia. Digestion. 1980;20:379–82.
59. Perry A, Molberg K, Albores-Saavedra J. Physiologic versus neoplastic C-cell hyperplasia of the thyroid: separation of distinct histologic and biologic entities. Cancer. 1996;77:750–6.
60. Komminoth P, Roth J, Saremaslani P, Matias-Guiu X, Wolfe HJ, Heitz PU. Polysialic acid of the neural cell adhesion molecule in the human thyroid: a marker for medullary thyroid carcinoma and primary C-cell hyperplasia. An immunohistochemical study on 79 thyroid lesions. Am J Surg Pathol. 1994;18:399–411.
61. Karanikas G, Moameni A, Poetzi C, et al. Frequency and relevance of elevated calcitonin levels in patients with neoplastic and nonneoplastic thyroid disease and in healthy subjects. J Clin Endocrinol Metab. 2004;89:515–9.
62. Barbot N, Calmettes C, Schuffenecker I, et al. Pentagastrin stimulation test and early diagnosis of medullary thyroid carcinoma using an immunoradiometric assay of calcitonin: comparison with genetic screening in hereditary medullary thyroid carcinoma. J Clin Endocrinol Metab. 1994;78:114–20.
63. Ichimura T, Kondo S, Okushiba S, Morikawa T, Katoh H. A calcitonin and vasoactive intestinal peptide-producing pancreatic endocrine tumor associated with the WDHA syndrome. Int J Gastrointest Cancer. 2003;33:99–102.
64. Mian C, Perrino M, Colombo C, et al. Refining calcium test for the diagnosis of medullary thyroid cancer: cutoffs, procedures, and safety. J Clin Endocrinol Metab. 2014;99:1656–64.
65. Hodak SP, Burman KD. The calcitonin conundrum--is it time for routine measurement of serum calcitonin in patients with thyroid nodules? J Clin Endocrinol Metab. 2004;89:511–4.
66. Deftos LJ. Should serum calcitonin be routinely measured in patients with thyroid nodules--will the law answer before endocrinologists do? J Clin Endocrinol Metab. 2004;89:4768–9. author reply 9–70
67. Elisei R, Bottici V, Luchetti F, et al. Impact of routine measurement of serum calcitonin on the diagnosis and outcome of medullary thyroid cancer: experience in 10,864 patients with nodular thyroid disorders. J Clin Endocrinol Metab. 2004;89:163–8.
68. Boi F, Maurelli I, Pinna G, et al. Calcitonin measurement in wash-out fluid from fine needle aspiration of neck masses in patients with primary and metastatic medullary thyroid carcinoma. J Clin Endocrinol Metab. 2007;92:2115–8.
69. Rosario PW, Calsolari MR. Basal serum calcitonin, after calcium stimulation, and in the needle washout of patients with thyroid nodules and mild or moderate basal hypercalcitoninemia. Horm Metab Res. 2017;49:129–34.
70. Busnardo B, Girelli ME, Simioni N, Nacamulli D, Busetto E. Nonparallel patterns of calcitonin and carcinoembryonic antigen levels in the follow-up of medullary thyroid carcinoma. Cancer. 1984;53:278–85.
71. Rougier P, Calmettes C, Laplanche A, et al. The values of calcitonin and carcinoembryonic antigen in the treatment and management of nonfamilial medullary thyroid carcinoma. Cancer. 1983;51:855–62.
72. Akbulut S, Sogutcu N. A high level of carcinoembryonic antigen as initial manifestation of medullary thyroid carcinoma in a patient with subclinical hyperthyroidism. Int Surg. 2011;96:254–9.

73. Baudin E, Bidart JM, Bachelot A, et al. Impact of chromogranin A measurement in the work-up of neuroendocrine tumors. Ann Oncol. 2001;12(Suppl 2):S79–82.
74. Barakat MT, Meeran K, Bloom SR. Neuroendocrine tumours. Endocr Relat Cancer. 2004;11:1–18.
75. Pacini F, Elisei R, Anelli S, Gasperini L, Schipani E, Pinchera A. Circulating neuron-specific enolase in medullary thyroid cancer. Int J Biol Markers. 1986;1:85–8.
76. Pacini F, Fugazzola L, Basolo F, Elisei R, Pinchera A. Expression of calcitonin gene-related peptide in medullary thyroid cancer. J Endocrinol Investig. 1992;15:539–42.
77. Wyon Y, Frisk J, Lundeberg T, Theodorsson E, Hammar M. Postmenopausal women with vasomotor symptoms have increased urinary excretion of calcitonin gene-related peptide. Maturitas. 1998;30:289–94.
78. Jaffe BM. Prostaglandins and serotonin: nonpeptide diarrheogenic hormones. World J Surg. 1979;3:565–78.
79. Elisei R, Lorusso L, Romei C, et al. Medullary thyroid cancer secreting carbohydrate antigen 19-9 (Ca 19-9): a fatal case report. J Clin Endocrinol Metab. 2013;98:3550–4.
80. Elisei R, Lorusso L, Piaggi P, et al. Elevated level of serum carbohydrate antigen 19.9 as predictor of mortality in patients with advanced medullary thyroid cancer. Eur J Endocrinol. 2015;173:297–304.
81. Milman S, Arnold JL, Price M, et al. Medullary thyroid cancer that stains negative for Ca 19-9 has decreased metastatic potential. Endocr Pract. 2015;21:590–4.
82. Sletten K, Westermark P, Natvig JB. Characterization of amyloid fibril proteins from medullary carcinoma of the thyroid. J Exp Med. 1976;143:993–8.
83. Rosai JCM, De Lellis RA. Tumors of the thyroid gland. In: Atlas of tumor pathology, 3rd series. Washington: Armed Forces Institute of pathology; 1992.
84. Matias-Guiu X. Mixed medullary and follicular carcinoma of the thyroid. On the search for its histogenesis. Am J Pathol. 1999;155:1413–8.
85. Biscolla RP, Ugolini C, Sculli M, et al. Medullary and papillary tumors are frequently associated in the same thyroid gland without evidence of reciprocal influence in their biologic behavior. Thyroid. 2004;14:946–52.
86. Vantyghem MC, Pigny P, Leteurtre E, et al. Thyroid carcinomas involving follicular and parafollicular C cells: seventeen cases with characterization of RET oncogenic activation. Thyroid. 2004;14:842–7.
87. Fluge O, Haugen DR, Akslen LA, et al. Expression and alternative splicing of c-ret RNA in papillary thyroid carcinomas. Oncogene. 2001;20:885–92.
88. Elisei R, Pinchera A, Romei C, et al. Expression of thyrotropin receptor (TSH-R), thyroglobulin, thyroperoxidase, and calcitonin messenger ribonucleic acids in thyroid carcinomas: evidence of TSH-R gene transcript in medullary histotype. J Clin Endocrinol Metab. 1994;78:867–71.
89. Katoh R, Miyagi E, Nakamura N, et al. Expression of thyroid transcription factor-1 (TTF-1) in human C cells and medullary thyroid carcinomas. Hum Pathol. 2000;31:386–93.
90. Ciampi R, Romei C, Pieruzzi L, et al. Classical point mutations of RET, BRAF and RAS oncogenes are not shared in papillary and medullary thyroid cancer occurring simultaneously in the same gland. J Endocrinol Investig. 2017;40:55–62.
91. Eng C, Smith DP, Mulligan LM, et al. Point mutation within the tyrosine kinase domain of the RET proto-oncogene in multiple endocrine neoplasia type 2B and related sporadic tumours. Hum Mol Genet. 1994;3:237–41.
92. Elisei R, Alevizaki M, Conte-Devolx B, Frank-Raue K, Leite V, Williams GR. 2012 European thyroid association guidelines for genetic testing and its clinical consequences in medullary thyroid cancer. Eur Thyroid J. 2013;1:216–31.
93. Romei C, Cosci B, Renzini G, et al. RET genetic screening of sporadic medullary thyroid cancer (MTC) allows the preclinical diagnosis of unsuspected gene carriers and the identification of a relevant percentage of hidden familial MTC (FMTC). Clin Endocrinol. 2011;74:241–7.
94. Romei C, Ugolini C, Cosci B, et al. Low prevalence of the somatic M918T RET mutation in micro-medullary thyroid cancer. Thyroid. 2012;22:476–81.
95. Sherman SI, Clary DO, Elisei R, et al. Correlative analyses of RET and RAS mutations in a phase 3 trial of cabozantinib in patients with progressive, metastatic medullary thyroid cancer. Cancer. 2016;122:3856–64.
96. Keiser HR, Beaven MA, Doppman J, Wells S Jr, Buja LM. Sipple's syndrome: medullary thyroid carcinoma, pheochromocytoma, and parathyroid disease. Studies in a large family. NIH conference. Ann Intern Med. 1973;78:561–79.
97. Cunliffe WJ, Hudgson P, Fulthorpe JJ, et al. A calcitonin-secreting medullary thyroid carcinoma associated with mucosal neuromas, marfanoid features, myopathy and pigmentation. Am J Med. 1970;48:120–6.
98. Farndon JR, Leight GS, Dilley WG, et al. Familial medullary thyroid carcinoma without associated endocrinopathies: a distinct clinical entity. Br J Surg. 1986;73:278–81.
99. Eng C, Mulligan LM, Smith DP, et al. Low frequency of germline mutations in the RET proto-oncogene in patients with apparently sporadic medullary thyroid carcinoma. Clin Endocrinol. 1995;43:123–7.
100. Wiench M, Wygoda Z, Gubala E, et al. Estimation of risk of inherited medullary thyroid carcinoma in apparent sporadic patients. J Clin Oncol. 2001;19:1374–80.
101. Jadoul M, Leo JR, Berends MJ, et al. Pheochromocytoma-induced hypertensive encephalopathy revealing MEN-IIa syndrome in a 13-year old boy. Implications for screening procedures and surgery. Horm Metab Res. 1989;21:46–9.

102. Lips KJ, Van der Sluys Veer J, Struyvenberg A, et al. Bilateral occurrence of pheochromocytoma in patients with the multiple endocrine neoplasia syndrome type 2A (Sipple's syndrome). Am J Med. 1981;70:1051–60.
103. Hamilton BP, Landsberg L, Levine RJ. Measurement of urinary epinephrine in screening for pheochromocytoma in multiple endocrine neoplasia type II. Am J Med. 1978;65:1027–32.
104. Miyauchi A, Masuo K, Ogihara T, et al. Urinary epinephrine and norepinephrine excretion in patients with medullary thyroid carcinoma and their relatives. Nihon Naibunpi Gakkai Zasshi. 1982;58:1505–16.
105. Plouin PF, Amar L, Dekkers OM, et al. European Society of Endocrinology Clinical Practice Guideline for long-term follow-up of patients operated on for a phaeochromocytoma or a paraganglioma. Eur J Endocrinol. 2016;174:G1–G10.
106. Lenders JW, Keiser HR, Goldstein DS, et al. Plasma metanephrines in the diagnosis of pheochromocytoma. Ann Intern Med. 1995;123:101–9.
107. Weise M, Merke DP, Pacak K, Walther MM, Eisenhofer G. Utility of plasma free metanephrines for detecting childhood pheochromocytoma. J Clin Endocrinol Metab. 2002;87:1955–60.
108. DeLellis RA, Wolfe HJ, Gagel RF, et al. Adrenal medullary hyperplasia. A morphometric analysis in patients with familial medullary thyroid carcinoma. Am J Pathol. 1976;83:177–96.
109. Carney JA, Sizemore GW, Tyce GM. Bilateral adrenal medullary hyperplasia in multiple endocrine neoplasia, type 2: the precursor of bilateral pheochromocytoma. Mayo Clin Proc. 1975;50:3–10.
110. Sisson JC, Shapiro B, Beierwaltes WH. Scintigraphy with I-131 MIBG as an aid to the treatment of pheochromocytomas in patients with the multiple endocrine neoplasia type 2 syndromes. Henry Ford Hosp Med J. 1984;32:254–61.
111. Silverberg SJ, Shane E, Jacobs TP, Siris E, Bilezikian JP. A 10-year prospective study of primary hyperparathyroidism with or without parathyroid surgery. N Engl J Med. 1999;341:1249–55.
112. Heath H, Sizemore GW, Carney JA. Preoperative diagnosis of occult parathyroid hyperplasia by calcium infusion in patients with multiple endocrine neoplasia, type 2a. J Clin Endocrinol Metab. 1976;43:428–35.
113. Taillefer R, Boucher Y, Potvin C, Lambert R. Detection and localization of parathyroid adenomas in patients with hyperparathyroidism using a single radionuclide imaging procedure with technetium-99m-sestamibi (double-phase study). J Nucl Med. 1992;33:1801–7.
114. Elisei R, Romei C, Renzini G, et al. The timing of total thyroidectomy in RET gene mutation carriers could be personalized and safely planned on the basis of serum calcitonin: 18 years experience at one single center. J Clin Endocrinol Metab. 2012;97:426–35.
115. Ukkat J, Lorenz K, Hinze R, Thomusch O, Dralle H. Importance of early screening and prophylactic thyroidectomy in asymptomatic nonindex RET germline carriers. World J Surg. 2001;25:713–7.
116. Fugazzola L, Pinchera A, Luchetti F, et al. Disappearance rate of serum calcitonin after total thyroidectomy for medullary thyroid carcinoma. Int J Biol Markers. 1994;9:21–4.
117. Pellegriti G, Leboulleux S, Baudin E, et al. Long-term outcome of medullary thyroid carcinoma in patients with normal postoperative medical imaging. Br J Cancer. 2003;88:1537–42.
118. Franc S, Niccoli-Sire P, Cohen R, et al. Complete surgical lymph node resection does not prevent authentic recurrences of medullary thyroid carcinoma. Clin Endocrinol. 2001;55:403–9.
119. Giraudet AL, Vanel D, Leboulleux S, et al. Imaging medullary thyroid carcinoma with persistent elevated calcitonin levels. J Clin Endocrinol Metab. 2007;92:4185–90.
120. Baudin E, Lumbroso J, Schlumberger M, et al. Comparison of octreotide scintigraphy and conventional imaging in medullary thyroid carcinoma. J Nucl Med. 1996;37:912–6.
121. Szakall S Jr, Esik O, Bajzik G, et al. 18F-FDG PET detection of lymph node metastases in medullary thyroid carcinoma. J Nucl Med. 2002;43:66–71.
122. Arslan N, Ilgan S, Yuksel D, et al. Comparison of In-111 octreotide and Tc-99m (V) DMSA scintigraphy in the detection of medullary thyroid tumor foci in patients with elevated levels of tumor markers after surgery. Clin Nucl Med. 2001; 26(8):683.
123. Archier A, Heimburger C, Guerin C, et al. (18) F-DOPA PET/CT in the diagnosis and localization of persistent medullary thyroid carcinoma. Eur J Nucl Med Mol Imaging. 2016;43:1027–33.
124. Kauhanen S, Schalin-Jantti C, Seppanen M, et al. Complementary roles of 18F-DOPA PET/CT and 18F-FDG PET/CT in medullary thyroid cancer. J Nucl Med. 2011;52:1855–63.
125. Faggiano A, Grimaldi F, Pezzullo L, et al. Secretive and proliferative tumor profile helps to select the best imaging technique to identify postoperative persistent or relapsing medullary thyroid cancer. Endocr Relat Cancer. 2009;16:225–31.
126. Salavati A, Puranik A, Kulkarni HR, Budiawan H, Baum RP. Peptide receptor radionuclide therapy (PRRT) of medullary and nonmedullary thyroid cancer using radiolabeled somatostatin analogues. Semin Nucl Med. 2016;46:215–24.
127. Abdelmoumene N, Schlumberger M, Gardet P, et al. Selective venous sampling catheterisation for localisation of persisting medullary thyroid carcinoma. Br J Cancer. 1994;69:1141–4.
128. Frank-Raue K, Raue F, Buhr HJ, Baldauf G, Lorenz D, Ziegler R. Localization of occult persisting medullary thyroid carcinoma before microsurgical reoperation: high sensitivity of selective venous catheterization. Thyroid. 1992;2:113–7.
129. Ben Mrad MD, Gardet P, Roche A, et al. Value of venous catheterization and calcitonin studies in the treatment and management of clinically inapparent medullary thyroid carcinoma. Cancer. 1989;63:133–8.

130. Schlumberger MBL, Dralle H, Jarzab B, Pacini F, Smit JWA, The European Task Force. 2012 European thyroid association guidelines for metastatic medullary thyroid cancer. Eur Thyroid J. 2012;1:5–14.
131. Giuliani M, Brierley J. Indications for the use of external beam radiation in thyroid cancer. Curr Opin Oncol. 2014;26:45–50.
132. Fersht N, Vini L, A'Hern R, Harmer C. The role of radiotherapy in the management of elevated calcitonin after surgery for medullary thyroid cancer. Thyroid. 2001;11:1161–8.
133. Fife KM, Bower M, Harmer CL. Medullary thyroid cancer: the role of radiotherapy in local control. Eur J Surg Oncol. 1996;22:588–91.
134. Murray L, Menard C, Zadeh G, et al. Radiosurgery for brainstem metastases with and without whole brain radiotherapy: clinical series and literature review. J Radiat Oncol. 2017;6:21–30.
135. Ringe KI, Panzica M, von Falck C. Thermoablation of bone tumors. RoFo. 2016;188:539–50.
136. Eisele RM. Advances in local ablation of malignant liver lesions. World J Gastroenterol. 2016;22:3885–91.
137. Lencioni R, Crocetti L, Cioni R, et al. Response to radiofrequency ablation of pulmonary tumours: a prospective, intention-to-treat, multicentre clinical trial (the RAPTURE study). Lancet Oncol. 2008;9:621–8.
138. Ribechini A, Bottici V, Chella A, et al. Interventional bronchoscopy in the treatment of tracheal obstruction secondary to advanced thyroid cancer. J Endocrinol Investig. 2006;29:131–5.
139. Roche A, Girish BV, de Baere T, et al. Trans-catheter arterial chemoembolization as first-line treatment for hepatic metastases from endocrine tumors. Eur Radiol. 2003;13:136–40.
140. Orlandi F, Caraci P, Mussa A, Saggiorato E, Pancani G, Angeli A. Treatment of medullary thyroid carcinoma: an update. Endocr Relat Cancer. 2001;8:135–47.
141. Schlumberger M, Abdelmoumene N, Delisle MJ, Couette JE. Treatment of advanced medullary thyroid cancer with an alternating combination of 5 FU-streptozocin and 5 FU-dacarbazine. The Groupe d'Etude des Tumeurs a Calcitonine (GETC). Br J Cancer. 1995;71:363–5.
142. Nocera M, Baudin E, Pellegriti G, Cailleux AF, Mechelany-Corone C, Schlumberger M. Treatment of advanced medullary thyroid cancer with an alternating combination of doxorubicin-streptozocin and 5 FU-dacarbazine. Groupe d'Etude des Tumeurs a Calcitonine (GETC). Br J Cancer. 2000;83:715–8.
143. Yamaga LYI, Cunha ML, Campos Neto GC, et al. 68Ga-DOTATATE PET/CT in recurrent medullary thyroid carcinoma: a lesion-by-lesion comparison with 111In-octreotide SPECT/CT and conventional imaging. Eur J Nucl Med Mol Imaging. 2017;44:1695–701.
144. Lupoli GA, Fonderico F, Fittipaldi MR, et al. The role of somatostatin analogs in the management of medullary thyroid carcinoma. J Endocrinol Investig. 2003;26:72–4.
145. Vaisman F, Rosado de Castro PH, Lopes FP, et al. Is there a role for peptide receptor radionuclide therapy in medullary thyroid cancer? Clin Nucl Med. 2015;40:123–7.
146. Budiawan H, Salavati A, Kulkarni HR, Baum RP. Peptide receptor radionuclide therapy of treatment-refractory metastatic thyroid cancer using (90)Yttrium and (177)Lutetium labeled somatostatin analogs: toxicity, response and survival analysis. Am J Nucl Med Mol Imaging. 2013;4:39–52.
147. Wells SA Jr, Robinson BG, Gagel RF, et al. Vandetanib in patients with locally advanced or metastatic medullary thyroid cancer: a randomized, double-blind phase III trial. J Clin Oncol. 2012;30:134–41.
148. Elisei R, Schlumberger MJ, Muller SP, et al. Cabozantinib in progressive medullary thyroid cancer. J Clin Oncol. 2013;31:3639–46.
149. Fox E, Widemann BC, Chuk MK, et al. Vandetanib in children and adolescents with multiple endocrine neoplasia type 2B associated medullary thyroid carcinoma. Clin Cancer Res. 2013;19:4239–48.
150. Baudry C, Paepegaey AC, Groussin L. Reversal of Cushing's syndrome by vandetanib in medullary thyroid carcinoma. N Engl J Med. 2013;369:584–6.
151. Nella AA, Lodish MB, Fox E, et al. Vandetanib successfully controls medullary thyroid cancer-related Cushing syndrome in an adolescent patient. J Clin Endocrinol Metab. 2014;99(9):3055.
152. Pitoia F, Bueno F, Schmidt A, Lucas S, Cross G. Rapid response of hypercortisolism to vandetanib treatment in a patient with advanced medullary thyroid cancer and ectopic Cushing syndrome. Arch Endocrinol Metabol. 2015;59:343–6.
153. Paepegaey AC, Cochand-Priollet B, Louiset E, et al. Long-term control of hypercortisolism by vandetanib in a case of medullary thyroid carcinoma with a somatic RET mutation. Thyroid. 2017;27:587–90.

Familial Non-Medullary Thyroid Cancer

20

Joanna Klubo-Gwiezdzinska,
Yevgenia Kushchayeva, Sudheer Kumar Gara,
and Electron Kebebew

Introduction

Familial nonmedullary thyroid cancer (FNMTC) accounts for 3–9% of all nonmedullary thyroid cancer (NMTC) cases. FNMTC may occur as a minor component of inherited cancer syndromes (PTEN hamartoma tumor, Peutz-Jeghers syndrome, familial adenomatous polyposis AFP, Carney complex, Pendred syndrome, DICER1 syndrome, ataxia-telangiectasia, and Werner syndrome) or as a nonsyndromic familial disease [1]. The majority of patients with FNMTC (95%) have nonsyndromic disease [2]. There are well-defined genotype-phenotype associations in syndromic FNMTC, while the genetic background of nonsyndromic FNMTC and its association in clinical behavior is currently controversial and not well understood.

J. Klubo-Gwiezdzinska
Metabolic Disease Branch, National Institute of Diabetes and Digestive and Kidney Diseases, National Institutes of Health, Bethesda, MD, USA

Y. Kushchayeva
Diabetes, Obesity and Endocrinology Branch, National Institute of Diabetes and Digestive and Kidney Diseases, National Institutes of Health, Bethesda, MD, USA

S. K. Gara
Endocrine Oncology Branch, National Cancer Institute, National Institutes of Health, Bethesda, MD, USA

E. Kebebew (✉)
Endocrine Oncology Branch, National Cancer Institute, National Institutes of Health, Bethesda, MD, USA

Department of Surgery, The George Washington University School of Medicine and Health Sciences, Washington, DC, USA
e-mail: kebebew@stanford.edu

Syndromic FNMTC

PTEN Hamartoma Tumor Syndrome (PHTS)

Genetics of PTEN Hamartoma Tumor Syndrome

PTEN hamartoma tumor syndrome (PHTS) is a complex disorder that is inherited in an autosomal-dominant manner and caused by germline inactivating mutations in the *PTEN* (phosphatase and tensin homolog) tumor-suppressor gene, located on chromosome 10q23.3. PHTS includes Cowden syndrome (CS), Bannayan-Riley-Ruvalcaba syndrome (BRRS), *PTEN*-related Proteus syndrome (PS), and Proteus-like syndrome. The *PTEN* mutation is found in 85% of patients [3]. There are approximately 150 unique pathogenic *PTEN* variants found throughout the coding region of *PTEN*, according to the Human Gene Mutation database. The *PTEN* gene product is an enzyme responsible for removing the phosphate group from other proteins and lipids, thereby regulating the cell-division process. The *PTEN* mutation is not a solitary genetic etiology of PHTS. Another

U. K. Mallick et al. (eds.), *Practical Management of Thyroid Cancer*,
https://doi.org/10.1007/978-3-319-91725-2_20

well-recognized genetic alteration that occurs in *KLLN* (killin) is a gene promoter hypermethylation [4]. Killin is a TP53 target gene, upstream of *PTEN*, which shares a common promoter. Therefore, hypermethylation of *KLLN* down-regulates its transcription and disrupts the TP53 activation of killin [5]. The other genetic causes of *PTEN* hamartoma tumor syndrome observed in a small percentage of cases are mutations in succinate dehydrogenase (*SDH*) genes *SDHB* or *SDHD* [4]. Mutations in the *SDHx* genes activate the AKT and MAPK signaling pathways, much like *PTEN* mutations. Some studies have identified mutations in *PIK3CA* and *AKT1* as additional genetic alterations associated with this syndrome [6]. Using whole-exome sequencing across four generations in a family with negative *PTEN* and *SDHx* mutations and no *KLLN* promoter hypermethylation, Yehia and colleagues identified three new culprit genes: *C16ORF72*, *PTPN2*, and *SEC23B*. *SEC23B* is an important component in protein transport from the endoplasmic reticulum (ER) to the Golgi apparatus. Functional studies documented that a V594G mutation in *SEC23B* results in ER stress, which subsequently mediates cell-colony formation and stimulates growth and invasion. These data suggest that the variant can predispose to cancer potentially through the induction of ER stress [7].

Clinical Features of PTEN Hamartoma Tumor Syndrome

Cowden Syndrome

Cowden syndrome (CS) was described by Lloyd and Dennis in 1963. Cowden is the surname of the first family diagnosed with this condition [8]. CS is characterized by the presence of the following clinical features:

- pathognomonic criteria: (a) dysplastic cerebellar gangliocytoma (also known as Lhermitte-Duclos disease), (b) facial trichilemmomas, (c) acral keratosis, and (d) papillomatous lesions.
- major criteria: (a) macrocephaly, (b) breast cancer, (c) NMTC, (d) endometrial cancer.
- minor criteria: (a) hamartomas, (b) thyroid lesions (adenoma, multinodular goiter (MNG)), (c) mental retardation, (d) fibrocystic breast disease, (e) lipomas, (f) fibromas, (g) uterine fibroids, and (h) renal cell carcinoma (RCC) [9, 10] (Table 20.1).

Cowden-like syndrome includes patients with features of CS that don't meet the diagnostic criteria for CS [11].

Thyroid diseases, including adenomatoid nodules, lymphocytic thyroiditis, follicular adenomas/carcinomas, and papillary thyroid cancer (PTC), are the most common extracutaneous manifestations of CS and are found in 50–68% of patients with CS [12, 13]. MNG and/or adenoma can be seen in up to 68% of patients [12, 13]. NMTC is the second-most-common cancer after breast cancer in patients with CS and has been reported in 3–14% of cases [12, 14]. The lifetime risk for thyroid cancer may be as high as 35.2% [10].

CS/CS-like patients have a higher risk of follicular thyroid cancer (FTC) due to *PTEN* mutations and a higher risk of PTC due to *SDH*x and *KLLN* alterations [4]. Analysis of *SDHx*-positive CS/CS-like patients showed NMTC in 5 of 10 cases (50%) compared to 15 of 206 cases (7.2%) among *PTEN*-positive patients with CS; however, this finding needs to be validated due to the small number of patients who were *SDHx*-mutation positive [11].

In patients from CS-like kindred who have concomitant thyroid and breast cancers, no *PTEN* mutations have been found [15]. Ni and associates found that 2 of 10 patients who had thyroid and breast cancers were positive for the *SDHD* mutation (Gly12Ser and His50Arg) [11].

Follicular thyroid cancer (FTC) has been reported to be more common than PTC, most likely because the *PTEN* mutation associated with FTC is the most common mutation observed in this group of patients [12, 13, 16]. Epidemiological data document female predominance with an average age of diagnosis in the third decade of life. However, an earlier onset between 7 and 13 years old has also been reported [4, 13, 16–19]. Based on analysis of 664 patients with CS and CS-like, 2.9% were diagnosed before 18 years of age [4].

Table 20.1 Familial syndromes associated with non-medullary thyroid cancer

Syndrome	Inheritance	Susceptibility gene	Chromosome location	Clinical features
APC-associated polyposis: FAP Attenuated polyposis Gardner Turcot syndrome II	AD	*APC*	5q21-q22	• At least 100 colorectal adenomatous polyps occurring before age 40 or fewer than 100 adenomatous polyps and a relative with FAP associated with fibromas, desmoid tumors, epithelial cysts, hypertrophic retinal pigment epithelium, upper GI tract hamartomas, supernumerary teeth, hepatoblastoma, benign and malignant thyroid disease • No family member with >100 polyps before age 30 AND at least two individuals with 10–99 adenomas after age 30 OR one member with 10–99 polyps after 30yo and a first-degree relative with colorectal cancer with a few adenomas • Colonic polyposis associated with osteomas and epidermoid cysts, desmoid tumors • Colonic polyps associated with CNS tumors, usually medulloblastoma
PTEN hamartoma tumor syndrome: Cowden Bannayan-Riley-Ruvalcaba PTEN-related Proteus Proteus-like	AD	*PTEN*—80% *SDHB/D*—10% Other: *KILLIN, PIK3CA, AKT*	10q23.31	• *Pathognomonic criteria* such as Lhermitte-Duclos disease, facial trichilemmomas, acral keratosis, papillomatous lesions; *major criteria* such as macrocephaly, breast cancer, NMTC, endometrial cancer, and *minor criteria* such GI hamartomas, thyroid lesions (adenoma, MNG), mental retardation, breast fibrocystic breast disease, lipomas, fibromas uterine fibroids, RCC, lipomas, fibromas • Macrocephaly, hamartomatous intestinal polyposis, lipomas, and pigmented macules of the glans penis • Distorting, progressive overgrowth, cerebriform connective tissue nevi, linear verrucous epidermal nevus, adipose dysregulation. Mosaic distribution, highly variable • Significant clinical features of PS, but do not meet the diagnostic criteria
Peutz-Jeghers syndrome	AD	*STK11/LKB1*	19p13.3	• Two or more PJS-type (hamartomatous gastrointestinal polyp) intestinal polyps[a], mucocutaneous macules, gynecomastia in males as a result of estrogen-producing Sertoli cell testicular tumor, h/o intussusception, especially in a child or young adult
Werner	AR	*WRN*	8p11-p12	• Premature aging, scleroderma-like skin changes, cataracts, subcutaneous calcifications, muscular atrophy, osteoporosis, atherosclerosis, DM, skin ulcers, melanoma, sarcomas, MDS
Pendred syndrome	AR	*SLC26A4 (PDS)*	7q21–34	• Hearing impairment and thyroid abnormalities, including benign and malignant lesions
Carney's complex	AD	*PRKA1A* *"CNC2"*	17q22-24 2p16	• Myxomas of soft tissue, lentiginosis, blue nevi, Sertoli cell testicular tumors, psammomatous melanotic schwannomatosis, pituitary adenoma, PPNAD, and endocrine overactivity secondary to pituitary adenomas, ACTH-independent Cushing syndrome due to primary pigmented nodular adrenocortical disease (PPNAD), and thyroid abnormalities, including benign and malignant tumors

(continued)

Table 20.1 (continued)

Syndrome	Inheritance	Susceptibility gene	Chromosome location	Clinical features
Papillary renal neoplasia	Unknown	*PRN1*	1q21	• Papillary renal neoplasia, PTC, benign thyroid nodules
DICER 1	AD	*DICER 1*	14q32.13	• Phenotypes including pleuropulmonary blastoma, ovarian sex cord-stromal tumors • (Sertoli-Leydig cell tumor, juvenile granulosa cell tumor, gynandroblastoma), cystic nephroma, thyroid gland neoplasia including MNG, adenomas, or DTC; ciliary body medulloepithelioma, botryoid-type embryonal rhabdomyosarcoma of the cervix or other sites, nasal chondromesenchymal hamartoma, pituitary blastoma, pineoblastoma
Ataxia-telangiectasia	AR	*ATM*	11q22-23	• Progressive cerebellar ataxia with onset between ages one and 4 years, oculomotor apraxia, choreoathetosis, telangiectasias of the conjunctivae, immunodeficiency, frequent infections, and an increased risk for malignancy, particularly leukemia and lymphoma

[a]Histopathologically characterized by distinctive interdigitating smooth muscle bundles in a characteristic arborizing (branching tree) appearance throughout the lamina propria, particularly of small bowel polyps, and lobular organization, particularly of colonic crypts

Bannayan-Riley-Ruvalcaba Syndrome (BRRS)

BRRS is a disease with a wide spectrum of phenotypic traits [20, 21]. BRRS was first described in 1971 as a congenital syndrome with lipomatosis, angiomatosis, and macrocephaly [22]. Features of the disease include macrocephaly, hamartomatous intestinal polyps, increased linear growth, dysmorphic features, joint hyperextensibility, pectus excavatum, scoliosis, café au lait spots, lipomas, and pigmented penile macules. Additional features include developmental delay, large birth weight, and proximal muscles myopathy [21, 22] (Table 20.1).

BRRS has been associated with MNG, follicular/Hürthle cell adenomas, FTC, and PTC, with a higher prevalence of FTC than PTC [21, 23]. The average FTC tumor size was 0.6–4.5 cm with minimal invasion. The average age at presentation was 14 years old. There were only two cases of micro-PTC that coexisted with FTC or follicular adenomas (FA) [23].

Management of Thyroid Cancer Associated with PTEN Hamartoma Tumor Syndrome

Given the rarity of PHTS, there are no high-quality data to use as a basis for evidence-based recommendations. Instead, clinical care is guided by the natural history of the case series described in the literature. The high prevalence of thyroid pathology in patients with CS warrants routine thyroid screening with ultrasound (US) [24]. A physical exam as well as a baseline and annual thyroid US have been recommended for surveying at-risk patients [10, 18]. For *PTEN* mutation–positive patients baseline thyroid US and annual US evaluation is recommended after 18 years of age. However, for families with a history of a particular cancer type at an early age, screening may be initiated five to 10 years prior to the youngest age of diagnosis in the family [25]. In addition, based on analysis of *SDHx*-positive *PTEN*-negative CS/CS-like patients who may have a significantly increased risks of breast, thyroid, and kidney cancers, active screening based on *SDHx* testing has been recommended [11]. In contrast, some experts recommend screening young patients with PHTS and unusual thyroid pathology such as MNG, multifocal, or bilateral disease [23].

The evaluation of thyroid nodules greater than 1 cm with US-guided fine-needle aspiration biopsy should be performed, and the indication and extent of the thyroidectomy should be based on the cytologic diagnosis and extent of disease if it is found to be thyroid cancer per established guidelines [26].

Peutz-Jeghers Syndrome

Genetics of Peutz-Jeghers Syndrome

Peutz-Jeghers syndrome (PJS) is an autosomal-dominant disorder caused by germline mutations in the *STK11* gene (also known as *LKB1*) located on chromosome 19p13.3 [27]. *STK11* is a tumor-suppressor gene with inactivating mutations disrupting its ability to restrain cell division. This increased cellular proliferation signal leads to the development of non-cancerous hamartomatous polyps in the gastrointestinal tract. In particular, mutations spanning the STK11 protein kinase domain are associated with a higher incidence (9 of 10, 90%) of gastrointestinal polyp dysplasia compared to 2 of 17 (11.8%) for polyp dysplasia in individuals with pathogenic variants in other regions of the gene [28]. Some studies suggested that the *STK11* pathogenic variant is not associated with an increased incidence of cancer [29, 30], while the others found that patients with pathogenic variants of *STK11*, apart from having a higher polyp count, also had a greater risk of melanoma [31, 32].

Clinical Features of Peutz-Jeghers Syndrome

Peutz-Jeghers syndrome (PJS) is characterized by the presence of small bowel hamartomatous polyposis, mucocutaneous hyperpigmentation, and, most likely, a predisposition to a wide variety of epithelial malignancies including in the pancreas, breast, uterus, ovary, and testes [33] (Table 20.1). The initial presentation is typically associated with complications of growing intestinal polyps predominantly resulting in a mechanical obstruction of the gastrointestinal tract, occurring in the first decade of the life [27].

NMTC is not a part of the known typical PJS spectrum. However, there are seven reported cases of differentiated thyroid cancer (DTC) in patients with PJS [27, 33–38]. The age of DTC diagnosis ranged between 21 and 30 years, with the youngest age of presentation being 6 years old [27, 33–38]. The most common histopathological subtype was PTC (five of seven cases) [27, 33–38]. Furthermore, elderly patients harboring an *STK11* mutation without clinical features of PJS have been described, indicating that *STK11* may play a role in DTC [39].

Management of Thyroid Cancer Associated with Peutz-Jeghers Syndrome

There is insufficient data to recommend for or against screening for thyroid cancer in patients with PJS. Some authors suggest that thyroid US might be recommended early because thyroid cancer, if present, occurs early in PJS patients [33]. Once a diagnosis is established, treatment would follow the current guidelines or the standard management of thyroid cancer and thyroid nodules [40].

Familial Adenomatous Polyposis (FAP)

Genetics of FAP

FAP was first described by Lockhart-Mummery in 1925 as a disease with a clear dominant inheritance pattern. It was later demonstrated as an autosomal-dominant syndrome caused by germline mutations in the adenomatous polyposis coli (*APC*) gene on chromosome 5q21 [41, 42]. The majority of the *APC* mutations are either frameshift or nonsense mutations leading to a truncated protein [43]. The APC protein is part of the regulatory beta-catenin destruction complex in the canonical Wnt/beta-catenin pathway. Upon binding with the ligand, the destruction complex dissociates, allowing beta catenin to enter the nucleus and promote gene transcription, which leads to cell proliferation. The *APC* inactivating mutations led to the loss of the beta-catenin destruction complex, therefore promoting beta-catenin translocation into the nucleus [44, 45]. An autosomal-recessive inheritance pattern of this disease was observed in patients with mutations in the *MUTYH* gene [46]. Mutations in this gene affect the ability of cells to correct the errors made during DNA replication. Two mutations (Y165C or G382D) are common in people of European descent. There are three subtypes of FAP: [1] Gardner syndrome, caused by mutations in the *APC* tumor suppressor gene; [2] Turcot syndrome type 1, a rare autosomal recessive disorder caused by a mutation in two DNA mismatch repair genes, *MLH1* and *PMS 2*; and [3] Turcot syndrome type 2 (Crail's syndrome), an autosomal-dominant syndrome secondary to the mutations in the *APC* gene. The MLH1 and PMS2 proteins form a complex that coordinates with other proteins to repair mistakes that arise during DNA replication.

Clinical Presentation of FAP

APC-associated polyposis includes the overlapping, often indistinguishable phenotypes of FAP, attenuated FAP, Gardner syndrome, and Turcot syndrome [47]. FAP is a prototypical intestinal polyposis syndrome with a nearly 100% lifetime risk of colorectal cancer [48]. Extra-colonic manifestations include hepatoblastoma, medulloblastoma, osteomas, supernumerary teeth or missing teeth, congenital hypertrophy of retinal pigment epithelium, desmoid tumors, fibromas, and thyroid abnormalities (Table 20.1). Gardner's syndrome (GS) is a clinical variant of FAP and is characterized by the association of FAP with the characteristic triad of desmoid tumors, osteomas, and epidermoid cysts (Table 20.1). Thyroid nodules can be found in 38% of patients with FAP [49]. Patients with FAP who had thyroid cancer were first described by Crail in 1949 [50]. PTC is the most common type of NMTC among FAP/GS patients, with a frequency of 0.7–12% [49, 51–54]. On average, NMTC has been estimated to occur about ten times more frequently than expected for sporadic PTC [51]. However, based on a summary of 62 registries of 3727 patients with FAP worldwide, the prevalence of PTC was reported to be 1.2% (44 women, 1 man) [55]. Similar results (1.3%) were found based on an analysis of almost 1200 patients by Truta and colleagues [56]. The same risk of NMTC has been described for attenuated FAP with *MUTYH* mutations [57, 58], which has a similar FAP phenotype but fewer polyps [52].

A diagnosis of NMTC can precede a diagnosis of FAP in one-third of patients. The most common age of presentation is in the second to third decade of life, with an age range between 18 and 40 years [18], [52]. GS/FAP patients are predominantly female (86% of cases), and the female-to-male ratio is between 10:1 and 20:1. Patients have an estimated 100–160-fold higher risk of NMTC compared to the general population [54, 59–61]. Furthermore, the risk for NMTC might be race-dependent. Based on an analysis of the Japanese population, the risk of PTC in women with FAP was 23-fold greater compared to non-Japanese women with FAP [62].

NMTC in patients with FAP is usually multifocal and bilateral, with rare metastases and a prognosis similar to sporadic PTC [51, 52, 63]. Based on a case series, multifocal tumors were found in 66–100% of patients, and bilateral involvement was noted in 42–66.6% [53, 56, 64]. There are distinct histologic features in NMTC associated with FAP, including a cribriform pattern with solid areas and a spindle-cell component with marked fibrosis [51, 65]. The cribriform-morular variant represents more than 90% of PTC in patients with FAP despite being a very rare variant in sporadic PTC (0.1–0.2%) [51]. The typical histologic features of sporadic PTC, such as nuclear grooving, overlapping, intranuclear inclusions, and clear nuclei, are rare or absent in the cribriform-morular type [63, 65, 66]. Isolated FTC can be found in 9% of FAP patients, and concomitant PTC and FTC have also been described in 5 of 36 cases. A case of medullary thyroid cancer has also been reported in a patient with FAP [52]. The prognosis for FAP-related NMTC after surgical treatment is excellent. Only one case of distant metastasis to the spine was observed among 36 patients with FAP-related NMTC (2.7%) [52]. In another study, NMTC was described as a cause of death in one of 45 patients with FAP [11].

Turcot syndrome includes patients with FAP who have central nervous system (CNS) tumors, usually medulloblastoma [24]. In 1959, Turcot and associates described two teenaged siblings with numerous adenomatous colorectal polyps and CNS malignant tumors. Turcot syndrome type 2 accounts for two-thirds of all cases, and most of these families harbor a germline *APC* gene mutation [67, 68]. There is limited data on the frequency and NMTC in patients with Turcot syndrome. There is a single case report of a 23-year-old woman with Turcot syndrome type II with multifocal PTC [69].

Management of Thyroid Cancer Associated with FAP

There are no clear recommendations regarding NMTC screening among patients with APC-associated polyposis. Annual surveillance with a physical exam or thyroid US for all patients with FAP has been recommended [48, 49, 53, 54]. According to the American College of Gastroenterology [18], an annual thyroid US is recommended in individuals with *FAP*, *MUTYH*-associated polyposis, and attenuated polyposis (a conditional recommendation, low quality of evidence). Septer and colleagues recommended annual US examination in female patients 18 years of age and older with a *FAP* germline mutation at codon 1061 or any mutation proximal to codon 528, followed by fine-needle aspiration biopsy if indicated [48]. Based on an observation from a small cohort study, which documented that 13 of 15 patients (87%) had germline mutations in the genomic region associated with congenital hypertrophy of the retinal pigment epithelium 5′ region of exon 15, it has been suggested that this mutation may direct PTC screening in patients with FAP [48, 70]. On the other hand, since the cribriform-morular form of PTC is very rare and associated with FAP, each patient with this variant of PTC should be screened for FAP [24] (Table 20.2). Once a diagnosis of NMTC associated with FAP is made, the treatment would follow the current guidelines or the standard management of sporadic thyroid cancer, as there is no data to suggest that the outcome (as compared to sporadic NMTC) is different [40].

Table 20.2 Characteristics of syndromic familial nonmedullary thyroid cancer (FNMTC)

Syndrome	Frequency of TC	Type of TC	Clinical characteristics, prognosis	Screening based on literature data	References
APC-associated polyposis: • FAP • Attenuated FAP • Gardner • Turcot syndrome, type 2	0.7–12%; 100–160-fold risk of TC compared to normal individuals	PTC, cribriform morular or classical PTC with sclerosis	Female predominance; 2nd–3rd decade of life; TC: Multifocal, bilateral, rare metastases; prognosis is similar to sporadic PTC	Annual thyroid US exam for all patients; annual thyroid US in female patients, 18 years of age and older with FAP harboring mutation at codon 1061, or any mutation proximal to codon 528, followed by FNA when indicated; in patients with mutation in genomic region associated with CHRPE, 5′region of exon 1, PTC screening can be suggested	[18, 48, 49, 53, 54, 70]
PTEN-Hamartoma Tumor syndrome[a]: • Cowden • Bannayan-Riley Ruvalcaba Cowden-like syndrome	3–14%, lifetime risk: 35.2%	FTC associated with numerous adenomatous nodules and FAs	Female predominance; 3rd decade of life; possible early onset in childhood at 7–13yo; prognosis is unknown	*For patients with known PHTS:* Exam, baseline and annual thyroid US; baseline thyroid ultrasound for patients <18yo and annual US evaluation in adults was recommended; for families with history of a particular cancer type at an early age, screening may be initiated 5–10 y before the earliest known TC in the family	[10, 18, 25]
				For patients with unknown history of PHTS: In young patients with unusual thyroid pathology such as MNG, multifocal or bilateral disease with LT, PHTS should be ruled out	[23]
Werner	Relative risk of TC 8.9% among Japanese WS patients	PTC, FTC, ATC, especially increased FTC and ATC	In Japanese WS patients: average age 39 years; F:M ratio 2.3:1	At least annual physical examination	[110]

Table 20.2 (continued)

Syndrome	Frequency of TC	Type of TC	Clinical characteristics, prognosis	Screening based on literature data	References
Carney's complex	Up to 10%	FTC, PTC	Up to 60% have TNs; 2/3 among children and adolescents; TNs appear during the first 10 years of life	Thyroid ultrasound is recommended as baseline examination for determining thyroid involvement in pediatric and young adults and may be repeated as needed. FNA is recommended in suspicious cases with treatment of TC appropriate for histologic phenotype	[71, 82, 86]
Papillary renal neoplasia	Prevalence unknown	PTC, classic variant	Limited data	Unknown due to rarity of the disease	[104]
DICER 1	Prevalence unknown	PTC, FTC	Young age; not aggressive features in TC	Annual thyroid physical examination Thyroid US in case of thyroid asymmetry and/or nodule(s) detected on physical examination, or if the patient has previously received, or will receive chemotherapy/repeated upper-body radiological imaging. A thyroid US could be repeated every 3–5 years if no nodule is detected Annual thyroid US during childhood/adolescence with appropriate endocrine referral for young *DICER1* mutation carriers	[97, 99]
Pendred syndrome	1%	FTC	Prognosis is unknown	Thyroid US evaluation and routine thyroid examination in a patient with hypothyroidism for early identification of TC	[24]
Ataxia-telangiectasia	Prevalence unclear	PTC, FTC	Only females were described; age 9.3–35.8 years; prognosis unknown	No screening recommendations have been established, but clinicians should have low threshold for thyroid evaluation	[11]

(continued)

Table 20.2 (continued)

Syndrome	Frequency of TC	Type of TC	Clinical characteristics, prognosis	Screening based on literature data	References
Peutz-Jeghers syndrome[b]	Prevalence is unknown	PTC	Age 21–30 years; prognosis is unknown	Thyroid US can be recommended to PJS patients even without clinical signs of thyroid disease due to early disease appearance	[33]
Screening recommendations based on current thyroid cancer guidelines					[40]
I. American Thyroid Association management guidelines for adult patients with thyroid nodules and differentiated thyroid cancer, 2015: • Syndromes associated with DTC (e.g., Cowden's disease, FAP, Carney's complex, Werner syndrome/progeria in a first-degree relative) warrant screening based on various components of that syndrome. However, the panel cannot recommend for or against US screening since there is no evidence that this would lead to reduced morbidity or mortality *II. British thyroid association guidelines for the Management of Thyroid Cancer, 2014:* • Cowden's syndrome, FAP; and familial TC are considered to be risk factors for thyroid cancer. In a case of strong familial incidence of TC or association with other cancers, genetic advice should be considered • No screening is recommended for patients with Cowden's syndrome and FAP					
III. Management guidelines for children with thyroid nodules and differentiated thyroid cancer, 2015: • Patients at increased risk of developing familial DTC should be referred to centers of excellence (recommendation 4C) • For children with tumor syndromes, thyroid US as a routine screening tool was not recommended. However, they do encounter children who have incidental nodules identified via screening thyroid US, and nodules detected in this setting should be interrogated by US performed by an experienced ultrasonographer. FNA should be performed if the nodule has concerning sonographic features or growth over time • In all children with FTC, consideration should be given to genetic counseling and genetic testing for germline PTEN mutations, particularly in a child with macrocephaly or with a family history suggestive of the PTEN hamartoma tumor syndrome (recommendation 32C) *IV. US preventive service task force:* The USPSTF recommends against screening asymptomatic adults for thyroid cancer, however, this recommendation does not apply to persons who are at increased risk of TC, including people with inherited genetic syndromes associated with thyroid cancer (https://www.uspreventiveservicestaskforce.org)					

DTC differentiated thyroid cancer, *TC* thyroid cancer, *NMTC* non-medullary thyroid cancer, *FA* follicular adenomas, *TN* thyroid nodules, *FNA* fine-needle aspiration

[a]PTEN-related Proteus syndrome and Proteus-like syndrome are not included due to limited literature data about association with TC

[b]It remains unclear if these tumors are a direct result of the underlying genetic defect in McCune–Albright syndrome and Peutz–Jeghers syndrome patients as well as in patients with Beckwith–Wiedemann syndrome, the familial paraganglioma syndromes, and Li–Fraumeni Syndrome, where DTC has also been reported

Carney Complex

Genetics of Carney Complex

Carney complex is an autosomal-dominant disease most commonly caused by a germline mutation in the *PRKAR1A* gene located on either chromosome 17q24.2 (type 1) or chromosome 2p16 (type 2) [71–74]. The *PRKAR1A* gene codes for a regulatory alpha subunit of protein kinase A, an enzyme that promotes cell growth. Protein kinase A remains turned off when the regulatory subunits are bound to the enzyme and becomes active when the subunits break away. Most *PRKAR1A* gene mutations (82%) produce nonsense mRNA, which is eventually degraded through a nonsense-mediated mRNA decay process [75, 76]. There are also studies demonstrating, based on linkage analysis, that a linkage site on the chromosome 2p16 locus is associated with this disease—though no candidate gene has been identified [77, 78].

Clinical Presentation of Carney Complex

Dr. J. Aidan Carney, a pathologist, first described the coexistence of "myxomas, spotty pigmentation, and endocrine overactivity" in 1985 [79]. Clinically, Carney complex is characterized by lentigines, atrial myxoma, mucocutaneous myxoma, blue nevi or nevi, myxoid neurofibroma, ephelide, and endocrinopathies such as growth hormone–secreting pituitary adenomas, ACTH-independent Cushing syndrome due to primary pigmented nodular adrenocortical disease, and thyroid abnormalities [80].

Either the presence of NMTC (at any age) or multiple hypoechogenic nodules on thyroid US in a prepubertal child are the major diagnostic criteria for Carney complex [81]. Up to 60% of all individuals with Carney complex may have thyroid nodules detected by US, and two-thirds of them occur in children and adolescents [71, 82]. Thyroid nodules appear during the first 10 years of life [83]. Nonspecific cystic disease can be seen in up to 75% of cases, and follicular adenomas can be seen in 25% of patients [75, 82, 84]. Both PTC and FTC are present in about 10% of patients with Carney complex [81, 85]. In general, the life span is decreased in patients with Carney complex, with the major cause of death (57%) being cardiovascular complications from the disease. Fourteen percent of patients die of cancer progression, but thyroid cancer as a cause of death has not been reported [81].

Management of Thyroid Cancer Associated with Carney Complex

In patients with Carney complex, screening thyroid US is recommended as a baseline examination and is a satisfactory, cost-effective method for determining thyroid involvement in pediatric and young adult patients. Thyroid US may be repeated in regular intervals as needed [81]. However, the value of thyroid US is questionable in older individuals [71, 86]. A fine-needle aspiration biopsy is recommended when a thyroid US feature is suspicious, and NMTC management should follow those as in sporadic NMTC based on standard of care treatment approach [82].

Pendred Syndrome

Genetics of Pendred Syndrome

Pendred syndrome is an autosomal-recessive disorder that is primarily caused by germline mutations in three genes: *SLC26A4, FOXI1,* and *KCNJ10*. More than half of the patients with Pendred syndrome are likely to harbor pathogenic variants in the *SLC26A4* gene [87, 88]. SLC26A4 is a cell membrane transport protein for negatively charged ions. Mutations in *SLC26A4* disrupt ion transport, leading to an imbalance of ions. Variants in the other two genes, *FOXI1* and *KCNJ10*, are less common, accounting for less than 1% of cases in this syndrome [89].

Clinical Features of Pendred Syndrome

Pendred syndrome is a disease of "deaf-mutism and goiter" first described by Pendred in 1896 [24]. Thyroid involvement ranges from minimal enlargement to large MNG and thyroid cancer [24]. The prevalence of NMTC in Pendred syndrome is estimated to be 1%, with FTC being the most common histologic subtype [90]. A follicular variant of papillary thyroid carcinoma and metastatic FTC and anaplastic transformation from FTC have been reported [91–94]. It has been proposed that the association of NMTC and Pendred syndrome may be due to untreated congenital hypothyroidism and chronic stimulation by thyroid-stimulating hormone [24]. Genetic analysis of the Pendred-associated follicular variant of papillary thyroid cancer showed a TP53 somatic mutation, supporting the idea that NMTC arising from goiter requires additional genetic alteration in addition to thyroid-stimulation hormone overstimulation [92].

Management of Thyroid Cancer Associated with Pendred Syndrome

Thyroid US evaluation and routine thyroid examination in a patient with hypothyroidism and Pendred syndrome may be recommended for early identification of NMTC. There is no role for routine prophylactic thyroidectomy in patients with Pendred syndrome. Thyroidectomy should be considered in hypothyroid patients with thyroid nodules [24]. Once diagnosed, NMTC should be managed according to the current treatment guidelines of sporadic NMTC [40].

DICER1 Syndrome

Genetics of DICER1 Syndrome

DICER1 syndrome is an autosomal-dominant disorder caused by germline mutations in the *DICER1* gene, located on chromosome 14q32.13. Somatic and germline mutations in this gene have been found in PTC [95]. Germline *DICER1* mutations are associated with dysregulated gene expression of five miRNAs (miR-345, let-7a, miR-99b, miR-133, and miR-194) [96].

Clinical Features of DICER1 Syndrome

DICER1 syndrome, or the pleuropulmonary blastoma (PPB) familial tumor and dysplasia syndrome, is a disease characterized by PPB, cystic nephroma, Sertoli-Leydig cell tumors, embryonal rhabdomyosarcomas, MNG, Wilms tumors (WT), and other very rare entities [97] (Table 20.1).

MNG is common in patients with *DICER1* germline mutations [95, 96]. DTC has also been described in DICER1 patients, though very infrequently [95, 97]. The development of a somatic RNase IIIb *DICER1* mutation in patients with *DICER1* germline mutations is suggested as a second hit for thyroid carcinogenesis [97]. Some authors have suggested that treatment of DICER1 patients with chemotherapy and/or bone marrow transplantation for pleuropulmonary blastomas can also be a predisposing risk factor for DTC [97, 98]. Five cases of DTC associated with a history of high-dose chemotherapy have been reported [95, 97]. However, DTC unrelated to chemotherapy or radiation therapy that developed at a young age has also been documented. Pathology was significant for distinct PTC foci developing within an encapsulated follicular nodule without extrathyroidal extension, infiltrative growth, or vascular invasion and negative somatic mutation in *BRAF, NRAS, HRAS, KRAS*, and *RET/PTC* 1 and 3 rearrangements. One patient had minimally invasive FTC [95].

Management of Thyroid Cancer Associated with DICER1 Syndrome

Guidelines for baseline and routine surveillance thyroid US screening in patients with germline *DICER1* mutations have not been established. Recommendations from the International PPB registries suggest that a thyroid physical examination should be performed annually [99]. Thyroid US is recommended if thyroid gland asymmetry and/or a nodule is detected during physical examination, or if the patient has previously received or is anticipated to receive chemotherapy or repeated upper-body radiological imaging for PPB or another DICER1-related malignancy [99]. A thyroid US could be repeated every three to 5 years if no nodule is detected [99]. Other investigators recommend annual thyroid US during childhood and adolescence, together with appropriate endocrine referral for these young *DICER1* mutation carriers [97]. NMTC, once detected, should be treated according to the standard guidelines as in sporadic NMTC [40].

Ataxia-Telangiectasia

Genetics of Ataxia-Telangiectasia

Ataxia-telangiectasia is a rare autosomal-recessive disorder caused by mutations in the

ATM (ataxia-telangiectasia mutated) gene, which is located on chromosome 11q22-23 [100]. Mutations in this gene disrupt the function of the serine-threonine kinase of ATM, which is associated with cell-cycle checkpoint defects and chromosomal instability. The *ATM* gene is critical for normal development and activity of the nervous system and immune system. More than 800 unique pathogenic variants of *ATM* have been identified, and many of them are known to be associated with a higher risk of cancer [101].

Clinical Features of Ataxia-Telangiectasia

Ataxia-telangiectasia is characterized by early-onset progressive cerebellar ataxia, progressive apraxia of eye movements, oculo-cutaneous telangiectasia, the absence or the rudimentary appearance of a thymus, immunodeficiency, lymphoid tumors, insulin-resistant diabetes, and radiosensitivity [102]. The rate of cancer is approximately 100-times higher than the general population [103]. Five cases of DTC have been reported in patients with ataxia-telangiectasia. All patients were females with an age at diagnosis ranging from 9.3 to 35.8 years. Four of five patients had PTC and one patient had FTC [103].

Management of Thyroid Cancer Associated with Ataxia-Telangiectasia

It is unclear if the risk of NMTC is higher in patients with ataxia-telangiectasia than the general population, but the early age of onset of NMTC reported suggests that it may be high. While there is a lack of data regarding screening results and the prognosis of ataxia-telangiectasia associated NMTC, we believe clinicians should have a low threshold for thyroid evaluation, and if NMTC is diagnosed, it should be treated according to standard guidelines and recommendations as for sporadic NMTC [11].

Papillary Renal Neoplasia (PRN)

Genetic Background of PRN

The genetic cause as well as the mode of inheritance is not known. This syndromic FNMTC is based on a single report with no additional studies reporting this association or a genetic basis for it.

Clinical Features of PRN

The association of PTC with PRN has been described based on analysis of one kindred with five family members diagnosed with PTC, two with PRN, and one with renal oncocytoma [104]. PTC associated with PRN was a classical variant of PTC. Interestingly, PRN has similar histologic features to PTC [104]. Immunostaining for thyroglobulin can distinguish PTC from PRN metastases if this is suspected. Based on an analysis of one family, all identified family members with PTC were characterized by a tumor larger than 3 cm, and many had coexisting benign thyroid nodules [104].

Management of Thyroid Cancer Associated with PRN

Due to the extreme rarity of this disease, there are neither management nor screening recommendations for patients with PRN. Thus, no recommendations for screening and follow-up can be made. The diagnostic evaluation and treatment of thyroid nodules and NMTC associated with PRN should be similar to sporadic thyroid nodules and NMTC.

Werner Syndrome

Genetics of Werner Syndrome

Werner syndrome, or adult progeria, is an autosomal-recessive disorder that is associated with mutations of the *WRN* gene, located on chromosome 8p11-p12 [105]. The *WRN* gene is critical in replicating and repairing DNA. Mutations in the *WRN* gene often lead to truncated non-functional WRN proteins, which lead to slower, decreased cell division.

Clinical Features of Werner Syndrome

Werner syndrome is a disease characterized by premature aging that starts in the third decade, with a median life expectancy of 54 years [80, 106, 107]. Initially, Dr. Werner reported four siblings with scleroderma in association with cataracts, described progeric manifestation, and even assumed a genetic origin for this condition [11]. Clinical presentation includes thin skin, wrinkles, alopecia, muscle atrophy, short stature due to an absence of pubertal growth period, age-related disorders such as diabetes, osteoporosis, cataracts, and peripheral vascular disease, and different types of malignant tumors (Table 20.1) [106, 107].

Werner syndrome patients have an increased risk of thyroid involvement, including benign and malignant thyroid diseases [51]. In Japanese descent, PTC has been associated with an N-terminal variant in *WNT*, whereas FTC is more frequently observed with a C-terminal variant [108]. Based on Japanese registry data, there is evidence that the age of DTC diagnosis is 10 years earlier than in the general Japanese population [108]. The female-to-male ratio is also different than the general population (2.3:1 in Werner syndrome and 6.6:1 in the general population) [108]. Moreover, the type of NMTC reveals a higher prevalence of histological subtypes of thyroid cancer rarely observed in the general population, such as FTC (48% in Werner syndrome vs. 14% in the general Japanese population) and anaplastic thyroid cancer (13% vs. 2%, respectively), and a lower rate of classic PTC (35% vs. 78%, respectively) [108]. A systematic review of published Werner syndrome cases showed the frequency of thyroid neoplasms being 16.1% among all patients diagnosed [109]. The relative risk of developing NMTC was estimated to be 8.9% for Japanese residents with Werner syndrome [109].

Management of Thyroid Cancer Associated with Werner Syndrome

Given the high prevalence of NMTC in Werner syndrome and the high rate of more aggressive histological subtypes such as FTC and ATC, screening and surveillance for thyroid nodule and NMTC by thyroid US or annual physical examination is justified [110]. The diagnostic evaluation and treatment of thyroid nodules and NMTC associated with Werner syndrome should be similar to sporadic thyroid nodules and NMTC.

Clinical Uncertainties in Syndromic FNMTC

Many syndromic NMTC have the cardinal features of inherited cancer syndromes such as early-age onset and a high rate of multifocal and bilateral disease [51, 111]. While for most syndromic FNMTC there appears to be an increased risk of NMTC, the penetrance is low, and there is great phenotypic heterogeneity. Moreover, there is limited data on screening and surveillance for NMTC, as well as the clinical course and prognosis of NMTC compared to sporadic NMTC. With future studies addressing these critical issues, including the discovery of any genotype-phenotype association, it may be possible to refine the management of syndromic FNMTC and optimize patient outcome.

Nonsyndromic FNMTC

The first description of nonsyndromic FNMTC was reported in 1955 by Robinson and Orr in monozygotic twins, and since then, numerous case reports and case series have led to its recognition as a distinct clinical entity [110]. Nonsyndromic FNMTC is defined as the presence of thyroid cancer of follicular-cell origin in two or more first-degree relatives, in the absence of other predisposing hereditary or environmental causes [112]. FNMTC is characterized by an autosomal-dominant pattern of inheritance with incomplete penetrance. Environmental factors such as low-dose radiation may affect the penetrance of disease in genetically predisposed individuals [113]. Patients with FNMTC also have an increased rate of benign thyroid diseases such as follicular adenoma, MNG, and Hashimoto thyroiditis, up to 45–55% [112, 114–118].

Genetics of Nonsyndromic FNMTC

Several different genetic susceptibility loci and genes have been reported, but few causative genes have been found that account for most cases of nonsyndromic FNMTC.

FOXE1

The forkhead box E1 (*FOXE1*) gene is located at chromosome 9q22.33 and encodes for the FOXE1 transcription factor. This gene is also known as thyroid transcription factor 2 (*TTF2*), which regulates thyroid morphogenesis and promotes thyroid precursor migration from the pharynx to the neck. A genome-wide association study in both sporadic PTC and FTC cases identified two single nucleotide polymorphisms, rs944289 and rs965513, and was subsequently validated by target sequencing in an independent cohort [119, 120]. Sequencing of the whole *FOXE1* gene revealed several germline variants in the promoter region and coding sequence [121, 122]. The functional studies using an A248G variant of *FOXE1* documented increased cell proliferation in rat normal thyroid and human PTC cell lines compared with the wild type, thus further supporting the role of *FOXE1* as a susceptibility gene for nonsyndromic FNMTC [122].

HABP2

The Hyaluronan-binding protein 2 (*HABP2*) gene is located on chromosome 10q25.3. It was identified as a susceptibility gene for FNMTC by a study utilizing whole-exome sequencing in large kindred with seven affected members (six PTC and one follicular adenoma) [123]. The G534E variant of HABP2 segregated with all seven affected members. Functional studies suggested that the *HABP2* G534E variant could act as a dominant negative tumor-suppressor gene. The study findings were validated by one group, which identified the same germline variant (G534E) of *HABP2* in four kindred with FNMTC out of 29 kindred tested by target sequencing [124]. However, other studies have either found incomplete segregation of the *HABP2* G534E variant in affected members with FNMTC or no difference in the presence of the variant between those with NMTC and "control" groups [125–131].

Tumor Cell Oxyphilia 1 (TCO1)

The tumor cell oxyphilia 1 locus on chromosome 19p13.2 was found to be a linkage site in a single French family with FNMTC (six MNG, two PTC) [132]. Subsequent analysis in 22 families confirmed the involvement of the *TCO1* locus in one French Canadian family [133]. Additionally, loss of heterozygosity has been shown at the *TCO1* locus in cases of sporadic thyroid cancer as well as FNMTC, suggesting the presence of a tumor-suppressor gene in this region [134, 135].

Telomere-Telomerase Complex

It was reported that FNMTC cases had a significantly shorter germline telomere length, higher *hTERT* gene amplification, and higher hTERT mRNA expression compared to patients with sporadic PTC [136]. The neoplastic and non-neoplastic thyroid tissue in FNMTC cases have a reportedly shorter telomere length compared with sporadic thyroid cancer cases. However, these observations have not been observed by other investigators. There were no differences in telomere length, *TERT* gene copy number, or mRNA expression level in affected FNMTC cases compared with unaffected family members and sporadic PTC cases. Only shorter germline telomere length was observed in affected members with FNMTC [137, 138].

Locus 4q32

Genome-wide linkage analysis using SNP arrays in a family pedigree with 13 affected members (11 PTC, 2 ATC) across three generations identified a locus on chromosome 4q32 on multipoint non-parametric linkage analysis [139]. An enhancer element that is critical to regulate gene expression upon binding to specific transcription factors was found to be at the linkage peak. Functional studies revealed that the 4q32 A > C mutation affected the binding of transcription factors POU2F1 and YY1 [139].

Multinodular Goiter 1 (MNG1)

The multinodular goiter 1 (*MNG1*) locus was identified as a potential susceptibility locus candidate on chromosome 14q32 in a Canadian family with 18 cases of MNG and two cases of PTC. It was inherited in an autosomal-dominant pattern [140]. However, other investigators have not found any linkage at the *MNG1* locus and FNMTC [133, 141–143].

Familial PTC/PRN Locus

The familial *PTC/PRN* locus on chromosome 1q21 was identified in large, three-generation kindred with five cases of PTC and two cases of PRN [104]. The same locus was independently validated in a separate cohort of FNMTC but without PRN [144]. However, other investigators have not found any association between this locus and FNMTC [133, 145].

NMTC1 Locus

A genome-wide scan followed by a haplotype analysis in a large Tasmanian pedigree with eight cases of NMTC (four classical PTC, four follicular-variant PTC) identified a locus on 2q21 [146]. Subsequent studies in 80 pedigrees also showed significant linkage at the 2q21 locus with FNMTC, particularly for the follicular variant of PTC [146]. In another study focused on 10 FNMTC, the locus was also found to be a linkage site [147]. However, other investigators did not find linkage at this locus and FNMTC [143, 145].

8p22-23.1 Locus

Genetic linkage analysis identified a locus at 8q22-23.1 as significantly associated with FNMTC by using single nucleotide polymorphism analysis followed by microsatellite analysis in a family with 11 cases of benign thyroid disease and five cases of NMTC (four PTC, one follicular variant of PTC) [145]. None of the variants in the 17 genes identified in this region were potentially pathogenic. Further studies in an additional six kindred by the same group did not find any linkage association with this locus [145].

6q22 Locus

A genome-wide single nucleotide polymorphism array in 38 FNMTC kindred with 49 PTC cases identified a linkage site at chromosomal locus 6q22 [144]. However, the specific candidate susceptibility genes are unknown, and this chromosomal locus has not been identified by other investigators.

SRGAP1

A genome-wide linkage analysis using SNP genotyping in 38 families with PTC identified a 12q14 locus in 21 families with a 30% probability of linkage to FNMTC [148]. The identified region contains a SNP rs2168411 spanning the gene Slit-Robo Rho GTPase-activating protein 1 (*SRGAP1*) [149]. Four germline missense variants (Q149H, A275T, R617C, and H875R) co-segregated in one FNMTC family each [148]. Functional studies demonstrated that two variants (Q149H and R617C) of *SRGAP1* were unable to inactivate its target protein, CDC42, which plays a role in cell mobility [148].

TTF-1/NKX2.1

Targeted DNA sequencing studies in 20 PTC patients with a history of MNG and 329 controls revealed the presence of a germline mutation (A339V) in *TTF-1/NKX2*.1 on chromosome 14q13 in four PTC patients [150]. TTF is a thyroid transcription factor that regulates the transcription of thyroglobulin, thyroperoxidase, and thyrotropin receptor. However, this association was not found by other groups [151].

Clinical Features of Nonsyndromic FNMTC

FNMTC is present in 3.2–9.6% of all the thyroid cancer patients [1, 112, 152, 153]. However, the true prevalence and incidence of FNMTC is not known, as it is estimated that sporadic NTMC accounts for as much as 45–69% of NMTC cases in families with only two affected family members [154]. The likelihood of a truly inherited cancer, rather than a chance occurrence of a common cancer in family members, is increased when three or more first-degree relatives are affected by NMTC [118, 154]. The most common histologic subtype of FNMTC is PTC similar to sporadic NMTC. Women are affected by FNMTC approximately two to three times more frequently than men [154, 155]. The age at diagnosis of patients with FNMTC tends to be less than that of sporadic cases (39–43 years vs. 46–49 years) (Figs. 20.1 and 20.2) [112, 114, 152]. However, it is not clear if the age difference is caused by the difference in cancer biology or increased active screening of the family members. Capezzone and associates found "clinical anticipation" with the second generation developing more aggressive disease at an earlier age, a finding that would support a more aggressive manifestation due to cancer biology [156]. On the other hand, there are several reports that did not find a difference in age at diagnosis between sporadic and familial NMTC [115, 153, 157–159].

Diagnosis

The American Thyroid Association guidelines in Recommendation one state that "Screening people with familial follicular cell–derived differentiated thyroid cancer may lead to an earlier diagnosis of thyroid cancer, but the panel cannot recommend for or against ultrasound screening since there is no evidence that this would lead to reduced morbidity or mortality. (No recommendation, insufficient evidence)" [40]. To critically review the rationale for screening, it's worthwhile to address the following questions:

1. Are family members truly at risk of cancer?
2. Is FNMTC more aggressive than sporadic FNMTC?
3. What is the optimal screening method?
4. Is screening resulting in detection of disease at an earlier stage and, as such, does it affect morbidity, mortality, and quality of life?
5. Is screening cost-effective?

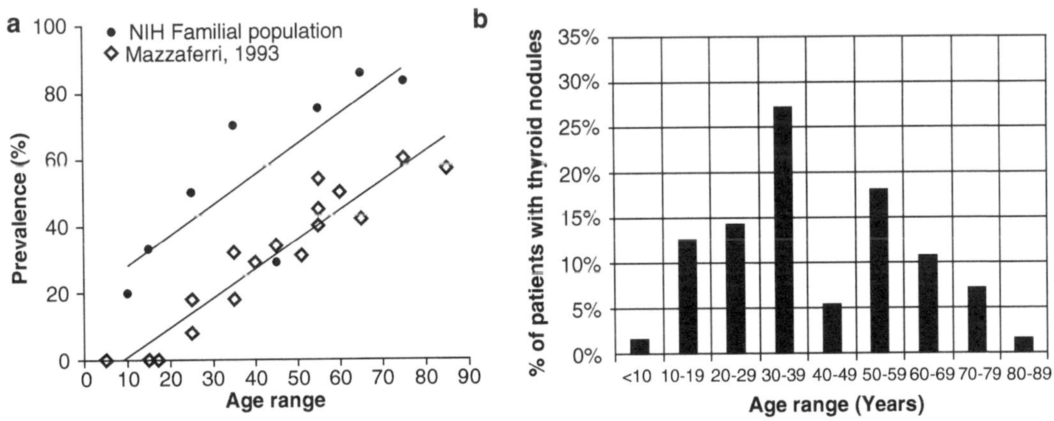

Fig. 20.1 Rate of thyroid nodule detected and age on screening thyroid ultrasound in kindred with nonsyndromic familial non-medullary thyroid cancer (FNMTC). (**a**) Prevalence of thyroid nodule by age in FNMTC kindred and general United States population. Data from Sadowski et al. [162]. (**b**) Age at thyroid nodule detection on screening thyroid ultrasound. Data from a cohort of at risk family members enrolled in a clinical protocol at the National Institutes of Health, National Cancer Institutes. The main inclusion criterion was the presence of at least two first-degree relatives with nonmedullary thyroid cancer in the kindred. All patients age of >7 years underwent screening. Twenty-five kindred were enrolled in the clinical protocol: 69 had an established diagnosis of thyroid cancer before enrollment, and 183 unaffected at risk relatives among whom 109 underwent screening with physical exam and thyroid ultrasound. Individuals with syndromic familial non-medullary thyroid cancer were excluded from the study and a family history questionnaire was obtained from all kindred

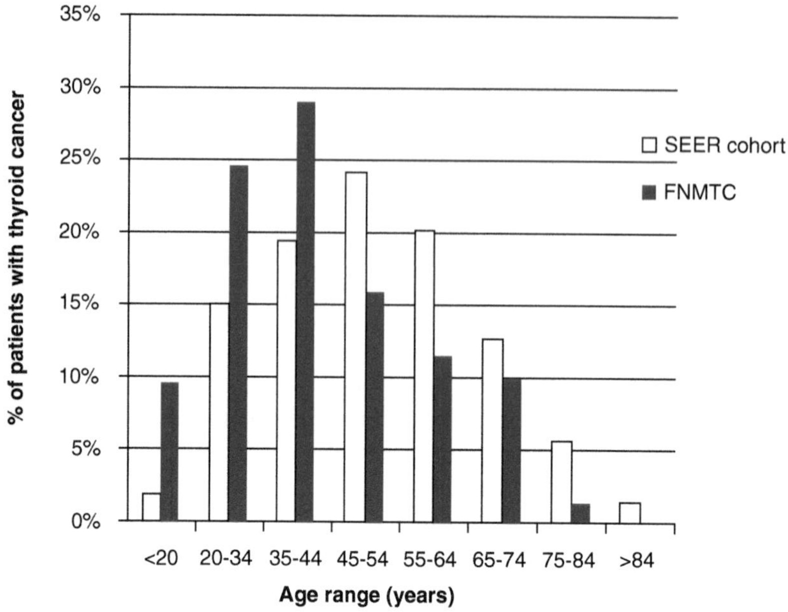

Fig. 20.2 Age at diagnosis in nonsyndromic familial nonmedullary thyroid cancer (FNMTC) compared to general population. The age of thyroid cancer diagnosis was earlier as compared to the general United States population ($p < 0.001$) as reported in the Surveillance, Epidemiology and End Result (SEER) data on NMTC. The comparison was made in 61,523 cases of nonmedullary thyroid cancer from the SEER data to 25 kindred with nonsyndromic FNMTC kindred enrolled in a clinical protocol at the National Institutes of Health, National Cancer Institute

1. Are the family members truly at increased risk of cancer?

As heritability of FNMTC is relatively high, screening all first-degree relatives of affected patients has been proposed; some authors even suggest expanding screening to second-degree relatives [160]. To the best of our knowledge, there is only one prospective cohort study, involving 25 kindred, focused on the benefits of screening in families with FNMTC [118, 161]. The study included 165 individuals—56 patients with an established diagnosis of thyroid cancer and 109 at-risk family members who underwent yearly thyroid US screening. Based on this study, PTC was detected by screening at a significantly lower rate in kindred with two first-degree relatives affected at enrollment compared to kindred who had at least three first-degree relatives affected (4.6% (2/43) vs. 22.7% (15/66), $p = 0.01$, respectively) [118]. This study confirms Charkes' probability estimates that, in kindred with two first-degree family members affected, the probability that the disease is sporadic is as high as 62%, but that decreases to less than 6% when three or more members are affected [154]. Several retrospective studies support this observation. McDonald et al. suggested that the more aggressive behavior is evident in families with three or more members affected by FNMTC as compared with families with two members affected [162].

2. Is FNMTC characterized by more aggressive clinical behavior than sporadic NMTC?

Several, but not all studies (Table 20.3) have suggested that FNMTC is associated with earlier age of onset, higher rate of multifocality, extrathyroidal extension, lymph node metastases, higher recurrence rate, and decreased disease-free survival [114, 115, 153, 163–167]. As mentioned earlier, Capezzone and colleagues found that the tumor is more aggressive in the second generation, in which it tends to be diagnosed on average 29.3 years earlier [156]. The prospective

Table 20.3 Comparison of clinicopathological characteristics, therapy, and outcome between patients with familial non-medullary thyroid cancer (FNMTC) and sporadic NMTC

Study design	Number of participants	Age at diagnosis (years mean ± SD)	Gender	Histology	Extent of surgery	RAI treatment	Duration of follow-up (years mean ± SD)	Recurrence rate FNMTC vs SDTC (OR ± CI)	Decreased DSS FNMTC vs SDTC (HR ± CI)
Cohort study [116]	FNMTC 258	49.1 ± 13.9	Female 88%	PTC 87.6%	TT/NTT 62.5%[a] LND 72%	n/a	11.7 ± 10	1.82 (1.3–2.57)	2.5 (2.05–2.95)
	SDTC 6200	48.5 ± 14	Female 90.7%	PTC 84.6%	TT/NTT 52.5%[a] LND 66%	n/a	12.2 ± 10		
Cohort study [164]	FNMTC 37	43.3 ± 3[a]	Female 78.4%	PTC 100%	TT/NTT 100% LND n/a	n/a	n/a	2.47 (1.1–5.63)	n/a
	SDTC 321	49 ± 1[a]	Female 71.3%	PTC 89.4%	TT/NTT 100% LND n/a	n/a	n/a		
Cohort study [154]	FNMTC 318	47 ± 11	Female 85.8%	PTC 96.2%	TT/NTT n/a LND n/a	n/a	6.2 ± 6.6	1.7 (1.31–2.20)	2.6 (2.21–3.04)
	SDTC 2733	47 ± 12	Female 82.5%	PTC 94.8%	TT/NTT n/a LND n/a	n/a	6.2 ± 6.2		
Cohort study [174]	FNMTC 113	45.3 ± 12.9	Female 85.8%	PTC 100%	TT/NTT 100% LND 99%	93.8%	8 (entire cohort)	n/a	1.7 (1.03–2.69)
	SDTC 1149	45.2+/12.4	Female 88.1%	PTC 100%	TT/NTT 100% LND 97%	95%			

(continued)

Study design	Number of participants	Age at diagnosis (years mean ± SD)	Gender	Histology	Extent of surgery	RAI treatment	Duration of follow-up (years mean ± SD)	Recurrence rate FNMTC vs SDTC (OR ± CI)	Decreased DSS FNMTC vs SDTC (HR ± CI)
Cohort study [157]	FNMTC 34	47.9 ± 18.2	Female 73.5%	PTC 100%	TT/NTT 100% LND n/a	n/a	4.2 ± 2.7	3.8 (1.07–13.3)	n/a
	SDTC 235	47.5 ± 16.6	Female 77%	PTC 100%	TT/NTT 100% LND n/a	n/a	4.7 ± 3.8		
Cohort study [163]	FNMTC 91	41.5 ± 1.9	Female 79.1%	PTC 100%	TT/NTT n/a LND n/a	n/a	5.1 ± 0.8	n/a	n/a
	SDTC 521	44.3 ± 0.6	Female 79.5%	PTC 100%	TT/NTT n/a LND n/a	n/a	4.2 ± 0.2		
Cohort study [153]	FNMTC 12	43[a]	Female 83.3%	PTC 100%	TT/NTT n/a LND n/a	n/a	1.58 (entire cohort)	n/a	n/a
	SDTC 124	48[a]	Female 73.4%	PTC 92.7%	TT/NTT n/a LND n/a	n/a			
Cohort study [160]	FNMTC 273	n/a	n/a	PTC 100%	TT/NTT 69%[a] LND 97%[a]	n/a	7.6 ± 5	1.0 (0.63–1.58)	1.2 (0.93–1.63)
	SDTC 5742	n/a	n/a	PTC 100%	TT/NTT 50%[a] LND 94%[a]	n/a			
Case-control study [158]	FNMTC 67	42.8 ± 16.8	Female 89.6%	PTC 88.8%	TT/NTT 86.2% LND 22%	80.6%	8.6 ± 10	1.5 (0.59–3.85)	n/a
	SDTC 375	47.2 ± 16.1	Female 80%	PTC 91%	TT/NTT 89.1% LND 15%	88%	8.4 ± 9		

Table 20.3 (continued)

Study design	Number of participants	Age at diagnosis (years mean ± SD)	Gender	Histology	Extent of surgery	RAI treatment	Duration of follow-up (years mean ± SD)	Recurrence rate FNMTC vs SDTC (OR ± CI)	Decreased DSS FNMTC vs SDTC (HR ± CI)
Case-control study [115]	FNMTC 48	39 ± 11[a]	n/a	n/a	TT/NTT 73%[a] LND 46%[a]	60.4%[a]	8	3.9 (1.89–7.98)	n/a
	SDTC 144	46 ± 15[a]	n/a	n/a	TT/NTT 94%[a] LND 22%[a]	84.7%	7		
Case-control study [159]	FNMTC 24	54.6 ± 18.5	Female 79.2%	PTC 70.8%	TT/NTT 91.7% LND 71%[a]	n/a	>2 (entire cohort)	0.7 (0.09–5.43)	1.2 (0.10–15.4)
	SDTC 519	57.8 ± 16	Female 80.7%	PTC 63%	TT/NTT 87.1% LND 30%	n/a			
Case-control study [175]	FNMTC 107	46.1	Female 76.6%	PTC 66.4%	TT/NTT 93.5% LND 28%	80.4%	n/a	1.2 (0.56–2.42)	1.0 (0.41–2.54)
	SDTC 107	46.2	Female 76.6%	PTC 66.3%	TT/NTT 94.4% LND 36%	74.8%	n/a		
Meta-analysis [173]	FNMTC 1256	n/a	n/a	n/a	n/a	n/a	n/a	1.7 (1.34–2.20)	1.8 (1.34–2.52)
	SDTC 16902	n/a	n/a	n/a	n/a	n/a	n/a		

PTC papillary thyroid cancer, *DSS* disease-specific survival, *OR* odds ratio, *HR* hazard ratio, *CI* confidence intervals, *SD* standard deviation, *TT/NTT* total thyroidectomy/near-total thyroidectomy, *LND* lymph node dissection

[a]Denotes statistically significant difference

cohort study of 25 FNMTC families revealed that the youngest patient found to have a thyroid nodule was 7 years old, and the youngest patient with PTC was 18 years old [118, 161]. Nine percent of screened subjects were diagnosed with NMTC between the ages of 18 and 20 years old [118]. Similar results were observed in several [153, 168] but not all [157] studies. In addition, results from several published reviews are conflicting [169–171].

A recent meta-analysis that included 12 studies with a total of 12,741 patients who were followed for 1.5–12.1 years tried to solve these discrepancies [172]. The analysis was based on retrospective studies, including eight cohort studies and four case-control studies, of which five were conducted in Asia [115, 153, 157, 159, 173], four in North America [152, 158, 162, 163], two in Europe [156, 174], and one in a combined U.S. and Japanese cohort [114]. Based on the data extracted from six eligible studies, the authors reported an increased rate of recurrence (OR 1.72, 95% CI: 1.34–2.20) and decreased disease-free survival (HR 1.83, 95% CI: 1.34–2.52) in comparison with sporadic DTC patients [172]. The meta-analysis also documented more aggressive biological features of FNMTC compared with sporadic DTC, with younger age at diagnosis (2.4 years lower on average for FNMTC patients compared with the sporadic cases), higher risk of multifocal tumor growth (OR 1.50, 95% CI: 1.32–1.71), bilateral disease (OR 1.29, 95% CI: 1.00–1.66), extrathyroidal invasion (OR 1.20, 95% CI: 1.02–1.41), and lymph node metastases (OR 1.18, 95% CI: 1.01–1.38) [172]. They reported no difference in tumor diameter [172]. Taken together, we believe most of the evidence suggests that FNMTC is characterized by more aggressive behavior than sporadic NMTC.

3. What is the optimal screening method?

Since there are no known susceptibility genes that have been validated and that account for most cases of FNMTC, genetic testing cannot be used to identify at-risk individuals in kindred with FNMTC. Thus, screening is based on clinical and imaging exams. The neck examination with palpation of the thyroid is not a sufficient method for detection of thyroid cancer, as reported in a large screening study of 18,000 women. Only 0.19% of thyroid nodules were diagnosed by clinical examination, whereas the incidence of US-detected thyroid nodules in healthy adults is estimated to be about 20% [175]. In the prospective cohort study focused on screening in FNMTC families, thyroid nodules were detected by physical examination in just 12.7% of patients compared to 50.5% by neck US [118]. Therefore, the use of thyroid US had been proposed as a useful and cost-effective tool for screening of asymptomatic family members of kindred with FNMTC, as it enables an earlier detection of non-palpable thyroid nodules [176]. Moreover, several studies have shown excellent specificity (95.7–100%) and reasonable sensitivity (83.3–92.6%) of neck US for identifying cervical lymph node metastases in the lateral neck [177, 178].

US-guided fine-needle aspiration biopsy and cytologic examination is the most accurate diagnostic tool for thyroid nodules. However, it has been suggested that the accuracy of fine-needle aspiration biopsy may be lower in patients with FNMTC, where a false-negative rate of up to 12% has been observed compared with 4% in matched controls [179]. Patients with FNMTC and a thyroid nodule greater than 1 cm should have US-guided fine-needle aspiration [40].

4. Is screening resulting in detection of disease at an earlier stage and, as such, does it affect morbidity, mortality, and quality of life?

The only prospective study to date utilizing screening in family members of patients with FNMTC documented that FNMTC detected by screening was characterized by a smaller tumor size (0.7 cm ± 0.5 vs. 1.5 cm ± 1.1, $p = 0.006$), a lower rate of central neck lymph node metastases (17.6% vs. 51.1%, $p = 0.02$) compared with the index cases, which was associated with less aggressive initial treatment (hemi-thyroidectomy 23.5% vs. 0%, $p = 0.002$, respectively) and a lower rate of radioactive iodine therapy (23.5%

vs. 79%, $p < 0.001$, respectively) [118, 161]. There was no statistically significant difference in complications associated with treatment between those patients diagnosed by screening and those patients with an established thyroid cancer diagnosis at the time of enrollment. However, there was no permanent hypoparathyroidism or vocal cord paralysis in the patients diagnosed by screening, while in one of the patients with an established diagnosis of thyroid cancer at enrollment, the recurrent laryngeal nerve was sacrificed due to invasion of the nerve. Excellent response to initial treatment was more frequently achieved in patients with FNMTC detected by screening compared with the index cases [93.3% vs. 68.3%, $p = 0.045$], while longer-term outcome data was not available because of a follow-up time of 18 ± 11 months after thyroid cancer diagnosis [118]. In a retrospective study of a subgroup of FNMTC patients, Uchino and colleagues reported that screening was associated with a small primary tumor size (9.1 ± 5.4 mm vs. 0.8 ± 0.6 mm) and a lower rate of multifocal tumors (47% vs. 53.3%) [176].

Sporadic PTC is characterized by overall five- and 10-year survival rates of 97% and 95%, respectively. Given the low mortality rate in sporadic PTC and the rarity of FNMTC, it is difficult to perform a study with adequate power to detect potential differences in mortality in sporadic versus FNMTC. Triponez and associates compared 139 affected family members with 757 unaffected ones and showed that survival was significantly shorter for patients from families with three or more affected members [180]. However, this study lacked a direct comparison to matched sporadic controls [180].

5. Is screening cost-effective?

There are no studies addressing the cost-effectiveness of screening in kindred with FNMTC. There is insufficient evidence to strongly recommend for or against screening, as data on its potential long-term beneficial effects on survival and cost-effectiveness are still lacking. However, several studies do suggest that screening results in the detection of an earlier stage of disease, which may be associated with a lower cost of treatment and better long-term outcomes. We believe screening with thyroid US should be performed in FNMTC kindred with at least three first-degree relatives affected. We believe the most optimal age to start screening is in the teenage years, as almost 10% of patients with FNMTC are diagnosed between the age of 18 and 20 years old [118].

Management of FNMTC

No national or international thyroid management guidelines specifically address screening and surveillance, optimal surgical procedures, adjuvant treatment, and follow-up for patients with FNMTC [40]. Therefore, the therapeutic approach to patients with FNMTC has been very variable, as summarized in Table 20.3. Any management recommendations regarding patients with FNMTC would be largely "expert opinion" grade C, because they rely on case-control studies (level III), retrospective studies (level IV), or expert opinions (level V). In general, management recommendations should be tailored to each patient and guided by the individual clinic-pathological characteristics as well as the number of family members affected and the disease nature within the family. Total thyroidectomy is usually recommended for patients found to have FNMTC; however, some authors offer hemithyroidectomy with close follow-up for patients with unilateral micro-PTC detected by screening [118]. As there is some evidence for increased lymph node involvement in patients with FNMTC, central lymph node dissection should be strongly considered [112, 171, 181]. A therapeutic central neck lymph node dissection should be performed in patients with suspected nodal involvement on US.

There are no specific data on postoperative radioactive iodine ablation results in FNMTC vs. sporadic disease. However, given that some data suggests higher recurrence rates, it might be reasonable to choose more aggressive adjuvant treatment with radioactive iodine ablation in patients with more aggressive FNMTC. All patients should be placed on levothyroxine treatment with appropriate levels of thyroid-stimulating hormone suppression [112, 171, 181].

Patients should not have a prophylactic thyroidectomy, as FNMTC has incomplete penetrance, and no susceptibility gene has been identified that would allow for such preventative intervention knowing that the patient would develop NMTC. Some investigators, however, have advocated total thyroidectomy for every FNMTC patient with a thyroid nodule because of the higher false-negative rate of fine-needle aspiration biopsy and the higher rate of incidental PTC in FNMTC families [171].

References

1. Vriens MR, Suh I, Moses W, Kebebew E. Clinical features and genetic predisposition to hereditary nonmedullary thyroid cancer. Thyroid. 2009;19(12):1343–9.
2. Peiling Yang S, Ngeow J. Familial non-medullary thyroid cancer: unraveling the genetic maze. Endocr Relat Cancer. 2016;23(12):R577–R95.
3. Marsh DJ, Coulon V, Lunetta KL, Rocca-Serra P, Dahia PL, Zheng Z, et al. Mutation spectrum and genotype-phenotype analyses in Cowden disease and Bannayan-Zonana syndrome, two hamartoma syndromes with germline PTEN mutation. Hum Mol Genet. 1998;7(3):507–15.
4. Ngeow J, Mester J, Rybicki LA, Ni Y, Milas M, Eng C. Incidence and clinical characteristics of thyroid cancer in prospective series of individuals with Cowden and Cowden-like syndrome characterized by germline PTEN, SDH, or KLLN alterations. J Clin Endocrinol Metab. 2011;96(12):E2063–71.
5. Bennett KL, Mester J, Eng C. Germline epigenetic regulation of KILLIN in Cowden and Cowden-like syndrome. JAMA. 2010;304(24):2724–31.
6. Orloff MS, He X, Peterson C, Chen F, Chen JL, Mester JL, et al. Germline PIK3CA and AKT1 mutations in Cowden and Cowden-like syndromes. Am J Hum Genet. 2013;92(1):76–80.
7. Yehia L, Niazi F, Ni Y, Ngeow J, Sankunny M, Liu Z, et al. Germline heterozygous variants in SEC23B are associated with Cowden syndrome and enriched in apparently sporadic thyroid cancer. Am J Hum Genet. 2015;97(5):661–76.
8. Lloyd KM, Dennis M. Cowden's disease. A possible new symptom complex with multiple system involvement. Ann Intern Med. 1963;58:136–42.
9. Pilarski R, Burt R, Kohlman W, Pho L, Shannon KM, Swisher E. Cowden syndrome and the PTEN hamartoma tumor syndrome: systematic review and revised diagnostic criteria. J Natl Cancer Inst. 2013;105(21):1607–16.
10. Ngeow J, Eng C. PTEN hamartoma tumor syndrome: clinical risk assessment and management protocol. Methods. 2015;77–78:11–9.
11. Thyroid Cancer. A comprehensive guide to clinical management. Third edition. Anticancer Res. 2017;37(1):361.
12. Pilarski R. Cowden syndrome: a critical review of the clinical literature. J Genet Couns. 2009;18(1): 13–27.
13. Starink TM, van der Veen JP, Arwert F, de Waal LP, de Lange GG, Gille JJ, et al. The Cowden syndrome: a clinical and genetic study in 21 patients. Clin Genet. 1986;29(3):222–33.
14. Eng C. Cowden syndrome. J Genet Couns. 1997;6(2):181–92.
15. Marsh DJ, Dahia PL, Caron S, Kum JB, Frayling IM, Tomlinson IP, et al. Germline PTEN mutations in Cowden syndrome-like families. J Med Genet. 1998;35(11):881–5.
16. Hanssen AM, Fryns JP. Cowden syndrome. J Med Genet. 1995;32(2):117–9.
17. Milas M, Mester J, Metzger R, Shin J, Mitchell J, Berber E, et al. Should patients with Cowden syndrome undergo prophylactic thyroidectomy? Surgery. 2012;152(6):1201–10.
18. Syngal S, Brand RE, Church JM, Giardiello FM, Hampel HL, Burt RW, et al. ACG clinical guideline: genetic testing and management of hereditary gastrointestinal cancer syndromes. Am J Gastroenterol. 2015;110(2):223–62. quiz 63.
19. Smith JR, Marqusee E, Webb S, Nose V, Fishman SJ, Shamberger RC, et al. Thyroid nodules and cancer in children with PTEN hamartoma tumor syndrome. J Clin Endocrinol Metab. 2011;96(1):34–7.
20. Marsh DJ, Kum JB, Lunetta KL, Bennett MJ, Gorlin RJ, Ahmed SF, et al. PTEN mutation spectrum and genotype-phenotype correlations in Bannayan-Riley-Ruvalcaba syndrome suggest a single entity with Cowden syndrome. Hum Mol Genet. 1999;8(8):1461–72.
21. Peiretti V, Mussa A, Feyles F, Tuli G, Santanera A, Molinatto C, et al. Thyroid involvement in two patients with Bannayan-Riley-Ruvalcaba syndrome. J Clin Res Pediatr Endocrinol. 2013;5(4):261–5.
22. Bannayan GA. Lipomatosis, angiomatosis, and macrencephalia. A previously undescribed congenital syndrome. Arch Pathol. 1971;92(1):1–5.
23. Laury AR, Bongiovanni M, Tille JC, Kozakewich H, Nose V. Thyroid pathology in PTEN-hamartoma tumor syndrome: characteristic findings of a distinct entity. Thyroid. 2011;21(2):135–44.
24. Richards ML. Familial syndromes associated with thyroid cancer in the era of personalized medicine. Thyroid. 2010;20(7):707–13.
25. Eng C. In: Pagon RA, Adam MP, Ardinger HH, Wallace SE, Amemiya A, LJH B, et al., editors. PTEN hamartoma tumor syndrome. Seattle: GeneReviews(R); 1993.

26. Haugen BRM, Alexander EK, Bible KC, Doherty G, Mandel SJ, Nikiforov YE, et al. 2015 American Thyroid Association Management Guidelines for Adult Patients with Thyroid Nodules and Differentiated Thyroid Cancer. Thyroid. 2015;26(1):1–133.
27. Zirilli L, Benatti P, Romano S, Roncucci L, Rossi G, Diazzi C, et al. Differentiated thyroid carcinoma (DTC) in a young woman with Peutz-Jeghers syndrome: are these two conditions associated? Exp Clin Endocrinol Diabetes. 2009;117(5):234–9.
28. Wang Z, Wu B, Mosig RA, Chen Y, Ye F, Zhang Y, et al. STK11 domain XI mutations: candidate genetic drivers leading to the development of dysplastic polyps in Peutz-Jeghers syndrome. Hum Mutat. 2014;35(7):851–8.
29. Lim W, Olschwang S, Keller JJ, Westerman AM, Menko FH, Boardman LA, et al. Relative frequency and morphology of cancers in STK11 mutation carriers. Gastroenterology. 2004;126(7):1788–94.
30. Hearle N, Schumacher V, Menko FH, Olschwang S, Boardman LA, Gille JJ, et al. STK11 status and intussusception risk in Peutz-Jeghers syndrome. J Med Genet. 2006;43(8):e41.
31. Amos CI, Keitheri-Cheteri MB, Sabripour M, Wei C, McGarrity TJ, Seldin MF, et al. Genotype-phenotype correlations in Peutz-Jeghers syndrome. J Med Genet. 2004;41(5):327–33.
32. Salloch H, Reinacher-Schick A, Schulmann K, Pox C, Willert J, Tannapfel A, et al. Truncating mutations in Peutz-Jeghers syndrome are associated with more polyps, surgical interventions and cancers. Int J Color Dis. 2010;25(1):97–107.
33. Triggiani V, Guastamacchia E, Renzulli G, Giagulli VA, Tafaro E, Licchelli B, et al. Papillary thyroid carcinoma in Peutz-Jeghers syndrome. Thyroid. 2011;21(11):1273–7.
34. Yamamoto M, Hoshino H, Onizuka T, Ichikawa M, Kawakubo A, Hayakawa S. Thyroid papillary adenocarcinoma in a woman with Peutz-Jeghers syndrome. Intern Med. 1992;31(9):1117–9.
35. Yalcin S, Kirli E, Ciftci AO, Karnak I, Resta N, Bagnulo R, et al. The association of adrenocortical carcinoma and thyroid cancer in a child with Peutz-Jeghers syndrome. J Pediatr Surg. 2011;46(3):570–3.
36. Spigelman AD, Murday V, Phillips RK. Cancer and the Peutz-Jeghers syndrome. Gut. 1989;30(11):1588–90.
37. Reed MW, Harris SC, Quayle AR, Talbot CH. The association between thyroid neoplasia and intestinal polyps. Ann R Coll Surg Engl. 1990;72(6):357–9.
38. Boardman LA, Thibodeau SN, Schaid DJ, Lindor NM, McDonnell SK, Burgart LJ, et al. Increased risk for cancer in patients with the Peutz-Jeghers syndrome. Ann Intern Med. 1998;128(11):896–9.
39. Wei S, LiVolsi VA, Brose MS, Montone KT, Morrissette JJ, Baloch ZW. STK11 mutation identified in thyroid carcinoma. Endocr Pathol. 2016;27(1):65–9.
40. Haugen BR, Alexander EK, Bible KC, Doherty GM, Mandel SJ, Nikiforov YE, et al. 2015 American Thyroid Association Management Guidelines for Adult Patients with Thyroid Nodules and Differentiated Thyroid Cancer: The American Thyroid Association Guidelines Task Force on Thyroid Nodules and Differentiated Thyroid Cancer. Thyroid. 2016;26(1):1–133.
41. Cottrell S, Bicknell D, Kaklamanis L, Bodmer WF. Molecular analysis of APC mutations in familial adenomatous polyposis and sporadic colon carcinomas. Lancet. 1992;340(8820):626–30.
42. Nagase H, Nakamura Y. Mutations of the APC (adenomatous polyposis coli) gene. Hum Mutat. 1993;2(6):425–34.
43. Beroud C, Soussi T. APC gene: database of germline and somatic mutations in human tumors and cell lines. Nucleic Acids Res. 1996;24(1):121–4.
44. Veeman MT, Axelrod JD, Moon RT. A second canon. Functions and mechanisms of beta-catenin-independent Wnt signaling. Dev Cell. 2003;5(3):367–77.
45. Giannelli SM, McPhaul L, Nakamoto J, Gianoukakis AG. Familial adenomatous polyposis-associated, cribriform morular variant of papillary thyroid carcinoma harboring a K-RAS mutation: case presentation and review of molecular mechanisms. Thyroid. 2014;24(7):1184–9.
46. Claes K, Dahan K, Tejpar S, De Paepe A, Bonduelle M, Abramowicz M, et al. The genetics of familial adenomatous polyposis (FAP) and MutYH-associated polyposis (MAP). Acta Gastroenterol Belg. 2011;74(3):421–6.
47. Jasperson KW, Burt RW. In: Pagon RA, Adam MP, Ardinger HH, Wallace SE, Amemiya A, LJH B, et al., editors. APC-associated polyposis conditions. Seattle: GeneReviews(R); 1993.
48. Septer S, Slowik V, Morgan R, Dai H, Attard T. Thyroid cancer complicating familial adenomatous polyposis: mutation spectrum of at-risk individuals. Hered Cancer Clin Pract. 2013;11(1):13.
49. Jarrar AM, Milas M, Mitchell J, Laguardia L, O'Malley M, Berber E, et al. Screening for thyroid cancer in patients with familial adenomatous polyposis. Ann Surg. 2011;253(3):515–21.
50. Crail HW. Multiple primary malignancies arising in the rectum, brain, and thyroid; report of a case. U S Nav Med Bull. 1949;49(1):123–8.
51. Nose V. Familial thyroid cancer: a review. Mod Pathol. 2011;24(Suppl 2):S19–33.
52. Punatar SB, Noronha V, Joshi A, Prabhash K. Thyroid cancer in Gardner's syndrome: case report and review of literature. South Asian J Cancer. 2012;1(1):43–7.
53. Herraiz M, Barbesino G, Faquin W, Chan-Smutko G, Patel D, Shannon KM, et al. Prevalence of thyroid cancer in familial adenomatous polyposis syndrome and the role of screening ultrasound examinations. Clin Gastroenterol Hepatol. 2007;5(3):367–73.
54. Plail RO, Bussey HJ, Glazer G, Thomson JP. Adenomatous polyposis: an association with carcinoma of the thyroid. Br J Surg. 1987;74(5):377–80.

55. Bulow S, Holm NV, Mellemgaard A. Papillary thyroid carcinoma in Danish patients with familial adenomatous polyposis. Int J Color Dis. 1988;3(1):29–31.
56. Truta B, Allen BA, Conrad PG, Kim YS, Berk T, Gallinger S, et al. Genotype and phenotype of patients with both familial adenomatous polyposis and thyroid carcinoma. Familial Cancer. 2003;2(2):95–9.
57. Burt RW, Leppert MF, Slattery ML, Samowitz WS, Spirio LN, Kerber RA, et al. Genetic testing and phenotype in a large kindred with attenuated familial adenomatous polyposis. Gastroenterology. 2004;127(2):444–51.
58. Jasperson KW, Tuohy TM, Neklason DW, Burt RW. Hereditary and familial colon cancer. Gastroenterology. 2010;138(6):2044–58.
59. Adams MS, Bronner-Fraser M. Review: the role of neural crest cells in the endocrine system. Endocr Pathol. 2009;20(2):92–100.
60. Cetta F, Curia MC, Montalto G, Gori M, Cama A, Battista P, et al. Thyroid carcinoma usually occurs in patients with familial adenomatous polyposis in the absence of biallelic inactivation of the adenomatous polyposis coli gene. J Clin Endocrinol Metab. 2001;86(1):427–32.
61. Cetta F, Olschwang S, Petracci M, Montalto G, Baldi C, Zuckermann M, et al. Genetic alterations in thyroid carcinoma associated with familial adenomatous polyposis: clinical implications and suggestions for early detection. World J Surg. 1998;22(12):1231–6.
62. Iwama T, Mishima Y, Utsunomiya J. The impact of familial adenomatous polyposis on the tumorigenesis and mortality at the several organs. Its rational treatment. Ann Surg. 1993;217(2):101–8.
63. Soravia C, Sugg SL, Berk T, Mitri A, Cheng H, Gallinger S, et al. Familial adenomatous polyposis-associated thyroid cancer: a clinical, pathological, and molecular genetics study. Am J Pathol. 1999;154(1):127–35.
64. Perrier ND, van Heerden JA, Goellner JR, Williams ED, Gharib H, Marchesa P, et al. Thyroid cancer in patients with familial adenomatous polyposis. World J Surg. 1998;22(7):738–42. discussion 43.
65. Harach HR, Williams GT, Williams ED. Familial adenomatous polyposis associated thyroid carcinoma: a distinct type of follicular cell neoplasm. Histopathology. 1994;25(6):549–61.
66. Cameselle-Teijeiro J, Chan JK. Cribriform-morular variant of papillary carcinoma: a distinctive variant representing the sporadic counterpart of familial adenomatous polyposis-associated thyroid carcinoma? Mod Pathol. 1999;12(4):400–11.
67. Hampel H, Panescu J, Lockman J, Sotamaa K, Fix D, Comeras I, et al. Comment on: screening for Lynch Syndrome (hereditary nonpolyposis colorectal cancer) among endometrial cancer patients. Cancer Res. 2007;67(19):9603.
68. Taylor MD, Perry J, Zlatescu MC, Stemmer-Rachamimov AO, Ang LC, Ino Y, et al. The hPMS2 exon 5 mutation and malignant glioma. Case report. J Neurosurg. 1999;90(5):946–50.
69. Gadish T, Tulchinsky H, Deutsch AA, Rabau M. Pinealoblastoma in a patient with familial adenomatous polyposis: variant of Turcot syndrome type 2? Report of a case and review of the literature. Dis Colon Rectum. 2005;48(12):2343–6.
70. Cetta F, Montalto G, Gori M, Curia MC, Cama A, Olschwang S. Germline mutations of the APC gene in patients with familial adenomatous polyposis-associated thyroid carcinoma: results from a European cooperative study. J Clin Endocrinol Metab. 2000;85(1):286–92.
71. Stratakis CA, Courcoutsakis NA, Abati A, Filie A, Doppman JL, Carney JA, et al. Thyroid gland abnormalities in patients with the syndrome of spotty skin pigmentation, myxomas, endocrine overactivity, and schwannomas (Carney complex). J Clin Endocrinol Metab. 1997;82(7):2037–43.
72. Matyakhina L, Pack S, Kirschner LS, Pak E, Mannan P, Jaikumar J, et al. Chromosome 2 (2p16) abnormalities in Carney complex tumours. J Med Genet. 2003;40(4):268–77.
73. Pan L, Peng L, Jean-Gilles J, Zhang X, Wieczorek R, Jain S, et al. Novel PRKAR1A gene mutations in Carney complex. Int J Clin Exp Pathol. 2010;3(5):545–8.
74. Kirschner LS, Sandrini F, Monbo J, Lin JP, Carney JA, Stratakis CA. Genetic heterogeneity and spectrum of mutations of the PRKAR1A gene in patients with the carney complex. Hum Mol Genet. 2000;9(20):3037–46.
75. Bertherat J, Horvath A, Groussin L, Grabar S, Boikos S, Cazabat L, et al. Mutations in regulatory subunit type 1A of cyclic adenosine 5′-monophosphate-dependent protein kinase (PRKAR1A): phenotype analysis in 353 patients and 80 different genotypes. J Clin Endocrinol Metab. 2009;94(6):2085–91.
76. Almeida MQ, Stratakis CA. Carney complex and other conditions associated with micronodular adrenal hyperplasias. Best Pract Res Clin Endocrinol Metab. 2010;24(6):907–14.
77. Stratakis CA, Carney JA, Lin JP, Papanicolaou DA, Karl M, Kastner DL, et al. Carney complex, a familial multiple neoplasia and lentiginosis syndrome. Analysis of 11 kindreds and linkage to the short arm of chromosome 2. J Clin Invest. 1996;97(3):699–705.
78. Casey M, Mah C, Merliss AD, Kirschner LS, Taymans SE, Denio AE, et al. Identification of a novel genetic locus for familial cardiac myxomas and Carney complex. Circulation. 1998;98(23):2560–6.
79. Carney JA, Gordon H, Carpenter PC, Shenoy BV, Go VL. The complex of myxomas, spotty pigmentation, and endocrine overactivity. Medicine (Baltimore). 1985;64(4):270–83.
80. Son EJ, Nose V. Familial follicular cell-derived thyroid carcinoma. Front Endocrinol (Lausanne). 2012;3:61.
81. Stratakis CA, Kirschner LS, Carney JA. Clinical and molecular features of the Carney complex: diagnos-

tic criteria and recommendations for patient evaluation. J Clin Endocrinol Metab. 2001;86(9):4041–6.
82. Correa R, Salpea P, Stratakis CA. Carney complex: an update. Eur J Endocrinol. 2015;173(4):M85–97.
83. Rothenbuhler A, Stratakis CA. Clinical and molecular genetics of Carney complex. Best Pract Res Clin Endocrinol Metab. 2010;24(3):389–99.
84. Sandrini F, Stratakis C. Clinical and molecular genetics of Carney complex. Mol Genet Metab. 2003;78(2):83–92.
85. Bossis I, Voutetakis A, Bei T, Sandrini F, Griffin KJ, Stratakis CA. Protein kinase A and its role in human neoplasia: the Carney complex paradigm. Endocr Relat Cancer. 2004;11(2):265–80.
86. Stratakis CA, Kirschner LS, Carney JA. Carney complex: diagnosis and management of the complex of spotty skin pigmentation, myxomas, endocrine overactivity, and schwannomas. Am J Med Genet. 1998;80(2):183–5.
87. Taylor JP, Metcalfe RA, Watson PF, Weetman AP, Trembath RC. Mutations of the PDS gene, encoding pendrin, are associated with protein mislocalization and loss of iodide efflux: implications for thyroid dysfunction in Pendred syndrome. J Clin Endocrinol Metab. 2002;87(4):1778–84.
88. Pera A, Villamar M, Vinuela A, Gandia M, Meda C, Moreno F, et al. A mutational analysis of the SLC26A4 gene in Spanish hearing-impaired families provides new insights into the genetic causes of Pendred syndrome and DFNB4 hearing loss. Eur J Hum Genet. 2008;16(8):888–96.
89. Yang T, Gurrola JG, Wu H, Chiu SM, Wangemann P, Snyder PM, et al. Mutations of KCNJ10 together with mutations of SLC26A4 cause digenic nonsyndromic hearing loss associated with enlarged vestibular aqueduct syndrome. Am J Hum Genet. 2009;84(5):651–7.
90. Nose V. Thyroid cancer of follicular cell origin in inherited tumor syndromes. Adv Anat Pathol. 2010;17(6):428–36.
91. Sakurai K, Hata M, Hishinuma A, Ushijima R, Okada A, Taeda Y, et al. Papillary thyroid carcinoma in one of identical twin patients with Pendred syndrome. Endocr J. 2013;60(6):805–11.
92. Tong GX, Chang Q, Hamele-Bena D, Carew J, Hoffman RS, Nikiforova MN, et al. Targeted next-generation sequencing analysis of a pendred syndrome-associated thyroid carcinoma. Endocr Pathol. 2016;27(1):70–5.
93. Snabboon T, Plengpanich W, Saengpanich S, Sirisalipoch S, Keelawat S, Sunthornyothin S, et al. Two common and three novel PDS mutations in Thai patients with Pendred syndrome. J Endocrinol Investig. 2007;30(11):907–13.
94. Camargo R, Limbert E, Gillam M, Henriques MM, Fernandes C, Catarino AL, et al. Aggressive metastatic follicular thyroid carcinoma with anaplastic transformation arising from a long-standing goiter in a patient with Pendred's syndrome. Thyroid. 2001;11(10):981–8.
95. Rutter MM, Jha P, Schultz KA, Sheil A, Harris AK, Bauer AJ, et al. DICER1 mutations and differentiated thyroid carcinoma: evidence of a direct association. J Clin Endocrinol Metab. 2016;101(1):1–5.
96. Rio Frio T, Bahubeshi A, Kanellopoulou C, Hamel N, Niedziela M, Sabbaghian N, et al. DICER1 mutations in familial multinodular goiter with and without ovarian Sertoli-Leydig cell tumors. JAMA. 2011;305(1):68–77.
97. de Kock L, Sabbaghian N, Soglio DB, Guillerman RP, Park BK, Chami R, et al. Exploring the association between DICER1 mutations and differentiated thyroid carcinoma. J Clin Endocrinol Metab. 2014;99(6):E1072–7.
98. Rome A, Gentet JC, Coze C, Andre N. Pediatric thyroid cancer arising as a fourth cancer in a child with pleuropulmonary blastoma. Pediatr Blood Cancer. 2008;50(5):1081.
99. Doros L, Schultz KA, Stewart DR, Bauer AJ, Williams G, Rossi CT, et al. In: Pagon RA, Adam MP, Ardinger HH, Wallace SE, Amemiya A, LJH B, et al., editors. DICER1-related disorders. Seattle: GeneReviews(R); 1993.
100. McConville CM, Stankovic T, Byrd PJ, McGuire GM, Yao QY, Lennox GG, et al. Mutations associated with variant phenotypes in ataxia-telangiectasia. Am J Hum Genet. 1996;59(2):320–30.
101. Concannon P, Gatti RA. Diversity of ATM gene mutations detected in patients with ataxia-telangiectasia. Hum Mutat. 1997;10(2):100–7.
102. Lavin MF. Ataxia-telangiectasia: from a rare disorder to a paradigm for cell signalling and cancer. Nat Rev Mol Cell Biol. 2008;9(10):759–69.
103. Brasseur B, Beauloye V, Chantrain C, Daumerie C, Vermylen C, Waignein F, et al. Papillary thyroid carcinoma in a 9-year-old girl with ataxia-telangiectasia. Pediatr Blood Cancer. 2008;50(5):1058–60.
104. Malchoff CD, Sarfarazi M, Tendler B, Forouhar F, Whalen G, Joshi V, et al. Papillary thyroid carcinoma associated with papillary renal neoplasia: genetic linkage analysis of a distinct heritable tumor syndrome. J Clin Endocrinol Metab. 2000;85(5):1758–64.
105. Yu CE, Oshima J, Fu YH, Wijsman EM, Hisama F, Alisch R, et al. Positional cloning of the Werner's syndrome gene. Science. 1996;272(5259):258–62.
106. Nehlin JO, Skovgaard GL, Bohr VA. The Werner syndrome. A model for the study of human aging. Ann N Y Acad Sci. 2000;908:167–79.
107. Muftuoglu M, Oshima J, von Kobbe C, Cheng WH, Leistritz DF, Bohr VA. The clinical characteristics of Werner syndrome: molecular and biochemical diagnosis. Hum Genet. 2008;124(4):369–77.
108. Ishikawa Y, Sugano H, Matsumoto T, Furuichi Y, Miller RW, Goto M. Unusual features of thyroid carcinomas in Japanese patients with Werner syndrome and possible genotype-phenotype relations to cell type and race. Cancer. 1999;85(6):1345–52.
109. Lauper JM, Krause A, Vaughan TL, Monnat RJ Jr. Spectrum and risk of neoplasia in Werner syndrome: a systematic review. PLoS One. 2013;8(4):e59709.

110. Oshima J, Martin GM, Hisama FM. In: Pagon RA, Adam MP, Ardinger HH, Wallace SE, Amemiya A, LJH B, et al., editors. Werner syndrome. Seattle: GeneReviews(R); 1993.
111. Bano G, Hodgson S. Diagnosis and management of hereditary thyroid cancer. Recent Results Cancer Res. 2016;205:29–44.
112. Sturgeon C, Clark OH. Familial nonmedullary thyroid cancer. Thyroid. 2005;15(6):588–93.
113. Nikiforova MN, Stringer JR, Blough R, Medvedovic M, Fagin JA, Nikiforov YE. Proximity of chromosomal loci that participate in radiation-induced rearrangements in human cells. Science. 2000;290(5489):138–41.
114. Alsanea O, Wada N, Ain K, Wong M, Taylor K, Ituarte PH, et al. Is familial non-medullary thyroid carcinoma more aggressive than sporadic thyroid cancer? A multicenter series. Surgery. 2000;128(6):1043–50. discussion 50–1.
115. Uchino S, Noguchi S, Kawamoto H, Yamashita H, Watanabe S, Yamashita H, et al. Familial nonmedullary thyroid carcinoma characterized by multifocality and a high recurrence rate in a large study population. World J Surg. 2002;26(8):897–902.
116. Pal T, Vogl FD, Chappuis PO, Tsang R, Brierley J, Renard H, et al. Increased risk for nonmedullary thyroid cancer in the first degree relatives of prevalent cases of nonmedullary thyroid cancer: a hospital-based study. J Clin Endocrinol Metab. 2001;86(11):5307–12.
117. Musholt TJ, Musholt PB, Petrich T, Oetting G, Knapp WH, Klempnauer J. Familial papillary thyroid carcinoma: genetics, criteria for diagnosis, clinical features, and surgical treatment. World J Surg. 2000;24(11):1409–17.
118. Joanna Klubo-Gwiezdzinska LY, Merkel R, Patel D, Nilubol N, Skarulis MC. Samira Mercedes Sadowski and Electron Kebebew screening in Familial Non-Medullary Thyroid Cancer (FNMTC) results in detection of low risk papillary thyroid cancer – a Prospective Cohort Study. 2016.
119. Gudmundsson J, Sulem P, Gudbjartsson DF, Jonasson JG, Sigurdsson A, Bergthorsson JT, et al. Common variants on 9q22.33 and 14q13.3 predispose to thyroid cancer in European populations. Nat Genet. 2009;41(4):460–4.
120. Landa I, Ruiz-Llorente S, Montero-Conde C, Inglada-Perez L, Schiavi F, Leskela S, et al. The variant rs1867277 in FOXE1 gene confers thyroid cancer susceptibility through the recruitment of USF1/USF2 transcription factors. PLoS Genet. 2009;5(9):e1000637.
121. Tomaz RA, Sousa I, Silva JG, Santos C, Teixeira MR, Leite V, et al. FOXE1 polymorphisms are associated with familial and sporadic nonmedullary thyroid cancer susceptibility. Clin Endocrinol. 2012;77(6):926–33.
122. Pereira JS, da Silva JG, Tomaz RA, Pinto AE, Bugalho MJ, Leite V, et al. Identification of a novel germline FOXE1 variant in patients with familial non-medullary thyroid carcinoma (FNMTC). Endocrine. 2015;49(1):204–14.
123. Gara SK, Jia L, Merino MJ, Agarwal SK, Zhang L, Cam M, et al. Germline HABP2 mutation causing familial nonmedullary thyroid cancer. N Engl J Med. 2015;373(5):448–55.
124. Zhang T, Xing M. HABP2 G534E mutation in familial nonmedullary thyroid cancer. J Natl Cancer Inst. 2016;108(6):djv415.
125. Sahasrabudhe R, Stultz J, Williamson J, Lott P, Estrada A, Bohorquez M, et al. The HABP2 G534E variant is an unlikely cause of familial non-medullary thyroid cancer. J Clin Endocrinol Metab. 2015;21:jc20153928.
126. Cantara S, Marzocchi C, Castagna MG, Pacini F. HABP2 G534E variation in familial non-medullary thyroid cancer: an Italian series. J Endocrinol Investig. 2016;21:557–60.
127. Weeks AL, Wilson SG, Ward L, Goldblatt J, Hui J, Walsh JP. HABP2 germline variants are uncommon in familial nonmedullary thyroid cancer. BMC Med Genet. 2016;17(1):60.
128. Ruiz-Ferrer M, Fernandez RM, Navarro E, Antinolo G, Borrego S. G534E variant in HABP2 and nonmedullary thyroid cancer. Thyroid. 2016;26(7):987–8.
129. Bohorquez ME, Estrada AP, Stultz J, Sahasrabudhe R, Williamson J, Lott P, et al. The HABP2 G534E polymorphism does not increase nonmedullary thyroid cancer risk in Hispanics. Endocr Connect. 2016;5(3):123–7.
130. Alzahrani AS, Murugan AK, Qasem E, Al-Hindi H. HABP2 gene mutations do not cause familial or sporadic non-medullary thyroid cancer in a highly inbred middle eastern population. Thyroid. 2016;26(5):667–71.
131. Tomsic J, Fultz R, Liyanarachchi S, He H, Senter L, de la Chapelle A. HABP2 G534E variant in papillary thyroid carcinoma. PLoS One. 2016;11(1):e0146315.
132. Canzian F, Amati P, Harach HR, Kraimps JL, Lesueur F, Barbier J, et al. A gene predisposing to familial thyroid tumors with cell oxyphilia maps to chromosome 19p13.2. Am J Hum Genet. 1998;63(6):1743–8.
133. Bevan S, Pal T, Greenberg CR, Green H, Wixey J, Bignell G, et al. A comprehensive analysis of MNG1, TCO1, fPTC, PTEN, TSHR, and TRKA in familial nonmedullary thyroid cancer: confirmation of linkage to TCO1. J Clin Endocrinol Metab. 2001;86(8):3701–4.
134. Stankov K, Pastore A, Toschi L, McKay J, Lesueur F, Kraimps JL, et al. Allelic loss on chromosomes 2q21 and 19p 13.2 in oxyphilic thyroid tumors. Int J Cancer. 2004;111(3):463–7.
135. Prazeres HJ, Rodrigues F, Soares P, Naidenov P, Figueiredo P, Campos B, et al. Loss of heterozygosity at 19p13.2 and 2q21 in tumours from familial clusters of non-medullary thyroid carcinoma. Familial Cancer. 2008;7(2):141–9.
136. Capezzone M, Cantara S, Marchisotta S, Filetti S, De Santi MM, Rossi B, et al. Short telomeres, telom-

erase reverse transcriptase gene amplification, and increased telomerase activity in the blood of familial papillary thyroid cancer patients. J Clin Endocrinol Metab. 2008;93(10):3950–7.
137. He M, Bian B, Gesuwan K, Gulati N, Zhang L, Nilubol N, et al. Telomere length is shorter in affected members of families with familial nonmedullary thyroid cancer. Thyroid. 2013;23(3):301–7.
138. Jendrzejewski J, Tomsic J, Lozanski G, Labanowska J, He H, Liyanarachchi S, et al. Telomere length and telomerase reverse transcriptase gene copy number in patients with papillary thyroid carcinoma. J Clin Endocrinol Metab. 2011;96(11):E1876–80.
139. He H, Li W, Wu D, Nagy R, Liyanarachchi S, Akagi K, et al. Ultra-rare mutation in long-range enhancer predisposes to thyroid carcinoma with high penetrance. PLoS One. 2013;8(5):e61920.
140. Bignell GR, Canzian F, Shayeghi M, Stark M, Shugart YY, Biggs P, et al. Familial nontoxic multinodular thyroid goiter locus maps to chromosome 14q but does not account for familial nonmedullary thyroid cancer. Am J Hum Genet. 1997;61(5):1123–30.
141. McKay JD, Williamson J, Lesueur F, Stark M, Duffield A, Canzian F, et al. At least three genes account for familial papillary thyroid carcinoma: TCO and MNG1 excluded as susceptibility loci from a large Tasmanian family. Eur J Endocrinol. 1999;141(2):122–5.
142. Lesueur F, Stark M, Tocco T, Ayadi H, Delisle MJ, Goldgar DE, et al. Genetic heterogeneity in familial nonmedullary thyroid carcinoma: exclusion of linkage to RET, MNG1, and TCO in 56 families. NMTC consortium. J Clin Endocrinol Metab. 1999;84(6):2157–62.
143. Tsilchorozidou T, Vafiadou E, Yovos JG, Romeo G, McKay J, Lesueur F, et al. A Greek family with a follicular variant of familial papillary thyroid carcinoma: TCO, MNG1, fPTC/PRN, and NMTC1 excluded as susceptibility loci. Thyroid. 2005;15(12):1349–54.
144. Suh I, Filetti S, Vriens MR, Guerrero MA, Tumino S, Wong M, et al. Distinct loci on chromosome 1q21 and 6q22 predispose to familial nonmedullary thyroid cancer: a SNP array-based linkage analysis of 38 families. Surgery. 2009;146(6):1073–80.
145. Cavaco BM, Batista PF, Martins C, Banito A, do Rosario F, Limbert E, et al. Familial non-medullary thyroid carcinoma (FNMTC): analysis of fPTC/PRN, NMTC1, MNG1 and TCO susceptibility loci and identification of somatic BRAF and RAS mutations. Endocr Relat Cancer. 2008;15(1):207–15.
146. McKay JD, Lesueur F, Jonard L, Pastore A, Williamson J, Hoffman L, et al. Localization of a susceptibility gene for familial nonmedullary thyroid carcinoma to chromosome 2q21. Am J Hum Genet. 2001;69(2):440–6.
147. McKay JD, Thompson D, Lesueur F, Stankov K, Pastore A, Watfah C, et al. Evidence for interaction between the TCO and NMTC1 loci in familial non-medullary thyroid cancer. J Med Genet. 2004;41(6):407–12.
148. He H, Bronisz A, Liyanarachchi S, Nagy R, Li W, Huang Y, et al. SRGAP1 is a candidate gene for papillary thyroid carcinoma susceptibility. J Clin Endocrinol Metab. 2013;98(5):E973–80.
149. Wong K, Ren XR, Huang YZ, Xie Y, Liu G, Saito H, et al. Signal transduction in neuronal migration: roles of GTPase activating proteins and the small GTPase Cdc42 in the Slit-Robo pathway. Cell. 2001;107(2):209–21.
150. Ngan ES, Lang BH, Liu T, Shum CK, So MT, Lau DK, et al. A germline mutation (A339V) in thyroid transcription factor-1 (TITF-1/NKX2.1) in patients with multinodular goiter and papillary thyroid carcinoma. J Natl Cancer Inst. 2009;101(3):162–75.
151. Cantara S, Capuano S, Formichi C, Pisu M, Capezzone M, Pacini F. Lack of germline A339V mutation in thyroid transcription factor-1 (TITF-1/NKX2.1) gene in familial papillary thyroid cancer. Thyroid Res. 2010;3(1):4.
152. Moses W, Weng J, Kebebew E. Prevalence, clinicopathologic features, and somatic genetic mutation profile in familial versus sporadic nonmedullary thyroid cancer. Thyroid. 2011;21(4):367–71.
153. Park YJ, Ahn HY, Choi HS, Kim KW, Park DJ, Cho BY. The long-term outcomes of the second generation of familial nonmedullary thyroid carcinoma are more aggressive than sporadic cases. Thyroid. 2012;22(4):356–62.
154. Charkes ND. On the prevalence of familial nonmedullary thyroid cancer in multiply affected kindreds. Thyroid. 2006;16(2):181–6.
155. Malchoff CD, Malchoff DM. Familial nonmedullary thyroid carcinoma. Cancer Control. 2006;13(2):106–10.
156. Capezzone M, Marchisotta S, Cantara S, Busonero G, Brilli L, Pazaitou-Panayiotou K, et al. Familial non-medullary thyroid carcinoma displays the features of clinical anticipation suggestive of a distinct biological entity. Endocr Relat Cancer. 2008;15(4):1075–81.
157. Robenshtok E, Tzvetov G, Grozinsky-Glasberg S, Shraga-Slutzky I, Weinstein R, Lazar L, et al. Clinical characteristics and outcome of familial nonmedullary thyroid cancer: a retrospective controlled study. Thyroid. 2011;21(1):43–8.
158. Maxwell EL, Hall FT, Freeman JL. Familial nonmedullary thyroid cancer: a matched-case control study. Laryngoscope. 2004;114(12):2182–6.
159. Ito Y, Kakudo K, Hirokawa M, Fukushima M, Yabuta T, Tomoda C, et al. Biological behavior and prognosis of familial papillary thyroid carcinoma. Surgery. 2009;145(1):100–5.
160. Navas-Carrillo D, Rios A, Rodriguez JM, Parrilla P, Orenes-Pinero E. Familial nonmedullary thyroid cancer: screening, clinical, molecular and genetic findings. Biochim Biophys Acta. 2014;1846(2):468–76.
161. Sadowski SM, He M, Gesuwan K, Gulati N, Celi F, Merino MJ, et al. Prospective screening in familial nonmedullary thyroid cancer. Surgery. 2013;154(6):1194–8.

162. McDonald TJ, Driedger AA, Garcia BM, Van Uum SH, Rachinsky I, Chevendra V, et al. Familial papillary thyroid carcinoma: a retrospective analysis. J Oncol. 2011;2011:948786.
163. Mazeh H, Benavidez J, Poehls JL, Youngwirth L, Chen H, Sippel RS. In patients with thyroid cancer of follicular cell origin, a family history of nonmedullary thyroid cancer in one first-degree relative is associated with more aggressive disease. Thyroid. 2012;22(1):3–8.
164. Jiwang L, Zhendong L, Shuchun L, Bo H, Yanguo L. Clinicopathologic characteristics of familial versus sporadic papillary thyroid carcinoma. Acta Otorhinolaryngol Ital. 2015;35(4):234–42.
165. Leux C, Truong T, Petit C, Baron-Dubourdieu D, Guenel P. Family history of malignant and benign thyroid diseases and risk of thyroid cancer: a population-based case-control study in New Caledonia. Cancer Causes Control. 2012;23(5):745–55.
166. Pitoia F, Cross G, Salvai ME, Abelleira E, Niepomniszcze H. Patients with familial non-medullary thyroid cancer have an outcome similar to that of patients with sporadic papillary thyroid tumors. Arq Bras Endocrinol Metabol. 2011;55(3):219–23.
167. Tavarelli M, Russo M, Terranova R, Scollo C, Spadaro A, Sapuppo G, et al. Familial non-medullary thyroid cancer represents an independent risk factor for increased cancer aggressiveness: a retrospective analysis of 74 families. Front Endocrinol. 2015;6:117.
168. Hillenbrand A, Varhaug JE, Brauckhoff M, Pandev R, Haufe S, Dotzenrath C, et al. Familial nonmedullary thyroid carcinoma-clinical relevance and prognosis. A European multicenter study. ESES Vienna presentation. Langenbeck's Arch Surg. 2010;395(7):851–8.
169. Loh KC. Familial nonmedullary thyroid carcinoma: a meta-review of case series. Thyroid. 1997;7(1):107–13.
170. Mazeh H, Sippel RS. Familial nonmedullary thyroid carcinoma. Thyroid. 2013;23(9):1049–56.
171. Sippel RS, Caron NR, Clark OH. An evidence-based approach to familial nonmedullary thyroid cancer: screening, clinical management, and follow-up. World J Surg. 2007;31(5):924–33.
172. Wang X, Cheng W, Li J, Su A, Wei T, Liu F, et al. Endocrine tumours: familial nonmedullary thyroid carcinoma is a more aggressive disease: a systematic review and meta-analysis. Eur J Endocrinol. 2015;172(6):R253–62.
173. Lee YM, Yoon JH, Yi O, Sung TY, Chung KW, Kim WB, et al. Familial history of non-medullary thyroid cancer is an independent prognostic factor for tumor recurrence in younger patients with conventional papillary thyroid carcinoma. J Surg Oncol. 2014;109(2):168–73.
174. Pinto AE, Silva GL, Henrique R, Menezes FD, Teixeira MR, Leite V, et al. Familial vs sporadic papillary thyroid carcinoma: a matched-case comparative study showing similar clinical/prognostic behaviour. Eur J Endocrinol. 2014;170(2):321–7.
175. Miki H, Oshimo K, Inoue H, Kawano M, Tanaka K, Komaki K, et al. Incidence of ultrasonographically-detected thyroid nodules in healthy adults. Tokushima J Exp Med. 1993;40(1-2):43–6.
176. Uchino S, Noguchi S, Yamashita H, Murakami T, Watanabe S, Ogawa T, et al. Detection of asymptomatic differentiated thyroid carcinoma by neck ultrasonographic screening for familial nonmedullary thyroid carcinoma. World J Surg. 2004;28(11):1099–102.
177. Stulak JM, Grant CS, Farley DR, Thompson GB, van Heerden JA, Hay ID, et al. Value of preoperative ultrasonography in the surgical management of initial and reoperative papillary thyroid cancer. Arch Surg. 2006;141(5):489–94. discussion 94–6.
178. Roh JL, Park JY, Kim JM, Song CJ. Use of preoperative ultrasonography as guidance for neck dissection in patients with papillary thyroid carcinoma. J Surg Oncol. 2009;99(1):28–31.
179. Vriens MR, Sabanci U, Epstein HD, Ngai S, Duh QY, Siperstein AE, et al. Reliability of fine-needle aspiration in patients with familial nonmedullary thyroid cancer. Thyroid. 1999;9(10):1011–6.
180. Triponez F, Wong M, Sturgeon C, Caron N, Ginzinger DG, Segal MR, et al. Does familial non-medullary thyroid cancer adversely affect survival? World J Surg. 2006;30(5):787–93.
181. Alsanea O, Clark OH. Familial thyroid cancer. Curr Opin Oncol. 2001;13(1):44–51.

Part VII

Thyroid Cancer in Children

Pediatric Differentiated Thyroid Carcinoma

21

Steven G. Waguespack
and Jonathan D. Wasserman

Introduction

Differentiated thyroid carcinoma (DTC) is the most common endocrine malignancy, with papillary thyroid carcinoma (PTC) representing 90% or more of cases in children [1–5]. Similar to adults, children with PTC commonly present with a palpable thyroid nodule or may be identified incidentally in the context of imaging studies. Tumor size is larger in children compared with older patients (70% of children aged 0–9 years have a tumor ≥2 cm) [5–7]. In further contrast with adults, pediatric PTC is frequently associated with clinically apparent, malignant cervical lymphadenopathy and may present as a diffusely infiltrative carcinoma without a discrete nodule (Fig. 21.1). Rarely, children may also be diagnosed via imaging that demonstrates pulmonary metastases that may initially be attributed to an infectious etiology (Fig. 21.2). Symptoms related to neoplastic involvement of adjacent aerodigestive structures is rare (4% or less of pediatric PTC patients) [7]. Often multifocal and bilateral, PTC is associated with regional metastases in 80% or more of childhood cases at diagnosis in some retrospective series [4, 8–15]. Children with significant cervical lymph node disease are at the highest risk of hematogenously-spread lung metastases, [10, 11] (Fig. 21.2) which have been identified in up to 25% of patients in some published pediatric case series [3, 5, 12, 16–19]. Other sites of distant metastatic disease can include the brain, bones, and other solid organs but such events are exceedingly rare in children. Paradoxically, despite having more extensive disease at diagnosis, pediatric PTC is usually a well-differentiated tumor with an indolent clinical course, which translates to an extremely low disease-specific mortality [1, 17, 20–22].

Follicular thyroid carcinoma (FTC) represents a distinct histopathological entity from PTC. In children, the diagnosis of FTC is almost always made following the pathologic identification of capsular and/or vascular invasion in a nodule surgically removed after an indeterminate fine needle aspiration biopsy (FNAB). Given the rarity of FTC in children and because it remains poorly studied in this age group, the bulk of this chapter, especially the treatment algorithms, will focus on PTC.

The excellent prognosis of pediatric DTC, in concert with substantive concerns regarding the potential for long-term sequelae related to overaggressive treatment during childhood, make the optimal management of pediatric DTC a

S. G. Waguespack (✉)
Department of Endocrine Neoplasia and Hormonal Disorders, University of Texas MD Anderson Cancer Center, Houston, TX, USA
e-mail: swagues@mdanderson.org

J. D. Wasserman
Division of Endocrinology, Hospital for Sick Children, University of Toronto, Toronto, ON, Canada
e-mail: jonathan.wasserman@sickkids.ca

U. K. Mallick et al. (eds.), *Practical Management of Thyroid Cancer*,
https://doi.org/10.1007/978-3-319-91725-2_21

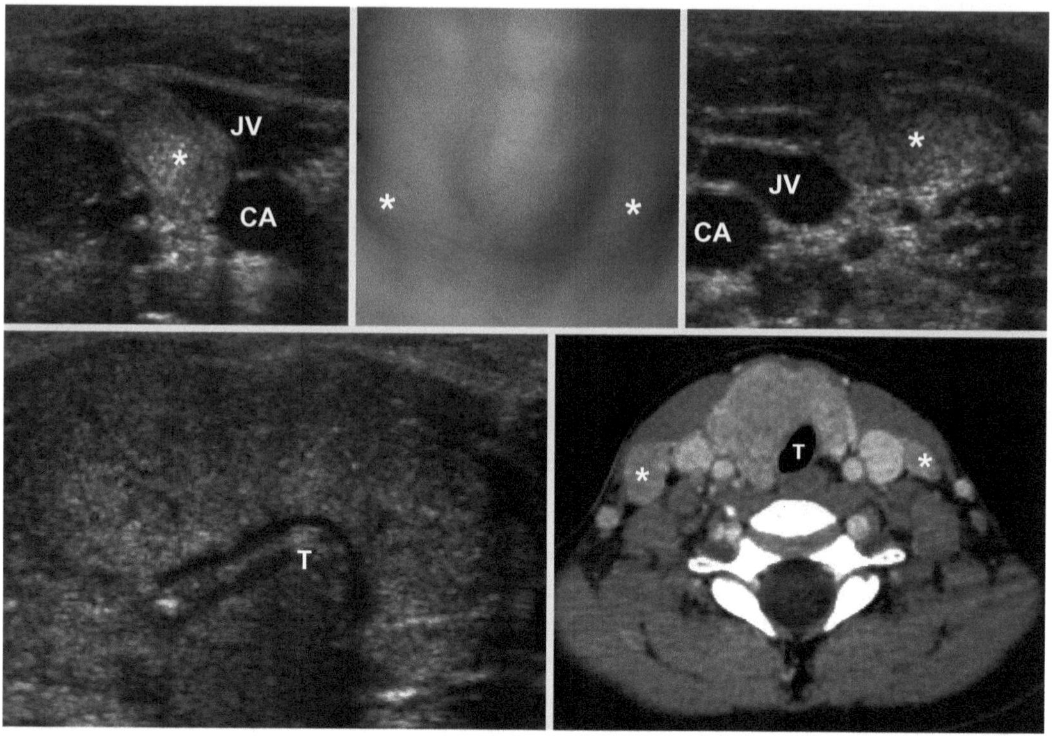

Fig. 21.1 Clinical presentation of pediatric papillary thyroid carcinoma. A 6-year-old boy with palpable cervical lymphadenopathy (asterisk) and a firm asymmetric goiter. Ultrasound demonstrates a primary tumor with scattered microcalcifications that is diffusely infiltrating both thyroid lobes and the isthmus (bottom left) as well as malignant neck lymphadenopathy (asterisk) in both the right (top left) and left (top right) lateral neck. CT neck with contrast obtained as part of pre-operative staging also documents the extent of disease and its anatomic relationship to underlying aerodigestive structures such as the trachea. *CA* carotid artery, *JV* jugular vein, *T* trachea

challenging endeavor. Moreover, the existence of a very small population of patients with advanced disease who may benefit from systemic therapy poses a further challenge to care, given that these agents remain largely untested in children with DTC. Only recently have formal guidelines for management been developed by the American Thyroid Association (ATA) [23].

Epidemiology and Prognosis

In 2017, it is estimated that there will be 56,870 new thyroid cancer diagnosed in the United States, [24] of which 1.4% are expected to occur in individuals <20 years of age [25]. Pediatric thyroid cancer incidence is significantly lower in blacks versus whites, and the diagnosis is much more common in females [1, 6, 22, 25]. From 2010 to 2014, the age-adjusted incidence rate for children ages 0–14 years was two case/million/year in males and five cases/million/year in females; adolescents (ages 15–19) are the most commonly affected pediatric age group (29 cases/million/year) and the female: male ratio is 5.4:1 in this population [25]. More broadly, thyroid cancer is the fifth most common cancer diagnosed in adolescence, representing 11% of all cancers [24]. In adolescents, incidence rates have been rising over the decades, [1, 6, 22, 25, 26] a trend that cannot solely be explained by an increased diagnosis of small tumors.

Children with DTC have an excellent prognosis and survival over decades is typical, even for those patients with distant metastases [1, 22]. Remission rates are high, especially in the current era of high-resolution neck ultrasonography and more comprehensive initial thyroid cancer surgery. In the pediatric population, 10-year survival is almost universally 100% [1, 19, 20, 27–32].

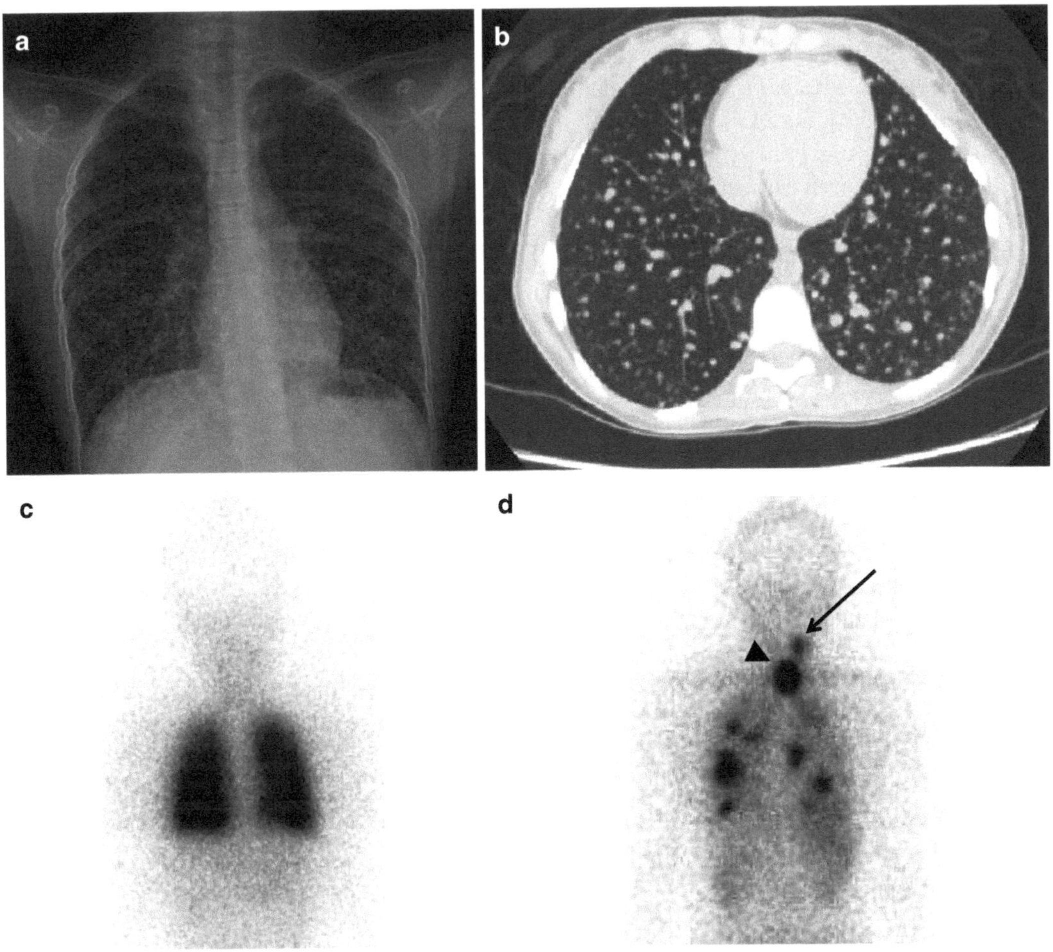

Fig. 21.2 Pulmonary metastases of pediatric papillary thyroid carcinoma. (**a**) Chest X-ray demonstrating a diffuse, miliary pattern of disease in a child; this pattern may initially be mistaken for an infectious etiology. (**b**) Axial post-contrast computed tomography image showing the micronodular pulmonary metastases typical of pediatric disease. (**c**) Post-treatment thyroid scan with diffuse and intense pulmonary uptake of ^{131}I. This pattern is associated with an increased risk of pulmonary fibrosis. (**d**) Post-treatment thyroid scan of a different patient showing multifocal nodular pulmonary uptake, thyroid bed uptake (arrowhead), and residual cervical lymph node disease (arrow)

Children diagnosed before age 10 years appear to have a higher risk of recurrence and ultimately death from their disease, [17, 21, 33–36] although a significant difference in tumor biology between the very young and older children has not been confirmed in other studies [7, 11, 37–39]. A subgroup of pediatric patients will ultimately die of their cancer or succumb to treatment-related complications [20, 28, 29, 40, 41]. For children with distantly metastatic disease, it is those with micronodular lung metastases and iodine-avid disease who maintain the best prognosis [29, 42]. Improved risk stratification that incorporates knowledge about clinical presentation, somatic mutational analysis, and response to treatment are needed to better identify those children who are at highest risk for ultimate disease-specific death and to avoid overzealous treatment of others who are unlikely to die from their cancer.

Risk Factors

Exposure of the thyroid to radiation (primarily in the context of medical therapy for cancer) is the major established risk factor for the development of thyroid carcinoma, although irradiation not including the thyroid region can also increase the risk [43]. Children, particularly those younger than age 5 years, appear to be especially sensitive to the tumorigenic effects of ionizing radiation [44]. Thyroid cancer is one of the most frequently diagnosed subsequent primary malignancies in childhood cancer survivors, with at least a five-fold increase in risk [45, 46]. This risk appears to decline once the thyroid dose exceeds 2000 cGy, [44, 47] suggesting that sublethal irradiation of the thyroid imparts the greatest risk. Radiation-induced tumors do not appear to be more aggressive compared with sporadic, non-radiation induced disease [48, 49]. The latency period between radiation exposure and diagnosis is typically long, with a median time to occurrence around 19 years [45]. Surprisingly, the risk of thyroid malignancy in childhood cancer survivors appears to be increased even in those who have not received therapeutic irradiation and this may reflect, at least in part, additional increased cancer risk among recipients of alkylating chemotherapy [50, 51].

Exposure to ionizing radiation can also occur via the ingestion of radionuclides, epitomized by the large environmental exposure to radioactive iodine (RAI) resulting from the Chernobyl, and possibly, the more recent Fukushima nuclear accidents [2, 52]. Additional environmental exposures may increase the risk of thyroid cancer in children living in geographic areas with volcanic activity [53]. The small activities of $^{123}I/^{131}I$ used for diagnostic studies and the treatment of hyperthyroidism appear to be below the threshold needed for tumorigenesis [54]. The use of ^{131}I-Metaiodobenzylguanidine (^{131}I-MIBG) to treat children with neuroblastoma has also been implicated in the development of benign and malignant thyroid neoplasia, [55] although common genetic factors and mechanisms of tumorigenesis between these two malignancies may also play a role [56, 57].

There has been some conjecture regarding a link between thyroid autoimmunity and the risk of DTC. However, whether or not a strong association between autoimmune thyroid disease and DTC exists in children remains unknown. The prevalence of PTC was 3% in one study of 375 children with autoimmune thyroiditis, [58] and another study of children with goiter did not clearly identify an increased risk of PTC in children with positive thyroid peroxidase antibodies compared with those with normal titers [59]. In a retrospective review of 32 children operated for Graves disease, DTC was identified in 22% of patients (including four diagnosed preoperatively); [60] three and two patients had lymph node and pulmonary metastases, respectively.

Although rare in the developed world, iodine deficiency is associated with an increased risk of thyroid neoplasia (specifically FTC) [61, 62] and, similar to many other cancers, obesity may be an additional risk factor [63]. Finally, although accounting for a small minority of pediatric DTC, germline variants in several genes have been associated with syndromic and non-syndromic hereditary DTC and are discussed in greater detail later in this chapter.

Histopathologic Variants

DTC comprises two major histopathologic variants, PTC and FTC, which differ in their clinical and metastatic presentations. Anaplastic (undifferentiated) thyroid carcinomas and poorly differentiated thyroid carcinomas are exceedingly rare in childhood, as are primary thyroid lymphomas and metastases to the thyroid gland.

Subtypes of PTC include classic/conventional, encapsulated, follicular (fvPTC), tall cell, oncocytic, columnar cell, diffuse sclerosing (dsPTC), hobnail, cribriform-morular and solid/trabecular variants [64, 65]. Recently, based on a retrospective analysis of clinical outcomes, the noninvasive encapsulated follicular variant of PTC has been reclassified in adults as a low risk tumor called NIFTP (noninvasive follicular thyroid neoplasm with papillary-like nuclear features [66]. It is unclear if these data can be extrapolated to pediatric patients with similar histology as no patients <age 21 years was in the NIFTP group.

In children, classic PTC is the most common variant (48%) followed by (in one recent study) dsPTC (16%), fvPTC (14.5%), encapsulated PTC (13%), tall cell PTC (13%), poorly differentiated (6.5%) and solid PTC (2%) [67]. In contrast with adults, histologic subtype does not appear to independently predict event-free survival, [67] although some studies have shown a higher risk of recurrence in children with classic PTC compared with fvPTC [18]. Solid variant PTC is more common in children with a history of radiation exposure [64]. The diffuse sclerosing variant, characterized by diffuse and often bilateral involvement of the thyroid, demonstrates extensive squamous metaplasia, abundant psammoma bodies, stromal fibrosis, and prominent lymphocytic infiltration. It is often accompanied by chronic lymphocytic thyroiditis in the background thyroid, extensive regional nodal metastases, and a higher frequency in younger patients [68, 69].

FTC is broadly divided into minimally invasive and widely invasive forms [70]. In 2017, the World Health Organization reclassified FTC into three groups: (1) minimally invasive (capsular invasion only) (2) encapsulated angioinvasive, and (3) widely invasive [65]. Similar to adults, minimally invasive FTC in children may be a low-risk malignancy, [30, 71] but bone and lung metastases have been described in minimally invasive tumors with vascular invasion, underscoring the fact that any degree of vacular invasion may confer a risk for metastatic disease in pediatric FTC [72]. The oncocytic (Hürthle-cell) variant of FTC is rare in the pediatric population [31, 71].

Molecular Mechanisms of Disease

Somatic Genomic Alterations

Abundant work over recent decades has established the primacy of aberrations in signaling through receptor tyrosine kinase (RTK) pathways, predominantly via the cognate RAS-RAF-MEK-ERK and PI3K-AKT-mTOR pathways, in the molecular pathogenesis of DTC. Recent genomic and transcriptome analyses [73, 74] have demonstrated that activating pathogenic variants in one of these two pathways are common, identified in 96.5% of PTCs [73] and 73% of follicular thyroid neoplasms (FTC and follicular adenomas) [74]. These somatic alterations typically are mutually exclusive and the mutational burden of DTC is low compared with other carcinomas. Moreover, the relative balance of RAF- versus RAS-mediated signaling has been linked to the extent of thyrocyte differentiation and differences in expression of genes responsible for iodine uptake and metabolism, which has potential treatment implications [73].

In pediatric PTC, gene rearrangements are the most common molecular event, especially after previous radiation exposure, [75–78] but they are not limited to children with that well-established risk factor [79–81]. Fusions involving the *RE*arranged during *T*ransfection (*RET*) proto-oncogene and the neurotropic tyrosine receptor kinase (*NTRK*) gene are the most common [77, 79–84]. Gene rearrangements of peroxisome proliferator-activated receptor gamma (*PPARG*) and paired box gene 8 (*PAX8*) and fusions involving the v-raf murine sarcoma viral oncogene homolog B (*BRAF*) and anaplastic lymphoma kinase (*ALK*) genes have also been identified, [77, 81, 84–87] although the *PAX8/PPARG* fusion is much more commonly associated with FTC [88]. $BRAF^{V600E}$ point mutations are also prevalent, [78–81, 86, 89, 90] although not as common as in adults. Rat sarcoma (*RAS*) mutations are also identified in pediatric PTC and FTC, [77, 78, 80, 81, 86, 90] although these have also been identified among benign follicular adenomas; [74] thus, at least from a diagnostic perspective, their relevance is debatable. *BRAF* mutations are more common in older pediatric patients, [84, 86, 87, 89] and it appears that *BRAF*-mutated PTC may not be more clinically aggressive in the pediatric population, as has been suggested for adult PTC [78, 79, 81, 86, 90, 91]. *TERT* promoter, *PIK3CA*, and *PTEN* mutations are rare [89–91].

Hereditary DTC

Hereditary DTC is rare and <5% of pediatric thyroid cancers are associated with an underlying germline mutation [78]. A family history of PTC is present in 4% of pediatric cases [7].

However, in the context of the high prevalence of PTC in the population at large, the presence of a single affected 1st degree relative with PTC does not indicate a familial etiology. Multiple genes and heritable tumor syndromes have been associated with both benign and malignant thyroid neoplasia: *APC*-Associated Polyposis (*APC* gene; OMIM[Online Mendelian Inheritance in Man®] #175100), Birt-Hogg-Dubé Syndrome (*FLCN* gene; OMIM #135150), the Carney complex (*PRKAR1A* gene; OMIM #160980), CHEK2-Related Cancer (*CHEK2* gene; OMIM #604373), DICER1-pleuropulmonary blastoma familial tumor predisposition syndrome (*DICER1* gene; OMIM #606241), familial nonmedullary thyroid carcinoma (FNMTC) (multiple genes; OMIM #188550), Li-Fraumeni syndrome (*TP53* gene; OMIM #151623), *PTEN* [phosphatase and tensin homolog] Hamartoma Tumor Syndrome (*PTEN* gene; OMIM #601728), Pendred syndrome (*SLC26A4* gene; OMIM #274600) and Werner syndrome (*WRN* gene; OMIM# 277700). Most recently, a germline compound heterozygous deletion in the *USF3* gene was identified in a Cowden syndrome-like kindred with PTC, suggesting that this gene may also be involved in the predisposition to thyroid cancer [92]. Comprehensive reviews on the individual syndromes are available elsewhere, [65, 78, 93–96] and it should be emphasized that the association of DTC with some of these tumor predisposition syndromes does not necessarily indicate causality.

The *PTEN* hamartoma tumor syndrome is one of the more common syndromic causes of multinodular goiter and DTC (primarily PTC and fvPTC, but FTC is overrepresented relative to the general population), [95, 97–99] and the youngest reported case of thyroid cancer associated with a *PTEN* mutation was in a 7-year-old [98]. A clue to this diagnosis in a child presenting with thyroid neoplasia is macrocephaly, present in 98% of children with a germline *PTEN* mutation, [99] although macrocephaly has also been reported in 42% of *DICER1* mutation carriers [100]. Multinodular goiter is predominant in patients with *DICER1* mutations, especially in females, and the risk of DTC is also increased [101, 102]. In contrast with children at risk for hereditary medullary thyroid carcinoma, it is *not* recommended that children at risk for DTC due to an underlying disease-predisposing gene mutation undergo prophylactic thyroidectomy. In these cases, screening ultrasounds may be considered (based on expert opinion) in the *DICER1*-Syndrome, *PTEN* hamartoma tumor syndrome, Carney complex, and *APC*-associated polyposis, [95, 102–106] noting that the latter syndrome is uniquely associated with the cribriform-morular variant of PTC [107].

Evaluation, Treatment, and Follow Up

Once described as a "fatal disease with few exceptions," [108] malignant thyroid disease is now recognized to have an excellent long-term prognosis in the majority of patients, especially in children. The evaluation and treatment of pediatric DTC has certainly evolved over the years. Historically, surgery was less-than comprehensive, relying more on palpation and limited by the lack of pre-operative high resolution ultrasonography and other cross-sectional imaging that are commonly utilized today. There has also shift in the utilization of RAI. It was once held that ^{131}I would "clean up" whatever disease was not removed surgically and RAI was used almost universally to treat children with DTC until the thyroid scan became negative or as long as the thyroglobulin (Tg) remained detectable (once this tumor marker became available for clinical use). More recently, the concept of iodine-refractory disease in pediatric DTC has been better appreciated and current guidelines suggest a more conservative approach to RAI treatment, even among those with iodine-avid cancer [23].

Initial Work Up and Staging (Fig. 21.3)

Once the diagnosis of thyroid cancer is established, a comprehensive pre-operative assessment is critical to understand the extent of cervical disease to facilitate the optimal surgical

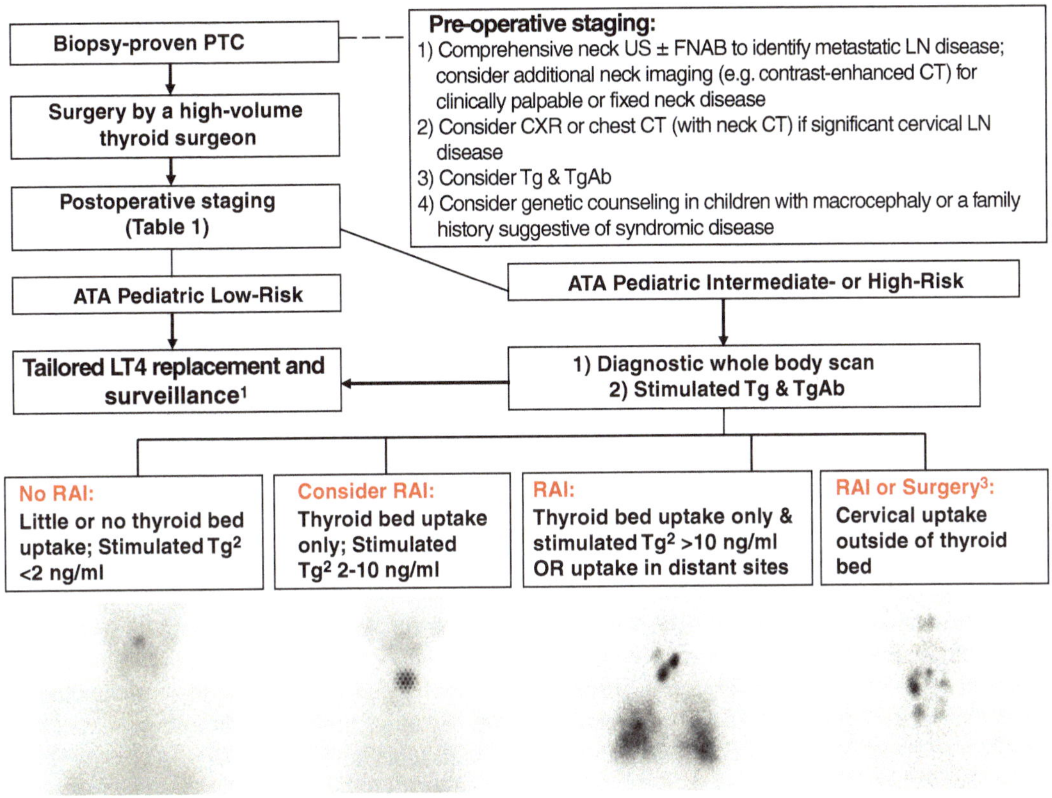

Fig. 21.3 Initial evaluation and treatment of biopsy-proven pediatric papillary thyroid carcinoma. [1]If residual/recurrent PTC is suspected during long-term follow up of low-risk patients, and assuming neck US is negative, further evaluation and treatment with RAI is recommended. [2]Assumes negative TgAb; if TgAb is positive and there is no evidence of iodine-avid disease on the diagnostic scan, consideration can be given to deferring RAI treatment, especially in intermediate-risk patients. [3]RAI only if surgery deemed unsafe or not feasible. *ATA* American Thyroid Association, *CT* computed tomography, *CXR* chest X-ray, *FNAB* fine needle aspiration biopsy, *LN* lymph node, *LT4* levothyroxine, *RAI* radioactive iodine (^{131}I), *Tg* thyroglobulin, *TgAb* thyroglobulin antibody, *TSH* thyroid stimulating hormone, *US* ultrasound

approach. Universally recommended, assuming it is not already done, is a high-resolution cervical ultrasound (US) performed by an experienced ultrasonographer to interrogate the thyroid and lateral neck lymph nodes [23, 109, 110]. If suspicious adenopathy is identified, US-guided FNAB should be undertaken to confirm disease and the extent of regional metastases. In the presence of cystic lymph nodes, which are highly suggestive of PTC metastases, measurement of Tg on fluid from the needle washout may help to secure the diagnosis of malignant involvement [111, 112]. In children with bulky cervical disease, a primary tumor that appears fixed to underlying aerodigestive structures, or vocal cord paralysis, contrast-enhanced computed tomography (CT) of the neck is recommended to help guide further the surgical approach [23, 109]. Only a minority of children will have pulmonary metastases, typically only those with bulky cervical disease, [10] and the detection of pulmonary metastatic disease does not change the initial therapeutic approach. In addition, postoperative staging with RAI, if indicated, will effectively identify most children with pulmonary metastases, even those with negative baseline radiographic imaging [16]. Therefore, current guidelines do not suggest routine chest imaging in all pediatric DTC patients, although some centers do obtain a preoperative CXR in high risk children because the finding of a significant disease burden may alter the approach to subsequent RAI therapy [109].

However, a CXR is not sensitive enough to identify small-volume micronodular pulmonary metastases, [16] and for that reason, some also consider chest CT, especially if neck CT is also planned. Although not recommended by all, some experts do obtain baseline Tg and thyroglobulin autoantibodies (TgAb) after confirmation of DTC [109].

Surgery

The surgical approach to pediatric DTC is not significantly different from adult cases and so will not be discussed in detail. In general, given the high rate of lymph node and pulmonary metastases, total thyroidectomy is recommended in most cases [23]. However, in children with small, incidentally discovered tumors, no previous radiation exposure, and no evidence of contralateral disease or cervical lymph node disease, thyroid lobectomy ± ipsilateral central neck dissection may result in similar long-term outcomes [7, 22, 32, 113, 114].

Current data suggest that the single most important factor for improving long-term disease-free survival is the extent of the initial surgery, with more complete surgery decreasing or eliminating persistent/recurrent disease and the need for additional treatment [11, 14, 17, 18, 20, 115–117]. Older studies, however, are confounded by the frequent prescription of RAI. Compartment-oriented neck dissection is advised for biopsy-proven lymph node disease and central neck dissection (CND), in the absence of documented lymph node metastases, can be selectively considered in children and determined by intraoperative findings, [23] recognizing that complication rates are higher with central neck dissection [118]. In the setting of a unifocal PTC > 1 cm, [119] an ipsilateral CND, with pursuit of contralateral CND only if intra-operative findings suggest central compartment disease, may help to balance the risks and benefits in pediatric patients. In every case, the decision to perform a CND should be driven by the experience of the surgeon and his or her ability to localize the parathyroid glands. Preservation of parathyroid function (including the liberal use of parathyroid autotransplantation) and avoidance of significant recurrent laryngeal nerve injury is paramount, even if it means leaving residual microscopic disease. Surgical complications are not insignificant in children with thyroid cancer, [2, 7, 19, 117, 118, 120] and there are lower complication rates and shorter hospital length of stay when surgery is performed by a high-volume thyroid surgeon [23, 121–125]. Therefore, it is strongly preferred that thyroid surgery, especially when lymph node dissection is required, always be performed by a surgeon experienced in the management of pediatric DTC.

Postoperative Staging

Several prognostic staging systems have been used for DTC, and a thorough discussion of this topic is beyond the scope of the current chapter. The pathological TNM (tumor-node-metastasis) classification developed by the American Joint Committee on Cancer (AJCC) and the Union for International Cancer Control (UICC) is the international reference staging system for thyroid cancer, [126] and this has recently been updated to the eighth edition, which will be implemented in January 2018. Underscoring the excellent prognosis, the highest TNM stage that anyone with pediatric-onset DTC can have is stage II, distinguished from stage I disease only by the presence of distant metastases. Therefore, most children, even those with extensive locoregional disease, are considered to have stage I disease. Another used staging system for PTC, the MACIS score, may also be useful in children and adolescents [127, 128].

Utilizing AJCC 7th edition TNM staging, a novel risk categorization for PTC (ATA Pediatric Low-, Intermediate-, and High-risk) was introduced in the inaugural ATA pediatric guidelines [23] (Table 21.1) and subsequently validated in other studies [4, 36, 39]. This risk stratification is intended to identify those at risk of persistent cervical disease and distant metastases in order to determine which patients would benefit from more intensive postoperative stag-

Table 21.1 ATA pediatric risk categories and recommendations for postoperative staging and clinical follow up[a]

ATA risk level	Definition[b]	Postoperative staging[c]	TSH target[d]	Surveillance of patients with no evidence of disease[e]
ATA pediatric low-risk	Disease grossly confined to the thyroid (T1-T3) with N0/Nx disease *or* patients with incidental N1a disease (metastasis <0.2 cm to ≤5 central neck lymph nodes)	Non-stimulated Tg[f] on LT4 therapy	0.5–1.0 mIU/L	US at 6 months post-operatively and then annually for 5 years Tg[f] on LT4 every 6 months for 2 years and then annually
ATA pediatric intermediate-risk	Extensive N1a (>5 central neck lymph nodes or lymph nodes >0.2 cm) or minimal N1b disease (≤5 lateral neck lymph nodes)	TSH-stimulated Tg[f] and diagnostic ^{123}I scan in most patients (see Fig. 21.3)	0.1–0.5 mIU/L	US at 6 months post-operatively, every 6–12 months for 5 years, and then every 2–3 years Tg[f] on LT4 every 6 months for 3 years and then annually Consider TSH-stimulated Tg[f] ± diagnostic ^{123}I scan after 1–2 years (or longer) in patients treated with ^{131}I
ATA pediatric high-risk	Regionally extensive disease (extensive N1b; >5 lateral neck lymph nodes) or locally invasive disease (T4 tumors); known distant metastasis	TSH-stimulated Tg[f] and diagnostic ^{123}I scan in all patients (see Fig. 21.3)	<0.1 mIU/L	US at 6 months post-operatively, every 6–12 months for 5 years, and then every 2–3 years Tg[f] on LT4 every 6 months for 3 years and then annually TSH-stimulated Tg[f] ± diagnostic ^{123}I scan after 1–2 years (or longer) in patients treated with ^{131}I

ATA American Thyroid Association, *LT4* levothyroxine, *Tg* thyroglobulin, *TSH* thyroid stimulating hormone, *US* ultrasound

[a]Adapted from the inaugural ATA pediatric thyroid nodule and DTC guidelines [23]. These recommendations apply to pediatric papillary thyroid carcinoma and not to follicular thyroid carcinoma or other rare pathologic variants

[b]Utilizing TNM staging from the American Joint Committee on Cancer, 7th edition, cancer staging manual [126]

[c]Postoperative staging that is done within 12 weeks after initial definitive thyroid surgery

[d]Initial targets for TSH suppression. These are subsequently adapted to the patient's disease status on long-term follow up. In higher risk patients who have no evidence of disease after 3–5 years, the TSH can be allowed to rise to the low normal range

[e]Surveillance after surgery ± radioactive iodine therapy in patients who are believed to be disease-free; these recommendations do not apply to patients with known or suspected residual disease who require additional imaging and possibly treatment (see Fig. 21.4)

[f]Assumes negative thyroglobulin autoantibodies (TgAb). In patients with elevated TgAb titers, serial monitoring of the antibody level (using the same assay at the same lab) may be used as a surrogate for disease trajectory, although elevated titers alone do not imply residual or recurrent disease

ing, management, and surveillance. Children with ATA Pediatric Intermediate- or High-risk PTC benefit from an initial postoperative diagnostic RAI scan and a TSH-stimulated Tg to identify persistent locoregional or distantly metastatic disease, [23, 109] whereas those in the ATA Pediatric Low-risk category can be more conservatively monitored, understanding that it is plausible for children initially identified in one risk category to move to a different risk level after appropriate surgery and RAI and during long-term follow up (Fig. 21.3). As increasingly employed in adults, [129] dynamic risk stratification based on the response to initial therapy may also predict outcomes in pediatric DTC [4]. Limitations of the ATA pediatric risk categorization is that it does not fully incorporate the identification of extrathyroidal extension, margin status, primary tumor and metastatic lymph node size, histologic variant or knowledge regarding tumor mutational status. Furthermore, the extent of pre-operative staging and the experience of the surgeon also impacts the validity of this system.

Radioactive Iodine Therapy

Employed for the treatment of thyroid cancer since the 1940s, RAI has had an important role in the evaluation and management of children with DTC. Almost universally administered in the past, the pendulum has now swung in the opposite direction and ^{131}I therapy is currently used much more selectively in children and only after incorporating new data obtained from initial postoperative staging [23, 109] (Fig. 21.3). This more conservative approach has, in part, arisen from knowledge that there are real long-term risks from the overzealous prescription of ^{131}I during childhood, such as pulmonary fibrosis in young children with a large lung disease burden and the potential for the late development of a second primary malignancy (primarily hematological and salivary gland malignancies) [20, 41, 42, 130–136]. Furthermore, better understanding that death from pediatric DTC remains quite rare, experts have come to realize that very aggressive treatment during childhood may not ultimately improve disease-specific survival, especially during an era when novel targeted therapeutics have become quickly incorporated into the treatment of advanced DTC.

RAI is no longer given exclusively to ablate normal remnant thyroid tissue, since the serum Tg can become undetectable within 5–7 years after no RAI therapy [137] and because the risks of routine remnant ablation largely outweigh the potential benefits in children, especially in those operated on by high-volume surgeons. Currently, surgery is preferred over RAI to treat residual/recurrent cervical disease that is amenable to surgical resection, [23, 109] and long-term control of cervical disease has been shown to be excellent in the reoperative setting [138].

The greatest challenge in pediatric DTC remains how to determine when additional ^{131}I therapy is warranted in children with iodine-avid, distantly metastatic disease and a previous response to RAI. Repeated courses of ^{131}I can induce remission in some, but not all children, with pulmonary metastases, of whom 50% or more will have persistent disease despite RAI [42, 139–141]. Children with small-volume, iodine-avid micronodular (<1 cm) lung disease are those most likely to respond to treatment, [142] and they may ultimately become disease-free whereas others, especially those with a more extensive metastatic disease burden, may never become cancer free as assessed by Tg levels [42, 139, 142, 143].

Furthermore, the Tg response to ^{131}I treatment may not be attained for up to 15–18 months [144] and studies have shown a continued decline in serum Tg levels years after the last dose of RAI has been administered [139, 143]. Recognizing these issues and asserting that an undetectable serum Tg level should no longer be the sole goal of treatment in children with pulmonary disease, the ATA guidelines have recommended longer intervals between ^{131}I courses, suggesting that treatment be given no sooner than 12 months after the last dose [23]. In all cases, the decision to prescribe ^{131}I to any child with DTC should be individualized and incorporate knowledge regarding prognosis, tumor avidity for RAI, and previous response to therapy (Fig. 21.4).

A diagnostic thyroid scan and a stimulated Tg level (assuming the patient is TgAb negative) are recommended for children with DTC who require such staging [23, 109] (Fig. 21.3). Obtaining these data can identify those children with no evidence of disease (defined as those with an undetectable serum Tg and the absence of structurally-apparent disease) who can avoid unnecessary RAI exposure, children with extensive RAI-avid cervical disease who may benefit from re-operation, and those with RAI-avid distant metastases, who may need to have their planned administered ^{131}I activity adjusted because of either the extent of disease or the intensity of the pulmonary uptake. Diagnostic thyroid scans using ^{123}I are generally preferred [145, 146]. One challenge in young patients is the fact that iodine-avid DTC may not be visualized

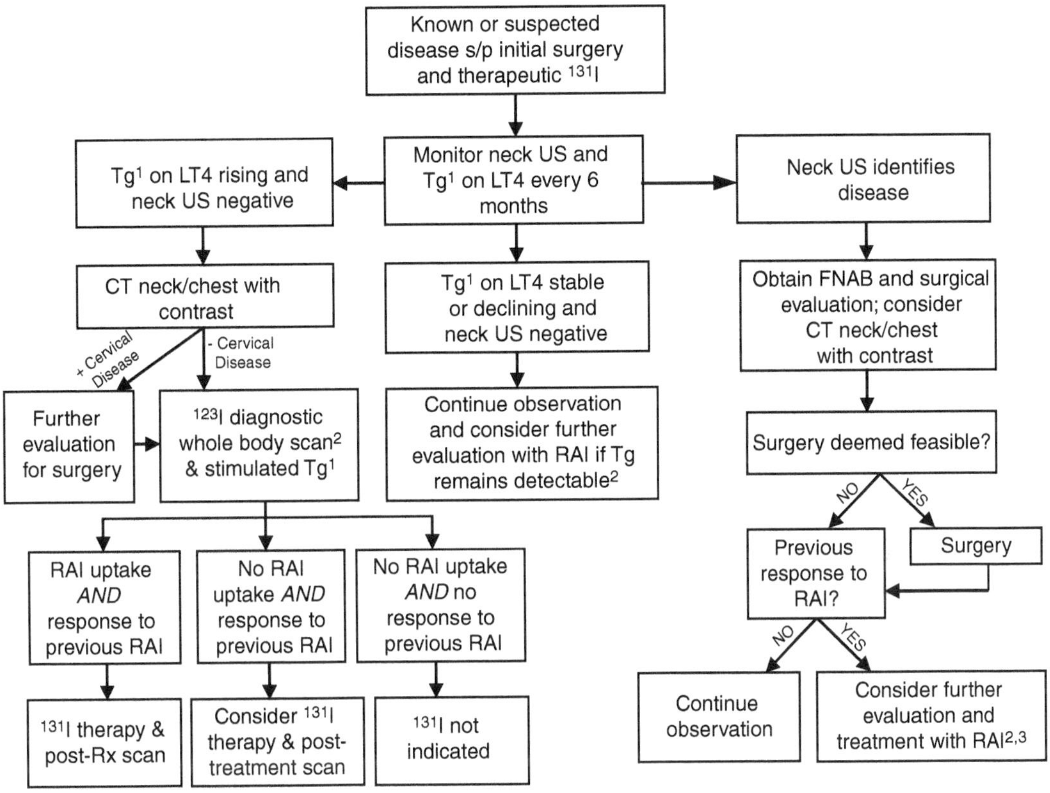

Fig. 21.4 Follow up of the pediatric patient with known or suspected residual/recurrent papillary thyroid carcinoma after initial surgery and RAI. [1] Assumes a negative TgAb; in TgAb-positive patients, the singular presence of TgAb cannot be interpreted as a sign of disease unless the titer is clearly rising over time; a declining TgAb titer would suggest ongoing response to treatment. [2]Further evaluation and treatment with RAI should only be considered after a reasonable period of time (1–2 years) has elapsed in order not to overtreat a patient who may have a delayed clinical response to prior RAI. [3]Repeated courses of ^{131}I should be considered only if iodine-avid disease is proven/suspected and there was a previous clinical response to ^{131}I therapy. *CT* computed tomography, *FNAB* fine needle aspiration biopsy, *LT4* levothyroxine, *RAI* radioactive iodine, *Tg* thyroglobulin, *TgAb* thyroglobulin antibody, *US* ultrasound

on the diagnostic scan [146] (Fig. 21.5). In these cases, the presence of disease is suggested by an elevated Tg out of proportion to the scan findings and what would be expected for normal remnant thyroid tissue. It has been proposed that a stimulated Tg is >10 ng/mL would be a reasonable cutoff for empirically treating patients at higher risk for residual/metastatic disease [23]. However, the exact Tg threshold above which treatment should be given has not been well studied in children. A recent study suggested that the novel application of a TSH/Tg ratio may help to inform the decision regarding ^{131}I treatment [147]. Another study in pediatric DTC patients, already treated with surgery and RAI, showed that all children with lung metastases had a stimulated Tg > 10 ng/mL. Thus, this cutoff may indeed be appropriate to identify higher risk patients who might benefit from further evaluation and treatment [148].

In order to facilitate RAI scanning and possible treatment, the TSH level should be above 30 mIU/mL and the ATA guidelines suggest an approach using short-term thyroid hormone withdrawal, except in select patients for whom recombinant human TSH (rhTSH) should be considered [23]. In children, an appropriately elevated TSH can almost always be achieved after 2–3 weeks of thyroid hormone withdrawal, [149, 150] which is usually extremely well-tolerated. The use of rhTSH for ^{131}I treatment may result in a lower

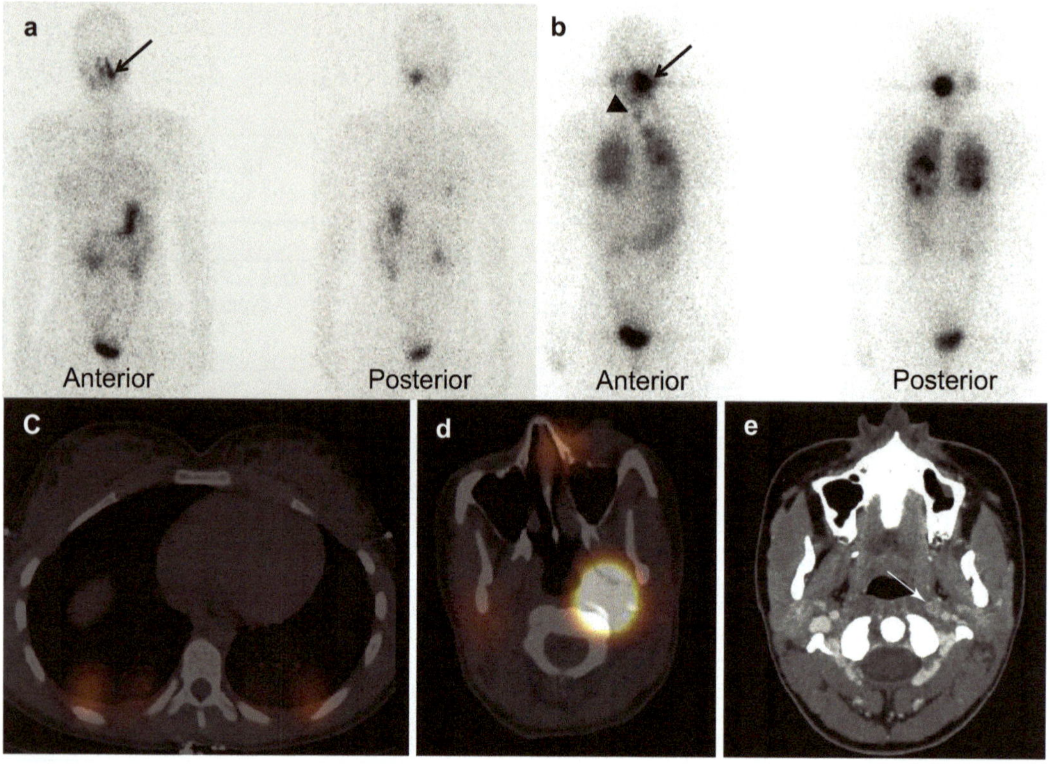

Fig. 21.5 Diagnostic (**a**) and post-treatment (**b**) radioactive iodine scans in a high-risk 15-year-old patient with a stimulated thyroglobulin of 229 ng/mL. The diagnostic ^{123}I scan (**a**) shows asymmetric upper cervical uptake (arrow) and subtle nodular uptake in the lungs on the posterior view. The scan obtained after treatment with high dose ^{131}I (**b**) demonstrates intense left upper cervical uptake with star artifact (arrow), subtle left thyroid bed uptake (arrowhead), and diffuse and nodular uptake in the lungs. The addition of SPECT/CT imaging documents the iodine-avidity of the pulmonary metastases (**c**) and confirms the location of the upper cervical uptake to be in a retropharyngeal lymph node (**d**), which is well demonstrated (arrow) on CT neck after intravenous contrast (**e**)

absorbed dose to the blood compared with withdrawal [151] and its efficacy appears to be noninferior to thyroid hormone withdrawal after 43 months of follow up [152]. A low iodine diet is generally advised for 1–2 weeks to facilitate uptake by remaining thyroid tissue; for children who received intravenous contrast during CT, it is advisable to wait 2–3 months or to confirm appropriate 24-h urine iodine levels first.

In pediatric DTC, there are no standardized approaches to determining the administered ^{131}I activity, which is generally based on a weight (child's weight in kg/70 kg) or body surface area (child's BSA m^2/1.6 m^2 for females or 1.9 m^2 for males) adjustment of the typical prescribed activity used in adults for a similar extent of disease [153–155]. For example, for empiric therapy, a child with pulmonary metastases would be administered an activity that is proportionately equivalent in an adult to a 150–200 mCi (5.55–7.4 GBq) dose (or less, if significant diffuse pulmonary uptake is present (Fig. 21.1), in order to minimize the risk of pulmonary fibrosis). Others determine the activity based on body weight alone (2.0–2.5 mCi/kg; 74–92.5 MBq/kg) [153]. Dosimetric studies to limit whole body retention at 48 h to less than 80 mCi (2.96 GBq) and blood/bone marrow exposure to less than 200 cGy should be considered in children anticipated to have significant diffuse lung uptake, patients with more widespread distant metastases, and children who may have limited bone marrow reserve due to prior cancer therapy [23, 145, 156, 157]. However, this approach is more time consuming, is not available at all centers, and has not yet been demonstrated to improve outcomes or minimize treatment-related morbidity.

In all children treated with ^{131}I, a post-treatment scan is advised 4–7 days subsequent to therapy to identify other sites of persistent disease that were not apparent on the diagnostic study [16, 157] (Fig. 21.5). The incorporation of single-photon emission computed tomography (SPECT)/CT with nuclear scintigraphy has substantially improved our ability to localize disease and distinguish benign from malignant sites of RAI uptake [158, 159] (Fig. 21.5). One must also be aware that 50% of children may have findings on the post-treatment thyroid scan, notably thymic uptake, that are not representative of iodine-avid disease [160]. Although the empiric treatment with ^{131}I of adults who have RAI scan-negative, structural disease or Tg positive, imaging negative disease has not been proven to be effective, [161, 162] whether or not similar empiric treatment of children with an abnormal Tg and a negative diagnostic scan results in similar long-term outcomes has not been studied.

Thyroid Stimulating Hormone Suppression and Follow Up

Thyroid stimulating hormone (TSH) is believed to be a thyrocyte mitogen. The role of exogenous thyroid hormone to treat thyroid cancer in children (by lowering TSH) was first reported in 1937, [163] and TSH suppression is universally employed in the management of DTC today. All children who have undergone total thyroidectomy for malignant thyroid disease are replaced with thyroid hormone at age-appropriate doses, [164] and the degree of initial TSH suppression depends on the child's ATA risk category [23] (Table 21.1). In general, the TSH goal can be loosened and the TSH allowed to rise to the low normal range in patients who have no evidence of disease after a 1–3 year period of follow up, depending on the original extent of disease. In children who have had thyroid lobectomy, the TSH is measured 4–6 weeks after surgery and supplementation considered if the TSH is in the upper half of the normal range or overtly elevated, understanding that thyroid hormone supplementation can be stopped and the TSH reevaluated after a period of follow up in the child who continues to have no evidence of cancer. The potential risks of TSH suppression in children (such as negative effects on growth and bone age, bone mineralization, cognition, behavior, and the heart) [165, 166] are unstudied but are assumed to be minimal in otherwise healthy children.

Follow-up of children with DTC should be lifelong, given that the probability of recurrence continues to increase over time and because clinical disease may not be identified until decades after initial treatment [20, 21, 32]. For those with persistent disease despite appropriate initial therapy, early recognition that thyroid cancer may become a chronic disease, albeit one with low morbidity and mortality, may justify a more restrained approach to treatment. In addition to tailored TSH suppression, and not dissimilar from adult recommendations, the long-term surveillance of pediatric DTC includes the periodic assessment of Tg and TgAb levels, routine neck US, and the selective use of diagnostic thyroid scans and other cross sectional imaging of the neck ± chest [23, 129] (Table 21.1 and Fig. 21.4). The intensity and type of follow up is primarily based on the postoperative ATA pediatric risk categorization and dynamic risk re-stratification, modifying the follow-up regimen as new data become available.

In adults, ^{18}F-fluorodeoxyglucose (FDG)-positron emission tomography (PET) imaging can be helpful in the prognostic evaluation of advanced disease and the determination of who would not benefit from empiric ^{131}I [167–169]. There are no similar published studies in children, who are more likely to have well-differentiated tumors and hence unlikely to have significant FDG-avid disease, although even in the presence of FDG-avid lung disease, younger adults are still likely to demonstrate RAI uptake [170].

Even if ^{131}I therapy is not utilized, Tg levels and their trend over time serve as a useful indicator of disease status, assuming there are no interfering TgAb [137, 171, 172]. Extrapolating from adult studies, children who have had only a lobectomy for low-risk disease should also be able to be followed similarly with Tg levels and cervical US [173]. If the TSH-suppressed Tg is undetectable after primary therapy has been completed, there appears to be very little added value in obtaining a TSH-stimulated Tg, [174–176] and there is now movement away from obtaining a routine TSH-stimulated Tg in children in the absence of other indicators of disease [23]. Nevertheless, as demonstrated in adult studies, [175–177] an undetectable TSH-stimulated Tg after initial treatment that includes total thyroidectomy and ^{131}I is highly predictive of long-term remission. Clinical recurrences primarily occur in cervical lymph nodes, [175, 176] underscoring the critical importance of cervical US during long-term disease surveillance [148] (Fig. 21.4). As alluded to earlier, the exact Tg values that indicate residual, clinically relevant disease in children that would warrant more intensive surveillance or treatment remains poorly studied in children, although a stimulated Tg >10 ng/mL is likely to represent an actionable threshold [23, 148].

In children with detectable TgAb, the antibody titer itself can be followed, and it is the trend of this analyte over time (using the same assay and lab) that is more important than its absolute value [178, 179]. Even with successful treatment of DTC, TgAb may persist for a median of 3 years after treatment [180]. Therefore, in patients with +TgAb, greater emphasis should be placed on structural and functional imaging to identify disease.

Systemic Therapy for Advanced Disease

In children, the development of progressive DTC that warrants systemic treatment outside of repeated courses of ^{131}I is very rare. The definition of RAI-refractory disease, better established in adults, [181] remains poorly defined in the pediatric population. It is now understood that RAI-refractory DTC does indeed occur in children, and contemporary guidelines clearly state that repeated courses of RAI should not be given when there was no documented response to previous ^{131}I therapy [23]. In such cases, disease may remain quite indolent for years while continuing TSH suppression. In the rare event of a child with progressive DTC needing alternative approaches to care, consultation with providers who are experienced in the use of systemic therapy in children is recommended. A review of the currently available, molecularly targeted agents for the treatment of DTC is beyond the purview of this chapter and is covered elsewhere. Of the FDA-approved therapies, single agent sorafenib has been studied in phase I and phase II clinical trials in pediatric patients with refractory solid tumors or leukemias, [182–185] but no children with DTC were enrolled into these trials and there is only limited and anecdotal experience using sorafenib to treat advanced PTC in children [186, 187]. Lenvatinib remains largely unstudied in the pediatric population and there have been no published reports on its use in children. Currently, a phase I/II study in children, including an expanded cohort with ^{131}I-refractory DTC, is recruiting (ClinicalTrials.gov Identifier NCT02432274).

Conclusion

Rare in children but increasing in incidence, pediatric DTC presents with more locally-advanced and distant disease compared with adults. Despite this more advanced clinical presentation, the prognosis for patients with pediatric-onset disease is excellent and disease-specific mortality remains low, even in the presence of pulmonary metastases. This is most likely due to the fact that DTC in children is typically a well-differentiated tumor that most often is iodine-avid and responsive to TSH suppression. Given the excellent prognosis and anticipated indolent nature of the cancer, therapy for pediatric DTC should be individualized and geared towards balancing goals of disease eradication with limiting treatment-related morbidity, particularly in non-progressive residual disease. It is preferred that, whenever possible, children with DTC be cared for at centers with established programs in the multidisciplinary management of this disease; most critical is the identification of a high-volume surgeon to undertake such cases, which should improve oncologic outcomes and minimize postoperative complications. Therapy with ^{131}I is becoming less frequently prescribed and is now tailored to the individual patient and based on the likelihood of having disease that is expected to respond to RAI therapy, recognizing that aggressive treatment may not improve the already low disease-specific mortality observed. Further research geared towards better understanding the optimal use of RAI and predicting long-term outcomes based on clinical presentation and tumor mutational status is needed.

References

1. Hogan AR, Zhuge Y, Perez EA, Koniaris LG, Lew JI, Sola JE. Pediatric thyroid carcinoma: incidence and outcomes in 1753 patients. J Surg Res. 2009;156(1):167–72.
2. Demidchik YE, Saenko VA, Yamashita S. Childhood thyroid cancer in Belarus, Russia, and Ukraine after Chernobyl and at present. Arq Bras Endocrinol Metabol. 2007;51(5):748–62.
3. Borson Chazot F, Causeret S, Lifante JC, Augros M, Berger N, Peix JL. Predictive factors for recurrence from a series of 74 children and adolescents with differentiated thyroid cancer. World J Surg. 2004;28(11):1088–92.
4. Sung TY, Jeon MJ, Lee YH, Lee YM, Kwon H, Yoon JH, et al. Initial and dynamic risk stratification of pediatric patients with differentiated thyroid cancer. J Clin Endocrinol Metab. 2017;102(3):793–800.
5. Silva-Vieira M, Santos R, Leite V, Limbert E. Review of clinical and pathological features of 93 cases of well-differentiated thyroid carcinoma in pediatric age at the Lisbon Centre of the Portuguese Institute of Oncology between 1964 and 2006. Int J Pediatr Otorhinolaryngol. 2015;79(8):1324–9.
6. Vergamini LB, Frazier AL, Abrantes FL, Ribeiro KB, Rodriguez-Galindo C. Increase in the incidence of differentiated thyroid carcinoma in children, adolescents, and young adults: a population-based study. J Pediatr. 2014;164(6):1481–5.
7. Spinelli C, Strambi S, Rossi L, Bakkar S, Massimino M, Ferrari A, et al. Surgical management of papillary thyroid carcinoma in childhood and adolescence: an Italian multicenter study on 250 patients. J Endocrinol Investig. 2016;39(9):1055–9.
8. Zimmerman D, Hay ID, Gough IR, Goellner JR, Ryan JJ, Grant CS, et al. Papillary thyroid carcinoma in children and adults: long-term follow-up of 1039 patients conservatively treated at one institution during three decades. Surgery. 1988;104(6):1157–66.
9. Frankenthaler RA, Sellin RV, Cangir A, Goepfert H. Lymph node metastasis from papillary-follicular thyroid carcinoma in young patients. Am J Surg. 1990;160(4):341–3.
10. Wada N, Sugino K, Mimura T, Nagahama M, Kitagawa W, Shibuya H, et al. Treatment strategy of papillary thyroid carcinoma in children and adolescents: clinical significance of the initial nodal manifestation. Ann Surg Oncol. 2009;16(12):3442–9.
11. Machens A, Lorenz K, Nguyen Thanh P, Brauckhoff M, Dralle H. Papillary thyroid cancer in children and adolescents does not differ in growth pattern and metastatic behavior. J Pediatr. 2010;157(4):648–52.
12. Newman KD, Black T, Heller G, Azizkhan RG, Holcomb GW 3rd, Sklar C, et al. Differentiated thyroid cancer: determinants of disease progression in patients <21 years of age at diagnosis: a report from the Surgical Discipline Committee of the Children's Cancer Group. Ann Surg. 1998;227(4):533–41.
13. Popovtzer A, Shpitzer T, Bahar G, Feinmesser R, Segal K. Thyroid cancer in children: management and outcome experience of a referral center. Otolaryngol Head Neck Surg. 2006;135(4):581–4.
14. Savio R, Gosnell J, Palazzo FF, Sywak M, Agarwal G, Cowell C, et al. The role of a more extensive surgical approach in the initial multimodality management of papillary thyroid cancer in children. J Pediatr Surg. 2005;40(11):1696–700.
15. Mao XC, Yu WQ, Shang JB, Wang KJ. Clinical characteristics and treatment of thyroid cancer in children and adolescents: a retrospective analysis of 83 patients. J Zhejiang Univ Sci B. 2017;18(5):430–6.
16. Bal CS, Kumar A, Chandra P, Dwivedi SN, Mukhopadhyaya S. Is chest x-ray or high-resolution computed tomography scan of the chest sufficient investigation to detect pulmonary metastasis in pediatric differentiated thyroid cancer? Thyroid. 2004;14(3):217–25.
17. Demidchik YE, Demidchik EP, Reiners C, Biko J, Mine M, Saenko VA, et al. Comprehensive clinical assessment of 740 cases of surgically treated thyroid cancer in children of Belarus. Ann Surg. 2006;243(4):525–32.
18. Handkiewicz-Junak D, Wloch J, Roskosz J, Krajewska J, Kropinska A, Pomorski L, et al. Total thyroidectomy and adjuvant radioiodine treatment independently decrease locoregional recurrence risk in childhood and adolescent differentiated thyroid cancer. J Nucl Med. 2007;48(6):879–88.
19. Klein Hesselink MS, Nies M, Bocca G, Brouwers AH, Burgerhof JG, van Dam EW, et al. Pediatric differentiated thyroid carcinoma in the Netherlands: a nationwide follow-up study. J Clin Endocrinol Metab. 2016;101(5):2031–9.
20. Hay ID, Gonzalez-Losada T, Reinalda MS, Honetschlager JA, Richards ML, Thompson GB. Long-term outcome in 215 children and adoles-

cents with papillary thyroid cancer treated during 1940 through 2008. World J Surg. 2010;34(6):1192–202.
21. Mihailovic J, Nikoletic K, Srbovan D. Recurrent disease in juvenile differentiated thyroid carcinoma: prognostic factors, treatments, and outcomes. J Nucl Med. 2014;55(5):710–7.
22. Golpanian S, Perez EA, Tashiro J, Lew JI, Sola JE, Hogan AR. Pediatric papillary thyroid carcinoma: outcomes and survival predictors in 2504 surgical patients. Pediatr Surg Int. 2016;32(3):201–8.
23. Francis GL, Waguespack SG, Bauer AJ, Angelos P, Benvenga S, Cerutti JM, et al. Management guidelines for children with thyroid nodules and differentiated thyroid cancer. Thyroid. 2015;25(7):716–59.
24. Siegel RL, Miller KD, Jemal A. Cancer statistics, 2017. CA Cancer J Clin. 2017;67(1):7–30.
25. Howlader N, Noone AM, Krapcho M, Miller D, Bishop K, Kosary CL, et al. SEER cancer statistics review, 1975-2014, based on November 2016 SEER data submission, posted to the SEER web site, April 2017. Bethesda: National Cancer Institute; 2017 [cited 2017 July 18]. Available from: https://seer.cancer.gov/csr/1975_2014/.
26. Pole JD, Zuk AM, Wasserman JD. Diagnostic and treatment patterns among children, adolescents, and young adults with Thyroid Cancer in Ontario: 1992–2010. Thyroid. 2017;27(8):1025–33.
27. Spoudeas HA, editor. Paediatric endocrine tumours. West Sussex: Novo Nordisk Ltd; 2005.
28. Vassilopoulou-Sellin R, Goepfert H, Raney B, Schultz PN. Differentiated thyroid cancer in children and adolescents: clinical outcome and mortality after long-term follow-up. Head Neck. 1998;20(6):549–55.
29. Durante C, Haddy N, Baudin E, Leboulleux S, Hartl D, Travagli JP, et al. Long-term outcome of 444 patients with distant metastases from papillary and follicular thyroid carcinoma: benefits and limits of radioiodine therapy. J Clin Endocrinol Metab. 2006;91(8):2892–9.
30. Ito Y, Miyauchi A, Tomoda C, Hirokawa M, Kobayashi K, Miya A. Prognostic significance of patient age in minimally and widely invasive follicular thyroid carcinoma: investigation of three age groups. Endocr J. 2014;61(3):265–71.
31. Golpanian S, Tashiro J, Sola JE, Allen C, Lew JI, Hogan AR, et al. Surgically treated pediatric nonpapillary thyroid carcinoma. Eur J Pediatr Surg. 2016;26(6):524–32.
32. Sugino K, Nagahama M, Kitagawa W, Shibuya H, Ohkuwa K, Uruno T, et al. Papillary thyroid carcinoma in children and adolescents: long-term follow-up and clinical characteristics. World J Surg. 2015;39(9):2259–65.
33. Landau D, Vini L, A'Hern R, Harmer C. Thyroid cancer in children: the Royal Marsden Hospital experience. Eur J Cancer. 2000;36(2):214–20.
34. Harach HR, Williams ED. Childhood thyroid cancer in England and Wales. Br J Cancer. 1995;72(3):777–83.
35. Alzahrani AS, Xing M. Impact of lymph node metastases identified on central neck dissection (CND) on the recurrence of papillary thyroid cancer: potential role of BRAFV600E mutation in defining CND. Endocr Relat Cancer. 2013;20(1):13–22.
36. Lazar L, Lebenthal Y, Segal K, Steinmetz A, Strenov Y, Cohen M, et al. Pediatric thyroid cancer: postoperative classifications and response to initial therapy as prognostic factors. J Clin Endocrinol Metab. 2016;101(5):1970–9.
37. O'Gorman CS, Hamilton J, Rachmiel M, Gupta A, Ngan BY, Daneman D. Thyroid cancer in childhood: a retrospective review of childhood course. Thyroid. 2010;20(4):375–80.
38. Lazar L, Lebenthal Y, Steinmetz A, Yackobovitch-Gavan M, Phillip M. Differentiated thyroid carcinoma in pediatric patients: comparison of presentation and course between pre-pubertal children and adolescents. J Pediatr. 2009;154(5):708–14.
39. Pires BP, Alves PA Jr, Bordallo MA, Bulzico DA, Lopes FP, Farias T, et al. Prognostic factors for early and long-term remission in pediatric differentiated thyroid carcinoma: the role of sex, age, clinical presentation, and the newly proposed American Thyroid Association Risk Stratification System. Thyroid. 2016;26(10):1480–7.
40. Schlumberger M, De Vathaire F, Travagli JP, Vassal G, Lemerle J, Parmentier C, et al. Differentiated thyroid carcinoma in childhood: long term follow-up of 72 patients. J Clin Endocrinol Metab. 1987;65(6):1088–94.
41. Hebestreit H, Biko J, Drozd V, Demidchik Y, Burkhardt A, Trusen A, et al. Pulmonary fibrosis in youth treated with radioiodine for juvenile thyroid cancer and lung metastases after Chernobyl. Eur J Nucl Med Mol Imaging. 2011;38(9):1683–90.
42. Pawelczak M, David R, Franklin B, Kessler M, Lam L, Shah B. Outcomes of children and adolescents with well-differentiated thyroid carcinoma and pulmonary metastases following (1)(3)(1)I treatment: a systematic review. Thyroid. 2010;20(10):1095–101.
43. Tucker MA, Jones PH, Boice JD Jr, Robison LL, Stone BJ, Stovall M, et al. Therapeutic radiation at a young age is linked to secondary thyroid cancer. The Late Effects Study Group. Cancer Res. 1991;51(11):2885–8.
44. Bhatti P, Veiga LH, Ronckers CM, Sigurdson AJ, Stovall M, Smith SA, et al. Risk of second primary thyroid cancer after radiotherapy for a childhood cancer in a large cohort study: an update from the childhood cancer survivor study. Radiat Res. 2010;174(6):741–52.
45. Turcotte LM, Liu Q, Yasui Y, Arnold MA, Hammond S, Howell RM, et al. Temporal trends in treatment and subsequent Neoplasm risk among 5-year survivors of childhood cancer, 1970–2015. JAMA. 2017;317(8):814–24.
46. Casagranda L, Oriol M, Freycon F, Frappaz D, Bertrand Y, Bergeron C, et al. Second malignant neoplasm following childhood cancer: a nested

case-control study of a recent cohort (1987–2004) from the childhood cancer registry of the Rhone-Alpes region in France. Pediatr Hematol Oncol. 2016;33(6):371–82.
47. Ronckers CM, Sigurdson AJ, Stovall M, Smith SA, Mertens AC, Liu Y, et al. Thyroid cancer in childhood cancer survivors: a detailed evaluation of radiation dose response and its modifiers. Radiat Res. 2006;166(4):618–28.
48. Naing S, Collins BJ, Schneider AB. Clinical behavior of radiation-induced thyroid cancer: factors related to recurrence. Thyroid. 2009;19(5):479–85.
49. Rose J, Wertheim BC, Guerrero MA. Radiation treatment of patients with primary pediatric malignancies: risk of developing thyroid cancer as a secondary malignancy. Am J Surg. 2012;204(6):881–6. discussion 6–7.
50. Inskip PD, Curtis RE. New malignancies following childhood cancer in the United States, 1973–2002. Int J Cancer. 2007;121(10):2233–40.
51. Veiga LH, Bhatti P, Ronckers CM, Sigurdson AJ, Stovall M, Smith SA, et al. Chemotherapy and thyroid cancer risk: a report from the childhood cancer survivor study. Cancer Epidemiol Biomark Prev. 2012;21(1):92–101.
52. Tsuda T, Tokinobu A, Yamamoto E, Suzuki E. Thyroid cancer detection by ultrasound among residents ages 18 years and younger in Fukushima, Japan: 2011 to 2014. Epidemiology. 2016;27(3):316–22.
53. Russo M, Malandrino P, Moleti M, D'Angelo A, Tavarelli M, Sapuppo G, et al. Thyroid cancer in the pediatric age in sicily: influence of the volcanic environment. Anticancer Res. 2017;37(3):1515–22.
54. Angusti T, Codegone A, Pellerito R, Favero A. Thyroid cancer prevalence after radioiodine treatment of hyperthyroidism. J Nucl Med. 2000;41(6):1006–9.
55. Clement SC, van Eck-Smit BL, van Trotsenburg AS, Kremer LC, Tytgat GA, van Santen HM. Long-term follow-up of the thyroid gland after treatment with 131I-Metaiodobenzylguanidine in children with neuroblastoma: importance of continuous surveillance. Pediatr Blood Cancer. 2013;60(11):1833–8.
56. de Vathaire F, Francois P, Schlumberger M, Schweisguth O, Hardiman C, Grimaud E, et al. Epidemiological evidence for a common mechanism for neuroblastoma and differentiated thyroid tumour. Br J Cancer. 1992;65(3):425–8.
57. Buryk MA, Picarsic JL, Creary SE, Shaw PH, Simons JP, Deutsch M, et al. Identification of unique, heterozygous germline mutation, STK11 (p.F354L), in a child with an encapsulated follicular variant of papillary thyroid carcinoma within six months of completing treatment for neuroblastoma. Pediatr Dev Pathol. 2015;18(4):318–23.
58. Corrias A, Cassio A, Weber G, Mussa A, Wasniewska M, Rapa A, et al. Thyroid nodules and cancer in children and adolescents affected by autoimmune thyroiditis. Arch Pediatr Adolesc Med. 2008;162(6):526–31.
59. Kambalapalli M, Gupta A, Prasad UR, Francis GL. Ultrasound characteristics of the thyroid in children and adolescents with goiter: a single center experience. Thyroid. 2015;25(2):176–82.
60. Kovatch KJ, Bauer AJ, Isaacoff EJ, Prickett KK, Adzick NS, Kazahaya K, et al. Pediatric thyroid carcinoma in patients with Graves' disease: the role of ultrasound in selecting patients for definitive therapy. Horm Res Paediatr. 2015;83(6):408–13.
61. Aydin Y, Besir FH, Erkan ME, Yazgan O, Gungor A, Onder E, et al. Spectrum and prevalence of nodular thyroid diseases detected by ultrasonography in the Western Black Sea region of Turkey. Med Ultrason. 2014;16(2):100–6.
62. Niedziela M, Korman E, Breborowicz D, Trejster E, Harasymczuk J, Warzywoda M, et al. A prospective study of thyroid nodular disease in children and adolescents in western Poland from 1996 to 2000 and the incidence of thyroid carcinoma relative to iodine deficiency and the Chernobyl disaster. Pediatr Blood Cancer. 2004;42(1):84–92.
63. Xu L, Port M, Landi S, Gemignani F, Cipollini M, Elisei R, et al. Obesity and the risk of papillary thyroid cancer: a pooled analysis of three case-control studies. Thyroid. 2014;24(6):966–74.
64. Lloyd RV, Buehler D, Khanafshar E. Papillary thyroid carcinoma variants. Head Neck Pathol. 2011;5(1):51–6.
65. Lloyd RV, Osamura RY, Klöppel G, Rosai J, editors. WHO classification of tumours of endocrine organs. Lyon: IARC Press; 2017.
66. Nikiforov YE, Seethala RR, Tallini G, Baloch ZW, Basolo F, Thompson LD, et al. Nomenclature revision for encapsulated follicular variant of papillary thyroid carcinoma: a paradigm shift to reduce overtreatment of indolent tumors. JAMA Oncol. 2016;2(8):1023–9.
67. Balachandar S, La Quaglia M, Tuttle RM, Heller G, Ghossein RA, Sklar CA. Pediatric differentiated thyroid carcinoma of follicular cell origin: prognostic significance of histologic subtypes. Thyroid. 2016;26(2):219–26.
68. Thompson LD, Wieneke JA, Heffess CS. Diffuse sclerosing variant of papillary thyroid carcinoma: a clinicopathologic and immunophenotypic analysis of 22 cases. Endocr Pathol. 2005;16(4):331–48.
69. Akaishi J, Sugino K, Kameyama K, Masaki C, Matsuzu K, Suzuki A, et al. Clinicopathologic features and outcomes in patients with diffuse sclerosing variant of papillary thyroid carcinoma. World J Surg. 2015;39(7):1728–35.
70. Sobrinho-Simoes M, Eloy C, Magalhaes J, Lobo C, Amaro T. Follicular thyroid carcinoma. Mod Pathol. 2011;24(Suppl 2):S10–8.
71. Vuong HG, Kondo T, Oishi N, Nakazawa T, Mochizuki K, Miyauchi A, et al. Pediatric follicular thyroid carcinoma – indolent cancer with low prevalence of RAS mutations and absence of PAX8-PPARG fusion in a Japanese population. Histopathology. 2017;71(5):760–8.

72. Enomoto K, Enomoto Y, Uchino S, Yamashita H, Noguchi S. Follicular thyroid cancer in children and adolescents: clinicopathologic features, long-term survival, and risk factors for recurrence. Endocr J. 2013;60(5):629–35.
73. Cancer Genome Atlas Research Network. Integrated genomic characterization of papillary thyroid carcinoma. Cell. 2014;159(3):676–90.
74. Yoo SK, Lee S, Kim SJ, Jee HG, Kim BA, Cho H, et al. Comprehensive analysis of the transcriptional and mutational landscape of follicular and papillary thyroid cancers. PLoS Genet. 2016;12(8):e1006239.
75. Leeman-Neill RJ, Kelly LM, Liu P, Brenner AV, Little MP, Bogdanova TI, et al. ETV6-NTRK3 is a common chromosomal rearrangement in radiation-associated thyroid cancer. Cancer. 2014;120(6):799–807.
76. Leeman-Neill RJ, Brenner AV, Little MP, Bogdanova TI, Hatch M, Zurnadzy LY, et al. RET/PTC and PAX8/PPARgamma chromosomal rearrangements in post-Chernobyl thyroid cancer and their association with iodine-131 radiation dose and other characteristics. Cancer. 2013;119(10):1792–9.
77. Ricarte-Filho JC, Li S, Garcia-Rendueles ME, Montero-Conde C, Voza F, Knauf JA, et al. Identification of kinase fusion oncogenes in post-Chernobyl radiation-induced thyroid cancers. J Clin Invest. 2013;123(11):4935–44.
78. Bauer AJ. Molecular genetics of thyroid cancer in children and adolescents. Endocrinol Metab Clin N Am. 2017;46(2):389–403.
79. Prasad ML, Vyas M, Horne MJ, Virk RK, Morotti R, Liu Z, et al. NTRK fusion oncogenes in pediatric papillary thyroid carcinoma in Northeast United States. Cancer. 2016;122(7):1097–107.
80. Cordioli MI, Moraes L, Cury AN, Cerutti JM. Are we really at the dawn of understanding sporadic pediatric thyroid carcinoma? Endocr Relat Cancer. 2015;22(6):R311–24.
81. Picarsic JL, Buryk MA, Ozolek J, Ranganathan S, Monaco SE, Simons JP, et al. Molecular characterization of sporadic pediatric thyroid carcinoma with the DNA/RNA ThyroSeq v2 next-generation sequencing assay. Pediatr Dev Pathol. 2016;19(2):115–22.
82. Romei C, Ciampi R, Elisei R. A comprehensive overview of the role of the RET proto-oncogene in thyroid carcinoma. Nat Rev Endocrinol. 2016;12(4):192–202.
83. Fenton CL, Lukes Y, Nicholson D, Dinauer CA, Francis GL, Tuttle RM. The ret/PTC mutations are common in sporadic papillary thyroid carcinoma of children and young adults. J Clin Endocrinol Metab. 2000;85(3):1170–5.
84. Cordioli MI, Moraes L, Bastos AU, Besson P, Alves MT, Delcelo R, et al. Fusion oncogenes are the main genetic events found in sporadic papillary thyroid carcinomas from children. Thyroid. 2016;27:182–8.
85. Cordioli MI, Moraes L, Carvalheira G, Sisdelli L, Alves MT, Delcelo R, et al. AGK-BRAF gene fusion is a recurrent event in sporadic pediatric thyroid carcinoma. Cancer Med. 2016;5(7):1535–41.
86. Nikita ME, Jiang W, Cheng SM, Hantash FM, McPhaul MJ, Newbury RO, et al. Mutational analysis in pediatric thyroid cancer and correlations with age, ethnicity, and clinical presentation. Thyroid. 2016;26(2):227–34.
87. Vanden Borre P, Schrock AB, Anderson PM, Morris JC, Heilmann AM, Holmes O, et al. Pediatric, adolescent, and young adult thyroid carcinoma harbors frequent and diverse targetable genomic alterations, including kinase fusions. Oncologist. 2017;22(3):255–63.
88. Raman P, Koenig RJ. Pax-8-PPAR-gamma fusion protein in thyroid carcinoma. Nat Rev Endocrinol. 2014;10(10):616–23.
89. Ballester LY, Sarabia SF, Sayeed H, Patel N, Baalwa J, Athanassaki I, et al. Integrating molecular testing in the diagnosis and management of children with thyroid lesions. Pediatr Dev Pathol. 2016;19(2): 94–100.
90. Alzahrani AS, Murugan AK, Qasem E, Alswailem M, Al-Hindi H, Shi Y. Single point mutations in pediatric differentiated thyroid cancer. Thyroid. 2017;27(2):189–96.
91. Onder S, Ozturk Sari S, Yegen G, Sormaz IC, Yilmaz I, Poyrazoglu S, et al. Classic architecture with multicentricity and local recurrence, and absence of TERT promoter mutations are correlates of BRAF (V600E) harboring pediatric papillary thyroid carcinomas. Endocr Pathol. 2016;27(2):153–61.
92. Ni Y, Seballos S, Fletcher B, Romigh T, Yehia L, Mester J, et al. Germline compound heterozygous poly-glutamine deletion in USF3 may be involved in predisposition to heritable and sporadic epithelial thyroid carcinoma. Hum Mol Genet. 2017;26(2):243–57.
93. Pagon RA, Adam MP, Ardinger HH, Wallace SE, Amemiya A, Bean LJH, et al.. GeneReviews® [Internet]. Seattle: University of Washington; 1993–2017 [cited 2017]. Available from: https://www.ncbi.nlm.nih.gov/books/NBK1116/.
94. Bauer AJ. Clinical behavior and genetics of nonsyndromic, familial nonmedullary thyroid cancer. Front Horm Res. 2013;41:141–8.
95. Schultz KAP, Rednam SP, Kamihara J, Doros L, Achatz MI, Wasserman JD, et al. PTEN, DICER1, FH, and their associated tumor susceptibility syndromes: clinical features, genetics, and surveillance recommendations in childhood. Clin Cancer Res. 2017;23(12):e76–82.
96. Nagy R, Ringel MD. Genetic predisposition for nonmedullary thyroid cancer. Horm Cancer. 2015;6(1):13–20.
97. Ngeow J, Mester J, Rybicki LA, Ni Y, Milas M, Eng C. Incidence and clinical characteristics of thyroid cancer in prospective series of individuals with cowden and cowden-like syndrome characterized by germline PTEN, SDH, or KLLN alterations. J Clin Endocrinol Metab. 2011;96(12):E2063–71.
98. Smith JR, Marqusee E, Webb S, Nose V, Fishman SJ, Shamberger RC, et al. Thyroid nodules and cancer in

children with PTEN hamartoma tumor syndrome. J Clin Endocrinol Metab. 2011;96(1):34–7.
99. Hansen-Kiss E, Beinkampen S, Adler B, Frazier T, Prior T, Erdman S, et al. A retrospective chart review of the features of PTEN hamartoma tumour syndrome in children. J Med Genet. 2017;54(7):471–8.
100. Khan NE, Bauer AJ, Doros L, Schultz KA, Decastro RM, Harney LA, et al. Macrocephaly associated with the DICER1 syndrome. Genet Med. 2016;19:244–8.
101. Rutter MM, Jha P, Schultz KA, Sheil A, Harris AK, Bauer AJ, et al. DICER1 mutations and differentiated thyroid carcinoma: evidence of a direct association. J Clin Endocrinol Metab. 2016;101(1):1–5.
102. Khan NE, Bauer AJ, Schultz KAP, Doros L, Decastro RM, Ling A, et al. Quantification of thyroid cancer and multinodular goiter risk in the DICER1 syndrome: a family-based cohort study. J Clin Endocrinol Metab. 2017;102(5):1614–22.
103. Doros L, Schultz KA, Stewart DR, Bauer AJ, Williams G, Rossi CT, et al. *DICER1*-related disorders Seattle: University of Washington; 2014. Available from: https://www.ncbi.nlm.nih.gov/books/NBK196157/.
104. Eng C. PTEN hamartoma tumor syndrome. Seattle: University of Washington; 2001 [Updated 2016 Jun 2]. Available from: https://www.ncbi.nlm.nih.gov/books/NBK1488/.
105. Jasperson KW, Patel SG, Ahnen DJ. APC-associated polyposis conditions. Seattle: University of Washington; 1998 [Updated 2017 Feb 2]. Available from: https://www.ncbi.nlm.nih.gov/books/NBK1345/.
106. Stratakis CA, Salpea P, Raygada M. Carney complex. Seattle: University of Washington; 2003 [Updated 2015 Jan 29]. Available from: https://www.ncbi.nlm.nih.gov/books/NBK1286/.
107. Lam AK, Saremi N. Cribriform-morular variant of papillary thyroid carcinoma: a distinctive type of thyroid cancer. Endocr Relat Cancer. 2017;24(4):R109–R21.
108. Schreiner BF, Murphy WT. Malignant neoplasms of the thyroid gland. Ann Surg. 1934;99(1):116–25.
109. Waguespack SG, Francis G. Initial management and follow-up of differentiated thyroid cancer in children. J Natl Compr Cancer Netw. 2010;8(11):1289–300.
110. Kim J, Sun Z, Adam MA, Adibe OO, Rice HE, Roman SA, et al. Predictors of nodal metastasis in pediatric differentiated thyroid cancer. J Pediatr Surg. 2017;52(1):120–3.
111. Landry CS, Grubbs EG, Busaidy NL, Monroe BJ, Staerkel GA, Perrier ND, et al. Cystic lymph nodes in the lateral neck as indicators of metastatic papillary thyroid cancer. Endocr Pract. 2011;17(2):240–4.
112. Wang Y, Zhao H, Wang YX, Wang MJ, Zhang ZH, Zhang L, et al. Improvement in the detection of cystic metastatic papillary thyroid carcinoma by measurement of thyroglobulin in aspirated fluid. Biomed Res Int. 2016;2016:8905916.
113. Kluijfhout WP, Pasternak JD, van der Kaay D, Vriens MR, Propst EJ, Wasserman JD. Is it time to reconsider lobectomy in low-risk paediatric thyroid cancer? Clin Endocrinol. 2017;86(4):591–6.
114. Jin X, Masterson L, Patel A, Hook L, Nicholson J, Jefferies S, et al. Conservative or radical surgery for pediatric papillary thyroid carcinoma: a systematic review of the literature. Int J Pediatr Otorhinolaryngol. 2015;79(10):1620–4.
115. Jarzab B, Handkiewicz Junak D, Wloch J, Kalemba B, Roskosz J, Kukulska A, et al. Multivariate analysis of prognostic factors for differentiated thyroid carcinoma in children. Eur J Nucl Med. 2000;27(7):833–41.
116. Sywak M, Cornford L, Roach P, Stalberg P, Sidhu S, Delbridge L. Routine ipsilateral level VI lymphadenectomy reduces postoperative thyroglobulin levels in papillary thyroid cancer. Surgery. 2006;140(6):1000–5. discussion 5–7.
117. Welch Dinauer CA, Tuttle RM, Robie DK, McClellan DR, Francis GL. Extensive surgery improves recurrence-free survival for children and young patients with class I papillary thyroid carcinoma. J Pediatr Surg. 1999;34(12):1799–804.
118. Machens A, Elwerr M, Thanh PN, Lorenz K, Schneider R, Dralle H. Impact of central node dissection on postoperative morbidity in pediatric patients with suspected or proven thyroid cancer. Surgery. 2016;160(2):484–92.
119. Lee KE, Chung IY, Kang E, Koo do H, Kim KH, Kim SW, et al. Ipsilateral and contralateral central lymph node metastasis in papillary thyroid cancer: patterns and predictive factors of nodal metastasis. Head Neck. 2013;35(5):672–6.
120. van Santen HM, Aronson DC, Vulsma T, Tummers RF, Geenen MM, de Vijlder JJ, et al. Frequent adverse events after treatment for childhood-onset differentiated thyroid carcinoma: a single institute experience. Eur J Cancer. 2004;40(11):1743–51.
121. Sosa JA, Tuggle CT, Wang TS, Thomas DC, Boudourakis L, Rivkees S, et al. Clinical and economic outcomes of thyroid and parathyroid surgery in children. J Clin Endocrinol Metab. 2008;93(8):3058–65.
122. Tuggle CT, Roman SA, Wang TS, Boudourakis L, Thomas DC, Udelsman R, et al. Pediatric endocrine surgery: who is operating on our children? Surgery. 2008;144(6):869–77. discussion 77.
123. Al-Qurayshi Z, Hauch A, Srivastav S, Aslam R, Friedlander P, Kandil E. A national perspective of the risk, presentation, and outcomes of pediatric thyroid cancer. JAMA Otolaryngol Head Neck Surg. 2016;142(5):472–8.
124. Thompson GB, Hay ID. Current strategies for surgical management and adjuvant treatment of childhood papillary thyroid carcinoma. World J Surg. 2004;28(12):1187–98.
125. Burke JF, Sippel RS, Chen H. Evolution of pediatric thyroid surgery at a tertiary medical center. J Surg Res. 2012;177(2):268–74.
126. AJCC. Chapter 8. Thyroid. In: Edge SB, Byrd DR, Compton CC, Fritz AG, Greene FL, Trotti A, editors.

AJCC cancer staging manual, 7th ed. New York: Springer; 2010. p. 87–96.
127. Powers PA, Dinauer CA, Tuttle RM, Francis GL. The MACIS score predicts the clinical course of papillary thyroid carcinoma in children and adolescents. J Pediatr Endocrinol Metab. 2004;17(3):339–43.
128. Jang HW, Lee JI, Kim HK, Oh YL, Choi YL, Jin DK, et al. Identification of a cut-off for the MACIS score to predict the prognosis of differentiated thyroid carcinoma in children and young adults. Head Neck. 2012;34(5):696–701.
129. Haugen BR, Alexander EK, Bible KC, Doherty GM, Mandel SJ, Nikiforov YE, et al. 2015 American Thyroid Association Management Guidelines for Adult Patients with Thyroid Nodules and Differentiated Thyroid Cancer: The American Thyroid Association Guidelines Task Force on Thyroid Nodules and Differentiated Thyroid Cancer. Thyroid. 2016;26(1):1–133.
130. Albano D, Bertagna F, Panarotto MB, Giubbini R. Early and late adverse effects of radioiodine for pediatric differentiated thyroid cancer. Pediatr Blood Cancer. 2017;64(11):26595.
131. Reiners C, Biko J, Haenscheid H, Hebestreit H, Kirinjuk S, Baranowski O, et al. Twenty-five years after Chernobyl: outcome of radioiodine treatment in children and adolescents with very high-risk radiation-induced differentiated thyroid carcinoma. J Clin Endocrinol Metab. 2013;98(7):3039–48.
132. Marti JL, Jain KS, Morris LG. Increased risk of second primary malignancy in pediatric and young adult patients treated with radioactive iodine for differentiated thyroid cancer. Thyroid. 2015;25(6):681–7.
133. Chen L, Shen Y, Luo Q, Yu Y, Lu H, Zhu R. Pulmonary fibrosis following radioiodine therapy of pulmonary metastases from differentiated thyroid carcinoma. Thyroid. 2010;20(3):337–40.
134. Iyer NG, Morris LG, Tuttle RM, Shaha AR, Ganly I. Rising incidence of second cancers in patients with low-risk (T1N0) thyroid cancer who receive radioactive iodine therapy. Cancer. 2011;117(19):4439–46.
135. Brown AP, Chen J, Hitchcock YJ, Szabo A, Shrieve DC, Tward JD. The risk of second primary malignancies up to three decades after the treatment of differentiated thyroid cancer. J Clin Endocrinol Metab. 2008;93(2):504–15.
136. Rubino C, de Vathaire F, Dottorini ME, Hall P, Schvartz C, Couette JE, et al. Second primary malignancies in thyroid cancer patients. Br J Cancer. 2003;89(9):1638–44.
137. Durante C, Montesano T, Attard M, Torlontano M, Monzani F, Costante G, et al. Long-term surveillance of papillary thyroid cancer patients who do not undergo postoperative radioiodine remnant ablation: is there a role for serum thyroglobulin measurement? J Clin Endocrinol Metab. 2012;97(8):2748–53.
138. Clayman GL, Agarwal G, Edeiken BS, Waguespack SG, Roberts DB, Sherman SI. Long-term outcome of comprehensive central compartment dissection in patients with recurrent/persistent papillary thyroid carcinoma. Thyroid. 2011;21(12):1309–16.
139. Dottorini ME, Vignati A, Mazzucchelli L, Lomuscio G, Colombo L. Differentiated thyroid carcinoma in children and adolescents: a 37-year experience in 85 patients. J Nucl Med. 1997;38(5):669–75.
140. Samuel AM, Rajashekharrao B, Shah DH. Pulmonary metastases in children and adolescents with well-differentiated thyroid cancer. J Nucl Med. 1998;39(9):1531–6.
141. Xu L, Liu Q, Liu Y, Pang H. Parameters influencing curative effect of 131I therapy on pediatric differentiated thyroid carcinoma: a retrospective study. Med Sci Monit. 2016;22:3079–85.
142. Bal CS, Garg A, Chopra S, Ballal S, Soundararajan R. Prognostic factors in pediatric differentiated thyroid cancer patients with pulmonary metastases. J Pediatr Endocrinol Metab. 2014;28(7–8):745–51.
143. Biko J, Reiners C, Kreissl MC, Verburg FA, Demidchik Y, Drozd V. Favourable course of disease after incomplete remission on (131)I therapy in children with pulmonary metastases of papillary thyroid carcinoma: 10 years follow-up. Eur J Nucl Med Mol Imaging. 2011;38(4):651–5.
144. Padovani RP, Robenshtok E, Brokhin M, Tuttle RM. Even without additional therapy, serum thyroglobulin concentrations often decline for years after total thyroidectomy and radioactive remnant ablation in patients with differentiated thyroid cancer. Thyroid. 2012;22(8):778–83.
145. Luster M, Lassmann M, Freudenberg LS, Reiners C. Thyroid cancer in childhood: management strategy, including dosimetry and long-term results. Hormones (Athens). 2007;6(4):269–78.
146. Schoelwer MJ, Zimmerman D, Shore RM, Josefson JL. The use of 123I in diagnostic radioactive iodine scans in children with differentiated thyroid carcinoma. Thyroid. 2015;25(8):935–41.
147. Livhits MJ, Pasternak JD, Xiong M, Li N, Gosnell JE, Yeh MW, et al. Pre-ablation thyroglobulin and thyroglobulin to thyroid-stimulating hormone ratio may be associated with pulmonary metastases in children with differentiated thyroid cancer. Endocr Pract. 2016;22(11):1259–66.
148. Vali R, Rachmiel M, Hamilton J, El Zein M, Wasserman J, Costantini DL, et al. The role of ultrasound in the follow-up of children with differentiated thyroid cancer. Pediatr Radiol. 2015;45(7):1039–45.
149. Kuijt WJ, Huang SA. Children with differentiated thyroid cancer achieve adequate hyperthyrotropinemia within 14 days of levothyroxine withdrawal. J Clin Endocrinol Metab. 2005;90(11):6123–5.
150. Turpin S, Lambert R, Deal C. Timing of hormone withdrawal in children undergoing 131I whole-body scans for thyroid cancer. Horm Res Paediatr. 2016;86(6):410–5.
151. Hanscheid H, Lassmann M, Luster M, Thomas SR, Pacini F, Ceccarelli C, et al. Iodine biokinetics and dosimetry in radioiodine therapy of thyroid cancer: procedures and results of a prospective international

controlled study of ablation after rhTSH or hormone withdrawal. J Nucl Med. 2006;47(4):648–54.
152. Handkiewicz-Junak D, Gawlik T, Rozkosz J, Puch Z, Michalik B, Gubala E, et al. Recombinant human thyrotropin preparation for adjuvant radioiodine treatment in children and adolescents with differentiated thyroid cancer. Eur J Endocrinol. 2015;173(6):873–81.
153. Jarzab B, Handkiewicz-Junak D, Wloch J. Juvenile differentiated thyroid carcinoma and the role of radioiodine in its treatment: a qualitative review. Endocr Relat Cancer. 2005;12(4):773–803.
154. Hung W, Sarlis NJ. Current controversies in the management of pediatric patients with well-differentiated nonmedullary thyroid cancer: a review. Thyroid. 2002;12(8):683–702.
155. Dinauer C, Francis GL. Thyroid cancer in children. Endocrinol Metab Clin N Am. 2007;36(3):779–806, vii.
156. Lassmann M, Hanscheid H, Verburg FA, Luster M. The use of dosimetry in the treatment of differentiated thyroid cancer. Q J Nucl Med Mol Imaging. 2011;55(2):107–15.
157. Verburg FA, Reiners C, Hanscheid H. Approach to the patient: role of dosimetric RAI Rx in children with DTC. J Clin Endocrinol Metab. 2013;98(10):3912–9.
158. Barwick TD, Dhawan RT, Lewington V. Role of SPECT/CT in differentiated thyroid cancer. Nucl Med Commun. 2012;33(8):787–98.
159. Lee M, Lee YK, Jeon TJ, Chang HS, Kim BW, Lee YS, et al. Frequent visualization of thyroglossal duct remnant on post-ablation 131I-SPECT/CT and its clinical implications. Clin Radiol. 2015;70(6):638–43.
160. Mostafa M, Vali R, Chan J, Omarkhail Y, Shammas A. Variants and pitfalls on radioiodine scans in pediatric patients with differentiated thyroid carcinoma. Pediatr Radiol. 2016;46(11).1579–89.
161. Sabra MM, Grewal RK, Tala H, Larson SM, Tuttle RM. Clinical outcomes following empiric radioiodine therapy in patients with structurally identifiable metastatic follicular cell-derived thyroid carcinoma with negative diagnostic but positive post-therapy 131I whole-body scans. Thyroid. 2012;22(9):877–83.
162. Rosario PW, Mourao GF, Dos Santos JB, Calsolari MR. Is empirical radioactive iodine therapy still a valid approach to patients with thyroid cancer and elevated thyroglobulin? Thyroid. 2014;24(3):533–6.
163. Hurley JR. Historical note: TSH suppression for thyroid cancer. Thyroid. 2011;21(11):1175–6.
164. Jonklaas J, Bianco AC, Bauer AJ, Burman KD, Cappola AR, Celi FS, et al. Guidelines for the treatment of hypothyroidism: prepared by the American Thyroid Association Task Force on thyroid hormone replacement. Thyroid. 2014;24(12):1670–751.
165. Bauer AJ. Approach to the pediatric patient with Graves' disease: when is definitive therapy warranted? J Clin Endocrinol Metab. 2011;96(3):580–8.
166. Rivkees SA. Pediatric Graves' disease: controversies in management. Horm Res Paediatr. 2010;74(5):305–11.
167. Robbins RJ, Wan Q, Grewal RK, Reibke R, Gonen M, Strauss HW, et al. Real-time prognosis for metastatic thyroid carcinoma based on 2-[18F]fluoro-2-deoxy-D-glucose-positron emission tomography scanning. J Clin Endocrinol Metab. 2006;91(2):498–505.
168. Ciarallo A, Marcus C, Taghipour M, Subramaniam RM. Value of fluorodeoxyglucose PET/computed tomography patient management and outcomes in thyroid cancer. PET Clin. 2015;10(2):265–78.
169. Leboulleux S, El Bez I, Borget I, Elleuch M, Deandreis D, Al Ghuzlan A, et al. Post-radioiodine treatment whole body scan in the era of fluorodesoxyglucose positron emission tomography for differentiated thyroid carcinoma with elevated serum thyroglobulin levels. Thyroid. 2012;22(8):832–8.
170. Isoda T, BaBa S, Maruoka Y, Kitamura Y, Tahara K, Sasaki M, et al. Impact of patient age on the iodine/FDG "flip-flop" phenomenon in lung metastasis from thyroid cancer. Ann Nucl Med. 2016;30(8):518–24.
171. Evans C, Tennant S, Perros P. Thyroglobulin in differentiated thyroid cancer. Clin Chim Acta. 2015;444:310–7.
172. Nascimento C, Borget I, Troalen F, Al Ghuzlan A, Deandreis D, Hartl D, et al. Ultrasensitive serum thyroglobulin measurement is useful for the follow-up of patients treated with total thyroidectomy without radioactive iodine ablation. Eur J Endocrinol. 2013;169(5):689–93.
173. Momesso DP, Vaisman F, Yang SP, Bulzico DA, Corbo R, Vaisman M, et al. Dynamic risk stratification in patients with differentiated thyroid Cancer treated without radioactive iodine. J Clin Endocrinol Metab. 2016;101(7):2692–700.
174. Dominguez JM, Nilo F, Contreras T, Carmona R, Droppelmann N, Gonzalez H, et al. Neck sonography and suppressed thyroglobulin have high sensitivity for identifying recurrent/persistent disease in patients with low-risk thyroid cancer treated with total thyroidectomy and radioactive iodine ablation, making stimulated thyroglobulin unnecessary. J Ultrasound Med. 2017;36(11):2299–307.
175. Castagna MG, Brilli L, Pilli T, Montanaro A, Cipri C, Fioravanti C, et al. Limited value of repeat recombinant human thyrotropin (rhTSH)-stimulated thyroglobulin testing in differentiated thyroid carcinoma patients with previous negative rhTSH-stimulated thyroglobulin and undetectable basal serum thyroglobulin levels. J Clin Endocrinol Metab. 2008;93(1):76–81.
176. Han JM, Kim WB, Yim JH, Kim WG, Kim TY, Ryu JS, et al. Long-term clinical outcome of differentiated thyroid cancer patients with undetectable stimulated thyroglobulin level one year after initial treatment. Thyroid. 2012;22(8):784–90.
177. Klubo-Gwiezdzinska J, Burman KD, Van Nostrand D, Wartofsky L. Does an undetectable rhTSH-stimulated Tg level 12 months after initial treat-

ment of thyroid cancer indicate remission? Clin Endocrinol. 2011;74(1):111–7.
178. Spencer C, Fatemi S. Thyroglobulin antibody (TgAb) methods – strengths, pitfalls and clinical utility for monitoring TgAb-positive patients with differentiated thyroid cancer. Best Pract Res Clin Endocrinol Metab. 2013;27(5):701–12.
179. Verburg FA, Luster M, Cupini C, Chiovato L, Duntas L, Elisei R, et al. Implications of thyroglobulin antibody positivity in patients with differentiated thyroid cancer: a clinical position statement. Thyroid. 2013;23(10):1211–25.
180. Chiovato L, Latrofa F, Braverman LE, Pacini F, Capezzone M, Masserini L, et al. Disappearance of humoral thyroid autoimmunity after complete removal of thyroid antigens. Ann Intern Med. 2003;139(5 Pt 1):346–51.
181. Cabanillas ME, McFadden DG, Durante C. Thyroid cancer. Lancet. 2016;388(10061):2783–95.
182. Kim A, Widemann BC, Krailo M, Jayaprakash N, Fox E, Weigel B, et al. Phase 2 trial of sorafenib in children and young adults with refractory solid tumors: a report from the Children's Oncology Group. Pediatr Blood Cancer. 2015;62(9):1562–6.
183. Widemann BC, Kim A, Fox E, Baruchel S, Adamson PC, Ingle AM, et al. A phase I trial and pharmacokinetic study of sorafenib in children with refractory solid tumors or leukemias: a Children's Oncology Group Phase I Consortium report. Clin Cancer Res. 2012;18(21):6011–22.
184. Karajannis MA, Legault G, Fisher MJ, Milla SS, Cohen KJ, Wisoff JH, et al. Phase II study of sorafenib in children with recurrent or progressive low-grade astrocytomas. Neuro-Oncology. 2014;16(10):1408–16.
185. Kim A, Dombi E, Tepas K, Fox E, Martin S, Wolters P, et al. Phase I trial and pharmacokinetic study of sorafenib in children with neurofibromatosis type I and plexiform neurofibromas. Pediatr Blood Cancer. 2013;60(3):396–401.
186. Iyer P, Mayer JL, Ewig JM. Response to sorafenib in a pediatric patient with papillary thyroid carcinoma with diffuse nodular pulmonary disease requiring mechanical ventilation. Thyroid. 2014;24(1):169–74.
187. Waguespack SG, Sherman SI, Williams MD, Clayman GL, Herzog CE. The successful use of sorafenib to treat pediatric papillary thyroid carcinoma. Thyroid. 2009;19(4):407–12.

Part VIII

Aggressive Thyroid Cancers

22 Anaplastic Thyroid Cancer

Robert C. Smallridge, John D. Casler,
and Michael E. Menefee

Anaplastic thyroid cancer is perhaps the most aggressive of all malignancies, with a median survival of 4–5 months. Time is critical, so the evaluation and treatment plan must be accomplished within a few days. The correct diagnosis is essential, so an adequate tissue sample (often from a core biopsy) must be obtained. Clinical evaluation includes examination of the airway, which is frequently compromised, and extensive imaging (preferably with a PET/CT scan) to accurately stage the patient. Those with Stage IVA disease (limited to the thyroid) have the most favorable outcomes and should have thyroidectomy with adjuvant radiation and chemotherapy. Stage IVB patients have locoregional extension and should be considered for surgery (if resectable) and chemo/radiation. Stage IVC patients have systemic metastases and a poor response rate to current therapies. Patients should be apprised of the risks/benefits of therapy and their values and preferences should be discussed. Palliative/hospice care should be part of the conversation when establishing goals of therapy.

Multimodal aggressive treatment has shown some success, but future treatments will require a better understanding of the extent of genomic and epigenetic disarray present in each patient's tumor.

R. C. Smallridge (✉)
Department of Internal Medicine, Division of Endocrinology and Metabolism, Mayo Clinic, Jacksonville, FL, USA
e-mail: smallridge.robert@mayo.edu

J. D. Casler
Department of Otorhinolaryngology—Head and Neck Surgery, Mayo Clinic, Jacksonville, FL, USA

M. E. Menefee
Department of Internal Medicine, Division of Hematology and Oncology, Mayo Clinic, Jacksonville, FL, USA

Background

Thyroid cancer incidence in the United States and other countries has increased dramatically in the past two decades. Many of these tumors are detected by medical imaging and are well differentiated papillary cancers of low metastatic potential [1]. In contrast, the frequency of anaplastic thyroid cancers (ATC) in the United States has remained low (~1.5%) [2] and has decreased in countries in response to iodine supplementation [2]. Unfortunately, due to the highly aggressive nature of ATC, deaths from this tumor comprise a disproportionate number of total thyroid cancer deaths every year.

Because of the small number of new cases annually, few medical centers have sufficient experience to perform prospective clinical trials. Most literature is retrospective and includes patients from many years or decades, during which time treatment options varied.

U. K. Mallick et al. (eds.), *Practical Management of Thyroid Cancer*,
https://doi.org/10.1007/978-3-319-91725-2_22

The American Thyroid Association (ATA) has published multiple versions of clinical management guidelines for both differentiated and medullary thyroid cancers, the most recent appearing in 2016 [3, 4]. The first such guidelines for ATC appeared in Nov 2012 [5]. Due to the behavior of this tumor, task force members were multidisciplinary, with representation by thyroidologists, surgeons, medical and radiation oncologists, endocrine pathologists, and a clinical bioethicist.

This chapter on ATC will utilize the framework of the ATA guidelines [5] to provide the reader with a practical approach to managing a patient who presents with ATC. There are several key points to remember: (1) Time is critical. ATC is perhaps the most aggressive of all malignancies, with a median survival of 4–5 months, so the evaluation and treatment plan must be completed within a few days; (2) The correct diagnosis must be made. There are several mimics of ATC, so an adequate tissue sample (often requiring a core biopsy, not just a fine needle aspirate) must be obtained. Secondary review by an experienced endocrine pathologist should be considered; (3) A treatment plan should be agreed upon by a multidisciplinary team and discussed with the patient and caregivers; (4) Palliative care should be discussed, particularly in the context of the patient's overall status and likelihood of multimodal therapy being beneficial; (5) Reassessment of goals after initial therapy should be performed.

Since publication of the ATA guidelines, new information has emerged and will be discussed. First, Next Generation Sequencing (NGS) has shed new light on the extent of genomic dysregulation in ATC, information which will inform the design of future treatments [6–15]. Second, several prospective trials have been completed or are in progress [16].

Clinical Presentation (Table 22.1)

Patients with ATC, as with other thyroid cancers, are predominantly female, and they are older and have larger tumors; they also frequently have a history of prior goiter or differentiated thyroid cancer (DTC). They typically present with the rapid growth of a neck mass (86%) and associated symptoms including voice change/hoarseness (33%), difficulty swallowing (37%), or shortness of breath (27%). Less common symptoms seen are pain (16%), cough (10%), hemoptysis (10%), or venous obstruction (8%) [2].

Table 22.1 Clinical characteristics of anaplastic thyroid cancer at onset

Gender: Female (66%); male (34%)
Age (median/mean): 69/66.5 years
Tumor size, median: 6.8 cm
Associated DTC: 27%
Distant metastasis: 42%

Adapted from Smallridge et al. [2]

Approach to ATC Evaluation

A recommended strategy for evaluating patients rapidly is depicted in Fig. 22.1.

Diagnosis

The correct diagnosis is critical to everything that follows, but may be difficult at times. Due to the undifferentiated features, necrosis, and lack of thyroid characteristics, ATC may be misidentified, particularly if performed on a fine needle aspirate. Therefore, a core biopsy may be required and an endocrine pathologist's second opinion should be strongly considered. The histologic variants include giant cell, fusiform (spindle cell), squamoid, and paucicellular [17]. Furthermore, there are a number of mimics that should be excluded, including squamous cell carcinoma, thyroid lymphoma, poorly differentiated thyroid cancer, thyroid sarcomas, medullary thyroid cancer, and metastases to the thyroid [5]. Immunohistochemical markers may be very helpful in arriving at the correct diagnosis. Histologic features that may favor longer survival include "presence of a pre-existing tumor, epithelial growth, a squamous cell carcinoma component, no neutrophilic infiltration and lymphocytic infiltration" [18].

Evaluation

The initial evaluation should include the patient's clinical assessment, laboratory testing, and imaging. Clinically, does the patient have or is at immediate risk of developing airway or esophageal obstruction? Do they have findings to suggest metastatic disease such as shortness of breath, bone pain, or recent onset of headache or other neurologic symptoms? Standard laboratory studies should include a CBC, comprehensive metabolic profile, and thyroid function. Of great importance is appropriate and extensive imaging. Unlike DTC, where preoperative imaging is often limited to neck ultrasound, patients with ATC should have an ^{18}FDG PET/CT scan. These tumors have an increase in both GLUT1 and GLUT3 glucose transport receptors, and the addition of PET to CT cross-sectional imaging increases detection of metastatic lesions and often alters both staging and subsequent management [19]. Neck CT should be performed with and without contrast, as detailed assessment of the extent of locoregional involvement will allow the surgeon to determine if the tumor is resectable (Fig. 22.2a). One of the most reliable predictors of prolonging survival is if the tumor is resectable [20]. The ATA guidelines Recommendation 19 states: "If locoregional disease is present and a grossly negative margin (R1 resection) can be achieved, surgical resection should be considered. (Furthermore) In patients with systemic disease, resection of

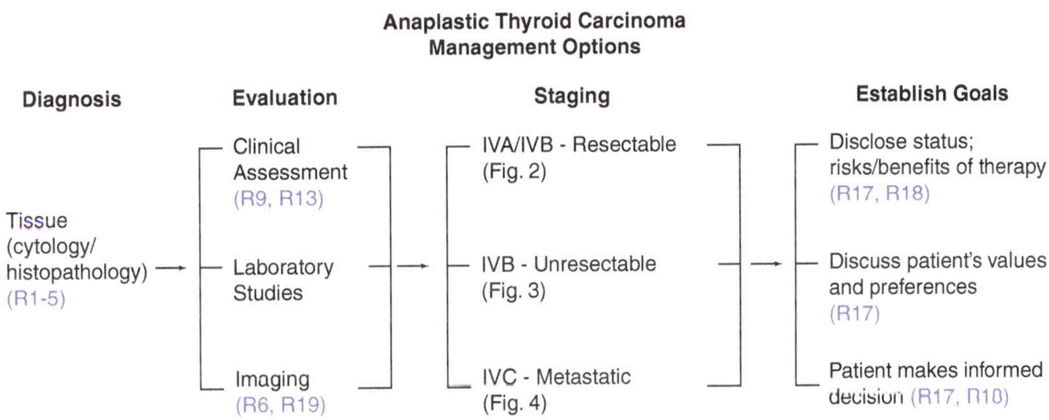

Fig. 22.1 Algorithm for the evaluation of patients with anaplastic thyroid carcinoma. Reproduced with permission from Smallridge et al. [5]

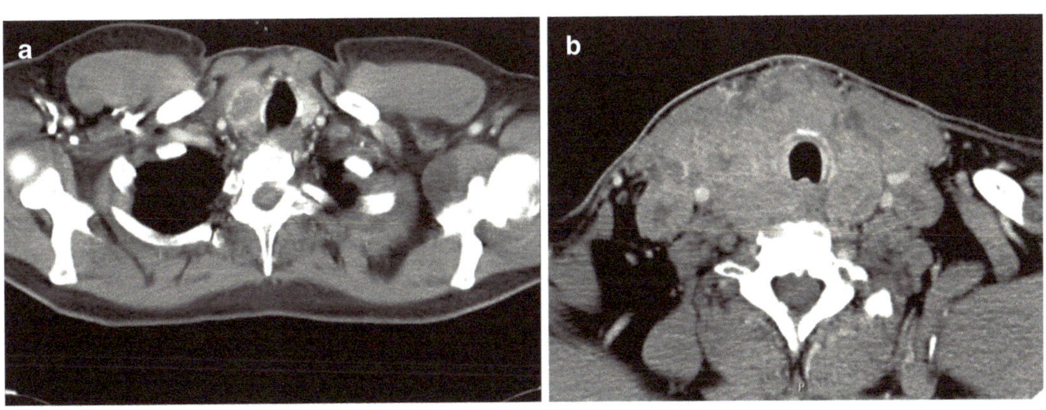

Fig. 22.2 Neck MRI scans of patients with (**a**) Stage IVB (resectable) and (**b**) Stage IVB (unresectable) disease

the primary tumor for palliation should be considered to avoid current or eventual airway or esophageal obstruction" [5].

Staging

Once the pathologic diagnosis is confirmed and extent of disease determined (ideally accomplished within 2 days), then the patient should be staged.

Thyroid cancers are staged using the TNM classification of the American Joint Committee on Cancer (AJCC/7th Edition), and ATC patients, even those with a small intrathyroidal tumor, are all classified as stage IV. Stage IVA requires that the tumor be intrathyroidal, IVB includes patients with local extension but no distant metastases, while IVC patients have distant metastases. Stage IVB patients are further subclassified depending upon whether or not the tumor is potentially surgically resectable.

The frequency of each stage of ATC in eight publications ($n = 961$ patients) (median %; range) was: Stage IVA = 10.2% (0–19); IVB = 40.2% (15.8–70); IVC = 45.8% (20–73.7) [20]. Almost half of patients have distant metastases at diagnosis and only 10% have localized disease, which helps explain the poor prognosis.

Establish Goals

Once staging is complete, the multidisciplinary team should meet with the patient and family/caregivers to establish treatment/care goals. First, the patient's status should be disclosed and the risks/benefits of therapy reviewed; second, the patient's values and preferences should be elicited; and third, the patient should then make an informed decision. A more detailed discussion of the issues related to patient decision-making capacity and informed consent, surrogate decision-making, patient autonomy, beneficent care, advance directives, and code status is available [5].

Surgical Considerations

There are three roles for surgery in the management of anaplastic thyroid carcinoma. When the diagnosis cannot be firmly established through fine needle aspiration (FNA) or core biopsy, surgery may be elected to obtain a more definitive tissue sample. It is important that the site for biopsy be chosen well so as not to put the patient at increased risk of airway compromise or to expose the patient to unnecessary risks that would delay initiation of other treatment modalities. Such risks would include hematoma formation or wound infection. The most superficial and most accessible part of the tumor should be chosen. The isthmus may serve well in this regard. An added benefit of isthmusectomy would be potential protection of the airway.

Protecting or establishing an airway is the second role for surgery in the management of ATC. As mentioned, isthmusectomy may not only help establish the diagnosis, but may be beneficial in decompressing the anterior tracheal wall if the tumor is encroaching on the airway. Tracheotomy is required on occasion to stabilize the airway that is compromised by ATC. Tracheotomy may be complicated by "seeding" of the tracheotomy site with tumor, however, and must be considered in that light. Patients who have suffered bilateral vocal cord paralysis from tumor invasion may have no other option than tracheotomy in order to secure their airway.

Lastly, surgery (thyroidectomy with or without neck dissection) may play a therapeutic role in the management of patients with Stage IVA and in some patients with Stage IVB disease. The goal of surgery should be complete resection of all gross disease. Surgery can be considered if there is a reasonable chance that complete resection can be performed and that the patient will not experience an undue delay in beginning adjuvant treatment as a result of the surgery. Complications like extensive wound breakdown, extensive chylous leakage, or pharyngo-cutaneous fistula should be avoided if possible. "Heroic" surgical procedures like total laryngectomy, esophagectomy, or mediastinal tracheotomy should probably not be attempted as they are unlikely to enhance survival, and will likely have a negative impact on quality of life.

Anaplastic thyroid carcinoma often incites an aggressive local tissue response with marked inflammatory and desmoplastic changes that obscure tissue planes making dissection difficult. Identification of normal structures such as the recurrent laryngeal nerves and parathyroid glands may be difficult if the tumor has spread laterally or posteriorly. Nerve monitoring may be beneficial in this circumstance. Identification of the nerves inferiorly in the neck in an uninvolved area may also be helpful.

Management

Treatment and palliative care options are guided by patient stage, patient general health status, and patient preferences. The general approach is summarized in Table 22.2.

Stage IVA

Thyroidectomy is recommended, followed by definitive external beam radiotherapy (possibly with chemotherapy) in patients with good performance status to achieve maximum benefit [5, 21]. Recently, Brierley and Tsang [22] recommended "accelerated hyperfractionated radiation without chemotherapy, 60 Gy in 40 fractions over 4 weeks, with 2 fractions of 1.5 Gy per day." Many other studies have supported the benefits of high-dose radiotherapy [21, 23].

The only situation where the ATA task force had differences of opinion was when a small incidental ATC was identified during thyroid surgery for another lesion—some members, but not all, felt postoperative radiotherapy (±) chemotherapy should be included. The reason for such concern is that some patients with only a microscopic primary tumor have developed distant metastases later, indicating the potential for systemic disease even in those felt most likely to be cured by surgery. Radiotherapy (preferably Intensity-Modulated Radiation Therapy or IMRT) should be administered as soon as the surgeon gives approval; this could be as soon as 2–3 weeks postoperatively.

The improved survival of patients with IVA disease has been reported by many authors. As examples, Akaishi et al. [24] found that in 100 stage IVA, B, and C patients, respectively, the median survival was 33.5, 6.1, and 2.5 months, while 6-month survival was 100, 49.6, and 22.4%; 1-year was 72.7, 24.8, and 8.2%; and 2-year survival was 62.3, 10.6, and 0%. In a review of 241 ATC patients in the SEER database, patients with tumor confined to the thyroid vs. those with adjacent structures invaded vs. those with further extension/distant metastases had a median survival of 9, 6, and 3 months, respectively. Further, the 1-year survival was 50.0, 27.6, and 7.4%; 2-year survival was 32.7, 16.2, and 2.1%; and 3-year survival was 22.9, 10.1, and 0% in the same categories [25].

Table 22.2 Initial treatment recommendations in anaplastic thyroid cancer

Stage IVA	Surgery → Radiotherapy ± chemotherapy
Stage IVB (resectable)	Surgery → Radiotherapy ± chemotherapy
Stage IVB (unresectable)	Radiotherapy ± chemotherapy → ? Surgery
Stage IVC Aggressive Rx Supportive care	Neck/locoregional radiotherapy (high dose or palliative)
	Systemic chemotherapy (cytotoxics/clinical trial)
	Palliative radiotherapy
	Focal lesion control
	Hospice/palliative care

Adapted from Smallridge et al. [5]

Stage IVB (Table 22.2)

For patients with locoregional disease but no distant metastases, and who have good performance status and want aggressive therapy, a contrast-enhanced CT of the neck is critical to determine whether the tumor is potentially operable with the goal to achieve an R0 or R1 (grossly negative margin) resection. Most studies suggest that complete removal of tumor prolongs disease-free and/or overall survival [5, 20, 26, 27]. In a large Japanese cohort, Sugitani [28] showed that in 242 stage IVB patients, 1-year survival increased from 12 to 41% in those receiving radical vs. no or palliative surgery; the Hazard Ratio = 0.39 (95% CI = 0.28–0.53). In a follow-up report [29], these authors found that "super-radical" surgery (laryngectomy, tracheal, or esophageal resection, etc.) did not improve survival vs. restricted radical surgery, given that the former patients more commonly needed tracheostomy and were less likely to receive radiation or chemotherapy. When patients are deemed unresectable initially then undergo external beam radiotherapy and/or chemotherapy, some may have such a beneficial response that surgery can be performed subsequently.

A second critical component of therapy is external beam radiation (preferably IMRT if available). For patients desiring aggressive therapy, high-dose radiotherapy (RT) $\geq$ 60–70 Gy should be given within 2–3 weeks of surgery. Even if the tumor is unresectable, RT can reduce the risk of severe locoregional complications and may prolong survival [26]. For those with poor performance status or who decline aggressive treatment for other reasons, a palliative dose of 2000 cGy given over 5 days is recommended [22].

ATC is almost always a systemic disease, even though only 40-50% of patients present with detectable distant metastases. Therefore, patients with stage IVA and IVB disease should strongly consider adjuvant systemic therapy in addition to surgery and radiation. The current first-line regimen recommended by both the ATA and NCCN guidelines [5, 30], is cytotoxic, either single or dual agent (Table 22.3). Several small non-randomized studies have documented prolonged survival in patients who undergo such aggressive multimodal therapy [31–33]. There have been a few clinical trials, the largest being with the microtubule disrupting agent, fosbretabulin [34], as well as individual patient responses to a variety of targeted agents including EGFR antagonists [27], BRAF-inhibitors [35–39], and receptor kinase [40, 41], ALK [42], mTOR inhibitors [43] and a combination of tyrosine kinase inhibitors [44]. At present, caution is advised as response times have been brief and serious side effects reported [45]. With the recent appearance of several reports utilizing Next Gen Sequencing which have shown multiple dysregulated genes, it is apparent that future studies will require combination therapies. Immunotherapeutics need to be examined also, as PDL-1 is highly expressed in a minority of patient tumors and infiltrating immune cells [46].

Stage IVC

Of all solid tumors, stage IVC anaplastic thyroid cancer is arguably the most devastatingly aggres-

Table 22.3 Examples of adjuvant/radiosensitizing chemotherapy regimens in anaplastic thyroid carcinoma

Regimen	Agents/dosages	Frequency
Paclitaxel/carboplatin	Paclitaxel 50 mg/m^2, carboplatin AUC 2 mg/m^2 IV	Weekly
Docetaxel/doxorubicin	Docetaxel 60 mg/m^2 IV, doxorubicin 60 mg/m^2 IV (w/pegfilgrastim); *or*	q3–4 weeks
	Docetaxel 20 mg/m^2 IV, doxorubicin 20 mg/m^2	Weekly
Paclitaxel	Paclitaxel 30–60 mg/m^2 IV	Weekly
Cisplatin	Cisplatin 25 mg/m^2 IV	Weekly
Doxorubicin	Doxorubicin 60 mg/m^2 IV	q3 weeks
Doxorubicin	Doxorubicin 20 mg/m^2 IV	Weekly

IV intravenously
Adapted from Smallridge et al. 2012 [5]

sive. Almost half of patients with ATC have distant metastases at presentation, and one-year survival is generally less than 10% [24, 25]. Should the patient embark upon a course of aggressive multi-model therapy when the response rate is so low, or should supportive care be favored? Establishing the extent of disease with ^{18}FDG-PET/CT imaging (a few oligometastases vs. widespread disease), extent of neck involvement, and general overall health status should all be considered when establishing goals of therapy. While brain metastases are uncommon, an MRI prior to pursuing aggressive therapy is advised [5].

Aggressive therapy entails definitive radiation and systemic chemotherapy (Table 22.2). First-line therapy has been single or combination cytotoxic agents, while second-line therapy has been either systemic chemotherapy or a clinical trial [34, 40, 41]. Single agent targeted therapy based upon individual responses has also been reported [27, 35–38, 42, 43]. Onoda et al. [47] studied weekly paclitaxel (80 mg/m^2 IV) in 52 ATC patients (IVA = 11; IVB = 19; IVC = 22) and reported a median overall survival of 14.1, 8.0, and 5.3 months, with a 6-month survival of 80.8%, 57.9%, and 40.9%, respectively. Recently, more trials have become available (www.clinicaltrials.gov) and, given the poor response rate to traditional drugs, earlier participation in a clinical trial could be considered. Supportive care should also be prominently discussed with the patient, and could include palliative radiotherapy, focal lesion ablations, and hospice/palliative care (discussed in the next chapter) to assist patients in symptom and pain relief for the rest of their lives.

Future Directions

Numerous genes and pathways are over- or underexpressed [6], and Next Gen Sequencing studies have recently established that ATC tumors have many mutations and gene rearrangements—far more than seen in differentiated thyroid cancers [7–14, 44]. Given the extensive dysregulation of the molecular landscape of ATC at the genetic and epigenetic levels as well as profound alterations in the tumor microenvironment, it is likely that more effective treatments will require an individualized characterization of each patient's tumor.

References

1. Brito JP, Hay ID, Morris JC. Low risk papillary thyroid cancer. BMJ. 2014;348:g3045.
2. Smallridge RC, Abate E. Anaplastic thyroid carcinoma: clinical aspects. In: Wartofsky L, Van Nostrand D, editors. Thyroid cancer: a comprehensive guide to clinical management. 3rd ed. New York: Springer; 2016. p. 929–32.
3. Haugen BR, Alexander EK, Bible KC, et al. 2015 American Thyroid Association management guidelines for adult patients with thyroid nodules and differentiated thyroid cancer: the American Thyroid Association Guidelines Task Force on thyroid nodules and differentiated thyroid cancer. Thyroid. 2016;26(1):1–133.
4. Wells SA Jr, Asa SL, Dralle H, et al. Revised American Thyroid Association guidelines for the management of medullary thyroid carcinoma. Thyroid. 2015;25(6):567–610.
5. Smallridge RC, Ain KB, Asa SL, et al. American Thyroid Association guidelines for management of patients with anaplastic thyroid cancer. Thyroid. 2012;22(11):1104–39.
6. Smallridge RC, Marlow LA, Copland JA. Anaplastic thyroid cancer: molecular pathogenesis and emerging therapies. Endocr Relat Cancer. 2009;16(1):17–44.
7. Jonker PK, van Dam GM, Oosting SF, et al. Identification of novel therapeutic targets in anaplastic thyroid carcinoma using functional genomic mRNA-profiling: paving the way for new avenues? Surgery. 2017;161(1):202–11.
8. Kasaian K, Wiseman SM, Walker BA, et al. The genomic and transcriptomic landscape of anaplastic thyroid cancer: implications for therapy. BMC Cancer. 2015;15:984.
9. Kunstman JW, Juhlin CC, Goh G, et al. Characterization of the mutational landscape of anaplastic thyroid cancer via whole-exome sequencing. Hum Mol Genet. 2015;24(8):2318–29.
10. Landa I, Ibrahimpasic T, Boucai L, et al. Genomic and transcriptomic hallmarks of poorly differentiated and anaplastic thyroid cancers. J Clin Invest. 2016;126(3):1052–66.
11. Lee J, Hwang JA, Lee EK. Recent progress of genome study for anaplastic thyroid cancer. Genomics Inform. 2013;11(2):68–75.
12. Pinto N, Black M, Patel K, et al. Genomically driven precision medicine to improve outcomes in anaplastic thyroid cancer. J Oncol. 2014;2014:936285.
13. Espinal-Enriquez J, Munoz-Montero S, Imaz-Rosshandler I, et al. Genome-wide expression analysis suggests a crucial role of dysregulation of matrix

metalloproteinases pathway in undifferentiated thyroid carcinoma. BMC Genomics. 2015;16:207.
14. Jeon M, Chun SM, Kim D, et al. Genomic alterations of anaplastic thyroid carcinoma detected by targeted massive parallel sequencing in a BRAFV600E mutation-prevalent area. Thyroid. 2016;26(5):683–90.
15. Weinberger P, Ponny SR, Xu H, et al. Cell cycle M-phase genes are highly upregulated in anaplastic thyroid carcinoma. Thyroid. 2017;27(2):236–52.
16. Clinical Trials.gov www.clinicaltrials.gov.
17. Baloch ZW, LiVolsi VA. Pathology of anaplastic carcinoma. In: Wartofsky L, Van Nostrand D, editors. Thyroid cancer: a comprehensive guide to clinical management. 3rd ed. New York: Springer; 2016. p. 935–8.
18. Hirokawa M, Sugitani I, Kakudo K, et al. Histopathological analysis of anaplastic thyroid carcinoma cases with long-term survival: a report from the Anaplastic Thyroid Carcinoma Research Consortium of Japan. Endocr J. 2016;63(5):441–7.
19. McDougall IR, Iagaru A. PET/CT in anaplastic cancer of the thyroid. In: Wartofsky L, Van Nostrand D, editors. Thyroid cancer: a comprehensive guide to clinical management. 3rd ed. New York: Springer; 2016. p. 939–42.
20. Smallridge RC, Abate E. Anaplastic thyroid carcinoma: prognosis. In: Wartofsky L, Van Nostrand D, editors. Thyroid cancer: a comprehensive guide to clinical management. 3rd ed. New York: Springer; 2016. p. 953–8.
21. Smallridge RC, Copland JA. Anaplastic thyroid carcinoma: pathogenesis and emerging therapies. Clin Oncol. 2010;22(6):486–97.
22. Brierley JD, Tsang RW. External radiation therapy for anaplastic thyroid cancer. In: Wartofsky L, Van Nostrand D, editors. Thyroid cancer: a comprehensive guide to clinical management. 3rd ed. New York: Springer; 2016. p. 943–6.
23. Glaser SM, Mandish SF, Gill BS, et al. Anaplastic thyroid cancer: prognostic factors, patterns of care, and overall survival. Head Neck. 2016;38(Suppl 1):E2083–90.
24. Akaishi J, Sugino K, Kitagawa W, et al. Prognostic factors and treatment outcomes of 100 cases of anaplastic thyroid carcinoma. Thyroid. 2011;21:1183–9.
25. Chen J, Tward JD, Shrieve DC, et al. Surgery and radiotherapy improves survival in patients with anaplastic thyroid carcinoma: analysis of the surveillance, epidemiology, and end results 1983-2002. Am J Clin Oncol. 2008;31(5):460–4.
26. Lee DY, Won JK, Lee SH, et al. Changes of clinicopathologic characteristics and survival outcomes of anaplastic and poorly differentiated thyroid carcinoma. Thyroid. 2016;26(3):404–13.
27. Smallridge RC. Approach to the patient with anaplastic thyroid carcinoma. J Clin Endocrinol Metab. 2012;97(8):2566–72.
28. Sugitani I, Miyauchi A, Sugino K, et al. Prognostic factors and treatment outcomes for anaplastic thyroid carcinoma: ATC Research Consortium of Japan cohort study of 677 patients. World J Surg. 2012;36(6):1247–54.
29. Sugitani I, Hasegawa Y, Sugasawa M, et al. Super-radical surgery for anaplastic thyroid carcinoma: a large cohort study using the Anaplastic Thyroid Carcinoma Research Consortium of Japan database. Head Neck. 2014;36(3):328–33.
30. National Comprehensive Cancer Network (NCCN). Thyroid cancer (Version 1.2016). https://www.nccn.org/professionals/physician_gls/f_guidelines.asp#thyroid. Accessed 21 Feb 2017.
31. Foote RL, Molina JR, Kasperbauer JL, et al. Enhanced survival in locoregionally confined anaplastic thyroid carcinoma: a single-institution experience using aggressive multimodal therapy. Thyroid. 2011;21(1):25–30.
32. Derbel O, Limem S, Segura-Ferlay C, et al. Results of combined treatment of anaplastic thyroid carcinoma (ATC). BMC Cancer. 2011;11:469.
33. Nachalon Y, Stern-Shavit S, Bachar G, et al. Aggressive palliation and survival in anaplastic thyroid carcinoma. JAMA Otolaryngol Head Neck Surg. 2015;141(12):1128–32.
34. Sosa JA, Elisei R, Jarzab B, et al. Randomized safety and efficacy study of fosbretabulin with paclitaxel/carboplatin against anaplastic thyroid carcinoma. Thyroid. 2014;24(2):232–40.
35. Agarwal R, Wang J, Wilson K, et al. Response to targeted therapy in BRAF mutant anaplastic thyroid cancer. J Natl Compr Cancer Netw. 2016;14(10):1203–7.
36. Lim AM, Taylor GR, Fellowes A, et al. BRAF inhibition in BRAFV600E-positive anaplastic thyroid carcinoma. J Natl Compr Cancer Netw. 2016;14(3):249–54.
37. Prager GW, Koperek O, Mayerhoefer ME, et al. Sustained response to vemurafenib in a BRAFV600E-mutated anaplastic thyroid carcinoma patient. Thyroid. 2016;26(10):1515–6.
38. Rosove MH, Peddi PF, Glaspy JA. BRAF V600E inhibition in anaplastic thyroid cancer. N Engl J Med. 2013;368(7):684–5.
39. Marten K, Gudena V. Use of vemurafenib in anaplastic thyroid carcinoma: a case report. Cancer Biol Ther. 2015;16(10):1430–3.
40. Savvides P, Nagaiah G, Lavertu P, et al. Phase II trial of sorafenib in patients with advanced anaplastic carcinoma of the thyroid. Thyroid. 2013;23(5):600–4.
41. Ha HT, Lee JS, Urba S, et al. A phase II study of imatinib in patients with advanced anaplastic thyroid cancer. Thyroid. 2010;20(9):975–80.
42. Godbert Y, Henriques de Figueiredo B, Bonichon F, et al. Remarkable response to crizotinib in woman with anaplastic lymphoma kinase-rearranged anaplastic thyroid carcinoma. J Clin Oncol. 2015;33(20):e84–7.
43. Wagle N, Grabiner BC, Van Allen EM, et al. Response and acquired resistance to everolimus in anaplastic thyroid cancer. N Engl J Med. 2014;371(15):1426–33.
44. Gibson W, Ruan D, Paulson V, et al. Genomic heterogeneity and exceptional response to dual pathway inhi-

bition in anaplastic thyroid cancer. Clin Cancer Res. 2017;23(9):2367–73. https://doi.org/10.1158/1078-0432.CCR-16-2154-T. Published 9 February 2017.
45. Gonfiotti A, Jaus MO, Barale D, et al. Extensive tracheal necrosis after treatment of anaplastic thyroid cancer with vascular endothelial growth factor inhibitors. Ann Thorac Surg. 2013;95(6):2181.
46. Ahn S, Kim T, Kim S, et al. Comprehensive screening for PD-L1 expression in thyroid cancer. Endocr Relat Cancer. 2107;24(2):97–106.
47. Onoda N, Sugino K, Higashiyama T, et al. The safety and efficacy of weekly paclitaxel administration for anaplastic thyroid cancer patients: a nationwide prospective study. Thyroid. 2016;26(9):1293–9.

Palliative Care

23

Mary Comiskey

Pain

Pain in cancer patients may be related to the tumour, it's treatment or completely unrelated to cancer. One prospective study of cancer patients found that 30% of patients had one pain, 39% had two pains and 31% had three or more pains [1]. Nine percent of pains encountered in this group were not due to malignancy. Patients with recurrent and/or metastatic thyroid cancer more commonly suffer pain due to local tumour progression, bone metastases and nerve compression or infiltration (Table 23.1).

The key to successful pain management is

- accurate diagnosis of the cause;
- appropriate analgesia including disease modifying treatment(s);
- adequate explanation of the cause and treatment plan
- regular monitoring of response.

World Health Organization Analgesic Ladder Eighty to ninety percent of cancer pains are relieved by following the World Health Organization's analgesic ladder (Fig. 23.1) [2]. It provides a basis for the use of primary analgesics. The choice of primary analgesics is wide. Those commonly used and thus widely available are listed in Table 23.2. Analgesia should be given orally, regularly to prevent pain, and titrated or changed according to response. Thus if pain fails to respond to a non-opioid (step 1), a weak opioid (step 2) is added and should that fail, a strong opioid (step 3) substituted. If pain fails to respond to one

Table 23.1 Choice of primary analgesics

Analgesic class	First choice	Second choice
Non-opioid	Acetaminophen (paracetamol)	Non-steroidal anti-inflammatory drugs (NSAIDs), aspirin
Weak opioid	Codeine	Dihydrocodeine
Strong opioid	Morphine	Oxycodone, hydromorphone, fentanyl, methadone

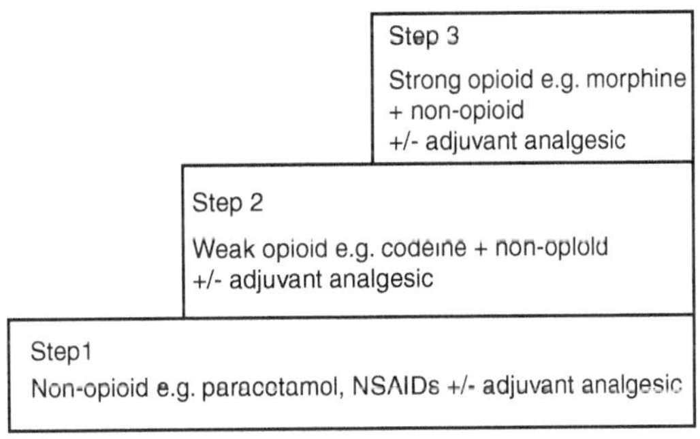

Fig. 23.1 The World Health Organization three-step analgesic stepladder for cancer pain relief [2]

M. Comiskey
Palliative Medicine, The Newcastle upon Tyne Hospitals NHS Foundation Trust, The Newcastle upon Tyne, UK
e-mail: Mary.Comiskey@nuth.nhs.uk

U. K. Mallick et al. (eds.), *Practical Management of Thyroid Cancer*,
https://doi.org/10.1007/978-3-319-91725-2_23

Table 23.2 Management of opioid intolerance

	Management options	
Problem	1	2
Gastric stasis	Switch opioid	Add prokinetic
Delirium/hallucinations	Reduce opioid dose	Switch opioid ± add major tranquilizer
Dysphoria	Reduce opioid	Switch opioid
Dry mouth	Switch opioid	
Vestibular stimulation	Switch opioid	Add antihistamine
Histamine release	Bronchodilator and antihistamine	Switch opioid
Generalised pruritus	Switch opioid	Consider 5HT3 antagonist, NSAID, gabapentin or mirtazapine
Myoclonus	Reduce opioid	Switch opioid

weak opioid a strong opioid should be used rather than trying an alternative weak opioid. Step 2 may be bypassed in favour of using a small dose of strong opioid. This is supported by a recently published randomised trial [3] which compared the weak opioids, codeine and tramadol, with morphine in moderate cancer pain. The study found that morphine provided earlier and better analgesia with no difference in adverse events between the two groups. In addition to regular preventative analgesia, patients with ongoing pain should also be provided with a rapid acting analgesic for breakthrough pain. This should be equivalent to 10–20% of their 24-h dose. They are currently separated by Fig. 23.1 and Table 23.2.

Prescribing Strong Opioids

NICE CG140 provides helpful information on strong opioid prescribing in palliative care patients [4]. Morphine is the oral strong opioid analgesic of choice [2]. This is based on its availability and familiarity rather than superiority over alternatives such as hydromorphone or oxycodone [5]. A typical starting dose in patients switching from a weak opioid (e.g. codeine 240 mg daily) is 30–60 mg daily. Smaller starting doses (e.g. 10–20 mg daily) should be considered in the elderly, and those who are opioid naïve. During the titration phase a sustained release or immediate acting preparation may be given and titrated regularly to response. Rescue doses of oral immediate release morphine, equivalent to 10–20% of the total daily dose, should be offered for breakthrough pain. It is advisable to seek specialist advice for patients with renal or hepatic impairment. Patients should be supervised during titration. It is reasonable to titrate daily in inpatients or every 3 days in outpatients. There is no ceiling dose for morphine. The same principles apply to oxycodone which is 50% more potent than morphine.

Common side effects of all strong opioids include:

- *Chemically mediated nausea and vomiting* occurs in approximately 30% of patients on commencement of opioids; it lasts 3–7 days, is mediated by dopamine and can be controlled by haloperidol 1.5–3 mg once daily. Haloperidol may be discontinued after 1 week. Nausea may recur with subsequent opioid dose escalation and should respond to the same intervention.
- *Constipation* affects most patients. Laxative therapy should be prescribed for all patients commenced on opioids unless there is a contraindication. The laxative dose requirement increases with opioid dose escalation. Most patients on higher opioid doses require a combination of softening and stimulating laxatives such as senna and docusate or codanthramer.
- *Transient drowsiness* lasts 3–5 days and may recur with subsequent opioid dose

increases. Patients should be advised of this possibility and counselled not to drive or operate mechanical equipment whilst affected.

Morphine Intolerance

Some patients are intolerant of morphine. Our understanding of opioid pharmacogenetics is incomplete and as yet there is no way of predicting which opioid will suit an individual patient. In addition there is significant inter-individual variation in bioavailability (Table 23.2).

Management strategies include:

1. Morphine dose reduction
2. Switching the patient to an alternative strong opioid
3. Addition of a drug treatment targeted at controlling the adverse effect. If opioid dose reduction fails to resolve the problem or results in recurrence of pain, switching the opioid is usually preferable to adding another pharmacological agent. The usual second line strong opioid of choice is oxycodone.

Clinical Presentation and Management of Morphine Intolerance

Morphine intolerance occurs in up to 30% of patients and can be managed by switching to an alternative strong opioid such as oxycodone. Table 23.3 details manifestations of opioid intolerance and suggested management strategies. It is important to distinguish between intolerance and opioid toxicity.

Alternative Strong Opioids

The more frequently used alternative strong opioid analgesics oxycodone and transdermal fentanyl are as effective as morphine [4–7]. They differ in their pharmacokinetic profiles [8] (Table 23.3). The recommended conversion ratios between some opioids vary between the UK and USA [9–11] (Table 23.4). More importantly, conversion ratios are merely an approximate guide. When switching opioids, it is essential to consider incomplete cross-tolerance, reduce the calculated conversion dose by 30–50% for patients on higher opioid doses and observe the patient closely for opioid toxicity.

Choice depends on: -

- Patient-related factors e.g. renal status, problems with constipation
- Disease/treatment related factors e.g. dysphagia, risk of mucositis or vomiting
- Cost

Table 23.5 may help with making a rational choice.

Table 23.4 Recommended conversion ratios for strong opioids USA and UK [9–11]

	Conversion ratio
Morphine → hydromorphone	5:1 USA 7.5: 1 UK
Hydromorphone → morphine	1:3.5–5 USA
Morphine → oxycodone	3:2 USA 3:2 UK
Morphine → methadone	10:1
Morphine → TD/SC fentanyl	100–150:1
Oral morphine → SC diamorphine	3:1
Oral → SC morphine	2:1
Oral → SC hydromorphone	2:1
Oral → SC oxycodone	2:1

Table 23.3 Pharmacokinetics of oral strong opioids [8–11]

	Morphine	Hydromorphone	Oxycodone	Methadone
Oral bioavailability	16–68%	37–62%	60-87%	40–96%
Onset of action (minutes)	20–30	20–30	20–30	30
Duration of action (hours)	3–6	4–5	4–6	4–24
Plasma half-life (hours)	1.5–4.5	2.5	3.5	8–75
Active metabolites	Yes	Yes	Yes	No

Table 23.5 Highlights the pros and cons of alternative strong opioids [4–11]

Drug	Pros	Cons
Oxycodone	Possibly less cognitive impairment and sedation; oral liquid available in UK	Accumulates in renal failure More constipating Risk of CNS side effects in CYP2D6 ultra-rapid metabolisers
Hydromorphone	Cheaper than equivalent higher doses of oxycodone in UK; injectable form is highly soluble	May accumulate in renal failure No oral liquid form in UK
Transdermal fentanyl	Safe in renal impairment Useful in patients with dysphagia, vomiting or mucositis Less constipating and possibly Less cognitive impairment	Unsuitable in unstable pain Patch allergy Most expensive—May save on laxative
Methadone	Least expensive Safe in renal and liver impairment NMDA receptor antagonist activity No active metabolites	Long half-life posing risk of fatal dose accumulation

Non-Oral Routes

In chronic pain management there is no analgesic benefit in giving strong opioids, available as oral formulations, by injection. Fentanyl and buprenorphine are available as transdermal patches and may be considered for management of chronic pain in patients with dysphagia, vomiting, or renal failure.

The indications for injectable analgesics are: -

- Vomiting;
- Need for rapid analgesic effect;
- Progressive or severe dysphagia;
- Last hours or days of life where swallowing is inconvenient for the patient.

Adjuvant Analgesics

Some pains, typically neuropathic pain, skin pain, movement-related pain and colic are only partially responsive to or do not respond to opioids. Adjuvant analgesics, also called secondary analgesics or co-analgesics, should be considered. They are usually used along with but may be considered instead of primary analgesics (i.e. paracetamol (acetaminophen), NSAIDs and opioids).

- *Anticonvulsants* for example gabapentin 100–800 mg 8-hourly and/or *Tricyclic antidepressants* for example amitriptyline 10–75 mg at night are the mainstay of treatment for neuropathic pain. The evidence base for gabapentin is superior though both drug groups have similar efficacy, relieving neuropathic pain intensity by 50% in 25–30% of patients [12, 13]. Some patients benefit from a combined approach.
- *Antispasmodics* for example hyoscine butylbromide (not available in USA) 20 mg SC as required or 40–120 mg by continuous infusion and glycopyrronium (glycopyrrolate in USA) 200–400 μcg SC as required or 600–1200 μcg by continuous infusion, usually relieve colic.
- *Corticosteroids* may be used to reduce peritumor edema and thus relieve pain related to nerve compression or cerebral metastases.
- *Muscle relaxants* e.g. diazepam or baclofen are useful for muscle cramp and myofascial pain.
- *NMDA-receptor-channel-blockers* e.g. ketamine for neuropathic, mucosal, skin or incident pain (unlicensed indications). There is limited robust evidence of benefit in cancer pain. Ketamine should only be prescribed under specialist supervision.

Non-Drug Therapies

Some patients benefit greatly from physiotherapy including heat therapy, ultrasonic therapy, massage and transcutaneous electrical nerve stimulation (TENS). Trigger point injection and acupuncture can be particularly useful for myofascial pain. Other useful treatments include relaxation therapy, lifestyle management advice, nerve blockade, cognitive behavioural therapy and hypnosis.

Persistent Pain

When pain persists it is important to re-assess the patient. Common pitfalls in management include:-

- Failure to diagnose and treat co-existing anxiety and depression.
- Onset of new pain or presence of previously undiagnosed pain.
- Poor patient adherence to prescribed medications.
- Inadequate analgesic dosing or inappropriate dosing intervals.

Jane was aged 47 years when she presented with a 6 × 4 cm rapidly growing inoperable anaplastic carcinoma of her thyroid gland causing stridor. She was treated with high dose corticosteroids and immediate tracheal stenting to relieve airways obstruction and then commenced radiotherapy with palliative intent. Her course was complicated by painful mucositis, which responded to substitution of codeine 240 mg, originally initiated for neck pain, for morphine 40 mg daily (using a conversion ratio of 10:1) and subsequent dose titration to 120 mg daily.

She also developed progressive dysphagia due to mucositis and opted for nasogastric intubation for feeding and delivery of medication rather than the alternative option of gastrostomy feeding.

The formulation of morphine was changed from modified release tablets to an equal dose of a modified release liquid formulation.

She suffered a series of blackouts that were attributed to carotid sinus dysfunction secondary to tumour encroachment. They occurred without warning and required her to have constant companionship for safety.

Their frequency was greatly reduced following re-introduction of corticosteroids, which presumably reduced peritumor edema.

Four weeks following completion of treatment she complained of drowsiness and twitching which was due to opioid toxicity. Her morphine requirement had fallen as a result of tumor response to radiotherapy and improvement in mucositis.

Discussion Points

1. Mucositis—other treatment options include:
    - benzydamine 0·15% oral rinse 15 mL 2-hourly if required;
    - topical lidocaine as a 2% solution or made up as a frozen or sugar-free lozenge;
    - alcohol-free liquid morphine 10 mg in 5 mL taken 4-hourly as a mouth rinse or swallowed;
    - coating agents such as sucralfate suspension 10 mL 4–8 hourly as a rinse and/or swallowed 12-hourly;
    - Ketamine transmucosal, oral or parenteral under specialist supervision.
2. Changing opioid requirements: It is important to monitor patients for opioid toxicity following disease-modifying treatments or nerve blockade or introduction of opioid sparing drugs such as corticosteroids, NSAIDs and ketamine. Signs of toxicity include pinpoint pupils, drowsiness, jerking and respiratory depression. The opioid dose including breakthrough pain medication should be reduced by 25–50%.
3. Dysphagia:
    - Consult a speech and language therapist for advice on swallowing techniques. If likely to be progressive or protracted consider percutaneous endoscopic gastrostomy (PEG) or a nasogastric feeding tube to facilitate feeding and administration of medication.
    - Rationalize medication and use non-oral preparations if practicable. Jane required a nasogastric tube and thus a change in opioid formulation. Transdermal fentanyl could have been used. Her anticipated requirement would have been 25–50 μcg/h starting with the lower option. In a randomised crossover study of oral morphine and transdermal fentanyl [14] most patients required a higher fentanyl dose than the manufacturers' recommendations when switched to fentanyl from morphine.

4. Corticosteroids as interim palliation may prove valuable in reducing peritumor edema pending response to radiotherapy. In fact edema may be temporarily exacerbated by radiotherapy causing an increase in local symptoms.

Jane developed progression of local neck disease, widespread pulmonary, nodal and base of skull metastases despite radiotherapy and chemotherapy. She complained of increasing neck pain and tenderness, facial pain with associated allodynia involving the mandibular division of the right trigeminal nerve and odynophagia related to candidiasis and probable glossopharyngeal neuralgia. Her neuropathic pains responded to introduction of gabapentin 100 mg 8-hourly with dose titration to tolerance—400 mg 8-hourly—and supplementation with amitriptyline 10 mg at night. The inflammatory component of neck pain responded to NSAIDs and pain on swallowing resolved with treatment of candidiasis. She also complained of a dry cough that was eventually controlled by nebulized 2% lidocaine 4 mL 6-hourly; her occasional minor hemoptysis resolved with introduction of tranexamic acid 500 mg 8-hourly. Breathlessness initially responded to relaxation techniques and a 25% increase in her daily opioid dose. She subsequently required re-stenting of her original tracheal stent for recurrence of upper airways obstruction. She felt particularly anxious and frightened that she would choke and was also troubled by excessive oropharyngeal secretions and drooling.

Discussion Points

1. Breathlessness is a particularly frightening, distressing and challenging symptom. To manage:
   - correct reversible causes e.g. bronchospasm or pleural effusion;
   - ensure optimal environmental conditions e.g. cool ambient temperature and through airflow or fan;
   - position patient comfortably;
   - explain the cause and treatment plan;
   - involve a physiotherapist to teach breathing techniques;
   - treat associated anxiety using relaxation and cognitive behavioural therapy techniques;
   - prescribe oxygen for hypoxic patients;
   - consider benzodiazepines for panic and anxiety;
   - prescribe opioids to reduce the sensation of breathlessness—if the patient is opioid naïve start with a low dose e.g. morphine 2.5–5 mg 4-hourly and titrate as required. If the patient is already on opioids increase their 24-h dose by 10–25% and continue to adjust according to response;
   - prescribe helium 80% and oxygen 20% mixture, which is lighter than room air, for upper airways obstruction.
2. Dry cough—if there is no underlying reversible cause it may be suppressed by:
   - oral antitussives such as simple linctus 10 mL as required, codeine linctus 15–30 mg 6-hourly or methadone linctus 1–2 mg 6-hourly;
   - inhaled or nebulized steroids;
   - lidocaine 2% 4 mL nebulized for troublesome cough where other measures have failed. Patients should be advised to avoid eating or drinking for 90 min following treatment to avoid aspiration.
3. Fear and panic are understandably common in patients with compressive symptoms related to neck disease and also in patients facing death. It is important to:
   - explore the underlying causes and address any irrational fears;
   - seek help from a clinical psychologist for patients with complex problems;
   - consider benzodiazepines e.g. diazepam 2–5 mg 8-hourly or lorazepam 0.5–1 mg 12-hourly. Antidepressants with anti-panic actions such as the selective serotonin reuptake inhibitor (SSRI) sertraline 50 mg daily, the noradrenergic and specific serotonergic antidepressant (NaSSA) mirtazapine 15 mg daily or the tricyclic antidepressant clomipramine 25 mg daily may also help.
4. Excess oral secretions and salivary drooling can be particularly frustrating and embarrassing. Drugs with anticholinergic activity such as hyoscine hydrobromide 1.5 mg transdermal

(TD) patch or 150–300μg sublingually (SL)/ orally 6-hourly are effective. Alternatively, glycopyrronium (glycopyrrolate) 200–400 μg SC or 400–1200 μg/24 h by continuous SC infusion (CSCI) and hyoscine butylbromide 20 mg SC and 40–120 mg by CSCI should help.

5. Management of bleeding
   - Identify and treat underlying cause if appropriate.
   - Consider referring the patient for palliative radiotherapy.
   - Monitor for anaemia and transfuse if indicated.
   - Prescribe tranexamic acid 500–1000 mg 8-hourly or ethamsylate 500 mg 6-hourly to reduce bleeding.
   - For patients at risk of a major bleed in the terminal phase, ensure ready availability of sedative medication such as midazolam 10 mg via buccal/IV/intramuscular (IM)/ SC routes or diazepam 10 mg per rectum, and green towels or surgical cloths to minimize the visual impact of blood loss. If a major bleed occurs stay with and reassure the patient and family.
6. Lymphedema—the mainstay of management is:
   - good skin care;
   - regular exercise of the affected limb;
   - massage therapy;
   - compression therapy;
   - prevention and early treatment of infection in the lymphedematous area;
   - a short course of high dose corticosteroids, for example dexamethasone 16 mg daily for 1 week for acute lymphatic obstruction;
   - further radiotherapy or chemotherapy if appropriate.

Other Problems Seen in Advanced Thyroid Cancer

Fungating Malodorous Neck Tumor

This is fortunately rare. Affected patients often require continuous inpatient care to manage the associated anxiety and fear of bleeding or choking as well as frequent need for dressings. Specific management should include:

- radiotherapy if appropriate to reduce bleeding and discharge;
- regular change of dressings;
- use of topical metronidazole 0.75–1% gel with dressings, which will control malodor in most patients; some will require systemic metronidazole for deep-seated anaerobic infection;
- active management of aerobic infection.

Nausea and Vomiting

One year later John required re-introduction and titration of regular morphine to control further pain due to bone metastases from his longstanding medullary thyroid cancer. He later complained of continuous nausea but also large volume vomiting towards the end of the day. The nausea was due to constipation and responded to cyclizine, used as an interim measure whilst his constipation was addressed. However large volume vomiting coupled with early satiety persisted and was attributed to morphine induced gastric stasis. It responded to introduction of regular metoclopramide. Ultimately his pain settled following further radiotherapy allowing dose reduction of morphine and withdrawal of metoclopramide.

It is important to distinguish the cause(s) of nausea and vomiting and target anti-emetic treatment at the appropriate receptor(s) [15].

Commonly overlooked causes in this patient group include constipation, excessive pharyngeal secretions, cerebral metastases, oropharyngeal candidiasis, emetogenic drugs, and gastric stasis. It is often necessary to initiate parenteral anti-emetic therapy to gain control, switching to oral therapy after 24–48 h.

There are five main causes:

- Chemical causes include drugs such as opioids or metronidazole, or biochemical disturbances such as hypercalcemia and uremia.

They act via the chemoreceptor trigger zone (CTZ), which has a preponderance of dopamine receptors. Thus the treatment of choice is haloperidol, a dopamine (D2) antagonist, 1.5–3 mg oral/SC once daily.
- Impaired gastric motility which is characterized by epigastric fullness, early satiety, flatulence, reflux and large volume vomiting, may be treated with metoclopramide 10–20 mg 8-hourly or 30–90 mg by CSCI or domperidone 10–20 mg 8-hourly if extrapyramidal side effects are a risk.
- Chemotherapy or radiotherapy induced nausea and vomiting should be managed with oral or parenteral 5HT3 antagonists.
- Vestibular or direct stimulation of the vomiting centre due to intracranial disease or radiotherapy—see below.
- Vagal/autonomic afferent stimulation of the vomiting centre due to pharyngeal irritation, mediastinal or sub-diaphragmatic problems including metastases are common in patients with advanced cancer. The main neurotransmitters implicated are histamine1 (H1), acetylcholine (AChm), and 5HT2. Cyclizine blocks H1 and AChm receptors, hyoscine hydrobromide blocks AChm receptors and levomepromazine has broad-spectrum anti-emetic activity blocking 5HT2, D2, AChm and H1. The respective doses are: cyclizine 50 mg oral/SC 8-hourly or 150 mg by CSCI; levomepromazine 5–12.5 mg oral/SC once daily; hyoscine hydrobromide 1.5 mg TD patch or 150–300 μg SL/oral 6-hourly or 600–1200 μg by CSCI over 24 h.

End of Life Discussions

Healthcare professionals are reticent about initiating discussions with patients about end of life care, despite most patients wishing to be informed and involved [16]. Senior clinical involvement is important, as is the language used in discussions. Conversations should focus on what can be done to improve quality of life rather than solely on withdrawing treatment and futility.

Good forward planning [17] enables patients to:

- understand the limited reversibility of their condition;
- share decision-making about the goals and plans for future care including advance guidance on cardiopulmonary resuscitation;
- express their wishes including choice of place of care at the end of life;
- agree/consent to information sharing with those important to them;
- identify a proxy to support decision-making in the event of loss of mental capacity;

The outcome of discussions should be clearly recorded in the patient's clinical record and communicated with all those directly involved in the patient's care. Plans may be formally recorded in an Advance Care Plan, Advance Decision to Refuse Treatment (ADRT), Emergency Healthcare Plan (EHCP) or Do Not attempt Resuscitation (DNAR) Form [18].

End-of-Life Care

One month later Jane was admitted as an emergency from home with sudden onset of stridor and a large intra-pulmonary hemorrhage. She was given midazolam 10 mg IM during transfer from home and remained calm until she died peacefully a few hours later surrounded by family and friends. On arrival she had marked halitosis that resolved shortly after receiving IV metronidazole.

As death approaches, care should be focussed on quality of life [17]. Where the burden outweighs the benefit, unhelpful investigations and ineffective treatments should be avoided or discontinued. Medications to relieve pain, nausea, dyspnea, agitation or troublesome respiratory secretions should be prescribed in anticipation. Patients already on oral opioids or anti-emetics should have their medication continued by subcutaneous infusion. Assisted hydration should be considered regularly on an individual patient basis [19]. Regular review and monitoring of the patient's clinical condition, their goals and response to treatment, carer's concerns and also for signs of recovery are of paramount importance. Signs that a patient may be imminently dying include:

- Bedbound
- Drowsiness, impaired cognition
- Difficulty taking oral medications
- Reduced food and fluid intake
- Increasing symptom burden

Typical end-of –life drug regimes include:

- parenteral opioid by CSCI
- cyclizine 100–150 mg or levomepromazine 5–12.5 mg by CSCI to prevent emesis.
- midazolam 10–60 mg or levomepromazine 25–100 mg for terminal agitation
- glycopyrronium 600–1200µg, hyoscine hydrobromide 600–1200 µg or hyoscine butylbromide 60–120 mg to reduce troublesome respiratory secretions.

The Leadership Alliance for the Care of Dying People, an alliance of 21 UK organisations vested in delivering or ensuring high quality end of life care set out the following priorities for care of the dying person [20]:

1. The possibility of dying is recognised and communicated clearly, decisions about care are made in accordance with the person's needs and wishes, and these are reviewed and revised regularly.
2. Sensitive communication takes place between staff and the dying person and those identified as important to them.
3. The dying person, and those identified as important to them, are involved in decisions about treatment and care to the extent that the dying person wants.
4. The needs of families and others identified as important to the dying person are actively explored, respected and met as far as possible.
5. An individual plan of care, which includes food and drink, symptom control and psychological, social and spiritual support, is agreed, co-ordinated and delivered with compassion.

References

1. Grond S, Zech D, Diefenbach C, et al. Assessment of cancer pain: a prospective evaluation in 2266 cancer patients referred to a pain service. Pain. 1996;64(1):107–14.
2. World Health Organization. Cancer pain relief with a guide to opioid availability. 2nd ed. Geneva: WHO; 1996. Available at http://apps.who.int/iris/bitstream/10665/37896/1/9241544821.pdf
3. Bandieri E, Romero M, Ripamonti C, et al. Randomized trial of low-dose morphine versus weak opioids in moderate cancer pain. J Clin Oncol. 2016;34(5):436–42.
4. Nice Clinical Guideline 140 (CG140): Palliative care for adults: strong opioids for pain relief. Pub May 2012. Last updated August 2016. https://www.nice.org.uk/guidance/cg140
5. Caraceni A, Hanks G, Kaasa S, et al. Use of opioid analgesics in the treatment of cancer pain: evidence based recommendations from the EAPC. Lancet Oncol. 2012;13:e58–68.
6. Bekkering GE, Soares-Weiser K, Reid K, et al. Can morphine still be considered to be the standard for treating chronic pain? A systematic review including pair-wise and network meta-analyses. Curr Med Res Opin. 2011;27(7):1477–91.
7. Reid CM, Martin RM, Sterne JAC, et al. Oxycodone for cancer related pain – meta-analysis of randomised controlled trials. Arch Intern Med. 2006;166(8):837–43.
8. Smith HS. Opioid metabolism. Mayo Clin Proc. 2009;84(7):613–24.
9. Lawlor P, Turner K, Hanson J, Brucra E. Dose ratio between morphine and hydromorphone in patients with cancer pain: a retrospective study. Pain. 1997;72:79–85.
10. Moriarty M, McDonald CJ, Miller AJ. A randomised crossover comparison of controlled release hydromorphone tablets with controlled release morphine tablets in patients with cancer pain. J Drug Assess. 1999;2:1–8.
11. Twycross R, Wilcock A, Howard P (eds) Palliative Care Formulary (PCF5) 5th ed. UK: palliativedrugs.com, 2014. Territorial specific editions are available in Canada, Germany, Japan and the USA.
12. Wiffen PJ, Derry S, Bell RF, et al. Gabapentin for chronic neuropathic pain in adults. Cochrane Database Syst Rev. 2017;6:CD007938. https://doi.org/10.1002/14651858.CD007938.pub4.
13. Moore R, Derry S, Aldington D, et al. Amitriptyline for neuropathic pain in adults. Cochrane Database Syst Rev. 2015;7:CD008242. https://doi.org/10.1002/14651858.CD008242.
14. Allan L, Hays H, Jensen N-K, et al. Randomised crossover trial of transdermal fentanyl and sustained release oral morphine for treating chronic non-cancer pain. BMJ. 2001;322:1154–8.
15. Peroutka SJ, Snyder SH. Antiemetic neurotransmitter receptor binding predicts therapeutic actions. Lancet. 1982;1:658–9.

16. Parker SM, Clayton JM, Hancock K, et al. A systematic review of prognostic/end-of-life communication with adults in the advanced stages of a life-limiting illness: patient/caregiver preferences for the content, style, and timing of information. J Pain Symptom Manag. 2007;34:81–93.
17. GMC. Treatment and care towards the end of life: good practice in decision making (2010) (Online). http://www.gmc-uk.org/guidance/ethical_guidance/end_of_life_care.asp
18. www.necn.nhs.uk/common-themes/deciding-right/resources/. A suite of documents to support decision-making towards the end of life.
19. Good P, Richard R, Syrmis W, et al. Medically assisted hydration for adult palliative care patients. Cochrane Database Syst Rev. 2014;4:CD006273.
20. One Chance to Get It Right. Improving people's experience of care in the last few days and hours of life. 2014; The Leadership Alliance for the Care of Dying People. https://www.gov.uk/government/uploads/system/uploads/attachment_data/file/323188/One_chance_to_get_it_right.pdf

Further Reading

Smallridge RC, Ain KB, Asa SL, et al. American Thyroid Association. Guidelines for Management of Patients with Anaplastic Thyroid Cancer. Thyroid. 2012;22(11):1104–39. http://online.liebertpub.com/doi/pdfplus/10.1089/thy.2012.0302

Perros P, Colley S, Boelaert K, et al. British Thyroid Association. Guidelines for the Management of Thyroid Cancer. Clin Endocrinol. 2014;81:1–122. https://doi.org/10.1111/cen.12515

Wells SA, Asa SL, Dralle H, et al. Revised American Thyroid Association Guidelines for the Management of Medullary Thyroid Carcinoma. Thyroid. 2015;25(6):567–610. http://online.liebertpub.com/doi/pdf/10.1089/thy.2014.0335

Twycross R, Wilcock A, Howard P, editors. Palliative care formulary (PCF5). 5th ed. UK: palliativedrugs.com; 2014. Territorial specific editions are available in Canada, Germany, Japan and the USA.

Twycross RG, Wilcock A, Howard P, editors. Palliative care formulary (PCF6). 6th ed. UK: palliativedrugs.com; 2017.

Cherny N, Fallon M, Kassa S, Portenoy RK, Currow D, editors. Oxford textbook of palliative medicine. 5th ed. Oxford: Oxford University Press; 2015.

Gawande A. Being mortal: medicine and what matters in the end. New York: Metropolitan Books; 2014.

Useful Websites

http://www.palliativedrugs.com/ (Features access to a very useful on-line palliative care formulary by annual subscription, a bulletin board for professionals together with regular updates covering topical issues in palliative care).

https://www.nice.org.uk/guidance/ng31 (covering the clinical care of adults during the last few days of life including guidance on recognition of dying, communication with patients and those important to them, symptom management and, anticipatory prescribing).

https://www.nice.org.uk/guidance/cg140 (covering safe and effective prescribing of strong opioids for pain relief in adults with advanced progressive disease last updated Aug 2016).

http://www.nescn.nhs.uk/common-themes/deciding-right/ (website providing guidance on decision-making at the end of life and a suite of documents designed for use in documenting end of life decisions – NHS UK).

http://www.e-lfh.org.uk/programmes/end-of-life-care/ (e-learning modules on end of life care – requires registration or access via Open Athens).

http://www.sign.ac.uk/guidelines/fulltext/44/. Features evidence-based guideline on pain management.

http://www.palliativecareguidelines.scot.nhs.uk/guidelines/symptom-control/Pruritis.aspx

Part IX

Future Developments and Directions for Research in Thyroid Cancer

Translational Research and Genomics Driven Trials in Thyroid Cancer

24

Maria E. Cabanillas, Rebecca E. Schweppe, Ramona Dadu, Gilbert J. Cote, Thomas C. Beadnell, and Marie Claude Hofmann

Introduction

Molecular targeted therapy has revolutionized the treatment of most malignancies, including thyroid cancer. Currently there are four drugs and one drug combination approved for advanced thyroid cancer—sorafenib and lenvatinib for differentiated thyroid cancer; and vandetanib and cabozantinib for medullary thyroid cancer (MTC); and dabrafenib plus trametinib for *BRAF* V600E mutated anaplastic thyroid cancer (ATC). While there is little data supporting extension of overall survival in DTC and MTC [1], all four FDA approved drugs have shown significant improvement in progression-free survival [2–5]. These drugs are also anti-angiogenic multikinase inhibitors and do not target any particular mutation selectively. The only FDA approved, mutation-driven targeted therapy in thyroid cancer is indicated for BRAF mutated ATC, however, mutation-driven targeted therapies have been studied in DTC and MTC. Table 24.1 shows the various targets for each of the FDA approved drugs for DTC and MTC.

There is a need to discover efficacious drugs for DTC and MTC that utilize different mechanisms of action than the currently approved anti-angiogenic drugs, for several reasons. First, since these drugs have multiple targets, they also have a significant number of toxicities. Some of these toxicities affect quality of life (e.g. diarrhea, fatigue, weight loss) while others are potentially life-threatening. For example, in some cases, it may not be safe for some patients to be exposed to anti-angiogenic inhibitors due to the potential for complications such as tracheoesophageal fistula [6, 7], hemoptysis [8], poor wound healing, gastrointestinal perforation, hypertension, and congestive heart failure. Thus, specifically and selectively targeting a particular mutation or other components of the tumor microenvironment is a desirable strategy in thyroid cancer, as it could reduce toxicity. Second, while the approved drugs delay progression, they do not cure the patient and virtually all patients stop responding to these drugs. Thus, an alternative class of drugs for patients who have progressed on anti-angiogenics (or who are not able to take these drugs) is needed. Furthermore, understanding the mechanisms underlying the emergence of resistance is critical to discovering agents that will effectively treat these patients. Mechanisms of resistance to targeted therapies are not well understood in thyroid cancer, largely because

M. C. Hofmann · G. J. Cote · R. Dadu
M. E. Cabanillas (✉)
Department of Endocrine Neoplasia and Hormonal Disorders, University of Texas MD Anderson Cancer Center, Houston, TX, USA
e-mail: mcabani@mdanderson.org

T. C. Beadnell · R. E. Schweppe
Endocrinology, Metabolism and Diabetes, University of Colorado, Aurora, CO, USA

U. K. Mallick et al. (eds.), *Practical Management of Thyroid Cancer*,
https://doi.org/10.1007/978-3-319-91725-2_24

Table 24.1 Molecular targets for the FDA approved drugs for differentiated and medullary thyroid cancer

Drug	VEGFR1	VEGFR2	VEGFR3	RET	c-KIT	Other
Cabozantinib		x		x	x	MET, TrkA
Lenvatinib	x		x	x	x	FGFR1–3
Sorafenib		x	x	x	x	RAF
Vandetanib		x		x	x	EGFR

Table 24.2 Targets for thyroid cancer and the associated selective drugs

	Targets of interest	Commercially available, selective agents	Investigational agents
Select mutations and genetic alterations	BRAFV600E mutations	Vemurafenib Dabrafenib	PLX8394
	RET mutations or RET/PTC rearrangements	–	LOXO-292 BLU-667 RXDX-105
	NTRK rearrangements	–	Entrectinib Larotrectinib LOXO-195
	ALK rearrangements	Crizotinib, ceritinib	Entrectinib
Cell signaling molecules	MEK	Cobimetinib, trametinib	Selumetinib RO5126766
	mTOR	Everolimus, temsirolimus, sirolimus	MLN0128
	SRC/FAK	Dasatinib	Defactinib GSK2256098
Immune checkpoints	CTLA-4	Ipilimumab	Tremelimumab
	PD-1	Pembrolizumab, nivolumab	PDR001 CA-170
	PD-L1	Atezolizumab, avelumab, durvalumab	
	OX-40	–	PF-04518600 MEDI6469
	LAG3	–	BMS-936558 LAG525
	4-1BB	–	Utomilumab Urelumab
Antibody-drug conjugates			Rovalpituzumab tesirine

serial biopsies in this small subset of patients on systemic therapy are frequently not obtained. However, "liquid biopsy" utilizing blood-based testing, discussed in this chapter, may be one way to facilitate our knowledge in this field.

Table 24.2 shows a list of potential targets in thyroid cancer beyond anti-angiogenic multikinase inhibitors that will be discussed in this chapter. Identifying some of these mutations in the absence of available tumor is also an area of research interest in thyroid cancer and will be discussed. Figure 24.1 shows the relevant signaling pathways and genetic aberrations discussed in this chapter.

Gene-Driven Targeted Therapies

BRAF Directed Therapy for Thyroid Cancer

BRAFV600E mutations are considered an early event driver mutation and results in the constitutive activation of the MAPK pathway leading to proliferation [9]. This mutation is the most common mutation found in papillary thyroid cancer (PTC), accounting for 40–80% of cases, and these tumors are known to be more radioiodine

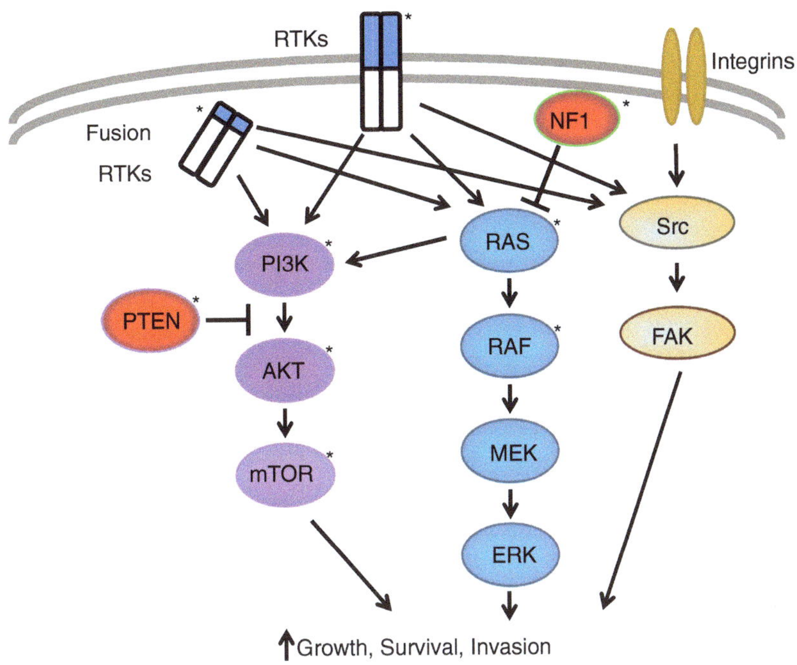

Fig. 24.1 Schematic overview of RTK, MAPK, PI3K, and Src/FAK signaling relevant to thyroid cancer. The asterick (*) indicate genetic alterations identified in thyroid cancer. RTKs (receptor tyrosine kinases) are typically activated by overexpression of the receptor itself or upstream growth factors. FAK and Src are activated by overexpression or by upstream integrin or RTK signaling. NF1 loss leads to activation of the RAS/MAPK pathway, and PTEN loss leads to activation of the PI3K pathway. Fusion RTKs, including NTRK, ALK, and RET, have the potential activate the PI3K, RAS, and Src/FAK signaling pathways

resistant [9]. The mutation is also fairly common in anaplastic thyroid cancer (ATC), present in approximately 25–50% of these tumors [10–12]. In ATC patients who have co-existing PTC in their tumor, the incidence of BRAF mutations would be expected to be much higher because PTC often transforms to ATC by accumulation of late event mutations [12]. Although BRAF mutations and fusions have been identified in MTC tumors [13–15], except for one series of Greek patients, the incidence appears to be very low.

Targeting BRAF mutations with selective BRAF inhibitors has been a successful strategy in melanoma patients who harbor this mutation [16–18]. Recently, the selective BRAF inhibitors, vemurafenib and dabrafenib, have been studied in both BRAF mutated PTC and ATC patients. Vemurafenib was studied in a phase 2 trial that included 51 BRAF-mutated PTC patients who had progression prior to trial entry [19]. Patients who were VEGFR inhibitor naïve (cohort 1) were analyzed separately from those who had been treated previously with a VEGFR inhibitor (cohort 2). Twenty-six patients were enrolled in cohort 1 and 25 in cohort 2. Partial responses were seen in 38.5% of patients in cohort 1 and 27.3% in cohort 2. The median progression-free survival (PFS) was 18.2 months in cohort 1 but significantly shorter in cohort 2, at 8.9 months. The most common grade 1–2 adverse event with vemurafenib were rash, fatigue, dysgeusia, weight loss, increased creatinine, and decrease appetite, nausea, arthralgias, hyperkeratosis, diarrhea, and photosensitivity. Squamous cell carcinomas of the skin were the most common grade 3–4 events.

Vemurafenib has also been studied as a neoadjuvant treatment prior to surgical resection in PTC (NCT01709292). Preliminary results for this clinical trial were presented at the European Thyroid Association in 2017 [20]. This trial enrolled BRAF mutated PTC patients who required either primary or revision surgery in the neck. Patients were treated for 56 days with single agent vemurafenib, were restaged on day 56 and then operated. It is important to note that progression was not a requirement for trial entry. Of 17 patients, 14 completed the 56 days on vemurafenib and were restaged. Of those restaged, 10 experienced stable disease (9 with regression of tumor, −6% to −26%), 3 partial responses, and 1 progression. Eleven of 17 (65%) patients underwent surgery on the trial. Six patients (35%) did not complete surgery due to toxicity (n = 4), progression (n = 1) or patient refusal (n = 1). Eight of the 11 operated patients had R0/R1 pathologic resection, while 3 had R2 resections. The investigators concluded that neoadjuvant vemurafenib was well tolerated and a reasonable strategy for patients with extensive, BRAF mutated PTC but that a randomized neoadjuvant trial to determine if this approach extends disease-free survival is needed.

Another study in BRAF mutated PTC using dabrafenib [NCT01723202] with or without trametinib (a selective MEK inhibitor) has completed enrollment and results were recently reported [21]. Progression was a requirement for trial entry. In this study, the effect of adding trametinib to dabrafenib either at start of treatment or at progression with dabrafenib alone was explored. Fifty three patients were randomized to either dabrafenib (total n = 26; 22 assessable) or dabrafenib + trametinib (total n = 27; 24 assessable). In the single agent dabrafenib arm, 45% of patients experienced a partial response and only 2 (9%) had progression as their best response. In the combination dabrafenib + trametinib arm, 37.5% of patients experienced a partial response with only 1 (4%) experiencing progression as their best response. Median PFS was 11.4 (single agent arm) and 15.1 months (combination arm; p = 0.27). The median duration of response was 15.6 and 13.3 months (p = 0.87) in the single agent and combination arms, respectively. Both arms showed reasonable tolerability but there was more alopecia, hyperglycemia, weight loss and skin/subcutaneous tissue disorders in the single agent arm, while there was more blurred vision, limb edema, liver function test abnormalities, and anorexia in the combination arm.

Dabrafenib was also studied to restore the ability of tumors to concentrate radioactive iodine in PTC patients [22]. Ten patients with BRAF mutated, RAI-refractory PTC were treated with dabrafenib for 25 days and then reimaged with whole body scan I-123. Those found to concentrate RAI were treated an additional 17 days before receiving 150 mCi of I-131. Six of the ten patients had new RAI uptake seen on WBS. After 3 months, 2 patients experienced partial response and 4 had stable disease by RECIST criteria. Other clinical trials with BRAF inhibitors to restore RAI uptake are ongoing (NCT02145143, NCT02456701).

In ATC, there are several case reports with selective BRAF inhibitors with or without MEK inhibitors that have shown impressive results [10, 23] and most recently, dabrafenib plus trametinib was approved for *BRAF* mutated ATC. The approval was based on the ongoing basket trial that included *BRAF* mutated ATC, studying dabrafenib plus trametinib [NCT02034110] [24]. Sixteen patients were enrolled at the first data cutoff. The median age was 72 years and all patients had a performance status of <2. All but one patient was confirmed to have a BRAFV600E mutation. Responses were confirmed independently in 63% of patients, and only 3 (19%) patients had a best response of progressive disease. Median PFS and overall survival (OS) were not reached due to lack of events at the time of data cutoff, however, 79% and 80% were without progression or death events at 1 year, respectively. There were no fatal adverse events, however in two patients, adverse events led to treatment discontinuation. The most common adverse events were fatigue (38%), pyrexia (37%) and nausea (35%).

RET Directed Therapies

Activation of the RET oncogene occurs in MTC and PTC. In MTC, RET point mutations are seen in approximately 50% of sporadic cases and 95% of hereditary cases [25]. In PTC, RET is activated due to RET/PTC rearrangements and is present in around 20% of these patients. This genetic rearrangement is more common in thyroid cancer patients with radiation exposure and in young patients [26–29].

There are four approved drugs for thyroid cancer that target RET, however, it is unknown if these drugs lead to responses via this mechanism, as they are also anti-angiogenic drugs. However, two selective RET inhibitors drugs, LOXO-292 [30] and BLU-667 [31], are undergoing clinical development. Both of these drugs have completed phase 1 and are in expansion phase [NCT03157128 and NCT03037385]. Both drugs target resistance mutations that emerge after multi-kinase inhibitor therapy and are being tested in all RET-driven tumors. The results of the phase 1 trials have recently been presented at national meetings [32, 33]. The response rate in RET mutated MTC for BLU-667 and LOXO-292 was 40% and 45%, respecively. The LOXO-292 response rate in the 7 patients with RET fusion DTC was 100%. A selective RET/BRAF inhibitor, RXDX-105, is being studied in a first-in-human study [NCT01877881l] [34]. Initial reports suggest that the drug may have efficacy in RET mutated or BRAF mutated thyroid cancer. Three BRAF mutated PTC patients were reported, of which the best response was stable disease in 2 and progression in 1 patient. One patient with RET918 mutated MTC achieved an unconfirmed partial response of −38%.

NTRK Directed Therapy

The NTRK 1, 2, and 3 genes encode for the tropomyosin receptor kinase receptor (Trk) family of proteins, Trk A, B, and C. Genetic rearrangements of the NTRK genes result in activation of the MAPK and PI3K/AKT pathways, leading to proliferation and growth of tumors. NTRK rearrangements occur in several adult and pediatric tumors, including approximately 2–5% of papillary thyroid carcinomas [26, 35–37]. These patients tend to be younger and do not typically harbor the other common mutations seen in PTC. Thus far, two clinical trials with the NTRK inhibitors, entrectinib and larotrectinib, have been reported, however only the larotrectinib trial included patients with NTRK fusion thyroid cancer. Compiled data from 3 larotrectinib clinical trials (NCT02576431, NCT02122913, and NCT02637687) that included a total of 55 patients were recently reported [38]. Of these 55 patients, 5 (9%) had thyroid cancer (histology not specified). The overall response rate was 78%, and all 5 of the thyroid cancer patients achieved an objective response—4 partial and 1 complete response. Median PFS was not reached. The drug was considered tolerable with the most common adverse events including fatigue, dizziness, anemia, and vomiting. Resistance mutations were observed in 6 patients (none of whom had thyroid cancer) and the first 2 patients were treated successfully with the second generation NTRK inhibitor, LOXO-195 [NCT03215511]. A recent, public presentation at the World Congress on Thyroid Cancer 2017 described a remarkable response in an ATC patients with NTRK3 fusion treated with entrectinib.

Anaplastic Lymphoma Kinase (ALK)-Rearrangements

ALK fusions are rare events in thyroid cancer. These are found in tumors that do not harbor the more common mutations such as BRAF, RAS, RET/PTC and are more common in poorly differentiated and ATC, but are also reported in very low frequency in PTC. Kelly et al. reported the frequency of ALK rearrangements to be 9% in PDTC, 4% in ATC and 1.6% in PTC [39]. One year after this publication, a case of an ATC patient with ALK fusion treated with crizotinib, a commercially available ALK inhibitor, was reported [40]. There was only short term follow up information published on this patient, however, she achieved a 90% reduction in target lesions by RECIST. One trial using ceritinib [19] in patients with ALK rearranged ATC is currently enrolling patients (NCT02289144). Other trials that are currently enrolling are basket trials that include thyroid cancer patients using entrectinib, an inhibitor of NTRK, ROS, and ALK (STARTRK-1 NCT02097810 and STARTRK-2

NCT02568267). Given the rarity of these fusions in thyroid cancer, it remains to be seen if sufficient ALK rearranged thyroid cancer patients can be enrolled to determine if this class of drugs is effective in this disease.

Pathway Inhibitors

MAPK Pathway: MEK Inhibitors

The MAP kinase pathway accounts for the majority of mutations found in thyroid cancer, with a high prevalence of *BRAF* and *RAS* mutations, making this pathway an attractive therapeutic target for thyroid cancer (Fig. 24.1). Agents targeting MEK1/2 were the first inhibitors developed to target this pathway, with PD98059 initially discovered [41, 42]. MEK1/2 inhibitors are allosteric inhibitors, and act independent of ATP, therefore allowing for higher selectivity [42, 43]. Despite promising preclinical results, it took 18 years for the first MEK1/2 inhibitor, trametinib, to be approved for BRAF-mutant melanoma [43]. Clinical development of MEK1/2 inhibitors has been hampered by low potency, thus, it is no surprise that a phase II trial with the MEK1/2 inhibitor, selumetinib (AZD6244) in RAI refractory papillary thyroid cancer resulted in only 3% of patients exhibiting a partial response, 54% with stable disease, and 28% with progressive disease, which failed to meet the 20% overall response rate criteria, and thus failed to meet the trial's primary endpoint [44]. With the exception of melanoma, the efficacy of targeting MEK1/2 in the clinic has been modest, likely due to weak inhibition of MEK1/2 itself, through the relief of negative feedback mechanisms, and rapid reprogramming of the kinome [45–48]. While newer generation MEK1/2 inhibitors, including trametinib (GSK1120212), CH5126766 (RO5126766), and GDC-0623, also have the limitation of inhibiting the negative feedback mechanism, this class of inhibitors result in sustained inhibition of ERK1/2 phosphorylation by reducing RAF phosphorylation of MEK1/2, resulting in higher efficacy in KRAS-mutant tumor models [48–51]. In contrast, the MEK1/2 inhibitor, cobimetinib (GDC-0973), does not block RAF phosphorylation of MEK, but has a higher binding affinity for activated MEK, likely accounting for its higher efficacy in BRAF-mutant tumors which require more potent inhibition of MEK1/2 [48–51]. Thus, it is important to understand the mechanisms of these MEK inhibitors in order to effectively target this pathway in the clinic.

As with BRAF inhibitors, MEK inhibitors have been explored in order to re-establish RAI uptake in DTC based on preclinical studies demonstrating that inhibition of the MAPK pathway promotes an increase in expression of the sodium iodide symporter (NIS) [52, 53]. The MEK1/2 inhibitor, selumetinib, was given for 4 weeks to patients who met criteria for RAI-refractory disease. If I-124 PET indicated restoration of RAI uptake, patients were treated with I-131. Of 20 evaluable patients, selumetinib increased the uptake in 12 patients, of which 8 reached dosimetry threshold and were treated with I-131. Of the 8 RAI treated patients, 5 achieved a partial response. Long-term follow up was not available in order to assess overall survival. Interestingly, both *BRAF*- and *RAS*-mutant tumors benefited from this therapy [54]. Two clinical trials (NCT01843062, NCT02393690) utilizing this strategy have since opened but results are not yet available.

More recently, Nagarajah and colleagues demonstrated that a sustained reduction of ERK1/2 phosphorylation, using the RO5126766 MEK1/2 inhibitor discussed above, correlates with enhanced uptake of RAI, indicating that only a short exposure to a more potent MEK1/2 inhibitor, such as RO5126766, may be sufficient to induce iodide uptake [52].

mTOR Pathway

Multiple studies in different tumor types have highlighted the efficacy of targeting both the MAPK and PI3K pathway [55–58]. There are three published phase 2 clinical trials using single agent everolimus in thyroid cancer. The first such publication was in a Korean population of patients with all subtypes of thyroid cancer [59]. Responses were mostly stable disease (76%) with only two partial responses (5%; one PTC, one FTC) and 7 (18%) patients experiencing progression as their best response. PFS was longest in the MTC patients (not reached) and shortest in ATC patients (10 weeks). DTC patients had a PFS of 43 weeks. A group of investigators in the Netherlands reported results in follicular-derived thyroid cancers (28 DTC, 7 ATC) [60]. There were no complete or partial responses, 65% showed stable disease and 39% showed progression as their best response. Median PFS and OS for the entire study group was 9 and 18 months, respectively. A group of investigators in the United States reported similar responses, however, this population of patients differed from the Korean and Dutch population in that patients had to have progression within 6 months prior to enrollment [61]. Thus, this group may have had more rapidly advancing disease. All subtypes of thyroid cancer were included in this trial. There were three responses among the 50 patients treated (one partial response in MTC and DTC and one very remarkable complete response in ATC which was later published as a case report [62]). PFS in the DTC and MTC cohorts was 12.9 and 13.1 months, respectively. In all three trials, the most common adverse events were stomatitis/mucositis and anorexia. A clinical trial in ATC with a second generation, pan-mTOR kinase inhibitor, MLN0128 is underway (NCT02244463).

Of importance, a recent salvage therapy case for a patient with ATC treated with the B-Raf inhibitor, dabrafenib, and the MEK1/2 inhibitor, trametinib, utilized rpS6 phosphorylation status as an indicator for a lack of responsiveness to the targeted therapies [63]. Importantly, upon observing rpS6 phosphorylation, post-treatment, the mTOR inhibitor, everolimus, was added to the therapeutic regimen, and a dramatic regression in tumor volume was observed [63]. This and another recent study supports the examination of rpS6 as a biomarker of response for the combined inhibition of the MAPK kinase and PI3K pathways in thyroid and other tumor types [64, 65].

SRC/FAK Pathway

The Src and Focal Adhesion Kinase (FAK) pathway play key roles in cancer progression, especially in relation to invasion and metastasis [66]. In addition, Src is a common point of convergence of many tyrosine kinase signaling pathways, thus targeting this pathway has the potential to block multiple pro-tumorigenic signaling pathways. Recent studies have shown that FAK is overexpressed and activated in thyroid patient tumor samples, and FAK mRNA expression may be correlated with a more aggressive phenotype [67–69]. In support of thyroid tumors being dependent on the Src-FAK pathway, preclinical studies have demonstrated targeting Src inhibits thyroid cancer growth, invasion, and metastasis [70–74]. Of interest, Schweppe et al. have shown that Src signals independently of the MAP kinase pathway, suggesting that the activation of Src represents an independent pro-tumorigenic pathway in thyroid cancer, which likely plays a key role in promoting tumor aggressiveness and metastasis [70].

There are currently four FDA approved inhibitors, which target Src, including dasatinib, bosutinib, ponatinib, and vandetanib [75]. With the exception of vandetanib, these inhibitors are clinically approved for the treatment of hematological malignancies [76]. While preclinical studies have demonstrated that Src inhibition results in the inhibition of cell growth, as well as invasion and metastasis, these studies have been difficult to translate to the clinic for solid tumors. Similar to early generation MEK1/2 inhibitors, the lack of efficacy of Src inhibitors in solid tumors may be due to insufficient inhibition of Src or due to the lack of biomarkers for targeting this pathway [77]. Nonetheless, promising results were recently observed in a phase II study of dasatinib in metastatic castrate resistant prostate cancer, in which 87% of patients had bone metastases, and dasatinib treatment resulted in 43% of patients exhibiting stable disease at 12 weeks, and 19% of patients exhibiting stable disease at 24 weeks [78, 79]. In addition, one non-small cell lung cancer patient exhibited a complete response to dasatinib, likely due to expression of a kinase impaired BRAF mutation [79]. Together, these studies highlight a need to better understand the role of Src in tumorigenesis, as well as key mechanisms of resistance to effectively target this pathway in the clinic. Indeed, recent studies by Beadnell et al. demonstrated a key role for the MAP kinase pathway in promoting resistance to Src-directed therapies, providing the necessary framework for a future clinical trial targeting Src and MEK1/2 in thyroid cancer [72].

Finally, whereas MAPK pathway regulation of NIS has primarily been demonstrated to function at the transcriptional level, it has also been demonstrated that the cellular localization of NIS can also be regulated by Src mediated phosphorylation of the pituitary tumor–transforming gene-binding factor (PBF) [80]. Specifically, Src mediated phosphorylation of PBF sequesters NIS from the plasma membrane, and results in a reduction in iodine uptake [81]. Taken together, both the MAPK and Src pathways may play important roles in regulating NIS expression and localization, as well as radioactive iodine uptake in thyroid cancers, and warrants further investigation.

Targeting the Microenvironment

Immune Checkpoint Therapy in Cancer

"Evading immune destruction" was recently introduced as one of the ten hallmarks of cancer [82]. It is now well understood that tumors are capable of escaping the immune response through a number of mechanisms. Specifically, the discovery of immune checkpoints has revolutionized the field of immunotherapy. Cytotoxic T-lymphocyte-associated protein 4 (CTLA-4) blocking antibodies were the first in class for checkpoint blockade. Ipilimumab was the first agent to demonstrate benefit in melanoma patients and was approved by the US Food and Drug Administration in 2011. Since, then the field of immune checkpoints has grown significantly. Several checkpoint therapies inhibiting the interaction between programmed death 1 (PD1) and its ligand programmed death-ligand 1 (PD-L1) have been approved. Other immune inhibitory (LAG3, TIM3, VISTA, BTLA, KIR, etc.) and costimulatory pathways (CD-40, OX-40, 4-1BB, GITR, etc.) have been discovered and antagonistic or agonistic antibodies are in clinical development. The use of these drugs as monotherapy or as part of combinational strategies enhance immunity with the potential to produce durable clinical responses and prolong survival. However, the exponential growth of clinical applications has not been paralleled by the discovery of a predictive biomarker of response. Although many studies demonstrated correlations between the degree of PD-L1 expression and response, there are patients with tumors negative for PD-L1 expression who responded to these therapies suggesting that PD-L1 expression alone should not be use as a sole predictive marker. Furthermore, there are growing data suggesting that PD-L1 expression in the tumor is most compelling when it is observed in the context of an active T cell response, and that the ongoing T cell response itself, not PD-L1 expression, is the key factor [83].

Immune Microenvironment and Experience with Immunotherapy in Thyroid Cancer

A growing body of literature has described the tumor-associated immune response in thyroid cancers. Similar to other cancer types, both an anti-tumor response (cytotoxic CD8+ T lymphocytes and natural killer cells) and immune evasion mechanisms (pro-inflammatory mast cells, tumor associated macrophages, regulatory T cells, PD1/PD-L1 mediated dysfunction) are present in thyroid cancer.

In DTC, several studies have shown that T cell dysfunction plays a role in DTC progression [84–92]. As PD-L1 expression is being considered as a potential biomarker for response of anti-PD1 or anti-PD-L1 drugs, several of these studies have also assessed the frequency of PD-L1 positivity. PD-L1 expression in DTC varies greatly depending on the study, ranging from

6% to 88%. Additionally, correlations between PD-L1 expression and outcomes are controversial. In the most recent study including a large number of samples, membranous PD-L1 expression on tumor cells of ≥1% was found in 6.1% of papillary and 7.6% of follicular thyroid cancer. In contrast with previous studies, no significant prognostic value of PD-L1 expression in predicting poorer cancer-specific survival or disease-free survival was observed [86]. Multiple factors may contribute to the wide range of PD-L1 positivity and outcome correlations reported across studies, including different patient populations, type of samples tested, antibodies used, methods of analysis, location of PD-L1 (membranous versus cytoplasmic) and thresholds. In clinical practice, single agent pembrolizumab (anti PD1 antibody) was tested in DTC in a phase 1b study (KEYNOTE-028) [93]. Of all patients screened for the trial, 71% had PD-L1 positive tumors (≥1% PD-L1 expression by immunohistochemistry). Despite enrolling only patients with PD-L1 positive tumors (≥ 1% expression), response rates were somewhat low, with PR in 2/22 (9%) patients, SD in 12/22 (55%) patients and PD in 8/22 (36%) patients. Median PFS was 6.8 months (95% CI, 1.9–14.1). Median OS had not yet been reached (95% CI, 18.6 months-NR). The 6- and 12-month OS rates were 100% and 89.9%, respectively [93]. In thyroid cancer, based on preclinical and clinical data, we predict that there will be several limitations in the use of immunotherapy and that combination strategies will almost certainly be needed. The VEGFR TKIs and molecular targeted therapy have dominated thyroid cancer therapeutics. This approach is likely to remain an important component in the treatment of this disease. However, the cure rates are low, the responses are only partial and short lived and patients remain on drug for prolonged periods of time causing long term toxicity. On the other hand, treatment with immunotherapy is typically associated with lower response rates, but they are durable. A clinical trial using combination lenvatinib plus pembrolizumab is underway (NCT02973997). Another approach is the use of immunotherapy and radiation. One trial with RAI and immunotherapy in DTC is ongoing (NCT03215095). Another trial with stereotactic body radiotherapy (SBRT) with immunotherapy is enrolling an extension cohort with all thyroid cancer subtypes (NCT02239900).

In ATC, small sample size studies showed that PD-1 and PD-L1 expressions were high and they appear to represent predictive markers for PFS and OS [86, 87, 94, 95]. Immunoprofiling of a large ATC cohort showed that both PD-L1 positive cells and tumor infiltrating lymphocytes (TILs) are present in high frequency. Additionally, strong positive correlations between tumor cells expressing PD-L1 and TILs exist. Although not statistically significant, higher PD-L1 expression was observed in BRAF positive tumors [96]. These data point to the presence of a "hot" immunogenic environment that can be targeted with immune based therapies. A clinical trial with single agent pembrolizumab is recruiting patients (NCT02688608). However, in an immunocompetent model of BRAF/p53 mutated ATC, it was shown that the combination of anti PD-L1 antibody with BRAF inhibitor dramatically reduced tumor volume compared to each agent alone. Additionally, immunohistochemistry analysis revealed intense CD8+ T cell infiltration and cytotoxicity with the combination compared to each individual treatment [97]. These data suggests that anti PD-L1 treatment potentiates the effect of BRAF inhibitor on tumor regression and intensifies antitumor immune response, leading to the conclusion that the combinational approach may be more beneficial. Clinically, the aggressiveness of ATC requires a therapy to provide significant decrease in the tumor burden in order for immunotherapy to work. A clinical trial using this approach is underway (NCT03181100). The study uses a backbone of atezolizumab (anti-PDL1 antibody). Depending on the mutation, patients will receive targeted therapy (vemurafenib/cobimetinib for BRAF mutated; cobimetinib for RAS mutated; bevacizumab for other) or cytotoxic chemotherapy (nab-paclitaxel) if they do not qualify for targeted therapy. Two clinical trials using combination radiotherapy with immunotherapy are recruiting patients with metastatic ATC (NCT03122496; NCT02239900).

In MTC, several small tumor vaccine and radioimmunotherapy studies were performed in the past with promising activity, but these approaches remain investigational [98–101]. Recent preclinical studies have attempted to characterize the expression of immune markers in MTC specimens, leading to the conclusion that most MTCs are "cold" non-immunogenic environments, with low PD-L1 expression and low frequency of TILs [102, 103]. Currently, there are no data on efficacy of immune checkpoint therapy in MTC. A clinical trial using pembrolizumab in patients with MTC divided in two groups based on prior treatment with immune stimulating vaccine is enrolling patients (NCT03072160). As in other types of cancers with similar "cold" nonimmunogenic tumor microenvironment, a combination strategy with kinase inhibitor drugs or radiotherapy that create an immunogenic environment and immune checkpoint therapy may result in durable clinical benefit. A thyroid cancer extension cohort is currently enrolling MTC patients (NCT02239900).

Antibody Drug Conjugates

Antibody drug conjugates (ADCs) combine the specificity of antibodies to the toxicity of agents such as cytotoxic drug or radionucleotides (such as yttrium-90). ADCs piggyback a toxin onto an antibody that is specific for a particular target. The antibody finds its target and the cell internalizes the toxin, leading to cell death. ADCs are a clever way to spare normal tissue and avoid the off-target effects of kinase inhibitors. This is not a new concept in oncology but the first ADC, gemtuzumab ozogamicin, was withdrawn due to lack of efficacy in phase III trials and cases of fatal liver toxicity. Since then, several other ADCs have been approved (ado-trastuzumab emtansine, brentuximab vedotin, ibritumomab tiuxetan) for various cancers. ADCs, have only recently been used in the thyroid cancer world with the initiation of a trial using rovalpituzumab tesirine for neuroendocrine tumors, including MTC (NCT02709889). Rovalpituzumab tesirine consists of a DLL3-specific IgG1 monoclonal antibody, conjugated to a DNA-damaging pyrrolobenzodiazepine dimer toxin. DLL3 is a member of the Notch receptor ligand family that appears to inhibit Notch receptor activation. DLL3 is upregulated in 64% of MTC tumors [104]. Reports of MTC patients treated with this drug are not available at this time.

Resistance Mechanisms

Overcoming Resistance to Targeted Therapies

Pharmacological inhibitors of BRAFV600E such as vemurafenib and dabrafenib increase PFS in thyroid cancer patients harboring the mutation [19, 105, 106]. While many patients will initially respond to treatment with these inhibitors, their responses are incomplete and the disease progresses within 8–18 months [105, 107]. Distant metastases are the major cause of tumor-related death. In an attempt to overcome this problem, BRAF V600E inhibitors have been combined with the MEK inhibitor, trametinib, however incidences of acquired resistance have already been reported [108, 109]. Resistance to kinase inhibitors presents a significant therapeutic challenge in thyroid cancer patients, and identifying the mechanisms that allow cancer cells to bypass targeted therapies is critical to improving patient outcomes.

Acquired resistance to BRAF inhibitors has been extensively studied in melanoma and colon cancers. Deep *BRAF* (exons 2–18) sequence analysis of vemurafenib-resistant melanoma tissues indicated that secondary BRAF V600E mutations responsible for vemurafenib-acquired resistance are rare [110], although a mutation in the kinase domain was recently found [111]. Secondary resistance to BRAF inhibitors can therefore mainly be attributed to other mechanisms. Some of them are epigenetic, as higher expression of *KIT, MET, EGFR, NRAS* and *PDGFRβ* at the mRNA and protein levels are not associated with genomic DNA copy number gain, nor mutational activation [110, 112–114]. Consequently overexpression of any receptor tyrosine kinase has the potential to reactivate the MAPK pathway [115, 116] or the PI3K pathway [117–120]. Further, growth factors production is often up-regulated in an autocrine manner in cancer cells, and experimental data have shown that most cells can be rescued from drug sensitivity by simply exposing them to one or more receptor tyrosine kinase (RTK) ligands [121]. These results indicate that changes in the microenvironment can account, at least in part, for drug resistance. Consequently, exposure to hepatocyte growth factor (HGF) from the stromal microenvironment for example will promote intrinsic resistance to BRAF inhibitors in cells overexpressing the MET receptor [122]. Vemurafenib resistance in melanoma can also be induced by over-expression of EPHA2, a member of the Ephrin receptor family of tyrosine kinases [123], which mediates cancer progression and cell migration. Finally, other mechanisms of acquired resistance in melanoma, colorectal cancers or derived cell lines can be attributed to additional mutations in the *NRAS* or *KRAS* genes [110, 124, 125], expression of a splice variant of BRAFV600E with enhanced dimerization properties [124, 126], and overexpression of MAP 3K8 (COT) [124, 127], a MAPK pathway agonist activating ERK through a MEK-dependent mechanism that does not require RAF activation.

Overcoming acquired resistance in BRAF-mutated PTC has been challenging because targeting MEK downstream of mutated BRAF with the MEK inhibitors selumetinib and trametinib, alone or in combination with BRAF inhibitors, may not necessarily prevent emergence of resistance. Multiple mechanisms have been proposed for how PTC cells escape the inhibitory control. Studies by Montero-Conde and colleagues demonstrated that BRAF-mutated PTC cell lines acquired resistance to vemurafenib by reactivating the MAPK pathway and over-expressing the ERBB or FGF receptor families [128]. Adaptive resistance to BRAF inhibitors can also depend on MET-mediated reactivation of the PI3K/AKT pathway in preclinical models [129]. Genomic alterations mediating acquired resistance have also been detected: in one patient, high copy number gain of the gene MCL1 and loss of CDKN2A (P16) have been associated with resistance to vemurafenib treatment [130]. Therefore, in addition to adaptive activation of alternate signaling or regulatory pathways, genomic heterogeneity of thyroid cancer cells under drug selection may lead to accelerated clonal evolution and emergence of more aggressive genotypes. So far, most translational studies aimed at elucidating mechanisms of resistance to BRAF inhibition in PTCs have used short-term *in vitro* experiments [128, 130]. In order to identify acquisition of secondary resistance mechanisms due to selective pressure through chronic inhibitor treatment, Danysh et al. recently investigated the consequences of long-term exposure of BRAFV600E PTC cells with different doses of vemurafenib (0, 0.5, 1.0 μg/mL) [131]. The fate of these cells was followed over a period of 5 months. Long-term vemurafenib treatment induced changes in gene expression associated with activation of PI3K/AKT and MAPK pathways dependent on up-regulation of MET, EGF AND ERBB receptors as previously described [128, 129]. However, the authors also identified a subpopulation of cells harboring a KRAS mutation (KRAS G12D) concurrent with BRAFV600E, which conferred significant proliferative and invasive advantages to the cells. Importantly, this same KRAS (G12D) mutation was recently found in a BRAF V600E PTC patient after dabrafenib treatment (clinical trial NCT01723202, personal communication from the trial leader Dr. M. Shah). Interestingly, KRAS (G12D)-mutated cells were also resistant to MEK inhibition. It is generally believed that genetic alterations in the *RAS* and *BRAF* genes are mutually exclusive in primary PTC tumors, and RAS and BRAF mutations in the same thyroid cancer cells have only been recently found in PDTC and ATC [132], confirming that the acquisition of RAS leads to more aggressive poorly differentiated disease. To elucidate whether the cell population already contained a small proportion of KRAS (G12D)-mutated cells selected by vemurafenib treatment, or whether vemurafenib itself induced the mutation possibly by downregulating normal DNA repair enzymes, the authors performed droplet-digital™ PCR (ddPCR). Result indicated that at passage 21 of long-term vemurafenib treatment, 50% of cells harbored the

KRAS G12D mutation, while control cells without BRAF inhibitors harbored the BRAF V600E mutation only. Therefore, this model confirmed that RAS-driven acquired resistance leads to progression of PTC, and demonstrated that selection of hot-spot mutations through BRAF inhibition is a plausible mechanism. Understanding PTC tumor heterogeneity and mutational patterns emerging under drug pressure is fundamental to improving clinical studies and will help investigate mechanisms of disease progression.

Because reactivation of ERK itself is a major mechanism of resistance in response to RAF and MEK inhibitors [133, 134], recent efforts have focused on the inhibition of ERK itself [135]. In support of ERK as a therapeutic target, pharmacologic inhibition of ERK with the novel SCH772984 compound has been shown to overcome resistance to RAF and MEK inhibitors, and is effective in a subset of RAS-mutant cancer cell lines [135–138]. Based on these studies, the first ERK inhibitor has entered human clinical trials (BVD-523 ERK inhibitor: NCT01781429; NCT02296242; NCT02608229). However, there is little known about ERK inhibition and potential resistance mechanisms, and whether these molecular responses will be similar to those observed in response to RAF or MEK inhibition. Thus, it will be of interest to evaluate ERK inhibitors in preclinical models of thyroid cancer. In summary, these studies indicate that through a better understanding of why thyroid tumors exhibit increased resistance to targeted therapies against the MAPK pathway, we will be able to define biomarkers that will better define which patients will respond to MAPK pathway targeted therapies, as well as potential combination therapies.

Circulating Tumor DNA as a Potential Thyroid Cancer Biomarker

As detailed in other chapters of this book circulating tumor biomarkers play a routine role in the care and management of thyroid cancer patient. For patients with differentiated thyroid cancer (DTC) circulating thyroglobulin serves as indirect measure of tumor burden, while calcitonin serves a similar role in MTC. Despite the central roles of these and other biomarkers their utility is not universal, can at times be uninformative, or in rare cases misleading. Examples include the absence of biomarkers for ATC, the interference of anti-thyroglobulin antibodies in DTC patients, and the limited correlations of biomarker expression level with tumor observed burden. Furthermore, with the expanded use of systemic therapy in thyroid cancer patients it becomes essential to understand how treatment impacts biomarker expression. Differentiating agents can lead to increased biomarker expression without tumor growth, while some treatments have been reported to have direct effects on biomarker gene expression [54, 139, 140].

In the search for the next generation of cancer biomarkers the measurement of circulating tumor DNA, more commonly referred to as "liquid biopsy", has perhaps garnered the most interest [141–143]. The concept is not new, and stems from the established observation that the level of cell free DNA (cfDNA) in circulation is increased under certain physiological conditions involving either tissue trauma, including cancer, or pregnancy. The primary driving forces behind the examination of circulating cfDNA is that it potentially provides a minimally invasive approach to obtain the mutation profile of a patient tumor, which in turn would allow for personalization of therapy. Compared with tissue biopsy, a blood-based biopsy provides an opportunity to study tumor when biopsy is not possible because of tumor location or previously removed specimens are not available for testing. Furthermore, there are clear advantages to using blood as a surrogate to study the tumors targeted for treatment rather than previously removed surgical specimens. For MTC there are examples where the mutation status of the metastatic lesions has diverged from that of their primary tumor counterpart [144, 145]. A recent study has brought to light the realization that such a difference may be even greater for nonmedullary thyroid cancer [146]. A particularly pertinent finding of this study was that rate of BRAF mutation in distant metastases was approximately half of what was observed in primary tumors. This would suggest that targeted therapy based solely on primary tumor tissue analysis would lead to a high percentage of inappropriate targeting of therapy. Thus the perceived benefits associated with therapeutic targeting alone are serving to drive the implementation of liquid biopsy into clinical practice. A role for liquid biopsy in thyroid cancer is currently largely exploratory. DTC and MTC studies have found a concordance less than 50% between mutations determined through liquid biopsy and tumor tissue raising questions as to how to implement clinical use [147–149]. By comparison a single study has demonstrated a high level of concordance in untreated ATC patients clearly highlighting the use of this approach where rapid initiation of treatment is essential [150].

The use of circulating cfDNA as a prognostic biomarker is a more recent undertaking, as it requires the ability to quantitatively distinguish tumor-specific DNA from normal circulating DNA with a high degree of specificity and sensitivity. This is where recent technological advances have come into play. Tumor DNA differs from normal DNA as a result of the somatic changes imparted to drive oncogenesis. While these can include epigenetic changes, gene rearrangements, and copy number changes, tumor-specific DNA point mutations are perhaps the most common approach to distinguishing tumor-derived DNA from normal DNA in the circulation. While several methods allow detection of tumor specific DNA mutations, next-generation sequencing and digital PCR provide a quantitative approach. The number of mutated versus unmutated genes can be compared by counting individual copies of each in a single patient sample. Based on the assumption that all mutated DNA is derived from tumor cells an allelic fraction is calculated. Therefore, the greater the contribution of tumor DNA, the higher the allelic fraction will be. While a complete understanding of the mechanisms contributing to the release of tumor DNA into the circulation is lacking, tumor cell death is thought to be the primary source. Therefore, the derived allelic fraction is dependent on both tumor burden and factors associated with cell death, with response to therapy being a key determinant. Thus for nearly all cancer types studied to date, strong correlations exist where larger allelic fractions are associated with worse prognosis and reductions in allelic fraction following treatment is associated with response [142, 143]. Unfortunately, there is a growing appreciation that allelic fraction is also dependent on portion of tumor cells harboring the specific DNA mutation being monitored. Thus in a PTC patient with an established BRAF V600E mutation in the primary tumor, a low allelic fraction could result from either slowly progressing tumor that is not seeing much cell death compared to a tumor where the major of cells have lost the mutated gene as a mechanism of either progression or resistance to therapy. These are nuances associated with using circulating tumor DNA as a biomarker that will need to be addressed with further study. At least for now a limited dataset suggests that detection of circulating tumor DNA in thyroid cancer patients is associated with worse prognosis and temporal reductions are predictive of response to treatment [147, 149–151].

Conclusions/Summary

While we currently approach advanced thyroid cancer based on histology, in the future we may approach the different types of thyroid cancers based on the molecular or microenvironment aberration driving tumor growth. In fact, the FDA recently approved pembrolizumab for adult and pediatric patients with unresectable or metastatic solid tumors with microsatellite instability—the first tissue/site agnostic indication. This will likely hold true for other drugs such as NTRK and selective RET inhibitors. Another approach in the future would be to construct patient derived xenografts from cultured cells taken from patients to truly personalize the therapy for patients. However, this approach is limited by the time and cost to make these models.

We have likely only begun to understand the drivers of aggressive tumor behavior. Liquid biopsy provides one avenue to be able to identify patients with these aggressive tumors and explore resistance mechanisms in real-time in order to make changes to treatment more efficiently. Along with the enormous number of targeted therapies that are being explored and a better understanding of possible targets and mechanisms of resistance, more effective therapeutic options for patients with thyroid cancer are on the horizon. Immunotherapy may also help to destroy tumor cells that have developed new mutations and have escaped control with targeted therapy. We are just starting to evaluate immunotherapy in thyroid cancer and, as in other solid tumors, this approach will surely continue to expand into vaccines, T-cell engineering, and ADCs in the near future.

Disclosures/Conflict of Interest Statement Dr. Cabanillas has received research funding from Roche, Exelixis and Eisai and has received compensation for participation on advisory boards for LOXO, Blueprint and Ignyta. Dr. Dadu has received research funding from Eisai and consulting fees from Bristol-Myers Squibb.

Drs. Hofmann, Schweppe, Beadnell and Cote have no conflicts of interest.

References

1. Brose MS, Schlumberger M, Tahara M, Wirth LJ, Robinson B, Elisei R, et al. Effect of age and lenvatinib treatment on overall survival for patients with 131I-refractory differentiated thyroid cancer in SELECT. J Clin Oncol. 2015;33(suppl):6048.
2. Schlumberger M, Tahara M, Wirth LJ, Robinson B, Brose MS, Elisei R, et al. Lenvatinib versus placebo in radioiodine-refractory thyroid cancer. N Engl J Med. 2015;372(7):621–30.
3. Brose MS, Nutting CM, Jarzab B, Elisei R, Siena S, Bastholt L, et al. Sorafenib in locally advanced or metastatic patients with radioactive iodine-refractory differentiated thyroid cancer: the phase III DECISION trial. J Clin Oncol. 2013;31(suppl):4.
4. Wells SA Jr, Robinson BG, Gagel RF, Dralle H, Fagin JA, Santoro M, et al. Vandetanib in patients with locally advanced or metastatic medullary thyroid cancer: a randomized, double-blind phase III trial. J Clin Oncol. 2012;30(2):134–41.
5. Elisei R, Schlumberger MJ, Muller SP, Schoffski P, Brose MS, Shah MH, et al. Cabozantinib in progressive medullary thyroid cancer. J Clin Oncol. 2013;31(29):3639.
6. Blevins DP, Dadu R, Hu M, Baik C, Balachandran D, Ross W, et al. Aerodigestive fistula formation as a rare side effect of antiangiogenic tyrosine kinase inhibitor therapy for thyroid cancer. Thyroid. 2014;24(5):918–22.
7. Song E, Song KM, Kim WG, Choi CM. Development of tracheoesophageal fistula after the use of Sorafenib in locally advanced papillary thyroid carcinoma: a case report. Int J Thyroidol. 2016;9(2):210–4.
8. Lamartina L, Ippolito S, Danis M, Bidault F, Borget I, Berdelou A, et al. Antiangiogenic tyrosine kinase inhibitors: occurrence and risk factors of hemoptysis in refractory thyroid cancer. J Clin Endocrinol Metab. 2016;101(7):2733–41.
9. Cabanillas ME, Patel A, Danysh BP, Dadu R, Kopetz S, Falchook G. BRAF inhibitors: experience in thyroid cancer and general review of toxicity. Horm Cancer. 2014;6(1):21–36.
10. Cabanillas ME, Busaidy N, Khan SA, Gunn GB, Dadu R, Rao SN, et al. Molecular diagnostics and anaplastic thyroid carcinoma: the time has come to harvest the high hanging fruit. Intl J Endocr Oncol. 2016;3(3):221–33.
11. Landa I, Ibrahimpasic T, Boucai L, Sinha R, Knauf JA, Shah RH, et al. Genomic and transcriptomic hallmarks of poorly differentiated and anaplastic thyroid cancers. J Clin Invest. 2016;126(3):1052–66.
12. Rao SN, Zafereo M, Dadu R, Busaidy NL, Hess K, Cote GJ, et al. Patterns of treatment failure in anaplastic thyroid carcinoma. Thyroid. 2017;27(5):672–81.
13. Goutas N, Vlachodimitropoulos D, Bouka M, Lazaris AC, Nasioulas G, Gazouli M. BRAF and K-RAS mutation in a Greek papillary and medullary thyroid carcinoma cohort. Anticancer Res. 2008;28(1a):305–8.
14. Kasaian K, Wiseman SM, Walker BA, Schein JE, Hirst M, Moore RA, et al. Putative BRAF activating fusion in a medullary thyroid cancer. Cold Spring Harb Mol Case Stud. 2016;2(2):a000729.
15. Cho U, Oh WJ, Bae JS, Lee S, Lee YS, Park GS, et al. Clinicopathological features of rare BRAF mutations in Korean thyroid cancer patients. J Korean Med Sci. 2014;29(8):1054–60.
16. Chapman PB, Hauschild A, Robert C, Haanen JB, Ascierto P, Larkin J, et al. Improved survival with vemurafenib in melanoma with BRAF V600E mutation. N Engl J Med. 2011;364(26):2507–16.
17. Flaherty KT, Infante JR, Daud A, Gonzalez R, Kefford RF, Sosman J, et al. Combined BRAF and MEK inhibition in melanoma with BRAF V600 mutations. N Engl J Med. 2012;367(18):1694–703.
18. Long GV, Stroyakovskiy D, Gogas H, Levchenko E, de Braud F, Larkin J, et al. Dabrafenib and trametinib versus dabrafenib and placebo for Val600 BRAF-mutant melanoma: a multicentre, double-blind, phase 3 randomised controlled trial. Lancet. 2015;386(9992):444–51.
19. Brose MS, Cabanillas ME, Cohen EE, Wirth LJ, Riehl T, Yue H, et al. Vemurafenib in patients with BRAF(V600E)-positive metastatic or unresectable papillary thyroid cancer refractory to radioactive

iodine: a non-randomised, multicentre, open-label, phase 2 trial. Lancet Oncol. 2016;17(9):1272–82.
20. Cabanillas ME, Busaidy NL, Zafereo M, Waguespack SG, Hu MI, Hofmann MC, et al. Neoadjuvant vemurafenib in patients with locally advanced papillary thyroid cancer (PTC). Eur Thyroid J. 2017;6(suppl 1). abstr OP-06-39.
21. Shah MH, Wei L, Wirth LJ, Daniels GH, De Souza JA, Timmers CD, et al. Results of randomized phase II trial of dabrafenib versus dabrafenib plus trametinib in BRAF-mutated papillary thyroid carcinoma. J Clin Oncol. 2017;35(suppl):6022.
22. Rothenberg SM, McFadden DG, Palmer E, Daniels GH, Wirth LJ. Re-differentiation of radioiodine-refractory *BRAF* V600E-mutant thyroid carcinoma with dabrafenib: a pilot study. J Clin Oncol. 2013;31(suppl):6025.
23. Rosove MH, Peddi PF, Glaspy JA. BRAF V600E inhibition in anaplastic thyroid cancer. N Engl J Med. 2013;368(7):684–5.
24. Subbiah V, Kreitman RJ, Wainberg ZA, Cho JY, Schellens JHM, Soria JC, et al. Efficacy of dabrafenib (D) and trametinib (T) in patients (pts) with BRAF V600E–mutated anaplastic thyroid cancer (ATC). J Clin Oncol. 2018;35(suppl):6023.
25. Wells SA Jr, Asa SL, Dralle H, Elisei R, Evans DB, Gagel RF, et al. Revised american thyroid association guidelines for the management of medullary thyroid carcinoma. Thyroid. 2015;25(6):567–610.
26. Nikiforov YE, Nikiforova MN. Molecular genetics and diagnosis of thyroid cancer. Nat Rev Endocrinol. 2011;7(10):569–80.
27. Nikiforov YE. RET/PTC rearrangement in thyroid tumors. Endocr Pathol. 2002;13(1):3–16.
28. Tallini G, Asa SL. RET oncogene activation in papillary thyroid carcinoma. Adv Anat Pathol. 2001;8(6):345–54.
29. Unger K, Zitzelsberger H, Salvatore G, Santoro M, Bogdanova T, Braselmann H, et al. Heterogeneity in the distribution of RET/PTC rearrangements within individual post-Chernobyl papillary thyroid carcinomas. J Clin Endocrinol Metab. 2004;89(9):4272–9.
30. Brandhuber BJ, Nanda N, Haas J, Bouhana K, Tuch B, Ebata K, et al. Identification and characterization of highly potent and selective RET kinase inhibitors for the treatment of RET-driven cancers. Clin Cancer Res. 2015;14(12):B192.
31. Rahal R, Evans EK, Hu W, Maynard M, Fleming P, DiPietro L, et al. The development of potent, selective RET inhibitors that target both wild-type RET and prospectively identified resistance mutations to multi-kinase inhibitors. Clin Cancer Res. 2016;76(14):2641.
32. Subbiah V. BLU-667 targets RET-altered cancers. Cancer Discov. 2018;8(6):OF8. https://doi.org/10.1158/2159-8290.CD-NB2018-050. Presented at: American Association for Cancer Research Annual Meeting; April 14–18, 2018; Chicago
33. Drilon A, Subbiah V, Oxnard G, Bauer T, Velcheti V, Lakhani N, et al. A phase 1 study of LOXO-292, a potent and highly selective RET inhibitor, in patients with RET-altered cancers. J Clin Oncol. 2018;36(15):102.
34. Patel MR, Fakih M, Olszanski AJ, Lockhart AC, Drilon AE, Fu S, et al. A phase 1 dose escalation study of RXDX-105, an oral RET and BRAF inhibitor, in patients with advanced solid tumors. J Clin Oncol. 2016;34(suppl):2574.
35. Cancer Genome Atlas Research Network. Integrated genomic characterization of papillary thyroid carcinoma. Cell. 2014;159(3):676–90.
36. Butti MG, Bongarzone I, Ferraresi G, Mondellini P, Borrello MG, Pierotti MA. A sequence analysis of the genomic regions involved in the rearrangements between TPM3 and NTRK1 genes producing TRK oncogenes in papillary thyroid carcinomas. Genomics. 1995;28(1):15–24.
37. Bongarzone I, Vigneri P, Mariani L, Collini P, Pilotti S, Pierotti MA. RET/NTRK1 rearrangements in thyroid gland tumors of the papillary carcinoma family: correlation with clinicopathological features. Clin Cancer Res. 1998;4(1):223–8.
38. Hyman DM, Laetsch TW, Kummar S, DuBois SG, Farago AF, Pappo AS, et al. The efficacy of larotrectinib (LOXO-101), a selective tropomyosin receptor kinase (TRK) inhibitor, in adult and pediatric TRK fusion cancers. J Clin Oncol. 2017;35(Suppl):LBA2501.
39. Kelly LM, Barila G, Liu P, Evdokimova VN, Trivedi S, Panebianco F, et al. Identification of the transforming STRN-ALK fusion as a potential therapeutic target in the aggressive forms of thyroid cancer. Proc Natl Acad Sci U S A. 2014;111(11):4233–8.
40. Godbert Y, Henriques de Figueiredo B, Bonichon F, Chibon F, Hostein I, Perot G, et al. Remarkable response to Crizotinib in woman with anaplastic lymphoma kinase-rearranged anaplastic thyroid carcinoma. J Clin Oncol. 2015;33(20):e84–7.
41. Sebolt-Leopold J, Dudley D, Herrera R, Van Becelaere K, Wiland A, Gowan R, et al. Blockade of MAP kinase pathway suppresses growth of colon tumors in vivo. Nat Med. 1999;5:810–6.
42. Dudley DT, Pang L, Decker SJ, Bridges AJ, Saltiel AR. A synthetic inhibitor of the mitogen-activated protein kinase cascade. Proc Natl Acad Sci U S A. 1995;92(17):7686–9.
43. Caunt CJ, Sale MJ, Smith PD, Cook SJ. MEK1 and MEK2 inhibitors and cancer therapy: the long and winding road. Nat Rev Cancer. 2015;15(10):577–92.
44. Hayes DN, Lucas AS, Tanvetyanon T, Krzyzanowska MK, Chung CH, Murphy BA, et al. Phase II efficacy and pharmacogenomic study of Selumetinib (AZD6244; ARRY-142886) in iodine-131 refractory papillary thyroid carcinoma with or without follicular elements. Clin Cancer Res. 2012;18(7):2056–65.
45. Duncan JS, Whittle MC, Nakamura K, Abell AN, Midland AA, Zawistowski JS, et al. Dynamic reprogramming of the kinome in response to targeted MEK inhibition in triple-negative breast cancer. Cell. 2012;149(2):307–21.

46. Leonowens C, Pendry C, Bauman J, Young GC, Ho M, Henriquez F, et al. Concomitant oral and intravenous pharmacokinetics of trametinib, a MEK inhibitor, in subjects with solid tumours. Br J Clin Pharmacol. 2014;78(3):524–32.
47. Friday BB, Yu C, Dy GK, Smith PD, Wang L, Thibodeau SN, et al. BRAF V600E disrupts AZD6244-induced abrogation of negative feedback pathways between extracellular signal-regulated kinase and Raf proteins. Cancer Res. 2008;68(15):6145–53.
48. Hatzivassiliou G, Haling JR, Chen H, Song K, Price S, Heald R, et al. Mechanism of MEK inhibition determines efficacy in mutant KRAS- versus BRAF-driven cancers. Nature. 2013;501(7466):232–6.
49. Gilmartin AG, Bleam MR, Groy A, Moss KG, Minthorn EA, Kulkarni SG, et al. GSK1120212 (JTP-74057) is an inhibitor of MEK activity and activation with favorable pharmacokinetic properties for sustained in vivo pathway inhibition. Clin Cancer Res. 2011;17(5):989–1000.
50. Lito P, Saborowski A, Yue J, Solomon M, Joseph E, Gadal S, et al. Disruption of CRAF-mediated MEK activation is required for effective MEK inhibition in KRAS mutant tumors. Cancer Cell. 2014;25(5):697–710.
51. Isshiki Y, Kohchi Y, Iikura H, Matsubara Y, Asoh K, Murata T, et al. Design and synthesis of novel allosteric MEK inhibitor CH4987655 as an orally available anticancer agent. Bioorg Med Chem Lett. 2011;21(6):1795–801.
52. Nagarajah J, Le M, Knauf JA, Ferrandino G, Montero-Conde C, Pillarsetty N, et al. Sustained ERK inhibition maximizes responses of BrafV600E thyroid cancers to radioiodine. J Clin Invest. 2016;126(11):4119–24.
53. Chakravarty D, Santos E, Ryder M, Knauf JA, Liao XH, West BL, et al. Small-molecule MAPK inhibitors restore radioiodine incorporation in mouse thyroid cancers with conditional BRAF activation. J Clin Invest. 2011;121(12):4700–11.
54. Ho AL, Grewal RK, Leboeuf R, Sherman EJ, Pfister DG, Deandreis D, et al. Selumetinib-enhanced radioiodine uptake in advanced thyroid cancer. N Engl J Med. 2013;368(7):623–32.
55. Hoeflich KP, O'Brien C, Boyd Z, Cavet G, Guerrero S, Jung K, et al. In vivo antitumor activity of MEK and phosphatidylinositol 3-kinase inhibitors in basal-like breast cancer models. Clin Cancer Res. 2009;15(14):4649–64.
56. Engelman JA, Chen L, Tan X, Crosby K, Guimaraes AR, Upadhyay R, et al. Effective use of PI3K and MEK inhibitors to treat mutant Kras G12D and PIK3CA H1047R murine lung cancers. Nat Med. 2008;14(12):1351–6.
57. Pitts TM, Newton TP, Bradshaw-Pierce EL, Addison R, Arcaroli JJ, Klauck PJ, et al. Dual pharmacological targeting of the MAP kinase and PI3K/mTOR pathway in preclinical models of colorectal cancer. PLoS One. 2014;9(11):e113037.
58. Jokinen E, Koivunen JP. MEK and PI3K inhibition in solid tumors: rationale and evidence to date. Ther Adv Med Oncol. 2015;7(3):170–80.
59. Lim SM, Chang H, Yoon MJ, Hong YK, Kim H, Chung WY, et al. A multicenter, phase II trial of everolimus in locally advanced or metastatic thyroid cancer of all histologic subtypes. Ann Oncol. 2013;24(12):3089–94.
60. Schneider TC, de Wit D, Links TP, van Erp NP, van der Hoeven JJ, Gelderblom H, et al. Everolimus in patients with advanced follicular-derived thyroid cancer: results of a phase II clinical trial. J Clin Endocrinol Metab. 2017;102(2):698–707.
61. Hanna GJ, Busaidy NL, Chau NG, Wirth LJ, Barletta JA, Calles A, et al. Genomic correlates of response to everolimus in aggressive radioiodine-refractory thyroid cancer: a phase II study. Clin Cancer Res. 2018;24(7):1546–53.
62. Wagle N, Grabiner BC, Van Allen EM, Amin-Mansour A, Taylor-Weiner A, Rosenberg M, et al. Response and acquired resistance to everolimus in anaplastic thyroid cancer. N Engl J Med. 2014;371(15):1426–33.
63. Gibson WJ, Ruan DT, Paulson VA, Barletta JA, Hanna GJ, Kraft S, et al. Genomic heterogeneity and exceptional response to dual pathway inhibition in anaplastic thyroid cancer. Clin Cancer Res. 2017;23(9):2367–73.
64. Axelrod MJ, Gordon V, Mendez RE, Leimgruber SS, Conaway MR, Sharlow ER, et al. p70S6 kinase is a critical node that integrates HER-family and PI3 kinase signaling networks. Cell Signal. 2014;26(8):1627–35.
65. Malaguarnera R, Chen KY, Kim TY, Dominguez JM, Voza F, Ouyang B, et al. Switch in signaling control of mTORC1 activity after oncoprotein expression in thyroid cancer cell lines. J Clin Endocrinol Metab. 2014;99(10):E1976–87.
66. Brunton VG, Frame MC. Src and focal adhesion kinase as therapeutic targets in cancer. Curr Opin Pharmacol. 2008;8(4):427–32.
67. Michailidi C, Giaginis C, Stolakis V, Alexandrou P, Klijanienko J, Delladetsima I, et al. Evaluation of FAK and Src expression in human benign and malignant thyroid lesions. Pathol Oncol Res. 2010;16(4):497–507.
68. Owens LV, Xu L, Craven RJ, Dent GA, Weiner TM, Kornberg L, et al. Overexpression of the focal adhesion kinase (p125FAK) in invasive human tumors. Cancer Res. 1995;55(13):2752–5.
69. Owens LV, Xu L, Dent GA, Yang X, Sturge GC, Craven RJ, et al. Focal adhesion kinase as a marker of invasive potential in differentiated human thyroid cancer. Ann Surg Oncol. 1996;3(1):100–5.
70. Schweppe RE, Kerege AA, French JD, Sharma V, Grzywa R, Haugen BR. Inhibition of Src with AZD0530 reveals the Src-focal adhesion kinase complex as a novel therapeutic target in papillary and anaplastic thyroid cancer. J Clin Endocrinol Metab. 2009;94:2199–203.

71. Chan CM, Jing X, Pike LA, Zhou Q, Lim DJ, Sams SB, et al. Targeted inhibition of SRC kinase with dasatinib blocks thyroid cancer growth and metastasis. Clin Cancer Res. 2012;18(13):3580–91.
72. Beadnell TC, Mishall KM, Zhou Q, Riffert SM, Wuensch KE, Kessler BE, et al. The mitogen-activated protein kinase pathway facilitates resistance to the Src inhibitor Dasatinib in thyroid cancer. Mol Cancer Ther. 2016;15(8):1952–63.
73. Chan D, Tyner JW, Chng WJ, BI C, Okamoto R, Said J, et al. Effect of dasatinib against thyroid cancer cell lines in vitro and a xenograft model in vivo. Oncol Lett. 2012;3:807–15.
74. Kim WG, Guigon CJ, Fozzatti L, Park JW, Lu C, Willingham MC, et al. SKI-606, an Src inhibitor, reduces tumor growth, invasion, and distant metastasis in a mouse model of thyroid cancer. Clin Cancer Res. 2012;18(5):1281–90.
75. Roskoski R Jr. Src protein-tyrosine kinase structure, mechanism, and small molecule inhibitors. Pharmacol Res. 2015;94:9–25.
76. Shah NP, Tran C, Lee FY, Chen P, Norris D, Sawyers CL. Overriding imatinib resistance with a novel ABL kinase inhibitor. Science. 2004;305(5682):399–401.
77. Herold CI, Chadaram V, Peterson BL, Marcom PK, Hopkins J, Kimmick GG, et al. Phase II trial of dasatinib in patients with metastatic breast cancer using real-time pharmacodynamic tissue biomarkers of Src inhibition to escalate dosing. Clin Cancer Res. 2011;17(18):6061–70.
78. Yu EY, Wilding G, Posadas E, Gross M, Culine S, Massard C, et al. Phase II study of dasatinib in patients with metastatic castration-resistant prostate cancer. Clin Cancer Res. 2009;15(23):7421–8.
79. Sen B, Peng S, Tang X, Erickson HS, Galindo H, Mazumdar T, et al. Kinase-impaired BRAF mutations in lung cancer confer sensitivity to dasatinib. Sci Transl Med. 2012;4(136):136–70.
80. Smith VE, Read ML, Turnell AS, Watkins RJ, Watkinson JC, Lewy GD, et al. A novel mechanism of sodium iodide symporter repression in differentiated thyroid cancer. J Cell Sci. 2009;122(Pt 18):3393–402.
81. Smith VE, Sharma N, Watkins RJ, Read ML, Ryan GA, Kwan PP, et al. Manipulation of PBF/PTTG1IP phosphorylation status; a potential new therapeutic strategy for improving radioiodine uptake in thyroid and other tumors. J Clin Endocrinol Metab. 2013;98(7):2876–86.
82. Hanahan D, Weinberg RA. Hallmarks of cancer: the next generation. Cell. 2011;144(5):646–74.
83. Sharma P, Allison JP. The future of immune checkpoint therapy. Science. 2015;348(6230):56–61.
84. Cunha LL, Marcello MA, Morari EC, Nonogaki S, Conte FF, Gerhard R, et al. Differentiated thyroid carcinomas may elude the immune system by B7H1 upregulation. Endocr Relat Cancer. 2013;20(1):103–10.
85. Angell TE, Lechner MG, Jang JK, Correa AJ, LoPresti JS, Epstein AL. BRAF V600E in papillary thyroid carcinoma is associated with increased programmed death ligand 1 expression and suppressive immune cell infiltration. Thyroid. 2014;24(9):1385–93.
86. Ahn S, Kim TH, Kim SW, Ki CS, Jang HW, Kim JS, et al. Comprehensive screening for PD-L1 expression in thyroid cancer. Endocr Relat Cancer. 2017;24(2):97–106.
87. Bastman JJ, Serracino HS, Zhu Y, Koenig MR, Mateescu V, Sams SB, et al. Tumor-infiltrating T cells and the PD-1 checkpoint pathway in advanced differentiated and anaplastic thyroid cancer. J Clin Endocrinol Metab. 2016;101(7):2863–73.
88. Chowdhury S, Veyhl J, Jessa F, Polyakova O, Alenzi A, MacMillan C, et al. Programmed death-ligand 1 overexpression is a prognostic marker for aggressive papillary thyroid cancer and its variants. Oncotarget. 2016;7(22):32318–28.
89. French JD, Bible K, Spitzweg C, Haugen BR, Ryder M. Leveraging the immune system to treat advanced thyroid cancers. Lancet Diabetes Endocrinol. 2017;5(6):469–81.
90. French JD, Kotnis GR, Said S, Raeburn CD, McIntyre RC Jr, Klopper JP, et al. Programmed death-1+ T cells and regulatory T cells are enriched in tumor-involved lymph nodes and associated with aggressive features in papillary thyroid cancer. J Clin Endocrinol Metab. 2012;97(6):E934–43.
91. Severson JJ, Serracino HS, Mateescu V, Raeburn CD, McIntyre RC Jr, Sams SB, et al. PD-1+Tim-3+ CD8+ T lymphocytes display varied degrees of functional exhaustion in patients with regionally metastatic differentiated thyroid cancer. Cancer Immunol Res. 2015;3(6):620–30.
92. French JD, Weber ZJ, Fretwell DL, Said S, Klopper JP, Haugen BR. Tumor-associated lymphocytes and increased FoxP3+ regulatory T cell frequency correlate with more aggressive papillary thyroid cancer. J Clin Endocrinol Metab. 2010;95(5):2325–33.
93. Mehnert JM, Varga A, Brose M, Aggarwal RR, Lin C-C, Prawira A, de Braud F, Tamura K, Doi T, Piha-Paul SA, Gilbert J, Saraf S, Thanigaimani P, Cheng JD, Keam B. Pembrolizumab for advanced papillary or follicular thyroid cancer: preliminary results from the phase 1b KEYNOTE-028 study. J Clin Oncol. 2016;34(suppl):6091.
94. Chintakuntlawar AV, Rumilla KM, Smith CY, Jenkins SM, Foote RL, Kasperbauer JL, et al. Expression of PD-1 and PD-L1 in anaplastic thyroid cancer patients treated with multimodal therapy: results from a retrospective study. J Clin Endocrinol Metab. 2017;102(6):1943–50.
95. Wu H, Sun Y, Ye H, Yang S, Lee SL. de las Morenas a. Anaplastic thyroid cancer: outcome and the mutation/expression profiles of potential targets. Pathol Oncol Res. 2015;21(3):695–701.
96. Dadu R, Para Cuentas E, Rodriguez Canales J, Wistuba I, Zhou S, Williams M, et al. Anaplastic

thyroid cancer is a hot immunogenic environment: immunoprofiling of a large cohort of ATC tumors. Thyroid. 2016;26(suppl. 1):A4–5. Presented at the 86th Annual Meeting of the American Thyroid Association, Denver, CO.

97. Brauner E, Gunda V, Vanden Borre P, Zurakowski D, Kim YS, Dennett KV, et al. Combining BRAF inhibitor and anti PD-L1 antibody dramatically improves tumor regression and anti tumor immunity in an immunocompetent murine model of anaplastic thyroid cancer. Oncotarget. 2016;7(13):17194–211.
98. Papewalis C, Wuttke M, Jacobs B, Domberg J, Willenberg H, Baehring T, et al. Dendritic cell vaccination induces tumor epitope-specific Th1 immune response in medullary thyroid carcinoma. Hormone Metab Res. 2008;40(2):108–16.
99. Bachleitner-Hofmann T, Friedl J, Hassler M, Hayden H, Dubsky P, Sachet M, et al. Pilot trial of autologous dendritic cells loaded with tumor lysate(s) from allogeneic tumor cell lines in patients with metastatic medullary thyroid carcinoma. Oncol Rep. 2009;21(6):1585–92.
100. Kraeber-Bodere F, Rousseau C, Bodet-Milin C, Ferrer L, Faivre-Chauvet A, Campion L, et al. Targeting, toxicity, and efficacy of 2-step, pretargeted radioimmunotherapy using a chimeric bispecific antibody and 131I-labeled bivalent hapten in a phase I optimization clinical trial. Journal of nuclear medicine : official publication. Soc Nucl Med. 2006;47(2):247–55.
101. Chatal JF, Campion L, Kraeber-Bodere F, Bardet S, Vuillez JP, Charbonnel B, et al. Survival improvement in patients with medullary thyroid carcinoma who undergo pretargeted anti-carcinoembryonic-antigen radioimmunotherapy: a collaborative study with the French endocrine tumor group. J Clin Oncol. 2006;24(11):1705–11.
102. Bongiovanni M, Rebecchini C, Saglietti C, Bulliard JL, Marino L, de Leval L, et al. Very low expression of PD-L1 in medullary thyroid carcinoma. Endocr Relat Cancer. 2017;24(6):L35–L8.
103. Dadu R, Canales JR, Wistuba I, Tian W, Lui H, Grubbs EG, Cote GJ, Ray G, Williams M, Cabanillas ME. Immune markers in medullary thyroid cancer (MTC) and their clinical significance. Thyroid. 2015;25(1):491.
104. Peng SL, Saunders L, Bheddah S, Williams S, Aggarwal RR, Shea JE, et al. Metastatic melanoma, glioblastoma and high-grade extrapulmonary neuroendocrine carcinomas (NECs) as novel indications for rovalpituzumab tesirine: a delta-like protein 3 (DLL3)-targeted antibody-drug conjugate (ADC). J Clin Oncol. 2016;34(suppl):11611.
105. Dadu R, Shah K, Busaidy NL, Waguespack SG, Habra MA, Ying AK, et al. Efficacy and tolerability of vemurafenib in patients with BRAF(V600E) -positive papillary thyroid cancer: M.D. Anderson cancer Center off label experience. J Clin Endocrinol Metab. 2015;100(1):E77–81.
106. Falchook GS, Millward M, Hong D, Naing A, Piha-Paul S, Waguespack SG, et al. BRAF inhibitor dabrafenib in patients with metastatic BRAF-mutant thyroid cancer. Thyroid. 2015;25(1):71–7.
107. Kim KB, Cabanillas ME, Lazar AJ, Williams MD, Sanders DL, Ilagan JL, et al. Clinical responses to vemurafenib in patients with metastatic papillary thyroid cancer harboring BRAF(V600E) mutation. Thyroid. 2013;23(10):1277–83.
108. Wagle N, Van Allen EM, Treacy DJ, Frederick DT, Cooper ZA, Taylor-Weiner A, et al. MAP kinase pathway alterations in BRAF-mutant melanoma patients with acquired resistance to combined RAF/MEK inhibition. Cancer Discov. 2014;4(1):61–8.
109. Fofaria NM, Frederick DT, Sullivan RJ, Flaherty KT, Srivastava SK. Overexpression of Mcl-1 confers resistance to BRAFV600E inhibitors alone and in combination with MEK1/2 inhibitors in melanoma. Oncotarget. 2015;6(38):40535–56.
110. Nazarian R, Shi H, Wang Q, Kong X, Koya RC, Lee H, et al. Melanomas acquire resistance to B-RAF(V600E) inhibition by RTK or N-RAS upregulation. Nature. 2010;468(7326):973–7.
111. Wagenaar TR, Ma L, Roscoe B, Park SM, Bolon DN, Green MR. Resistance to vemurafenib resulting from a novel mutation in the BRAFV600E kinase domain. Pigment Cell Melanoma Res. 2014;27(1):124–33.
112. Lidsky M, Antoun G, Speicher P, Adams B, Turley R, Augustine C, et al. Mitogen-activated protein kinase (MAPK) hyperactivation and enhanced NRAS expression drive acquired vemurafenib resistance in V600E BRAF melanoma cells. J Biol Chem. 2014;289(40):27714–26.
113. Prahallad A, Sun C, Huang S, Di Nicolantonio F, Salazar R, Zecchin D, et al. Unresponsiveness of colon cancer to BRAF(V600E) inhibition through feedback activation of EGFR. Nature. 2012;483(7387):100–3.
114. Corcoran RB, Ebi H, Turke AB, Coffee EM, Nishino M, Cogdill AP, et al. EGFR-mediated re-activation of MAPK signaling contributes to insensitivity of BRAF mutant colorectal cancers to RAF inhibition with vemurafenib. Cancer Discov. 2012;2(3):227–35.
115. Sanchez-Laorden B, Viros A, Girotti MR, Pedersen M, Saturno G, Zambon A, et al. BRAF inhibitors induce metastasis in RAS mutant or inhibitor-resistant melanoma cells by reactivating MEK and ERK signaling. Sci Signal. 2014;7(318):ra30.
116. Yadav V, Zhang X, Liu J, Estrem S, Li S, Gong XQ, et al. Reactivation of mitogen-activated protein kinase (MAPK) pathway by FGF receptor 3 (FGFR3)/Ras mediates resistance to vemurafenib in human B-RAF V600E mutant melanoma. J Biol Chem. 2012;287(33):28087–98.
117. Jiang CC, Lai F, Thorne RF, Yang F, Liu H, Hersey P, et al. MEK-independent survival of B-RAFV600E melanoma cells selected for resistance to apoptosis induced by the RAF inhibitor PLX4720. Clin Cancer Res. 2011;17(4):721–30.

118. Atefi M, von Euw E, Attar N, Ng C, Chu C, Guo D, et al. Reversing melanoma cross-resistance to BRAF and MEK inhibitors by co-targeting the AKT/mTOR pathway. PLoS One. 2011;6(12):e28973.
119. Greger JG, Eastman SD, Zhang V, Bleam MR, Hughes AM, Smitheman KN, et al. Combinations of BRAF, MEK, and PI3K/mTOR inhibitors overcome acquired resistance to the BRAF inhibitor GSK2118436 dabrafenib, mediated by NRAS or MEK mutations. Mol Cancer Ther. 2012;11(4):909–20.
120. Delmas A, Cherier J, Pohorecka M, Medale-Giamarchi C, Meyer N, Casanova A, et al. The c-Jun/RHOB/AKT pathway confers resistance of BRAF-mutant melanoma cells to MAPK inhibitors. Oncotarget. 2015;6(17):15250–64.
121. Wilson TR, Fridlyand J, Yan Y, Penuel E, Burton L, Chan E, et al. Widespread potential for growth-factor-driven resistance to anticancer kinase inhibitors. Nature. 2012;487(7408):505–9.
122. Straussman R, Morikawa T, Shee K, Barzily-Rokni M, Qian ZR, Du J, et al. Tumour micro-environment elicits innate resistance to RAF inhibitors through HGF secretion. Nature. 2012;487(7408):500–4.
123. Miao B, Ji Z, Tan L, Taylor M, Zhang J, Choi HG, et al. EPHA2 is a mediator of vemurafenib resistance and a novel therapeutic target in melanoma. Cancer Discov. 2015;5(3):274–87.
124. Monsma DJ, Cherba DM, Eugster EE, Dylewski DL, Davidson PT, Peterson CA, et al. Melanoma patient derived xenografts acquire distinct Vemurafenib resistance mechanisms. Am J Cancer Res. 2015;5(4):1507–18.
125. Kopetz S, Desai J, Chan E, Hecht JR, O'Dwyer PJ, Maru D, et al. Phase II pilot study of Vemurafenib in patients with metastatic BRAF-mutated colorectal cancer. J Clin Oncol. 2015;33(34):4032–8.
126. Poulikakos PI, Persaud Y, Janakiraman M, Kong X, Ng C, Moriceau G, et al. RAF inhibitor resistance is mediated by dimerization of aberrantly spliced BRAF(V600E). Nature. 2011;480(7377):387–90.
127. Johannessen CM, Boehm JS, Kim SY, Thomas SR, Wardwell L, Johnson LA, et al. COT drives resistance to RAF inhibition through MAP kinase pathway reactivation. Nature. 2010;468(7326):968–72.
128. Montero-Conde C, Ruiz-Llorente S, Dominguez JM, Knauf JA, Viale A, Sherman EJ, et al. Relief of feedback inhibition of HER3 transcription by RAF and MEK inhibitors attenuates their antitumor effects in BRAF-mutant thyroid carcinomas. Cancer Discov. 2013;3(5):520–33.
129. Byeon HK, Na HJ, Yang YJ, Kwon HJ, Chang JW, Ban MJ, et al. C-met-mediated reactivation of PI3K/AKT signaling contributes to insensitivity of BRAF(V600E) mutant thyroid cancer to BRAF inhibition. Mol Carcinog. 2016;55(11):1678–87.
130. Duquette M, Sadow PM, Husain A, Sims JN, Antonello ZA, Fischer AH, et al. Metastasis-associated MCL1 and P16 copy number alterations dictate resistance to vemurafenib in a BRAFV600E patient-derived papillary thyroid carcinoma preclinical model. Oncotarget. 2015;6(40):42445–67.
131. Danysh BP, Rieger EY, Sinha DK, Evers CV, Cote GJ, Cabanillas ME, et al. Long-term vemurafenib treatment drives inhibitor resistance through a spontaneous KRAS G12D mutation in a BRAF V600E papillary thyroid carcinoma model. Oncotarget. 2016;7(21):30907–23.
132. Costa AM, Herrero A, Fresno MF, Heymann J, Alvarez JA, Cameselle-Teijeiro J, et al. BRAF mutation associated with other genetic events identifies a subset of aggressive papillary thyroid carcinoma. Clin Endocrinol. 2008;68(4):618–34.
133. Lito P, Rosen N, Solit DB. Tumor adaptation and resistance to RAF inhibitors. Nat Med. 2013;19(11):1401–9.
134. Samatar AA, Poulikakos PI. Targeting RAS-ERK signalling in cancer: promises and challenges. Nat Rev Drug Discov. 2014;13(12):928–42.
135. Morris EJ, Jha S, Restaino CR, Dayananth P, Zhu H, Cooper A, et al. Discovery of a novel ERK inhibitor with activity in models of acquired resistance to BRAF and MEK inhibitors. Cancer Discov. 2013;3(7):742–50.
136. Hayes TK, Neel NF, Hu C, Gautam P, Chenard M, Long B, et al. Long-term ERK inhibition in KRAS-mutant pancreatic cancer is associated with MYC degradation and senescence-like growth suppression. Cancer Cell. 2016;29(1):75–89.
137. Jha S, Morris EJ, Hruza A, Mansueto MS, Schroeder G, Arbanas J, et al. Dissecting therapeutic resistance to ERK inhibition. Mol Cancer Ther. 2016;15(4):548–59.
138. Wong DJ, Robert L, Atefi MS, Lassen A, Avarappatt G, Cerniglia M, et al. Antitumor activity of the ERK inhibitor SCH772984 [corrected] against BRAF mutant, NRAS mutant and wild-type melanoma. Mol Cancer. 2014;13:194.
139. Akeno-Stuart N, Croyle M, Knauf JA, Malaguarnera R, Vitagliano D, Santoro M, et al. The RET kinase inhibitor NVP-AST487 blocks growth and calcitonin gene expression through distinct mechanisms in medullary thyroid cancer cells. Cancer Res. 2007;67(14):6956–64.
140. Dadu R, Shah K, Busaidy NL, Waguespack SG, Habra MA, Ying AK, et al. Efficacy and tolerability of Vemurafenib in patients with BRAF -positive papillary thyroid cancer: M.D. Anderson cancer Center off label experience. J Clin Endocrinol Metab. 2014;100(1):E77–81. jc20142246.
141. Leung F, Kulasingam V, Diamandis EP, Hoon DS, Kinzler K, Pantel K, et al. Circulating tumor DNA as a cancer biomarker: fact or fiction? Clin Chem. 2016;62(8):1054–60.
142. Siravegna G, Marsoni S, Siena S, Bardelli A. Integrating liquid biopsies into the management of cancer. Nat Rev Clin Oncol. 2017;14(9):531–48.

143. Wan JC, Massie C, Garcia-Corbacho J, Mouliere F, Brenton JD, Caldas C, et al. Liquid biopsies come of age: towards implementation of circulating tumour DNA. Nat Rev Cancer. 2017;17(4):223–38.
144. Eng C, Mulligan LM, Healey CS, Houghton C, Frilling A, Raue F, et al. Heterogeneous mutation of the RET proto-oncogene in subpopulations of medullary thyroid carcinoma. Cancer Res. 1996;56(9):2167–70.
145. Romei C, Ciampi R, Tacito A, Casella F, Ugolini C, Porta M, et al. Genetic heterogeneity of medullary thyroid carcinoma. Endocr Abstr. 2016;40:P1.
146. Melo M, Gaspar da Rocha A, Batista R, Vinagre J, Martins MJ, Costa G, et al. TERT, BRAF, and NRAS in primary thyroid cancer and metastatic disease. J Clin Endocrinol Metab. 2017;102(6):1898–907.
147. Pupilli C, Pinzani P, Salvianti F, Fibbi B, Rossi M, Petrone L, et al. Circulating BRAFV600E in the diagnosis and follow-up of differentiated papillary thyroid carcinoma. J Clin Endocrinol Metab. 2013;98(8):3359–65.
148. Chuang TC, Chuang AY, Poeta L, Koch WM, Califano JA, Tufano RP. Detectable BRAF mutation in serum DNA samples from patients with papillary thyroid carcinomas. Head Neck. 2010;32(2):229–34.
149. Evers C, Duose DY, Meenakshi M, Hai T, Houston MR, Hu PC, et al. Liquid biopsy: comparison of mutation detection methods for measurement of RET M918T circulating cell-free DNA in medullary thyroid cancer patients. Cancer Genet. 2016;209:287 a7.
150. Sandulache VC, Williams MD, Lai SY, Lu C, William WN, Busaidy NL, et al. Real-time genomic characterization utilizing circulating cell-free DNA in patients with anaplastic thyroid carcinoma. Thyroid. 2017;27(1):81–7.
151. Lubitz CC, Parangi S, Holm TM, Bernasconi MJ, Schalck AP, Suh H, et al. Detection of circulating BRAF(V600E) in patients with papillary thyroid carcinoma. J Mol Diagn. 2016;18(1):100–8.

Thyroid Cancer Trials

25

Allan Hackshaw

Introduction

The number of new cancer therapies and indications has increased over the years, particularly targeted and immunotherapeutic agents. The US Food and Drug Administration, for example, has approved four drugs for thyroid cancer alone since 2011 (vandetanib, cabozantinib, sorafenib and lenvatinib) (https://www.fda.gov/drugs/informationondrugs/approveddrugs/ucm279174.htm). These (commercial) trials represent a fraction of the research being undertaken in thyroid cancer, with many studies being conducted by research clinicians and scientists in non-commercial organisations.

Thyroid cancer differs from many other solid tumours, in that patients are often younger than 60 years, many are still in work, and some are still taking care of children. Even though this type of cancer is relatively uncommon, these features are of particular importance when developing interventions for thyroid cancer. There is also a wide range of prognoses, with a majority of patients being successfully treated and essentially cured (with no recurrence seen after 10 or 20 years), whilst a minority are diagnosed with advanced disease, whose prognoses can be poor, with overall survival (OS) of several months only.

Funding opportunities for clinical trials has improved substantially in the past 10 or so years, with pharmaceutical companies, public sector/governmental bodies and charitable organisations investing heavily in finding new treatments or combinations of therapies for treating all stages of thyroid cancer, as a consequence of greater interest in uncommon cancers. In the area of thyroid disease, cancer has had by far the most number of publications between 2006 and 2015 (~9000), compared to the next most prevalent field, thyrotoxicosis/eye disease (<5000) [1]. There has been a 1.8-fold increase in the number of publications per year [1]. Of the three most highly cited articles between 2013 and 2016, two were on clinical trials: cabozantinib for progressive medullary thyroid cancer [2] and selumetinib for enhancing uptake of radioactive iodine in advanced thyroid cancer [3].

A. Hackshaw
Cancer Research UK and UCL Cancer Trials Centre, University College London, London, UK
e-mail: a.hackshaw@ucl.ac.uk

U. K. Mallick et al. (eds.), *Practical Management of Thyroid Cancer*,
https://doi.org/10.1007/978-3-319-91725-2_25

Types of Clinical Trials and Main Design Features

Several types of trial designs have been used for many years in cancer research, and with more funding available for thyroid cancer the full range of designs have been applied (Box 25.1) [4].

Box 25.1 Types of Trials

Phase I

- First time a new drug, regimen or combination of therapies are tested in patients
- Few participants (usually <30)
- Aim is to find a dose with an acceptable level of safety, or that a new combination does not have unacceptable adverse events; and examine the biological and pharmacological effects

Phase II

- Not too large (e.g. 30–100 patients)
- Aim is to obtain a *preliminary* estimate of efficacy, relatively quickly
- Can be single arm or randomised with a control/placebo group, or randomised with several experimental arms
- Produces data to design a phase III trial
- Some phase II studies in rare subgroups can change practice directly, if there is clear unmet need, and a lack of current effective treatments

Phase III

- Must be randomised and with a comparison (control) group
- Relatively large, usually several hundred patients
- Aim is to provide a *definitive* answer on whether a new treatment is better than the control group (superiority trial), or is no worse/similarly effective but there are other advantages such as safer, better quality of life, easier to administer or cheaper (non-inferiority trial)

Whilst observational studies have well-established uses, and provide good evidence on, for example, trends in incidence or various features of managing patients, their value is limited when evaluating interventions. There is a wide variety of observational study designs, but most, if not all, are affected to some extent by inherent confounding and bias, and can have substantial missing data for important factors. An example is the use of radioiodine ablation for well-differentiated thyroid cancer. A systematic review of 16 prospective cohort or retrospective studies indicated that a low administered activity was associated with a 10% lower ablation success rate than the standard high activity ($p = 0.01$) [5]. However, two subsequent large randomised studies both confirmed that ablation success rates were not materially reduced with the low activity (1.1 GBq) compared to 3.7 GBq [6, 7]. This contrast in findings means that evidence from observational studies of treatments needs to be examined with care, to avoid making inappropriate conclusions.

Box 25.2 shows the key design features of clinical trials. The sections below provide examples of clinical trials, illustrating aspects of their design, analysis or interpretation that are of special interest but can be generalised to other studies.

Box 25.2 Key Design Features of Thyroid Cancer Trials

Design feature	General comments
Eligibility	• Ideally should be representative of the target patient population, but is often a selected group (who are interested in research). It might be useful to collect data on eligible patients who decline to participate, to see if and how their characteristics differ from those who enter the trial • Histopathology-related eligibility criteria require care when being defined in order to (1) be understood easily across many centres and (2) not be so strict that the patient group becomes too narrow, thus hampering recruitment • Diagnostic procedures also need to be reliable, and so should include imaging of the neck, at least
Interventions	• For advanced disease, typical systemic therapies are used (which need to be clearly defined: route of administration, dose and duration) • For low risk disease, new interventions tend to be associated with less treatment (but with similar efficacy outcomes), hence they need to have other benefits for patients
Randomisation	• Essential for phase III studies, but can be challenging when examining interventions in low risk patients where major recent trials aimed to reduce the amount of treatment patients receive (i.e. several patients do not wish to receive what they perceive to be an inferior intervention)
Blinding	• Placebo minimises the bias due to the placebo effect, which is especially important for progression-free survival (PFS), a common primary endpoint in phase III thyroid cancer trials • Whilst regulatory/licensing agencies seem to have a preference for placebo (where appropriate), health technology assessment agencies often prefer control groups that reflect current therapies available locally, if they exist
Sample size	• Can be quite challenging for many thyroid cancer trials, without national or international collaboration. For advanced disease (poor prognoses) the main issue is being able to recruit enough patients (e.g. medullary or anaplastic disease). For low risk patients (good prognoses) the main issue is seeing enough events, such as recurrences (e.g. for well-differentiated cancer)
Outcome measures	• For advanced thyroid cancer, PFS and overall survival (OS) are important endpoints, with tumour response rate and duration of response in addition for early phase trials. Whilst OS is feasible for cancers like anaplastic carcinoma, it might be limited for metastatic differentiated thyroid cancer which requires long follow up • For distant metastatic disease, endpoints will need to cover local control of the primary tumour, with treatment of the distant metastatic sites • For low risk disease, OS is not feasible, and only endpoints such as recurrence are associated with enough events • Toxicity and health-related quality of life (patient reported outcomes) are important, particularly for younger patients with families. The timing of the QoL assessments needs to be considered carefully, in order to capture patient-relevant time-points that reflect their exposure to the treatment
Follow up schedule and assessments	• Advanced disease typically requires relatively short follow up for PFS (e.g. 1–2 years), but phase II and III trials can require much longer to get enough events for OS • Low risk disease typically requires long follow up for recurrence, requiring hospitals to provide continuous resources to collect data for several years, including follow up scans (e.g. ultrasound) and/or blood tests (e.g. thyroglobulin)

Early Phase Trials

Phase I

Thyroid cancer is usually one of several cancer types in phase I trials of novel agents. Patients tend to have had relapsed disease, and after multiple lines of therapy. Such trials are most suitable for advanced or progressive forms of thyroid cancer.

Example 25.1 Cabozanitib for Medullary Thyroid Cancer [8]

Design: 3 + 3 dose escalation

Eligibility: Advanced solid tumours (metastatic/unresectable disease no longer responding to standard therapies, or no standard therapy available): 37 out of 85 patients had medullary thyroid cancer

Interventions: Oral cabozanitib, given in up to 13 different doses and schedules (suspension formulation given intermittently or continuously, or continuous dosing using capsules)

Outcomes: Dose-limiting toxicity (DLT)—Needs careful definition to avoid including adverse events that are likely to be disease-related

Findings:

- 2 of 6 patients who received the 250 mg capsule had a DLT, hence the maximum tolerated dose was the next lowest dose, 175 mg
- Phase I trials can also be used to examine signs of efficacy, usually tumour response, and here 29% of thyroid cancer patients had a confirmed partial response. But 41% had stable disease for ≥6 months, which can be an additional important outcome for early phase studies, particularly when few patients are expected to have a complete/partial response, and instead would normally progress relatively quickly

Example 25.1 has a typical design for dose-finding trials, i.e. a 3 + 3 ('rule based') design, in which patients are treated with the same dose in cohorts of three, then an assessment of toxicity is made to determine whether the following three patients receive the same dose, the next higher dose, or the next lower dose. The simplicity of this type of design has been very appealing to clinicians, because toxicity monitoring can be done by hand. The 3 + 3 design is probably acceptable with very few dose cohorts (1–3), particularly when the doses are fixed by the manufacturer, as is sometimes the case with tablets/capsules. However, in the example, there were 13 potential cohorts, making it more amenable to 'model-based' designs (e.g. Bayesian or continual reassessment methods) [9]. Such designs are now generally preferred, and perhaps more likely to be accepted by funding organisations when reviewing grant applications. They involve treating one to say three patients first, assessing toxicity, then using the observed data to fit a model between dose and toxicity rates. This model helps determine the next dose for the next cohort, and the model is re-fitted again and again as the data accumulate, therefore becoming more accurate and reliable. Model-based designs have the major potential advantages of (1) skipping doses that yield little information about toxicity and (2) requiring a fewer number of patients, hence the cabozanitib study which took 3 years to enrol 85 patients might have completed quicker had it not used a 3 + 3 design. The limitation of model-based designs is that they require statistical input (and the use of software) to monitor toxicity during the trial. However, the models can be flexible, and recently developed sophisticated model-based designs can examine two or more different therapies, or combinations of different doses and schedules; ideal for the example here.

Single Arm Phase II

For many years, the majority of phase II designs in oncology were single arm trials. All patients would receive the experimental therapy, making such studies simpler and often quicker to conduct than randomised trials. However, the main limitations of these types of designs had been:

- Using historical data on patients treated with the standard therapy as the comparator for the experimental treatment group, which can be unreliable because patient outcomes are completely confounded by time. Patients treated with a standard treatment could now have better outcomes than, for example 5–10 years before, just by improvement in patient management. Hence an experimental therapy might appear better than it really is when compared with historical instead of concurrent controls.
- Using tumour response rates as the main endpoint, which can often be poor surrogates for clinical outcomes such as OS. Some drugs might show an effect on response but not on survival, or vice versa.

The major consequence of using results from single arm trials is that new treatments or regimens that initially appear effective 'fail' when evaluated with randomised phase II or III trials: only about 40% of phase III oncology trials yield results that show benefit [10]. There is, therefore, a general preference for randomised phase II studies now, because they include concurrent controls [11]. Nevertheless, there is still a role for single arm trials (Box 25.3).

Box 25.3 Reasons Why Single Arm Trials Could Still Be of Value

- The historical control data is close in time to the trial of the experimental treatment, and ideally similar geographical location
- The trial provides initial evidence (proof of concept) of the efficacy of a new/novel single agent; particularly when few patients respond to current treatments, and the magnitude of benefit with the new therapy appears to be large
- The trial of a novel agent confirms a treatment class effect, and the benefit is much larger than expected and other types of drugs in the same class
- A combination of a novel agent with other therapies yields a benefit that is so large, that it is likely to be due to the new therapy, rather than the other active therapies in the combination
- The trial incorporates a biomarker that validates a mechanism of action, provides evidence for a promising new predictive marker, or could be used to select patients for a subsequent trial who are most likely to benefit from the experimental therapy

Based on [11].

Example 25.2 is a trial that fulfilled some of the reasons in Box 25.3. Although it only had 20 evaluable patients, the novel mechanism of action in addition to the much larger than expected effect made it appealing to a high impact factor journal [3].

Example 25.2 Selumetinib in Advanced Thyroid Cancer [3]

Design: Single arm trial

Eligibility: Patients with metastatic thyroid cancer that are refractory to radioiodine

Interventions: Oral selumetinib for 4 weeks, then an iodine-124 PET-CT scan to assess iodine uptake (to be compared to the same type of scan at baseline)

Outcomes: Iodine-124 uptake that was new, increased or both

Sample size: Very few patients usually show new/increased uptake (the investigators assume a historical control rate of **5%**), and the target was **25%** with selumetinib. They also specify a one-sided error rate of **5%** (statistical significance; i.e. there is a 5% chance they could claim an effect when there really is no effect), and power of **85%** (i.e. if there really is an improvement in uptake from 5 to 25% or higher, there is an 85% chance of finding it in a trial of a certain size). The four numbers in bold are incorporated into a formula to yield a sample size of 17 patients, of which at least 3 need to show new/increased uptake

Findings:

- 24 patients were recruited of which 20 were eligible and started selumetinib
- Of the 20, 12 showed new/increased uptake: 60%, much higher than the target of 25%
- Of these 12, eight patients met the dosimetry threshold for receiving radio-iodine therapy, of which 5 had a partial response and 3 had stable disease

The selumetinib example is a trial of an agent that may or may not have a direct anti-cancer mechanism, but instead is meant to enhance the effect of another (established) therapy, here radioiodine therapy. The historical control group effect (5%) is likely to still reflect patient outcomes at the time of the trial, because of limited other treatment options for this patient group. Another appeal of this trial and drug to both patients and clinicians, is that it only needs to be taken for a short time (4 weeks initially, then ending 2 days after iodine-131 therapy), and there were no serious side effects (grade ≥3) considered causally related to selumetinib. These attributes can be especially desirable when the youngest patient is only 44 years, up to a median of 61 years [3]. The appeal of a clinical trial can directly influence patient uptake, at a time when many patients wish to simply get on with their treatment, without the additional obligation to comply with trial-specific assessments and procedures.

Randomised Phase II

There is a wide range of randomised phase II trial designs: those with a control group receiving current standard therapy, use of a placebo control group, several experimental therapies/regimens of which one or more would proceed to phase III (often called 'pick the winner'), those that have formal interim analyses (two-stage designs, in which the trial stops if the first stage shows no/little efficacy), and those that could lead directly into a phase III trial. The main strengths of randomised studies that include a control group is that they should yield a more reliable estimate of treatment effect, increasing the chance that the experimental therapy 'succeeds' at phase III [10, 11]. They also provide initial evidence of the toxicity profile, particularly the *excess* toxicity over and above that seen with standard treatment/placebo, and the percentage of patients who agree to participate and be randomised could be examined when designing a subsequent phase III trial. The main limitations of randomised phase II trials is the requirement for a randomisation system, and more patients are needed than for single arm studies, hence the trial will usually be longer and more expensive to conduct.

Two common questions asked by investigators when designing randomised phase II trials are (1) is a placebo necessary and (2) is a 2:1 treatment allocation better than a 1:1 allocation?

Placebos are often expensive to manufacture, and they represent an added financial cost to trials, which may be prohibitive particularly when the funding organisation is not a commercial company (who would often be supplying the experimental agent anyway). The advantages of using placebo in phase III trials is well-established, and indeed a requirement in many instances in order to get a favourable review by licensing agencies or journals. Even in advanced thyroid cancer, there are some patients whose tumour(s) may partially regress spontaneously or remain stable, as observed in the placebo arms reported in a review of five randomised trials of TKI therapies for locally advanced or metastatic differentiated and medullary thyroid cancer [12]. Also, use of placebo can reliably identify adverse effects that are genuinely associated with the experimental agent [12]. However, when the aim of a phase II study is to only obtain a preliminary idea of the effect of a new treatment/regimen, the design strengths of having a placebo need to be weighed against costs and logistics.

A trial with a 1:1 random allocation is the most commonly used. But when designing a phase II study there are advantages to having more patients given the experimental therapy: (1) it is more appealing to patients if they know they have a two-thirds chance of receiving a potentially better treatment (instead of a ½ chance), and (2) if the toxicity profile of the control therapy is already well known, having more patients on the experimental treatment allows a more reliable assessment of toxicity in that group. The main disadvantage is that the sample size is larger. For example, to detect a difference in response rates of 10% vs 30% (with 80% power and one-sided 10% error rate) requires a trial of 90 patients with 1:1 allocation, but 102 (13% larger) with 2:1 allocation. The difference in study size varies according to size of effect, and can matter for trials of rare subgroups of thyroid cancer.

Example 25.3 illustrates some key features of a randomised phase II study. It is perhaps larger than typical phase II trials in oncology (which tend to have around 100 patients in total), but the main influence on study size is the expected (target) treatment effect, where the investigators have appropriately specified a moderate PFS hazard ratio of 0.71. A problem in trials (oncology or other disease area) is when investigators specify an overly large treatment effect in order to minimise the sample size. This short term apparent advantage comes at a cost later on if the observed effect is smaller (and was more realistic) than the target effect. The consequence is that results from studies like these tend to miss statistical significance [13]. It could be argued that phase II trials should aim for relatively large effects if the experimental therapy is worthwhile taking forwards to phase III. However, treatments could have moderate but still clinically important effects that are worth investigating further, and an unsatisfactory situation is terminating research too early, particularly in areas of unmet need or where there are no current effective treatments.

It is useful to be aware that the design of randomised phase II trials can be very similar to phase III, in that there is a control group and the main analysis involves a direct quantitative comparison between the trial arms. The design parameters are identical to phase III, and the key difference that leads to smaller sample sizes for phase II is the error rate (statistical significance; see Example 25.2 for definition). In superiority phase III trials, the error rate must be ≤5% and two-sided (unless there is a clear justification otherwise) to allow for the possibility that the experimental therapy could be less effective. With phase II trials, the error rate can be more relaxed, up to 20%, and be one-sided because at this stage we are only interested in the new therapy being more effective.

Example 25.3 Vandetanib for Advanced Differentiated Thyroid Cancer [14]

Design: Randomised phase II

Eligibility: Patients with locally advanced/metastatic differentiated thyroid cancer that are refractory to radioiodine

Interventions: Oral vandetanib or matching placebo until disease progression

Primary outcome: Progression-free survival (PFS) by RECIST

Sample size: 135 patients to get 100 events (progression or deaths, whichever occurred first), based on detecting a hazard ratio of **0.71**,[a] with one-sided error rate of **<20%** and **80%** power, **12** months accrual then **12** months follow up, and **10%** drop out. (The numbers in bold would be used in a formula to yield the target number of patients and events)

Findings:

- 145 patients were recruited, with 113 PFS events
- PFS hazard ratio 0.63, 95% CI 0.43–0.92, p = 0.017[b]
- Overall survival hazard ratio 0.83, p = 0.42

[a]A hazard ratio in a sample size section should be accompanied by the estimated/expected median PFS or PFS rate at a time point in either the control or experimental group

[b]The *p*-value threshold for statistical significance is the one used for the sample size (here 20%); it does not have to be 5% (as with phase III trials). Hence the result here is far below the pre-specified threshold

The trial was funded by a pharmaceutical company, making it easier to include placebo as the control group. Placebo is considered important when the main trial endpoint is PFS, because knowing the treatment allocation in an unblinded trial could influence (bias) clinicians/radiologists when assessing a patient's scan. Other key strengths of this trial were:

- Multi-centre and multi-country—which should help with generalisability (as well as ensuring that recruitment finishes on time, as occurred in this case)
- Two central independent reviewers who assessed patient scans—to confirm the date of RECIST progression specified by the local clinician. Ideally, the central reviewers should be unaware of the local clinician's assessment. Here, the central review showed a greater effect for PFS, with a hazard ratio of 0.49 (compared to 0.63 using the local assessment). There is greater interest in whether the central review yields a smaller treatment effect, as is often seen in oncology trials.

The observed hazard ratio was 0.63, which is a measure of *relative effect*, and can be converted to a percentage change in risk (technically hazards), which is interpreted as a 37% reduction. This is clinically important, and it exceeds the target of 0.71 (29% risk reduction). The hazard ratio for OS (0.83, $p = 0.42$) indicates no statistically significant effect (though the trial was not powered for this). However, many patients on placebo were allowed to cross over to vandetanib on disease progression or after 12 months with stable disease. One justification for having crossover is to allow the control patients to receive the potentially more effective therapy at some point. Whilst this has some merit, large numbers of crossover makes OS difficult to interpret reliably: it can substantially dilute the treatment effect.

Late Phase Trials

Whilst large scale phase III trials in other cancers have been established for decades, the idea of conducting similar studies in thyroid cancer many years ago, with its relatively low incidence, might have sounded overly ambitious. Nevertheless, with better networks of clinicians, scientists, statisticians and trial management within and between countries, and support from funding organisations, phase III studies in this cancer type are no longer considered unfeasible.

Superiority Phase III Studies (Suitable for Advanced Disease)

Patients with low risk disease, such as well-differentiated thyroid cancer, already have excellent outcomes, such that it is not feasible to find better treatments, when only a few patients relapse. Instead, superiority trials are of interest in poorer prognosis patients (advanced cancer), where there is much room for improvement in outcomes.

Example 25.4 shows a recent large trial. As with Example 25.3, key strengths include multi-centre and multi-country. Although clinical trials generally use 80% power and 5% error rate when estimating sample size, it is useful to note that the investigators here wanted a trial with even higher power (90%) and lower error rate (1%). This will always yield a larger, more expensive, and probably longer study, but the benefits are results that are highly reliable, which should making the findings appealing to regulatory agencies and payers.

Example 25.4 Lenvatinib for Progressive Thyroid Cancer, the SELECT Trial [15]
Design: Randomised phase III

Eligibility: Patients with evidence of disease progression and refractory to radio-iodine therapy

Interventions: Oral lenvatinib or matching placebo until disease progression or unacceptable side effects

Primary outcome: Progression-free survival (PFS) using independent radiological review

Sample size: 392 patients to get 214 events (progression or deaths, whichever occurred first), based on detecting an improvement in median PFS from **8** to **14** months, hazard ratio of **0.57**, with two-sided error rate of **1** and **90%** power. (The numbers in bold would be used in a formula to yield the target number of patients and events)

Findings:

- 392 patients were recruited (2:1 allocation), with 220 PFS events
- PFS hazard ratio 0.21, 99% CI 0.13–0.31, p < 0.001
- Median PFS 18.3 (lenvatinib) vs. 3.6 months (placebo)
- Overall survival hazard ratio 0.53, p = 0.005 [17]

In example 25.4, the treatment is specified to continue until progression rather than a fixed time period. There has been debate on this issue in oncology trials: i.e. exposing patients to a therapy with potential side effects for long periods of time and the financial cost of this, versus the cancer responds well and the therapy keeps it at bay, with the obvious benefits to patients. The latter argument might be preferred with a view that if long-duration therapy is effective, future trials might examine whether efficacy is compromised by reducing treatment duration.

When interpreting trials it is always useful to compare observed outcomes with those expected. This helps determine whether patients in the trial were fairly representative of the target population. In Example 25.4, the median PFS in the control group was anticipated to be 8 months, but it was only half of this in the actual trial (3.6 months). Sometimes the mix of patients (e.g. disease status) explains this, and it is worth examining the baseline characteristics table. Nevertheless, the observed *absolute* benefit (14.7 months improvement in median PFS) is much larger than expected (6 months). Similarly, the observed *relative* effect (hazard ratio 0.21; 79% reduction in risk) is much greater than expected (hazard ratio 0.57, 43% risk reduction). Both are arguably striking results.

The toxicity profile of all trials should be examined carefully, and balanced against the magnitude of the improvement in efficacy. In the SELECT trial, there was a large difference in the percentage of patients with any-treatment related toxicity of grade ≥3: 76% lenvatinib vs. 10% placebo, with notable specific effects on hypertension, diarrhoea, and weight loss. It is also worth considering the percentage of patients who discontinue treatment for toxicity in any trial, because this might affect efficacy if very unbalanced, though it reflects how well patients tolerate the treatment (14% lenvatinib vs. 2% placebo).

A major aspect of the SELECT study was that patients on placebo were allowed to cross over to lenvatinib if they progressed, which occurred for nearly 90% of these patients. This issue was raised in Example 25.3, but the decision to allow cross over is even more important for confirmatory phase III trials, where benefits on PFS only might lead to uncertainty over the value of the treatment to patients when considered by some clinicians but particularly payers (health technology assessment agencies). In the SELECT trial, the OS hazard ratio in the first report was 0.73, which became 0.62 after attempting to adjust for crossovers at that early analysis [15]. Fortunately, the final analysis showed an adjusted hazard ratio of 0.53 (p = 0.005), indicative of a large effect on survival [16]. However, some may question the validity of the statistical adjustment when there are so many crossovers.

Most phase III trials of thyroid cancer have PFS as the primary endpoint, which raises questions about it being used as a surrogate marker for OS. The topic of surrogate markers in oncology is ongoing, and there are relatively few very good surrogates for OS (a surrogate and OS need to be highly correlated) [17]. The key issue arises when there are clear benefits for PFS but not for OS. An example of this is the EXAM trial of cabozantinib for advanced medullary thyroid cancer: a phase III study [2] conducted after the promising findings from the phase I study (in Example 25.1) [8]. Whilst there was a substantial improvement for

PFS (hazard ratio 0.28, median PFS increased from 4 to 11.2 months, compared to placebo), the improvement in median OS was 5.5 months (from 21.1 to 26.6 months), which although is not negligible, it was nowhere near statistical significance ($p = 0.24$) [18]. This result could not be explained by crossovers because it was not allowed in the trial. There seemed to be an effect on OS within the subgroup of patients who had RET M918T mutations (median OS increased from 18.9 to 44.3 months, $p = 0.026$), but this may need further investigation/confirmation.

The importance of PFS to cancer patients continues to be the subject of research [19, 20]. Some patients do not understand PFS, [20] and it is suggested that improvements in PFS should ideally come with positive impacts on QoL [19]. A combined analysis of two trials of afatinib in lung cancer, for example, showed a clear positive correlation between PFS and QoL, and the authors concluded that PFS is a relevant endpoint for these patients [21]. It is therefore valuable for future thyroid cancer trials to collect data on QoL.

Non-Inferiority Phase III Studies (Suitable for Low Risk Disease)

The increasing number of trials of systemic therapies for patients with advanced thyroid cancers is very encouraging, with substantial impacts on clinical practice seen in recent years. In patients with low risk disease there have been several important unresolved research questions, usually associated with less interventions for patients. One major question was whether a low administered activity (dose) of radioiodine for ablation could be used instead of the standard high dose. Small underpowered randomised trials had been attempted, but without clear results that could change practice [5]. The issue is that non-inferiority trials are always larger than superiority studies, because the aim is to have a study size big enough to exclude the possibility of the smallest clinically important difference between two intervention arms, rather than just yield a statistically significant result [4]. Such studies require national collaborations, and two are shown in Example 25.5. Both trials (HiLo and ESTIMABL) had the same intention of determining whether patients could have the lower radioiodine dose, and they included another main objective: to determine whether preparing patients for ablation using Thyrogen affects ablation success. Trials with two main research questions are factorial studies, which are relatively uncommon in oncology, but is a very efficient approach, that can be appealing to funders, as was the case here.

One key design issue for non-inferiority trials is specifying the non-inferiority margin, i.e. the maximum allowable difference (Example 25.5). If it is set to be too large, patients, clinicians and payers would not accept the trial results, but the smaller the margin, the larger the trial (and longer and more expensive). In Example 25.5, a difference of 10% points was discussed and importantly had to be agreed by many investigators as well as the funding organisation, to ensure that the results would be acceptable for clinical practice.

Having two or more trials of the same intervention for the same cancer is not very common in oncology nowadays, unlike many years ago when it was usual practice for different researchers to conduct similar trials. Example 25.5 represents a good case where having two similar but not identical trials, and from different countries, produces the strongest evidence when they yield similar results. As a result, international practice changed [22–24]. Differences in design allow one trial to complement the other, particularly with the inclusion of T3 stage in HiLo, for which some UK investigators were unsure whether to include at the start of the trial, but were reassured when the subgroup analysis for T3 alone also showed no difference in ablation success between 1.1 and 3.7 GBq [6].

The trials in Example 25.5 aimed to avoid the limitations of previous randomised trials examining the same question, by having:

- Thyroid cancer confirmed by histopathology (plus central independent review in HiLo)
- Total thyroidectomy by specialist surgeons
- Central laboratory for measurement of thyroglobulin

Example 25.5 Radioiodine for Well-Differentiated Thyroid Cancer, the HiLo [6] and ESTIMABL Trials [7]

Design: Randomised factorial phase III

Eligibility: Patients T1–T2 disease at diagnosis with possible spread to the neck lymph nodes, but no metastases. They had to have had a total thyroidectomy. HiLo also included T3 disease

Interventions: Patients were randomised to be prepared for ablation using either thyroid hormone withdrawal (THW) or recombinant human thyroid stimulating hormone (Thyrogen), and in each of these groups, patients were randomised to have radioiodine ablation using either 1.1 vs. 3.7 GBq

Primary outcome: Ablation success rate 6–9 months after ablation using both negative scan and low thyroglobulin (HiLo used an iodine-131 scan, ESTIMABL used ultrasound).

Sample size: 421 patients for HiLo and 700 for ESTIMABL. Both had 80–82% power for a non-inferiority margin of 10% points (i.e. assuming the ablation success rate with 3.7 GBq is 80%, the true rate with 1.1 GBq can go down to 70% and be acceptable, but any lower would mean that 1.1 GBq is substantially less effective and should not be recommended). The same margin applied to the comparison of THW and Thyrogen. The difference in sample size is due to HiLo using a one-sided error rate of 5%, whilst ESTIMABL used 2.5%

Findings:

- HiLo recruited 428 patients. Ablation success was 85% (low) vs. 89% (high dose); and 87% (Thyrogen) vs. 87% (hormone withdrawal
- ESTIMABL recruited 752 patients. Ablation success was 91% (low) vs. 93% (high dose); and 92% (Thyrogen) vs. 93% (hormone withdrawal
- Importantly, the 95% confidence interval for the differences in ablation rates for each research question were within the allowable margin of 10% points; it is this that allows the conclusion of non-inferiority to be made

- Pre-ablation thyroglobulin, and in HiLo a pre-ablation scan to examine remnant size after surgery

Trials of low risk patients must be able to address important outcomes for patients, such as QoL and social impact. One of the main advantages of using 1.1 GBq for ablation was that patients require fewer days in hospital isolation. The trials in Example 25.5 also showed that patients prepared using Thyrogen had significantly better QoL than those who had to endure thyroid hormone withdrawal 2–4 weeks before ablation. Both of these aspects matter a great deal to younger patients with families [6, 25]. Established QoL questionnaires should be used, and HiLo and ESTIMABL both employed the Short-Form36. In addition the HiLo study collected information on social impact, such as difficulty in performing activities at home or work, and ability to take care of children (all showing positive results for Thyrogen), [6], and ESTIMABL collected data on patient travel costs and cost of sick leave [25].

The two research groups who conducted HiLo and ESTIMABL are currently conducting two similar, and again not identical, large randomised trials, which represent the next logical step after reducing the ablation dose from 3.7 GBq to 1.1 GBq. These are IoN (clinicaltrials.gov NCT01398085) and ESTIMABL2 (NCT01837745), which aim to show that suitable low risk patients do not require radioiodine ablation at all. Observational studies yield conflicting results, though the more recent ones indicate that ablation appears unnecessary [26].

However, this is another controversial issue, where only a randomised trial can fully address the question [26]. IoN and ESTIMABL involve randomising carefully selected low risk patients with well-differentiated thyroid cancer to receive either 1.1 GBq or no ablation. Recruitment to these two studies is more challenging than for HiLo and ESTIMABL, because of the possible perception by some patients that they could be receiving 'no treatment,' when in fact they have already had a total thyroidectomy and are on thyroid hormone therapy. For trials like these, it is therefore essential to get good support from clinical investigators (because they need to be able to explain the trial), but importantly also from patient support groups. IoN, for example, has had active involvement from the UK national thyroid cancer charity, Butterfly Thyroid Cancer Trust (http://www.butterfly.org.uk), from the point of inception through to grant application, then study conduct.

Immunotherapy Trials

There is substantial activity in immunotherapies for oncology in recent years, with major advances in melanoma and lung cancer. Understandably, there is growing interest in thyroid cancer, with ongoing early phase trials of pembrolizumab for advanced or radioiodine refractory tumours [27, 28]. Designs of immunotherapy trials are generally like most other systemic treatment trials (examples above), but notable features include selection of patients, timing of scans, and interpretation of results.

A key design consideration for immunotherapy trials is whether or not to select patients based on PD-L1 or PD-1 expression. The ongoing iPRIME trial of pembrolizumab combined with docetaxel for aggressive radioiodine refractory disease does not select on biomarker expression [27]. The advantage of this is the investigators will be able to examine whether efficacy is noticeably different between patients with PD-L1 positive or negative tumours, or that all patients benefit. A potential disadvantage is that if tumours with low/no expression do not respond well, including them will dilute the overall treatment effect, acknowledging that subgroup analyses according to expression status will be limited by sample size. The KEYNOTE-28 trial of pembrolizumab for advanced papillary or follicular thyroid cancer only includes patients whose tumours express PD-L1 in $\geq 1\%$ cells, with the advantage that this study might be more likely to find a treatment effect, but then they will be unable to make any conclusions about PD-L1 negative patients [28].

The timing of scans is partly related to interpretation of results. PFS is often used in thyroid cancer trials, and in immunotherapy studies the Kaplan-Meier curves for PFS sometimes appear as in Fig. 25.1, for example ipilimumab for melanoma [29]. It initially seems that immunotherapy is ineffective early on, but on closer inspection of the design the lack of early separation is due to the scheduling of imaging that defines PFS measurement. In the melanoma trial, the timing of the first radiological assessment scan for progression was 12 weeks, which coincides with the median PFS (2.8 months in both groups), making it appear that there is no difference. Hence, median PFS may not be a useful measure here, because the 'true' progression for many patients clearly occurred before 12 weeks.

Another problem with Kaplan-Meier curves as in Fig. 25.1 (whether for PFS or OS), is that the assumption of proportional hazards does not hold. Therefore, hazard ratios are inappropriate, despite still being reported in the literature [30]. There are more appropriate effect sizes, for example using the area under the curves (Life Expectancy Difference and Life Expectancy Ratio without progression), which can also provide two estimates of each measure, before and after the curves separate, reflecting that whilst some patients do not benefit, others derive greater (and potentially long-lasting) benefit [30].

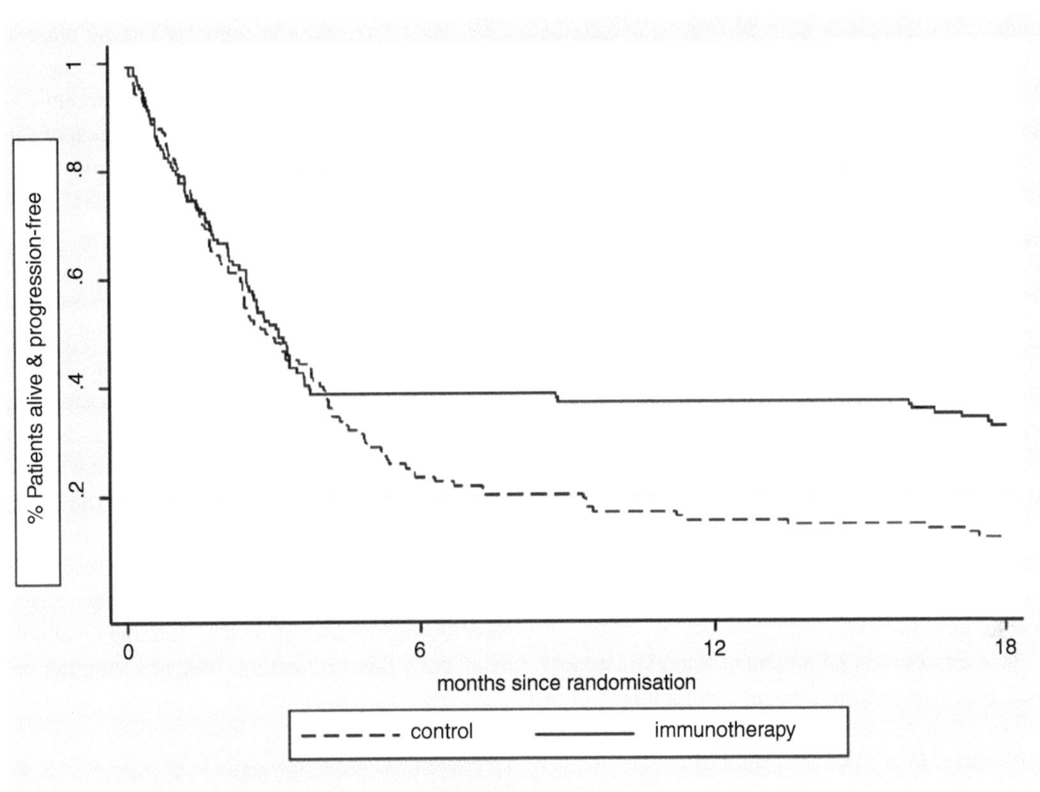

	Effect size
Incorrectly assuming proportional hazards	
Improvement in median PFS	0.4 months (3.2 immunotherapy vs. 2.8 control)
Relative effect (hazard ratio)	0.68
Alternative method (no assumption required) [31]	
Improvement in 'average' PFS*(LED)	2.4 months (7.7 vs 5.3 months)
Relative effect (LER)	1.46 (or 1/1.46=0.68 in same direction as HR)
Only after the curves separate	
Improvement in 'average' PFS* (LED)	2.3 months (5.0 vs 2.7 months)
Relative effect (LER)	1.83 (or 1/1.83=0.55 in same direction as HR)

*area under the curve LED: Life Expectancy Difference without progression LER: Life Expectancy Ratio without progression

Fig. 25.1 Kaplan-Meier curves typically seen for some trials of immunotherapy in solid tumours, and different types of effect sizes [30]

Surgical Trials

With more clinical trials of systemic and radioiodine interventions, there appears to be increasing attention to surgical trials. Surgeons can play a central role in thyroid cancer trials, including recruitment to treatment trials, and translational research because of their easy access to tissue sample collection [31]. Specific areas of interest for surgical trials are: [26, 32–34].

- the use of lobectomy instead of total thyroidectomy for low risk patients
- the value of prophylactic central compartment neck dissection (PCCND) in node-negative papillary thyroid cancer
- the role of robotic surgery instead of open thyroidectomy.

Current evidence for all of these are exclusively from observational studies, including large studies with long follow up. However, whilst, for example, several observational studies indicate that patients who have lobectomy have low recurrence rates and so could avoid a total thyroidectomy, others arrive at the opposite conclusion [35]. There have been occasions in medicine when surgical approaches have been introduced in expert centres, and then become more commonplace over time. Although the strength of evidence for the change is limited, conducting a randomised trial might be too challenging if practice already appears to have moved on. Furthermore, if a randomised study is perceived as being unfeasible at the start, the clinical community might never attempt such studies. For example, it has been estimated that 5840 patients are needed for a trial to evaluate PCCND, which would require major international long-term co-operation [36].

Recruitment to and conduct of surgical oncology trials have often been challenging. In a review of three such trials in head and neck cancer in the UK, the main barriers were: [37].

- Patient preference for one surgical arm over another
- Surgeon preference for one surgical arm over another (so they do not have equipoise)
- Lack of time in clinic for the surgeon to deal with the paperwork associated with the trial
- Lack of resources/staff and time to conduct the trial in the clinic

If surgical trials in thyroid cancer are to be successful, they need sufficient support and funding for surgeons and their research teams, with full engagement from patient support groups (as employed in other areas).

Future Trials

Thyroid cancer incidence has almost tripled in the USA from 1975 through 2009 from 4.9 to 14.3 cases per 100,000 individuals [38]. Similar trends are observed in the UK, where incidence has more than doubled since the 1970s, and is projected to rise by 74% between 2014 and 2035 [39]. Therefore, reducing exposure to radiation to a patient group that is increasing in size is important, in addition to finding other interventions that are safer, more convenient, or cheaper for patients and payers. Finding more effective therapies for advanced disease, particularly those with radioiodine refractory tumours, should also be a priority.

The sections in this chapter have covered a range of issues in relation to different trial phases and interventions. Clinicians who treat thyroid cancer often treat other tumours too, therefore the work associated with developing new trial ideas or conducting an existing trial in their centre can appear daunting. Also, individual centres are often reluctant to spend resources on the substantial bureaucratic procedures associated with setting up a trial, when they would only see a few cases. Nevertheless, with substantial funding available from both the commercial and non-commercial

Box 25.4 Some Ideal Features of Future Trials

- Larger trials with greater collaborations between networks of clinicians within and between countries
- Use of more sophisticated but efficient methods for designing phase I trials
- More use of phase II/III trials, in which patients from the phase II stage are included in the final assessment at phase II, rather than the common approach of separate phase II and III
- Attempts to design and conduct surgical trials associated with long-standing research questions
- Continue close collaboration with patient support groups and charities when designing and conducting trials
- Biomarker-embedded trials, where one or more biomarkers are used to direct treatment
- Genomic research, including the definition and clinical relevance of tumour heterogeneity, and how this influences response to treatment

- Better understanding of the value of PFS to thyroid cancer patients, because it will likely remain the most commonly used endpoint in therapy trials
- Non-invasive sensitive methods for diagnosing or monitoring thyroid cancer, including the relevance and application of circulating tumour cells

sector it is hoped that these issues can be overcome. Box 25.4 lists some general considerations for future trials.

The traditional approach to drug development has been to conduct separate phase II and III trials. This requires many patients and long duration in total. However, phase II/III studies have great appeal, whereby patients are analysed in the phase II stage to observe initial evidence of treatment efficacy, and if 'positive' the trial proceeds to phase III, and all are included together for the final analysis. This has been an efficient approach in other similarly uncommon cancers, for example biliary tract cancer [40], with special remark on designs like this in the editorial [41].

Two other important areas are the application of biomarkers [42] and sensitive/non-invasive methods of diagnosis or monitoring. Biomarkers in thyroid cancer are already used in some ongoing trials. A recent single arm phase II trial of vemurafenib for patients with BRAF mutation showed very promising results on tumour response [43]. These are the types of trials that are appealing, even though they are single arm (Box 25.3). Similarly, a randomised phase II trial of dabrafenib and dabrafenib plus trametinib had also preselected patients for inclusion based on having BRAF positive tumours, and showed response rates much higher than anticipated [44]. The collection of tumour and blood samples for translational research will become standard because of the opportunity to find novel insights into the mechanism of therapies, and to use new biomarkers for prognosis and to predict outcomes (tumour response and PFS) for specific treatments.

Technological advances, including cheaper next generation sequencing, means good potential for finding simple and cost-effective biomarkers for thyroid cancer patients. Liquid biopsy (identifying tumour cells or tumour DNA in blood, saliva, or urine) represents an opportunity to find more sensitive ways of diagnosing (earlier detection) and monitoring patients (during and after treatment), compared to traditional approaches such as using tumour tissue (invasive), thyroglobulin or calcitonin [45]. Such methods might also produce better prognostic or predictive models, and have particular value when it is not possible to obtain a biopsy of the tumour because of its location or patient fitness. Future trials could involve randomising patients to blood (non-invasive) monitoring tests followed by some intervention or closer monitoring when early signs of relapse are seen in liquid biopsies before there is of clinical/imaging evidence of relapse, or no monitoring and treat as usual practice when clinically indicated.

Summary

The successful conduct of a range of clinical trials in thyroid cancer has had major impacts on the management of these patients, and provides new insight into the biological mechanisms. With much interest by both commercial and non-commercial funding organisations, clinical trials of thyroid cancer, with its increasing incidence, should continue to be encouraged, with modern designs and ideally including surgical approaches and biomarkers embedded into the design.

References

1. Cooper DS, Anton B. The decade in clinical thyroid disease: an analysis of published literature. Thyroid. 2016;26(8):993–1003.
2. Elisei R, Schlumberger MJ, Müller SP, Schöffski P, Brose MS, Shah MH, Licitra L, Jarzab B, Medvedev V, Kreissl MC, Niederle B, Cohen EE, Wirth LJ, Ali H, Hessel C, Yaron Y, Ball D, Nelkin B, Sherman SI. Cabozantinib in progressive medullary thyroid cancer. J Clin Oncol. 2013;31(29):3639–46.
3. Ho AL, Grewal RK, Leboeuf R, Sherman EJ, Pfister DG, Deandreis D, Pentlow KS, Zanzonico PB,

Haque S, Gavane S, Ghossein RA, Ricarte-Filho JC, Domínguez JM, Shen R, Tuttle RM, Larson SM, Fagin JA. Selumetinib-enhanced radioiodine uptake in advanced thyroid cancer. N Engl J Med. 2013;368(7):623–32.
4. Hackshaw AK. A concise guide to clinical trials. 1st ed. Hoboken: Wiley-Blackwell, BMJ Books; 2009. isbn:9781405167741.
5. Hackshaw AK, Harmer C, Mallick U, Haq M, Franklyn J. ^{131}I activity for remnant ablation in patients with differentiated thyroid cancer: a systematic review. J Clin Endocrinol Metab. 2007;92(1):28–38.
6. Mallick U, Harmer C, Yap B, Wadsley J, Clarke S, Moss L, Nicol A, Clark PM, Farnell K, McCready R, Smellie J, Franklyn J, John R, Nutting C, Newbold K, Lemon C, Gerrard G, Abdel-Hamid A, Hardman J, Macias E, Roques T, Whitaker S, Vijayan R, Alvarez P, Beare S, Forsyth S, Kadalayil L, Hackshaw A. Ablation with low-dose radioiodine and thyrotropin alfa in thyroid cancer. N Engl J Med. 2012;366:1674–85.
7. Schlumberger M, Catargi B, Borget I, Deandreis D, Zerdoud S, Bridji B, Bardet S, Leenhardt L, Bastie D, Schvartz C, Vera P, Morel O, Benisvy D, Bournaud C, Bonichon F, Dejax C, Toubert ME, Leboulleux S, Ricard M, Benhamou E, Tumeurs de la Thyroïde Refractaires Network for the Essai Stimulation Ablation Equivalence Trial. Strategies of radioiodine ablation in patients with low-risk thyroid cancer. N Engl J Med. 2012;366(18):1663–73.
8. Kurzrock R, Sherman SI, Ball DW, Forastiere AA, Cohen RB, Mehra R, Pfister DG, Cohen EE, Janisch L, Nauling F, Hong DS, Ng CS, Ye L, Gagel RF, Frye J, Müller T, Ratain MJ, Salgia R. Activity of XL184 (Cabozantinib), an oral tyrosine kinase inhibitor, in patients with medullary thyroid cancer. J Clin Oncol. 2011;29(19):2660–6.
9. Love SB, Brown S, Weir CJ, Harbron C, Yap C, Gaschler-Markefski B, Matcham J, Caffrey L, McKevitt C, Clive S, Craddock C, Spicer J, Cornelius V. Embracing model-based designs for dose-finding trials. Br J Cancer. 2017;117(3):332–9.
10. Sharma MR, Stadler WM, Ratain MJ. Randomized phase II trials: a long-term investment with promising returns. J Natl Cancer Inst. 2011;103(14):1093–10.
11. Cannistra SA. Phase II trials in the journal of clinical oncology. J Clin Oncol. 2009;27(19):3073–6.
12. Llavero-Valero M, Guillén-Grima F, Zafon C, Galofré JC. The placebo effect in thyroid cancer: a meta-analysis. Eur J Endocrinol. 2016;174(4):465–72.
13. Hackshaw A, Kirkwood A. Research and methods: interpreting and reporting clinical trials with results of borderline statistical significance. BMJ. 2011;343:d3340. https://doi.org/10.1136/bmj.d3340.
14. Leboulleux S, Bastholt L, Krause T, de la Fouchardiere C, Tennvall J, Awada A, Gómez JM, Bonichon F, Leenhardt L, Soufflet C, Licour M, Schlumberger MJ. Vandetanib in locally advanced or metastatic differentiated thyroid cancer: a randomised, double-blind, phase 2 trial. Lancet Oncol. 2012;13(9):897–905.
15. Schlumberger M, Tahara M, Wirth LJ, Robinson B, Brose MS, Elisei R, Habra MA, Newbold K, Shah MH, Hoff AO, Gianoukakis AG, Kiyota N, Taylor MH, Kim SB, Krzyzanowska MK, Dutcus CE, de las Heras B, Zhu J, Sherman SI. Lenvatinib versus placebo in radioiodine-refractory thyroid cancer. N Engl J Med. 2015;372(7):621–30.
16. Haddad RI, Schlumberger M, Wirth LJ, Sherman EJ, Shah MH, Robinson B, Dutcus CE, Teng A, Gianoukakis AG, Sherman SI. Incidence and timing of common adverse events in Lenvatinib-treated patients from the SELECT trial and their association with survival outcomes. Endocrine. 2017;56(1):121–8.
17. Ciani O, Davis S, Tappenden P, Garside R, Stein K, Cantrell A, Saad ED, Buyse M, Taylor RS. Validation of surrogate endpoints in advanced solid tumors: systematic review of statistical methods, results, and implications for policy makers. Int J Technol Assess Health Care. 2014;30(3):312–24.
18. Schlumberger M, Elisei R, Muller S, et al. Final overall survival analysis of EXAM, an international, double-blind, randomized, placebo-controlled phase III trial of cabozantinib (Cabo) in medullary thyroid carcinoma (MTC) patients with documented RECIST progression at baseline. Proc Am Soc Clin Oncol. 2015;33(Suppl):6012 (abstr).
19. Fallowfield LJ, Fleissig A. The value of progression-free survival to patients with advanced-stage cancer. Nat Rev Clin Oncol. 2012;9:41–7.
20. Fallowfield LJ, Catt SL, May SF, Matthews L, Shilling VM, Simcock R, Westwell S, Jenkins VA. Therapeutic aims of drugs offering only progression-free survival are misunderstood by patients, and oncologists may be overly optimistic about likely benefits. Support Care Cancer. 2017;25(1):237–44.
21. Griebsch I, Palmer M, Fayers PM, Ellis S. Is progression-free survival associated with a better health-related quality of life in patients with lung cancer? Evidence from two randomised trials with afatinib. BMJ Open. 2014;4(10):e005762.
22. Haugen BR, Alexander EK, Bible KC, Doherty GM, Mandel SJ, Nikiforov YE, Pacini F, Randolph GW, Sawka AM, Schlumberger M, Schuff KG, Sherman SI, Sosa JA, Steward DL, Tuttle RM, Wartofsky L. 2015 American Thyroid Association management guidelines for adult patients with thyroid nodules and differentiated thyroid cancer: the American Thyroid Association guidelines task force on thyroid nodules and differentiated thyroid cancer. Thyroid. 2016;26(1):1–133.
23. Perros P, Boelaert K, Colley S, Evans C, Evans RM, Gerrard BA, Gilbert J, Harrison B, Johnson SJ, Giles TE, Moss L, Lewington V, Newbold K, Taylor J, Thakker RV, Watkinson J, Williams GR, British Thyroid Association. Guidelines for the management of thyroid cancer. Clin Endocrinol. 2014;81(Suppl 1):1–122.

24. US National Comprehensive Cancer Network. Clinical practice guidelines in oncology, version 2.2017. 2017.
25. Borget I, Bonastre J, Catargi B, Déandréis D, Zerdoud S, Rusu D, Bardet S, Leenhardt L, Bastie D, Schvartz C, Vera P, Morel O, Benisvy D, Bournaud C, Bonichon F, Kelly A, Toubert ME, Leboulleux S, Journeau F, Benhamou E, Schlumberger M. Quality of life and cost-effectiveness assessment of radioiodine ablation strategies in patients with thyroid cancer: results from the randomized phase III ESTIMABL trial. J Clin Oncol. 2015;33(26):2885–92.
26. McLeod DS, Sawka AM, Cooper DS. Controversies in primary treatment of low-risk papillary thyroid cancer. Lancet. 2013;381(9871):1046–57.
27. Seiwert TY, De Souza JA, Vokes EE, Agrawal N. A phase II study of pembrolizumab and docetaxel for aggressive RAI refractory thyroid carcinomas or salivary gland cancers: the iPRIME study. J Clin Oncol. 2017;35(Suppl 15):6099.
28. Mehnert JM, Varga A, Brose M, Aggarwal RR. Pembrolizumab for advanced papillary or follicular thyroid cancer: preliminary results from the phase 1b KEYNOTE-028 study. J Clin Oncol. 2016;34(Suppl):6091.
29. Hodi FS, O'Day SJ, McDermott DF, Weber RW, et al. Improved survival with ipilimumab in patients with metastatic melanoma. N Engl J Med. 2010;363(8):711–23.
30. Dehbi HM, Royston P, Hackshaw A. Life expectancy difference and life expectancy ratio: two measures of treatment effects in randomised trials with non-proportional hazards. BMJ. 2017;357:j2250.
31. You YN, Wells SA Jr. Role of surgeons in clinical trials for thyroid cancer. World J Surg. 2007;31(5):987–95.
32. Cabanillas ME, McFadden DG, Durante C. Thyroid cancer. Lancet. 2016;388(10061):2783–95.
33. Gambardella C, Tartaglia E, Nunziata A, Izzo G, Siciliano G, Cavallo F, Mauriello C, Napolitano S, Thomas G, Testa D, Rossetti G, Sanguinetti A, Avenia N, Conzo G. Clinical significance of prophylactic central compartment neck dissection in the treatment of clinically node-negative papillary thyroid cancer patients. World J Surg Oncol. 2016;14(1):247.
34. Son SK, Kim JH, Bae JS, Lee SH. Surgical safety and oncologic effectiveness in robotic versus conventional open thyroidectomy in thyroid cancer: a systematic review and meta-analysis. Ann Surg Oncol. 2015;22(9):3022–32.
35. Hwangbo Y, Kim JM, Park YJ, Lee EK, Lee YJ, Park DJ, Choi YS, Lee KD, Sohn SY, Kim SW, Chung JH, Lim DJ, Kim MH, Kim MJ, Jo YS, Shong MH, Koong SS, Hahm JR, Jung JH, Yi KH. Long-term recurrence of small papillary thyroid cancer and its risk factors in a Korean multicenter study. J Clin Endocrinol Metab. 2017;102(2):625–33.
36. Carling T, Carty SE, Ciarleglio MM, Cooper DS, Doherty GM, Kim LT, Kloos RT, Mazzaferri EL Sr, Peduzzi PN, Roman SA, Sippel RS, Sosa JA, Stack BC Jr, Steward DL, Tufano RP, Tuttle RM, Udelsman R, American Thyroid Association Surgical Affairs Committee. American Thyroid Association design and feasibility of a prospective randomized controlled trial of prophylactic central lymph node dissection for papillary thyroid carcinoma. Thyroid. 2012;22(3):237–44.
37. Kaur G, Hutchison I, Mehanna H, Williamson P, Shaw R, Tudur Smith C. Barriers to recruitment for surgical trials in head and neck oncology: a survey of trial investigators. BMJ Open. 2013;3(4):e002625.
38. Davies L, Welch H. Current thyroid cancer trends in the United States. JAMA Otolaryngol Head Neck Surg. 2014;140:317–22.
39. Cancer Research UK. Thyroid cancer statistics. http://www.cancerresearchuk.org/health-professional/cancer-statistics/statistics-by-cancer-type/thyroid-cancer.
40. Valle J, Wasan H, Palmer DH, Cunningham D, Anthoney A, Maraveyas A, Madhusudan S, Iveson T, Hughes S, Pereira SP, Roughton M, Bridgewater J, ABC-02 Trial Investigators. Cisplatin plus gemcitabine versus gemcitabine for biliary tract cancer. N Engl J Med. 2010;362(14):1273–81.
41. Wolpin BM, Mayer RJ. A step forward in the treatment of advanced biliary tract cancer. N Engl J Med. 2010;362:1335–7.
42. Xing M, Haugen BR, Schlumberger M. Progress in molecular-based management of differentiated thyroid cancer. Lancet. 2013;381(9871):1058–69.
43. Brose MS, Cabanillas ME, Cohen EE, Wirth LJ, Riehl T, Yue H, Sherman SI, Sherman EJ. Vemurafenib in patients with BRAF(V600E)-positive metastatic or unresectable papillary thyroid cancer refractory to radioactive iodine: a non-randomised, multicentre, open-label, phase 2 trial. Lancet Oncol. 2016;17(9):1272–82.
44. Shah MH, Wei L, Wirth LJ, Daniels GA, De Souza JA, Timmers CD, et al. Results of randomized phase II trial of dabrafenib versus dabrafenib plus trametinib in BRAF-mutated papillary thyroid carcinoma. J Clin Oncol. 2017;35(Suppl):6022.
45. Cote GJ, Evers C, Hu M, et al. Poster 74. Liquid biopsy of cfDNA as a predictor of survival in medullary thyroid carcinoma patients with somatic *RET* M918T mutations. Presented at American Thyroid Association Annual Meeting; Sept 21–25, 2016; Denver, Colorado.

26 The Barriers to Uniform Implementation of Clinical Practice Guidelines (CPG) for Thyroid Cancer

Ujjal K. Mallick and Fabián Pitoia

Introduction

Clinical Practice Guidelines (CPGs) provide recommendations about the current best practice likely to offer the best outcome based upon the most reliable scientific evidence available at the time, for relevant professionals, patients, and policy makers of healthcare organizations. National CPGs thus aim to standardize high quality care amongst all professionals, specialist units and hospitals of the country by reducing the variation and heterogeneity in practice.

They also might play an important role in providing good practice guidance for specialist professionals in other countries who can consider using some well researched respected CPGs appropriately adapted to their local priorities and needs, as a basis for discussion and developing their own.

The problems of implementation of CPG's in different countries based on the local needs and resources are beyond the scope of this chapter and no attempt is made to discuss these issues in detail here. But valuable opinion (unedited) of some experts commenting on the prevailing situation in their own country are included below. Because of lack of space and time it has been possible to include only selected examples with the help of colleagues who kindly contributed.

However, it is the observation of many clinicians and several studies that implementation of guidelines is less than optimal across different specialist centers in the same country. The various reasons for this and possible solutions are well documented in the literature [1–12]. Generally speaking, according to one of the authors of this chapter, it might be helpful to briefly mention the presumed difficulties to uniform CPG implementation in the following categories:

Generic Factors

1. Educational—Some clinicians may not be quite aware or well informed about all of the recommendations provided in the CPG for specific clinical scenarios. The situation should be hopefully quite rare now-a days among specialist multidisciplinary team (MDT) members due to continuing professional development (CPD), and continuing medical education (CME) programme requirements etc. But attempts such as providing an aide memoir in the clinic have been suggested. A computer based clinical decision making module support system (CDMM) of

U. K. Mallick (✉)
Chief Investigator UK National "IoN" and HiLo Trials, Past clinical oncologist and Chair Regional Thyroid MDT, Northern Centre for Cancer Care, Freeman Hospital, Newcastle upon Tyne, United Kingdom
e-mail: Ujjal.mallick@nuth.nhs.uk

F. Pitoia
Division of Endocrinology, Hospital de Clínicas, University of Buenos Aires, Buenos Aires, Argentina
e-mail: fpitoia@intramed.net

U. K. Mallick et al. (eds.), *Practical Management of Thyroid Cancer*,
https://doi.org/10.1007/978-3-319-91725-2_26

the Thyroid Cancer Care Collaborative (TCCC) has been proposed in the United States and might be tested in other countries.
2. Cultural—Clinicians may be well informed about the CPGs but for a variety of reasons are resistant or unable to change practice. Some of the reasons could be related to the interpretation of the recommendation provided in the CPG by individual professionals because of the inherent limitations of thyroid cancer specific CPGs mentioned below.
3. Organisational—Some clinicians in an organisation may be knowledgeable and prepared to change but the organisation as a whole may not be ready or unable to change in a timely manner for a number of reasons. However, professional organisations in most countries do play a significant role in implementing CPGs and in arranging regular audit of measurable outcomes after CPG implementation.
4. Resources—One of the common problems professionals might face is lack of adequate time for implementing guideline based practice particularly at the point of treatment delivery in a busy clinic. In addition, staffing or funding issues for implementation of new drugs or new techniques may also present as barriers to timely implementation of CPGs. In centres using international guidelines, obviously often these would have to be adapted to local priorities and available resources.

Thyroid CPG Specific Factor

The lack of high quality studies and trials in thyroid cancer, compared to other commoner solid tumors, might well be one of the important causes of poor adherence to thyroid cancer CPG.

Because of lack of high quality trials and studies in thyroid cancer the scientific evidence available to give clear recommendations about treatment for many key aspects of thyroid cancer are often of low quality. The majority of the guideline recommendations are thus based on consensus statements or expert opinions. Therefore, about 70–80% of the published guideline recommendations are not "Strong Recommendations" leaving areas of uncertainty and clinical equipoise [1]. Different clinicians and patients might interpret these in different ways. In such clinical situations, the clinician and the patient's "shared and individualized" decisions may well vary between different units; however they should usually should be one of the acceptable recommendations suggested by the CPG.

Implementation of Guidelines Across the World

In June 2014, the American Thyroid Association (ATA) Guidelines for the treatment and follow-up of patients with differentiated thyroid cancer were presented at the ENDO/ICE meeting in Chicago. After inputs from ATA members, they were finally published in Thyroid by the end of 2015 [1]. They clearly stated that "national clinical practice guidelines may not necessarily constitute a legal standard of care in all jurisdictions and that if important differences in practice settings present barriers to meaningful implementation of the recommendations of the guidelines, interested physicians or groups (in or outside of the USA) may consider adapting the guidelines using established methods" [1]. However, after the introduction of these new guidelines, several questions were raised on how some of these new approaches would be implemented in different care settings around the world.

One of the first changes addressed was the more conservative approach in small thyroid nodules (no indication for a fine needle aspiration biopsy [FNAB] in patients with suspicious thyroid nodules smaller than 1 cm in bigger diameter, if the patient has no other risk factors of aggressiveness such as: suspicious lymph nodes, a past history of familial non-medullary thyroid cancer, and/or radiation exposure, etc.). In western countries, routine FNAB used to be the common practice in these suspicious thyroid nodules and it has been suggested that this situation was probably generating an over diagnosis of incidental papillary microcarcinomas, which can reach almost 30–40% in most series [13]. A clear example of this, is what happened in South Korea, where the highest incidence of thyroid cancer in the world was reported [14]. This has raised public concern about the potential cause and also about the financial burden on the national healthcare system. Thyroid cancer related mortality has remained stable for several decades despite there being no major improvement in treatment, as exemplified by the trend in thyroid cancer incidence and mortality in South Korea [15, 16]. Further evidence shows a close correlation between the incidence rate of thyroid cancer and rates of screening for thyroid cancer by ultrasonography [17]. A recent study clearly showed how the widespread use of ultrasonography impacted adversely on the epidemics of diagnosis of thyroid cancer [18]. Between 1999 and 2008, the incidence of thyroid cancer increased 6.4-fold, from 6.4 (95% confidence interval 6.2–6.6) per 100,000 population to 40.7 (40.2–41.2) per 100,000 population [18]. These authors concluded that the current "epidemic" of thyroid cancer in South Korea would be due to an increase in the detection of small tumors, most likely as a result of over detection [18].

By moving to a selective indication of US and FNAB there will probably be a decrease in the diagnosis of incidental tumors that are not impacting on the survival of most patients. However, a difficult issue will be how to communicate this high probability of malignancy to patients without having a definitive diagnosis. In Kuma Hospital (Japan), Professor Akira Miyauchi had discussions with the doctors there on this issue in 1993 and they decided to perform FNAB on suspicious nodules to make diagnosis, reporting the result to the patients and letting them choose immediate surgery or active surveillance [19]. The Japanese studies have shown that only a minority of patients with papillary microcarcinomas will have tumor growth or appearance of lymph node metastasis during the long-term follow-up [1, 20]. One of the concerns with the new approach of not performing FNAB to suspicious thyroid nodules smaller than 1 cm will be how doctors will do the follow-up of their patients without making a diagnosis. Education for patients and doctors will be essential.

Although there is no published data until now about the implementation of this recommendation, it seems that with the epidemic of the diagnosis of DTC in South Korea, it is expected that the population of physicians move slowly to a lower use of US and probably, to the indication of FNAB on sub-centimetre thyroid nodules.

In Latin America, there are no available data on this subject. However, one of the author's impression is that the movement to perform thyroid US and FNAB in subcentimeter thyroid nodules will move even slower than in other parts of the world.

Another not minor change is the proposal for less than total thyroidectomy for most intrathyroidal thyroid cancers (the so called "low risk of recurrence patients"). Although this approach has shown to be very successful in many areas of the world, including Japan [21, 22], it is going to be harder to implement in Latin America for example, where endocrinologists have long been arguing with surgeons in order to make total thyroidectomy the treatment of choice every time a patient was diagnosed with a thyroid cancer. This has to do with the subsequent radioiodine remnant ablation usually performed in most low risk patients until not so long ago [23]. Although the bibliography is endorsing lobectomy for most low risk thyroid cancers [1], it will take a while for this new approach to be implemented in all occidental countries. On the other hand, the indication for hemithyroidectomy with paratracheal lymph node dissection is/was routinely done in most centers in Japan if papillary carcinoma 2 cm or smaller in maximum diameter is confined in one lobe without lymph node or in the presence of a distant metastasis or a massive extrathyroidal extension [21, 22]; the situation might be changing slightly in recent years.

One of the most novel things that have appeared in these last 5 years has been the approach of classifying every single patient with a diagnosis of thyroid cancer according to the risk of recurrence [1, 23–25]. This classification of patients was introduced in the 2009 ATA, ETA and LATS guidelines, and then validated in several cohorts of patients around the world [26–29]. This methodology would help to predict the long-term outcome of patients, allowing physicians to estimate the probability of structural persistent disease (3–13% for low risk patients; 17–45% for intermediate risk of recurrence patients and higher than 60% for high risk patients), also giving us the possibility to know in advance the probability of an excellent response to treatment [26]. The analysis of published studies led to a new re-classification of low and intermediate risk of recurrence in patients with DTC [1]. The ATA guidelines are now proposing that patients with less than 5 affected lymph nodes, or incidental metastasis smaller than 2 mm in diameter, or T3 tumors with minimal extrathyroidal extension might be considered as low risk of recurrence (Risk of Recurrence Stratification System) [1]. This is surely a big change that will help doctors to visualize the low probability of structural persistent disease in this group of patients and will allow to plan a more relaxed follow-up in this group of patients. However, it is not always possible to perform an accurate risk of recurrence classification of all patients. This is what in Argentina we have decided to call "the broken chair". We know that for performing a good risk stratification we need complete information about: [1] the surgical procedure (communication between the endocrinologist and the surgeon); [2] the exhaustive pathological examination; [3] the accuracy of images during follow-up (e.g. Post dose whole body scan, ultrasound, etc.) and; [4] the accuracy of the laboratory tests during the follow-up. These four "legs of the chair" should be strong enough to permit the stratification of patients according to the risk of recurrence (initial and ongoing risk of recurrence). However, although this information may not be complete when we first classify our patient, it can be overcome when we have the initial response to treatment during the first 2 years of follow-up (the so called "ongoing risk of recurrence" or "delayed risk stratification") [1, 26, 27].

Regarding remnant ablation, in most western countries, it used to be very frequent for patients with a thyroid cancer larger than 1 cm to receive radioiodine after surgery (usually radioiodine doses equal or higher than 100 mCi 131-I) [23]. New studies appeared in 2012 (ESTIMABL and HILO) showing that 30 mCi 131-I administered after recombinant human TSH or thyroid hormone withdrawal was enough and effective for low risk patients, and this new evidence slowly changed the approach for remnant ablation in most occidental countries [30, 31].

On the other side, in high risk M1 patients, the use of radioiodine has also its limitations and changes [1]. Currently, it is widely accepted that a cumulative activity higher than 600 mCi 131-I is one of the indicators of radioiodine refractory thyroid cancer [32], that when progressive or symptomatic should lead to further treatments. The new guidelines address that "when a patient with DTC is classified as refractory to radioiodine, there is no indication for further radioiodine treatment" [1]. Slight differences exist in the extent of neck surgery and RAI dosing regimens, but the approaches are similar in treatment guidelines from the ATA, ETA, LATS, and Japanese Society of Thyroid Surgeons (JSTS)/Japanese Association or Endocrine Surgeons (JAES) [1, 21–25]. Regional treatment guidelines are typically prepared by multidisciplinary teams chaired by medical oncologists or endocrinologists, except in Japan, where guidelines are written by surgeons. A multidisciplinary team approach to managing patients with advanced disease is recommended, to maximize patient care and outcomes; however, the team concept and members may vary across regions. MDT are typically composed of a surgeon, endocrinologist, nuclear medicine physician, and pathologist for most thyroid carcinomas; an oncologist is added for the treatment of radioiodine refractory thyroid cancer. In most cases, it is also helpful to have easy access to a radiotherapist. The specialties of the physicians primarily responsible for treating patients with refractory thyroid carcinoma differ between countries, depending on the structure of the health care system. In Western countries, a medical oncologist or endocrinologist functioning within the multidisciplinary team has primary contact with the patient and is responsible for establishing a treatment plan in collaboration with other team members [33]. The situation is different in Japan, where surgeons are responsible for the diagnosis and management of patients. There is also limited capacity to administer RAI due to legal restrictions [21, 22].

In France, all patients with refractory thyroid cancer are referred to the TUTHYREF (Tumeurs de la Thyroïde Réfractaires) network, composed of 34 centers and recognized by the French National Cancer Institute. All treatment decisions are made within the context of the network in one of the multidisciplinary teams, where an agreement must be reached prior to treating the patient. For patients with difficult or unusual presentation, the case is discussed during a Web conference that is organized every 2 weeks, with 190 cases being discussed in 2010. Indeed, the TUTHYREF network represents a unique situation, since in the majority of European centers a local multidisciplinary team is responsible for managing and treating these complicated cases.

Two multikinase inhibitors are approved for the treatment of locally advanced and/or progressive thyroid cancer: sorafenib and lenvatinib [34, 35]. These MKI are not widely available around the world to be used as first or second line treatments. For example, in Latin America, only sorafenib is available in most countries.

Comment on the Application of Thyroid Cancer and Thyroid Nodules Guidelines in Specific Countries

United Kingdom

In the UK National Health Service (NHS), the variation in CPG implementation across different units also exists to a degree but is much less likely in relation to cancer management. The National Health Service has got mandatory multidisciplinary team (MDT) management of cancer treatment for all cancer sites including thyroid cancer for many years. Because of this, the different specialists involved in the multi-disciplinary team have a collective responsibility for implementation of guidelines. At the present time, almost all non-surgical treatments are led by clinical oncologists; surgery is performed by specialist Head and Neck and/or endocrine surgeon member of the MDT.

As it happens in other countries, in specialist units in the UK, all thyroid cancer cases are discussed in MDT and guideline based individualized treatments are recommended. In areas of controversy, if there are any ongoing trials, it is also recommended in the MDT outcome, that available high quality national multicentre trial information is mentioned to the patient; it is then discussed in more detail if the patient expresses a desire to consider whether to take part or not.

The MDT has to take part in regular mandatory National peer review process where specific measures about guideline based protocols are discussed and reviewed.

The National Institute for Health and Care Excellence (NICE) provides national guidance and advice to improve health and social care and was set up in 1999 to reduce variation in the availability and quality of NHS treatments and care [5]. NICE has transformed the management of patients in the NHS over the last few years. There is a statutory requirement that clinicians and managers of all healthcare trusts implement all disease specific management guidelines developed by disease specific guideline development group selected by NICE after extensive, meticulous distillation and analysis of evidence including effectiveness, cost effectiveness and "Cost per QALY". The healthcare trusts also have a duty to make arrangements to use all NICE approved new technology and drugs made available in the NHS (following a very comprehensive and rigorous approval process) and within a specified time frame [5].

The British thyroid Association guidelines (BTA) CPG for thyroid cancer was developed by BTA supported by all other relevant professional organizations as the current national guideline [6]. Therefore, while there is no legal or statutory requirement for implementation of this but as in other countries all professional organizations support its implementation and recommend this as the good practice document to be followed nationally. Also, in UK, very active patient support groups accept this as such. Shared and individualized decision-making is largely followed for thyroid cancer in the UK due to many areas of uncertainty as dis cussed above; therefore both informed patients and clinicians expect discussions about treatment decisions where the guideline recommendations are weak. Despite this, some variation do exist, as usual, related to the reasons mentioned earlier in this chapter.

The professional specialist organizations such as British Association of Thyroid and Endocrine surgeons (BAETS), (BTA), some of the specialist groups of the Royal colleges, play an important role in advising members to implement these.

The UK has a very proactive National thyroid cancer research subgroup under the auspices of the National Cancer Research Institute (NCRI) and has successfully conducted National multi-center trials on thyroid cancer. In addition to well-designed national trials and studies addressing aspects of thyroid cancer management where there is clinical equipoise, more collaborative international studies are essential to have more high-quality evidence required to give strong recommendations in future guidelines within a more realistic time frame.

A recent and unique conference was arranged by the patient support group Butterfly Thyroid cancer trust (BTCT) in which most of the attendees (150 in number) were patients. Physicians and patients made presentations on thyroid cancer. What was concluded from this conference is that a collaborative approach with patients and doctors working together might help improve implementation of guidelines in every centre.

In conclusion, in the UK, high quality thyroid cancer CPG have been painstakingly developed by leading professionals under the auspices of the BTA which is largely followed nationally; the quality of care has been better standardized and has improved because of the CPG which hopefully will improve overall outcome. As expected there are some minor variation in implementation of CPG between units. The NHS MDT structure, research and trial focus by an active NCRI group, international collaboration and patient doctor partnership are continually trying to improve the situation.

Italy (Furio Pacini, MD)

Thyroid cancer is the human solid cancer with the highest increased incidence in the world. Prognosis for patients with thyroid cancer is highly variable with many small thyroid cancers having very little clinical impact and only a minority having aggressive behavior and poor prognosis. To help clinicians provide the most updated medical care, a number of societies have established clinical guidelines for thyroid nodules and thyroid cancer. These guidelines are composed of evidence-based recommendations for particular clinical scenarios after review of the literature data by experts from several specialties involved in the care of patients with thyroid cancer. Recent diagnostic procedures have been developed to better characterize thyroid nodules. An important effort has been implemented in providing new risk stratification systems that can be modified over time allowing for individualization of diagnosis, initial treatment, and subsequent follow-up strategies. Advances in surgical approaches and new treatments for patients with the most aggressive forms of thyroid cancer have all influenced management guidelines. Despite substantial similarities, there are important differences between recent guidelines according to country specific scenarios and facilities. Guidelines are not intended to give rules but rather recommendations in order to take evidence-based decision.

The uniform application of guidelines is far to be accomplished. Different approaches to the patient are still driven by the specific background of different specialists. Nuclear medicine physicians behave differently from endocrinologist, and oncologists have different approach compare to endocrinologist. For instance, some country still uses radioiodine as a routine practice, while others have reduced the use of radioiodine to metastatic patients. In some setting, surgery is still total thyroidectomy regardless of the individual risk of a particular patient, while in other realities the extent of surgery is modulated according to the real risk of recurrence. Reason for this discrepancy is mainly due to the lack of prospective studies in thyroid cancer. Until we will be able to set up multicentric, prospective studies in the hottest topics we will assist to the proliferation of different guidelines and different strategies for similar patients. This will vanish the utility of the guidelines and will continue to generate discrepancy among different countries and within individual countries.

Canada (J. Brierley)

Changes in use and geographical variations in the administration of RAI and in the management of differentiated thyroid cancer have been known about in Canada for some time. In a survey of thyroid practitioners in the US and Canada performed in 2006 Sawka et al. [36] presented a case of low risk thyroid cancer (a 38-year-old woman with a 1.6 cm papillary carcinoma). Sixty three percent of respondents strongly recommended the administration of remnant ablation (RRA) in this patient who would not now meet the American Thyroid Association criteria for remnant ablation. There were regional differences, the strongest support for RAI administration was in Quebec and the southern United States, intermediate support in eastern Canada and the northeastern United States, and the least support in western Canada and the western and Midwestern United States [36].

This regional variation has also been demonstrated in a prospective database [37]. The Canadian Collaborative Network for Cancer of the Thyroid (CANNECT) is a collaborative network of seven academic centers across Central and Eastern Canada. Prospective data was collected from year 2000 in 4 centers, by year 2006 in all seven academic centers. There was an even distribution of cases by histology and TNM stage across the population but there was a significant variation in the administration of RAI in low risk cancers. In one center 15% of patients with T1N0/NX tumours received RAI but it was up to 85% in another center. There was variation but not as great for T3 N0 patients ranging from 54% to 97%. In addition to this geographical variation there was variation over time with the use of RAI rising from 51% in all patients in 2000, peaking in 2005 at 82% and falling in back to 51% by 2010 [38].

Variations in all aspects of management of differentiated thyroid cancer over a more limited geographical area, Ontario, has also been described [38], using population based data rather than individual treatment center data for patients who had surgery between 2000 and 2008. As in other jurisdictions there was a significant rise in the incidence of thyroid cancer (from 10.19 to 18.89/100,000) and there was also a wide variation in incidence across the province. The authors link this rise and the geographical variation to the rise in diagnostic ultrasound usage. There was also a significant variation across the province of the type of initial surgery, total thyroidectomy being the initial surgery in 29% of cases in one region and 82% in other and the use of RAI ranged from 41% to 66%.

These three studies show a wide variation the management of differentiated thyroid cancer across time as well as geography. In the CANNECT study the fall in the use of RAI preceded the ATA guidelines change in recommendation for low risk thyroid cancer, but this was in academic centers and it could be speculated that this was due practice patterns changing based on the data that subsequently informed the ATA guidelines, although four of the centers stated they used the ATA guidelines [1]. In Ontario, although Cancer Care Ontario has a robust process of developing evidence based guidelines it does not currently have any on differentiated thyroid cancer, however in mid-2017 guidelines and diagnostic and treatment pathways with be available on line (https://www.cancercare.on.ca/toolbox/qualityguidelines/ and https://www.cancercare.on.ca/ocs/qpi/dispathmgmt/pathways/); we will have to wait and see if this results in any reduction in variability in diagnosis and management within the province.

India (Prof C.S. Bal)

There are dozens of National and International guidelines published by different societies and professional bodies in the management of differentiated thyroid cancer (DTC), however, ATA guideline is universally followed in most of the countries [1]. My comments shall be limited to ATA guidelines on the management of thyroid nodules and DTC in adults.

In India, for thyroid nodule evaluation, sonography and FNAB is universally performed. If blinded FNAC fails, US guided FNAB is repeated. For follicular neoplasm on cytology surgeons prefer hemithyroidectomy rather than asking for molecular methodologies on cytology samples. Molecular diagnostic tools are not available locally, and for sending samples abroad to get either “rule-in” or “rule-out” tests of DTC is prohibitively expensive. Regarding surgery, elective central compartment dissection for papillary thyroid cancer is highly debated; some surgeons based in academic centres meticulously follow 2009 ATA guidelines and the vast majority do not follow this recommendation for T3 tumors, due to large number of complications, particularly hypoparathyroidism. Now, everybody is happy that 2015 ATA guidelines made this elective central compartment dissection optional [1].

Near total thyroidectomy is the procedure of choice in India. In our own series, the percentage of surgically ablated patients have increased from 7% in early 2000s to 15%, currently. Interestingly, pathologists do not follow detailed histopathological report as recommended by 2015 ATA guideline [1].

A major difference in practice of DTC patients is the pre-ablation diagnostic ^{131}I-whole body scan (WBS) performed routinely in most centers in India. The ATA guideline does not recommend routine pre-ablation diagnostic scan; it only recommended the post-therapy WBS. In India, every DTC patient undergoes diagnostic ^{131}I-WBS for planning ^{131}I-therapy. If pre-ablation diagnostic scan shows no residual thyroid tissue or nodal or distant metastasis and stimulated thyroglobulin <10 ng/ml with negative AntiTgAb, no ^{131}I therapy is administered in low-risk, and even intermediate-risk DTC patients. We have now more than 900 low- and intermediate-risk DTC patients who did not undergo radioiodine administration. Our initial experience has been recently published [39, 40]. “Lobar ablation” i.e. ablation of intact lobe to differentiate it from remnant ablation is widely practiced at our centre. The 2009 ATA guidelines had negated this approach and favoured completion thyroidectomy. However, the 2015 ATA guidelines has suggested it could be ‘an alternative to completion thyroidectomy in some patients’ [1]. This is because no randomized controlled trial is currently available to make a strong recommendation against or for this procedure.

Other major difference is preparation of patients for remnant ablation- the ATA 2015 guidelines recommends rhTSH-stimulated ablation is an equally effective method of preparation compared to conventional thyroid hormone withdrawal. In India, rarely patients undergo rhTSH-stimulated ^{131}I- remnant ablation only because of the high cost of the rhTSH kit.

Difficult area is radioiodine refractory/non-iodine concentrating structural disease management in India. Tyrosine kinase inhibitors are widely available in India, For some reason, the hand-foot-syndrome is observed in 40–50% patients and rarely patients could tolerate 800 mg recommended daily dose of Sorafenib. The rest of the ATA guideline-based management recommendations of DTC are by-and –large followed universally in India.

USA (Prof Bryan R. Haugen)

The 2015 American Thyroid Association (ATA) Evidence-Based Guidelines for Management of Patients with Thyroid Nodules and Differentiated Thyroid Cancer (DTC) have significant changes from the previous 2006 and 2009 ATA guidelines [1]. The 2015 guidelines generated 8 new questions, 21 new recommendations and 21 significantly changed recommendations. There are a number of barriers which likely limit successful uniform implementation of CPG into practice. These include the supporting evidence, concern for disease recurrence by the provider and patient as well as entrenched practice patterns. There are also likely cultural and financial barriers that will not be discussed here.

Supporting Evidence for Recommendations

The 2015 ATA guidelines for patients with thyroid nodules and DTC has 101 recommendations and 175 specific subrecommendations (i.e.–Recommendation 8A, 8B, etc.). The recommendations are rated as *Strong* or *Weak* based on an adapted grading system from the American College of Physicians [41], citing high-quality, moderate-quality or low-quality evidence. Only 6 of the specific recommendations were Strong recommendations supported by high-quality evidence. A majority of the recommendations were Strong recommendations supported by moderate-quality evidence or Weak recommendations supported by low-quality evidence. A Strong recommendation is one in which the patient should receive or be offered the recommended course of action, while a Weak recommendation notes that different choices may be appropriate for different patients. It is difficult to expect practitioners to strictly adhere to a Weak recommendation based on low-quality evidence. One example is *Recommendation 23C* which states that patients with benign FNA cytology and a very low risk sonographic pattern thyroid nodule, do not need a repeat thyroid/neck US, but if done, it should be done at >24 months. Many practitioners may not be comfortable with this seemingly nihilistic approach for a patient with a 3 cm thyroid nodule, and may repeat the US at 6–12 months. Another example is *Recommendation 50D* which states that a "postoperative diagnostic RAI WBS may be useful when the extent of the thyroid remnant or residual disease cannot be accurately ascertained and the results may alter the decision to treat or the activity of RAI." Some practitioners still routinely use diagnostic WBS in all patients, while others rarely use this approach. Getting uniform implementation is difficult when more than 40% of the recommendations are Weak based on low-quality evidence.

Concern for Cancer Recurrence/Survival

I believe that concern for cancer recurrence or survival by the practitioner, patient or both tends to drive a lot of decision-making in care for patients with DTC, even when there is evidence showing that more aggressive care does not improve outcome. This can be a major barrier to uniform implementation of CPG even with Strong recommendations. One example is *Recommendation 51B* which is a Strong recommendation based on moderate-quality evidence recommending against routine use of RAI remnant ablation in patients with unifocal papillary microcarcinoma. This was also a similar recommendation against use of RAI based on fair evidence in the 2009 guidelines. It would seem that based on this guidance and evidence, most or all patients with micropapillary carcinoma should not receive RAI remnant ablation, yet a publication in 2013 showed that 28–47% of patients in the U.S. with micropapillary thyroid carcinoma were being treated with RAI in different regions of the country [42]. Another study noted that factors influencing whether a patient receives radioiodine for thyroid cancer included physician and patient worry about death from thyroid cancer, both of which rank highly in the consideration [43]. I believe that there is still a strong perception that radioiodine is virtually harmless and there is a concern that any patient with even low risk disease may have a poor outcome if not treated with radioiodine. Continued dissemination of evidence-based guidelines and multiple efforts for provider and patient education are needed to assure more uniform implementation of guidelines.

Conclusion

The changes proposed by the ATA and other guidelines will surely result in a more individualized approach in patients with differentiated thyroid cancer, which will probably improve their outcome, quality of life, decrease the anxiety related to their disease and diminish health related costs for the treatment of a disorder that seems to be indolent in the big majority of cases.

However uniform implementation of guidelines seems to be below the desired level both within individual countries and across different countries. The reasons for this are multifactorial. Generic and Thyroid cancer CPG specific causes have been well-documented in the literature and have been briefly mentioned here. These need addressing in order to improve the overall outcome of Thyroid Cancer globally.

It is suggested that in addition to all other efforts, the quest for high quality large, national and international randomised and non randomised clinical trials are continued. These trials should target the major areas of uncertainty that still remain in the clinical management of thyroid cancer in the first instance. The aim will be to provide level 1 and reliable scientific evidence which will help guidelines provide strong recommendations to clinicians and patients in the areas of clinical equipoise that exist currently. Parallelly translational studies must continue too with international collaboration in discovering new therapies. Much closer multidisciplinary national and international collaboration is required for these efforts to be successful. Patient participation in well-designed studies and trials must be encouraged as in other rare tumors such as pediatric cancer, etc.

Finally patient education and effective patient -doctor partnership can be an important and valuable driver for implementation of thyroid CPGs.

Contributors F Pacini (Italy), J Brierley (Canada), C S Bal (India), B Haugen (USA).

References

1. Haugen BR, Alexander EK, Bible KC, Doherty GM, Mandel SJ, Nikiforov YE, Pacini F, Randolph GW, Sawka AM, Schlumberger M, Schuff KG, Sherman SI, Sosa JA, Steward DL, Tuttle RM, Wartofsky L. 2015 American thyroid association management guidelines for adult patients with thyroid nodules and differentiated thyroid cancer: the American thyroid association guidelines task force on thyroid nodules and differentiated thyroid cancer. Thyroid. 2016;26(1):1–133.
2. Haymart MR, Banerjee M, Yang D, Stewart AK, Sisson JC, Koenig RJ, Doherty GM, Griggs JJ. Variation in the management of thyroid cancer. J Clin Endocrinol Metab. 2013;98(5):2001–8.
3. Famakinwa OM, Roman SA, Wang TS, Sosa JA. ATA practice guidelines for the treatment of differentiated thyroid cancer: were they followed in the United States? Am J Surg. 2010;199(2):189–98.
4. Harrison MB, Graham ID, van den Hoek J, Dogherty EJ, Carley ME, Angus V. Guideline adaptation and implementation planning: a prospective observational study. Implement Sci. 2013;8:49–63.
5. https://www.nice.org.uk/.
6. Perros P, Boelaert K, Colley S, Evans C, Evans RM, Gerrard Ba G, Gilbert J, Harrison B, Johnson SJ, Giles TE, Moss L, Lewington V, Newbold K, Taylor J, Thakker RV, Watkinson J, Williams GR, British Thyroid Association. Guidelines for the management of thyroid cancer. Clin Endocrinol. 2014;81(Suppl 1):1–122.
7. Phillips AW, Fenwick JD, Mallick UK, Perros P. The impact of clinical guidelines on surgical management in patients with thyroid cancer. Clin Oncol (R Coll Radiol). 2003;15(8):485–9.
8. Likhterov I, Tuttle RM, Haser GC, Su HK, Bergman D, Alon EE, Bernet V, Brett E, Cobin R, Dewey EH, Doherty G, Dos Reis LL, Klopper J, Lee SL, Lupo MA, Machac J, Mechanick JI, Milas M, Orloff L, Randolph G, Ross DS, Rowe ME, Smallridge R, Terris D, Tufano RP, Urken ML. Improving the adoption of thyroid cancer clinical practice guidelines. Laryngoscope. 2016;126(11):2640–5.
9. Institute of Medicine (US) Committee on Quality of Health Care in America. Crossing the quality chasm: a new health system for the 21st century. Washington, DC: National Academies Press (US); 2001.
10. Mehra S, Tuttle RM, Bergman D, Bernet V, Brett E, Cobin R, Doherty G, Klopper J, Lee S, Machac J, Milas M, Mechanick JI, Orloff L, Randolph G, Ross DS, Smallridge R, Terris D, Tufano R, Alon E, Clain J, Dos Reis L, Scherl S, Urken ML. Improving the quality of thyroid cancer care: how does the thyroid cancer care collaborative cross the institute of medicine's quality chasm? Thyroid. 2014;24(4):615–24.
11. Lewis C. Editorial: consent to treatment: supreme court discards Bolam principle. Med Leg J. 2015;83:59–61.
12. Lewis MH, Gohagan JK, Merenstein DJ. The locality rule and the physician's dilemma: local medical practices vs the national standard of care. JAMA. 2007;297:2633–7.
13. Davies L, Welch HG. Increasing incidence of thyroid cancer in the United States, 1973–2002. JAMA. 2006;295:2164–7.
14. Ferlay J, Soerjomataram I, Ervik M, et al. GLOBOCAN 2012 v1.0, cancer incidence and mortality worldwide: IARC Cancer Base No. 11. International Agency for Research on Cancer; 2013. http://globocan.iarc.fr.
15. La Vecchia C, Malvezzi M, Bosetti C, et al. Thyroid cancer mortality and incidence: a global overview. Int J Cancer. 2015;136:2187–95. https://doi.org/10.1002/ijc.29251.
16. Jung KW, Won YJ, Kong HJ, et al. Cancer statistics in Korea: incidence, mortality, survival, and prevalence in 2012. Cancer Res Treat. 2015;47:127–41. https://doi.org/10.4143/crt.2015.060.
17. Oh CM, Jung KW, Won YJ, Shin A, Kong HJ, Lee JS. Age-period-cohort analysis of thyroid cancer incidence in Korea. Cancer Res Treat. 2015;47:362–9. https://doi.org/10.4143/crt.2014.110.
18. Park S, Oh CM, Cho H, Lee JY, Jung KW, Jun JK, Won YJ, Kong HJ, Choi KS, Lee YJ, Lee JS. Association between screening and the thyroid cancer "epidemic" in South Korea: evidence from a nationwide study. BMJ. 2016;355:i5745. https://doi.org/10.1136/bmj.i5745.
19. Ito Y, Uruno T, Nakano K, Takamura Y, Miya A, Kobayashi K, Yokozawa T, Matsuzuka F, Kuma S, Kuma K, Miyauchi A. An observation trial without surgical treatment in patients with papillary microcarcinoma of the thyroid. Thyroid. 2003;13(4):381–7.
20. Ito Y, Miyauchi A, Kihara M, Higashiyama T, Kobayashi K, Miya A. Patient age is significantly

related to the progression of papillary microcarcinoma of the thyroid under observation. Thyroid. 2014;24:27–34.
21. Takami H, Ito Y, Okamoto T, Yoshida A. Therapeutic strategy for differentiated thyroid carcinoma in Japan based on newly established guideline managed by Japanese Society of Thyroid Surgeons and Japanese Association of endocrine surgeons. World J Surg. 2011;35:111–21.
22. Takami H, Ito Y, Okamoto T, Onoda N, Noguchi H, Yoshida A. Revisiting the guidelines issued by the Japanese Society of Thyroid Surgeons and Japan Association of endocrine surgeons: a gradual move towards consensus between Japanese and western practice in the management of thyroid carcinoma. World J Surg. 2014;38(8):2002–10.
23. Pitoia F, Ward L, Wohllk N, Friguglietti C, Tomimori E, Gauna A, Camargo R, Vaisman M, Harach R, Munizaga F, Corigliano S, Pretell E, Niepomniszcze H. Recommendations of the Latin American thyroid society on diagnosis and management of differentiated thyroid cancer. Arq Bras Endocrinol Metabol. 2009;53(7):884.
24. Cooper DS, Doherty GM, Haugen BR, Kloos RT, Lee SL, Mandel SJ, Mazzaferri EL, McIver B, Pacini F, Schlumberger M, Sherman SI, Steward DL, Tuttle RM. Revised American Thyroid Association management guidelines for patients with thyroid nodules and differentiated thyroid cancer. Thyroid. 2009;19(11):1167–214. https://doi.org/10.1089/thy.2009.0110. Erratum in: Thyroid. 2010 Jun;20(6):674-5.
25. Pacini F, Schlumberger M, Dralle H, Elisei R, Smit JW. Wiersinga W; European thyroid Cancer taskforce: European consensus for the management of patients with differentiated thyroid cancer of the follicular epithelium. Eur J Endocrinol. 2006;154:787–803.
26. Tuttle RM, Tala H, Shah J, Leboeuf R, Ghossein R, Gonen M, Brokhin M, Omry G, Fagin JA, Shaha A. Estimating risk of recurrence in differentiated thyroid cancer after total thyroidectomy and radioactive iodine remnant ablation: using response to therapy variables to modify the initial risk estimates predicted by the new American Thyroid Association staging system. Thyroid. 2010;20:1341–9.
27. Castagna MG, Maino F, Cipri C, Belardini V, Theodoropoulou A, Cevenini G, Pacini F. Delayed risk stratification, to include the response to initial treatment (surgery and radioiodine ablation), has better outcome predictivity in differentiated thyroid cancer patients. Eur J Endocrinol. 2011;165:441–6.
28. Vaisman F, Momesso D, Bulzico DA, Pessoa CH, Dias F, Corbo R, Vaisman M, Tuttle RM. Spontaneous remission in thyroid cancer patients after biochemical incomplete response to initial therapy. Clin Endocrinol. 2012;77:132–8.
29. Pitoia F, Bueno F, Urciuoli C, Abelleira E, Cross G, Tuttle RM. Outcomes of patients with differentiated thyroid cancer risk-stratified according to the American Thyroid Association and Latin American thyroid society risk of recurrence classification systems. Thyroid. 2013;23:1401–7.
30. Schlumberger M, Catargi B, Borget I, Deandreis D, Zerdoud S, Bridji B, Bardet S, Leenhardt L, Bastie D, Schvartz C, Vera P, Morel O, Benisvy D, Bournaud C, Bonichon F, Dejax C, Toubert ME, Leboulleux S, Ricard M, Benhamou E, Tumeurs de la Thyroïde Refractaires Network for the Essai Stimulation Ablation Equivalence Trial. Strategies of radioiodine ablation in patients with low-risk thyroid cancer. N Engl J Med. 2012;366(18):1663–73.
31. Mallick U, Harmer C, Yap B, Wadsley J, Clarke S, Moss L, Nicol A, Clark PM, Farnell K, McCready R, Smellie J, Franklyn JA, John R, Nutting CM, Newbold K, Lemon C, Gerrard G, Abdel-Hamid A, Hardman J, Macias E, Roques T, Whitaker S, Vijayan R, Alvarez P, Beare S, Forsyth S, Kadalayil L, Hackshaw A. Ablation with low-dose radioiodine and thyrotropin alfa in thyroid cancer. N Engl J Med. 2012;366(18):1674–85.
32. Schlumberger M, Brose M, Elisei R, Leboulleux S, Luster M, Pitoia F, Pacini F. Definition and management of radioactive iodine-refractory differentiated thyroid cancer. Lancet Diabetes Endocrinol. 2014;2(5):356–8. https://doi.org/10.1016/S2213-8587(13)70215-8.
33. Brose MS, Smit J, Capdevila J, Elisei R, Nutting C, Pitoia F, Robinson B, Schlumberger M, Shong YK, Takami H. Regional approaches to the management of patients with advanced, radioactive iodine-refractory differentiated thyroid carcinoma. Expert Rev Anticancer Ther. 2012;12(9):1137–47. https://doi.org/10.1586/era.12.96.
34. Brose MS, Nutting CM, Jarzab B, Elisei R, Siena S, Bastholt L, et al. Sorafenib in radioactive iodine-refractory, locally advanced or metastatic differentiated thyroid cancer: a randomised, double-blind, phase 3 trial. Lancet. 2014;384(9940):319–28.
35. Schlumberger M, Tahara M, Wirth LJ, Robinson B, Brose MS, Elisei R, et al. Lenvatinib versus placebo in radioiodine-refractory thyroid cancer. NEJM. 2015;372(7):621–30.
36. Sawka A, Rotstein L, Brierley J, et al. Regional differences in opinion on adjuvant radioactive iodine treatment in the United States and Canada. Thyroid. 2007;17(12):1235–42.
37. Rachinsky I, Rajaraman M, Leslie W, et al. Regional variation across Canadian centers in radiactive iodine administration for thyroid remnant ablation in well-differentiated thyroid cancer diagnosed in 2000–2010. J Thyroid Res. 2016;2016:2867916. https://doi.org/10.1155/2016/2867916.
38. Hall S, Irish J, Groome P, et al. Practice patterns in the management of patients with differentiated thyroid cancer in Ontario Canada 2000–2008. J Otolaryngol Head Neck Surg. 2014;43:29.
39. Ballal S, Soundararajan R, Garg A, Chopra S, Bal C. Intermediate-risk differentiated thyroid carcinoma patients who were surgically ablated do not need

adjuvant radioiodine therapy: long-term outcome study. Clin Endocrinol. 2016;84(3):408–16.
40. Bal C, Ballal S, Soundararajan R, Chopra S, Garg A. Radioiodine remnant ablation in low-risk differentiated thyroid cancer patients who had R0 dissection is an over treatment. Cancer Med. 2015;4(7):1031–8.
41. Qaseem A, Snow V, Owens DK, Shekelle P. The development of clinical practice guidelines and guidance statements of the American college of physicians: summary of methods. Ann Intern Med. 2010;153:194–9.
42. Haymart MR, Muenz DG, Stewart AK, Griggs JJ, Banerjee M. Disease severity and radioactive use for thyroid cancer. J Clin Endo Metab. 2013;98:678–86.
43. Papaleontiou M, Banerjee M, Yang D, Sisson JC, Koenig RJ, Haymart MR. Factor that influence radioactive iodine use for thyroid cancer. Thyroid. 2013;23:219–24.

27 Survivorship: The Role of the Clinical Psychologist and the Clinical Nurse Specialist in Thyroid Cancer Care

Katherine Kendell and Nicola Jane Armstrong

The Thyroid Cancer Multidisciplinary Team

Improving Outcomes Guidance for commissioning services for adults with thyroid cancer in England and Wales is incorporated within the guidance for head and neck cancer. The National Health Service Standard Contract for Head and Neck Cancer in adults, stipulates that for population bases of over one million, a specialist thyroid multi-disciplinary team (MDT) should treat patients with thyroid cancer and work closely with the specialist head and neck service [1]. The MDT should discuss every new patient and take responsibility for their management throughout the course of their disease and rehabilitation. Each MDT should have at least one Clinical Nurse Specialist (CNS) as a core member and a CNS should be present at every MDT meeting. The CNS plays a key role within the MDT, including co-ordination of patient care and psychosocial support. Every patient should have access to the CNS, during the decision making process regarding disease management and thereafter as a point of contact for information and support. The CNS supports both patients and carers in managing the practical, psychological and social consequences of treatment, roles which require excellent communication and psychosocial skills. The CNS also provides education and support to the wider nursing team and consultation and advice to other professionals. She/he works closely with patient support groups, with extended members of the MDT and other specialist teams. An important role is identifying those patients who might benefit from referral to other professionals such as the clinical psychologist, liaison psychiatrist, social worker or benefits advisor. The guidance advocates particularly close liaison between the CNS and psychological support services. A designated Clinical Psychologist (CP), with interest and experience in this patient group, should be an extended member of the MDT and available to assess patients' psychological needs and provide therapy as appropriate [2].

The Nature of Thyroid Cancer

Thyroid cancer is currently relatively rare. There were 3404 new cases of thyroid cancer diagnosed in the UK in 2014, representing 1% of total cancer cases for that year. It is much more common in women than men, with a male to female ratio of 4:10. Incidence rates for thyroid cancer have increased by 71% in the UK over the last decade, probably reflecting an increase in detection of

K. Kendell · N. J. Armstrong (✉)
The Newcastle upon Tyne Hospitals, NHS Foundation Trust, Freeman Hospital, Newcastle upon Tyne, UK
e-mail: Kate.Kendell@nuth.nhs.uk; nicola.armstrong2@nuth.nhs.uk

U. K. Mallick et al. (eds.), *Practical Management of Thyroid Cancer*,
https://doi.org/10.1007/978-3-319-91725-2_27

asymptomatic disease, due to greater use of medical imaging. Incidence rates for thyroid cancer are growing faster than for any other cancer and are projected to rise a further 74% between 2014 and 2035.

Of people diagnosed with any thyroid cancer in England, almost 90% will survive at least 5 years and 85% will survive at least 10 years. The most common thyroid cancers are papillary and follicular cancers, known as differentiated thyroid cancer (DTC). Ninety percent of all diagnosed thyroid cancers are DTC and have the most favourable prognoses, with 5 year survival rates between 80% and 100%. Medullary thyroid cancer, accounting for 3–12% of cases, has a 60% 5 year survival rate. Anaplastic thyroid cancer, accounting for only 1–3% of cases, carries a very poor prognosis with survival rates of only 5% and 10% for men and women respectively [3].

Although DTC survival rates may be considered favourable, the risk of recurrence is 20–40%, depending on age and tumour stage at initial treatment. Recurrence can occur decades after initial treatment, so lifelong follow-up and monitoring are necessary to detect recurrence as early as possible and to maintain optimum levels of thyroid hormones [4].

Survivorship

A cancer survivor is defined as 'an individual who has been diagnosed with a cancer, regardless of when diagnosis was received, and who is still living [5]. Survivorship is a three stage process and no specific timeframes exist for each stage, nor do all patients experience all stages [6]:

- Acute—time surrounding initial diagnosis and treatment (thyroid surgery and radio-iodine ablation). This period includes post-surgical recovery, and may involve sick leave from work and time away from children due to radiation risks;
- Extended—completion of treatment. Patients with thyroid cancer are re-assessed 6–9 months after completion of treatment and have to await results and dynamic risk stratification. This period may be characterised by anxiety due to uncertainty and the possibility of recurrence;
- Permanent—achievement of cure or extended long term survival, presumed to be permanent. The probability of recurrence is diminished but survivors may face long-term or late effects of disease and treatment including post-surgical changes to voice, fatigue, hypocalcaemia.

Increasing incidence rates, relatively young age at diagnosis and overall long survival times, mean that a growing number of people are living with a diagnosis of thyroid cancer. "It cannot be ignored that survival creates a multitude of problems, of which psychological and psychosocial issues are paramount" [7]. The Cancer Reform Strategy emphasised that greater consideration needs to be given to the requirements of those living with or 'surviving' cancer [8]. During recent years, there has been growing recognition of thyroid cancer patients' demand for more medical information on their disease and for more psychosocial support [9, 10]). However, these needs are not yet being adequately addressed.

Health Related Quality of Life

Due to the generally favourable prognosis associated with DTC "patients often report that they have been told that they have a "good" cancer but this does not reflect their personal experience with the disease". Health related quality of life (QOL) data were collected for 284 patients attending an Austrian nuclear medicine department, over 30 months, and compared to the general population. The authors found evidence that DTC patients experience detrimental sleep disturbance, fatigue and reduced ability to perform usual work and leisure activities as well as psychosocial distress [11]. In a German study of patients with thyroid cancer who opted for a period of inpatient rehabilitation, the authors again compared them to the general population and found strong evidence for decreased QOL particularly in the areas of insomnia, fatigue, role functioning and mental health [12].

A recent study using results from the large scale North American Thyroid Cancer Survivorship Study, compared survivors of thyroid cancer with survivors of other cancers carrying a worse prognosis (colon, glioma, breast, and gynaecological). Survivors of thyroid cancer reported similar or worse QOL to those with the other cancers. The authors concluded that prognosis alone should not be used to predict QOL in patients with cancer [13]. In a related study, the authors compared physician perceptions of QOL in thyroid cancer survivors to patient reports. They found that physicians significantly underestimated the physical problems experienced by patients, namely fatigue, weight gain, voice changes and heat/cold intolerance [14].

A large, multinational, survivor-initiated cross-sectional survey indicated that thyroid cancer survivors suffer frequent treatment morbidity and have considerable unmet need for information and psychosocial support [15]. The long term nature of impairment suffered by survivors was illustrated in a cross-sectional case-control study assessing QOL in 153 patients, considered cured of thyroid cancer, with two control groups. The authors found firstly that QOL was not related to serum TSH levels and secondly that QOL was only restored to normal approximately 12–20 years after cure [16]. The authors of a qualitative study of patients with DTC or stage one carcinoma of the larynx, both associated with a good prognosis, concluded that cancer should never be described as "good". Patient interviews illustrated that despite being given a favourable prognosis, patients "are still very shocked to hear the word cancer and react in similar ways to those with other forms of cancer" [17].

Psychological Distress in Patients with Cancer

It is now well recognised that patients with cancer, including long term survivors, are at increased risk of psychological distress and morbidity compared to the general population. Distress may be understood along a continuum from normal feelings of sadness and fear to disabling problems of clinical depression, anxiety and other diagnosable disorders [18]. Estimates of the prevalence of psychological/psychiatric disorder in a population with cancer vary widely, due to differences in the sub-groups studied and use of different criteria for defining disorder. However, the National Institute for Health and Care Excellence (NICE) concludes that following diagnosis, around 50% of patients experience clinically significant levels of anxiety and/or depression and that about 25% continue to do so during the next 6 months. Fifty percent of patients experiencing recurrence and 50% of those with advanced disease, suffer from clinically significant anxiety and/or depression. 10% of patients in the year following diagnosis and 10–15% of those with advanced disease have symptoms of anxiety and/or depression severe enough to merit intervention by specialist psychological or psychiatric services [19].

Walker and colleagues reported the first study of the prevalence of depression in patients with cancer based on a large-scale screening service, using standard diagnostic interviews, carried out by trained interviewers. They found the prevalence of depression was more than double the estimated point prevalence in the general population. Of those patients diagnosed with major depression, 73% were not receiving any potentially effective treatment. Patients who had been living with cancer for over 12 months were just as likely to be depressed as those within the first year of diagnosis. Patients treated with curative intent were also as likely to be depressed as those receiving only palliative treatment. Major depression was more common in younger patients, female patients and those with greater social deprivation [20]. (Although this study did not include patients with thyroid cancer, this finding is of interest as thyroid cancer is more prevalent among women and affects a younger population than many cancers.)

Anxiety and depression are the most common emotional problems in patients with cancer [21]. Other common diagnosable psychiatric disorders in this population include adjustment disorder, delirium, dementia, substance abuse and post-traumatic stress disorder [22]. However, limiting the study of psychological distress in patients with cancer to those with diagnosable psychiatric disorders, overlooks other important psychological dimensions related to poor coping and impaired quality of life, e.g.: giving up; hopelessness; anxious preoccupation; emotional repression [23]; health anxiety; demoralization; and alexithymia (lack of psychological understanding of one's own emotions and moods, which can be linked to psychosomatic symptoms) [24]. A survey carried out by Macmillan in 2006 found that 75% of patients reported having experienced problems with anxiety at some time during their cancer journey. However, within a population of patients with cancer, anxiety may not meet diagnostic criteria for a specific anxiety disorder. Instead it may present as generalised worry or fear in relation to treatment, side effects, changes to abilities and roles, effect on family and others, financial consequences or the future [25]. Fear of recurrence (FOR) is one of the most commonly reported problems and one of the most commonly cited areas of unmet need in both cancer survivors and their carers. FOR tends to remain stable over the cancer pathway and is strongly associated with younger age [26]. The end of treatment is often a psychologically vulnerable time as patients have less contact with healthcare professionals who have played an important role while they are going through a major life event. Patients may feel a sense of loss or abandonment at this stage [27].

Failure to recognise, identify and treat psychological morbidity has significant detrimental consequences for patients, their families and healthcare systems. Co-morbid depression and physical illness is associated with impaired quality of life. Patients with depression in addition to cancer suffer greater anxiety, pain, fatigue and suicidal ideation and also poorer functioning than those without depression [20]. They are also three times more likely not to adhere to their cancer treatment and they have increased risk of mortality from cancer. The incidence of suicide in patients with cancer is two times higher than for the general population [28, 29]. It is known that co-morbid mental illness and a long term physical illness increases the total cost of healthcare by at least 45% [30].

Psychological Distress in Thyroid Cancer

Research specifically relating to psychological wellbeing in patients with thyroid cancer has increased over the last decade. As with other types of cancer, depression and anxiety are the most common emotional problems in patients with thyroid cancer [31]. An Italian study used a standardized diagnostic instrument to identify the prevalence of anxiety and mood disorders in thyroid diseases, including thyroid cancer. Thyroid patients were shown to have higher rates of several psychiatric disorders (panic disorder; simple phobia; obsessive-compulsive disorder; major depressive disorder; bipolar disorder; and cyclothymia) than the general population. These authors suggest that underlying biochemical abnormalities may explain the co-occurrence of psychiatric disorder and thyroid diseases [32]. A number of studies have shown an association between thyroid cancer and poor sleep [33–35].

A Dutch study of 205 survivors of DTC, using well recognised screening instruments, identified 34.3% of the patients as suffering from clinically relevant distress. Levels of distress were not significantly correlated with either clinical or demographic variables, with the exception of employment status. Participants in full or part time employment showed significantly less distress [18]. Employment status was investigated in an Israeli historical prospective study, comparing 48 thyroid cancer survivors to matched healthy controls. Positive significant associations between thyroid cancer and unemployment at 2 years post diagnosis, and between thyroid cancer and decreased income at both 2 and 4 years post diagnosis, were found. The association between thyroid cancer and unemployment was no longer significant at 4 years and the authors concluded that this may be explained by a return to part time rather than full time work [36]. A study carried out in the USA, involving 64 survivors of thyroid cancer, included the Fear of Cancer Recurrence scale as an on-line self-report measure. Thyroid cancer survivors were shown to experience FOR which was related to a decrease in emotional, physical and overall well-being but not to knowledge of the disease [37]. A Canadian study conducted a cross-sectional, self-administered, written survey of members of the Thyroid Cancer Canada patient support group, using the Assessment of Survivor Concerns questionnaire used in a previously published study of a mixed cancer population. Thyroid cancer patients and survivors were found to suffer significant cancer related worry. The focus of worry was most frequently the individual's own health or their children's health rather than fear of death [38]. Anxious preoccupation and helplessness-hopelessness have both been identified as psychological factors related to distress in patients with thyroid cancer [39, 40].

A small qualitative study carried out in Canada investigated the psychosocial impact of further neck surgery for patients with DTC experiencing loco-regional recurrence of disease. The authors found that recurrence was associated with significant psychological distress. Confidence in health-care professionals and social support aided coping with recurrence. However, concerns about further recurrence remained at follow-up [41].

A large multinational cross-sectional survey of patients with thyroid cancer, identified that receiving a cancer diagnosis and anxiety/uncertainty about the future, were the two most difficult aspects of the disease, rated by 24.4% and 21.9% of respondents respectively. 15.5% of respondents cited lack of informational or psychological support as the most difficult aspect. The most commonly cited patient suggestion for improving care was more information on disease/treatment, cited by 45% of respondents; access to support from a psychologist was the second most common suggestion, cited by 43.1%. The authors called for an increase in availability of psychological and other trained professional support for those in need [15].

Another recent survey of unmet needs, in over 2000 Thyroid Cancer patients and survivors, found that the majority of them reported wanting information and support about medical and physical matters, practical issues and emotional/psychological concerns at the time of diagnosis. However <50% recalled having had these needs met [42].

There is clear and growing evidence of significant levels of psychological distress and concerns in patients and survivors of thyroid cancer. However, there is also some evidence of positive psychological consequences in this population. Post-traumatic growth may be defined as the success with which individuals coping with the aftermath of trauma reconstruct or strengthen their perceptions of self, others and the meaning of events; benefit finding is described as the acquisition of benefit from adversity [43]. Despite ongoing FOR after local-regional recurrence of thyroid cancer, qualitative interviews identified a theme of positive outlook and lifestyle changes, e.g.: heightened appreciation of life; enhancement of family relationships; increased self-confidence/motivation to make healthy life-style changes [41].

Effectiveness of Psychological Interventions in Cancer

A Cochrane review of psychosocial interventions to improve quality of life and emotional wellbeing for recently diagnosed cancer patients concluded that nurse-delivered interventions combining information and supportive attention may have a beneficial effect on mood [44]. There is now a substantial evidence base demonstrating the effectiveness of a range of interventions to address psychological distress, including anxiety and depression, for cancer patients and survivors. Interventions shown to be effective include: cognitive-behavioural therapy; acceptance and commitment therapy; problem-solving therapy; short-term psychodynamic therapy; supportive-expressive therapy; mindfulness-based therapy; psycho-education; and relaxation training [29].

In a climate of financial restraint and limited resources, it is important to be able to demonstrate cost-effectiveness in addition to clinical effectiveness. A systematic review of eight studies, suggested that offering information, emotional support and psychological care to cancer patients and survivors can be cost-effective and also efficiently integrated into health care, alongside medical treatment. The authors concluded that several psychosocial interventions, and in particular cognitive-behavioural interventions, have been identified as cost-effective in this population [45]. Another recent review of current evidence from studies of cost-effectiveness and cost-utility of psychosocial interventions in cancer care, concluded that psychosocial care is likely to be considered as cost-effective according to various criteria [46]. An earlier systematic review found psychosocial interventions to be inexpensive on a per patient basis [47].

A Psychological Model of Adjustment to Cancer

When someone first receives the news that they have any type of cancer, the greatest concern is usually survival and the main preoccupation is "am I going to die?" The individual then goes through a period of appraisal to make sense of what Moorey and Greer refer to as "the threat to survival". At some point after this initial threat has been processed, the wider implications of cancer and its treatment are considered and may become significant sources of distress. Moorey and Greer refer to this second threat as the "threat to self" in which they include: debilitating physical symptoms; inability to carry out former work, leisure or family roles; and disfigurement. The idiosyncratic appraisal of the twin threats to survival and self, result in the "personal meaning of cancer" which becomes an important determinant of the individual's adjustment to their disease [48].

Brennan provides a useful psychological model of the process of appraisal and adjustment to cancer (Fig. 27.1). Human brains have evolved to make sense of the physical and social world, by developing "mental maps". This process begins at birth and is largely pre-conscious. It enables humans to learn from past experiences, to make sense of present experiences and to have expectations of the future. Human beings each have a unique and idiosyn-

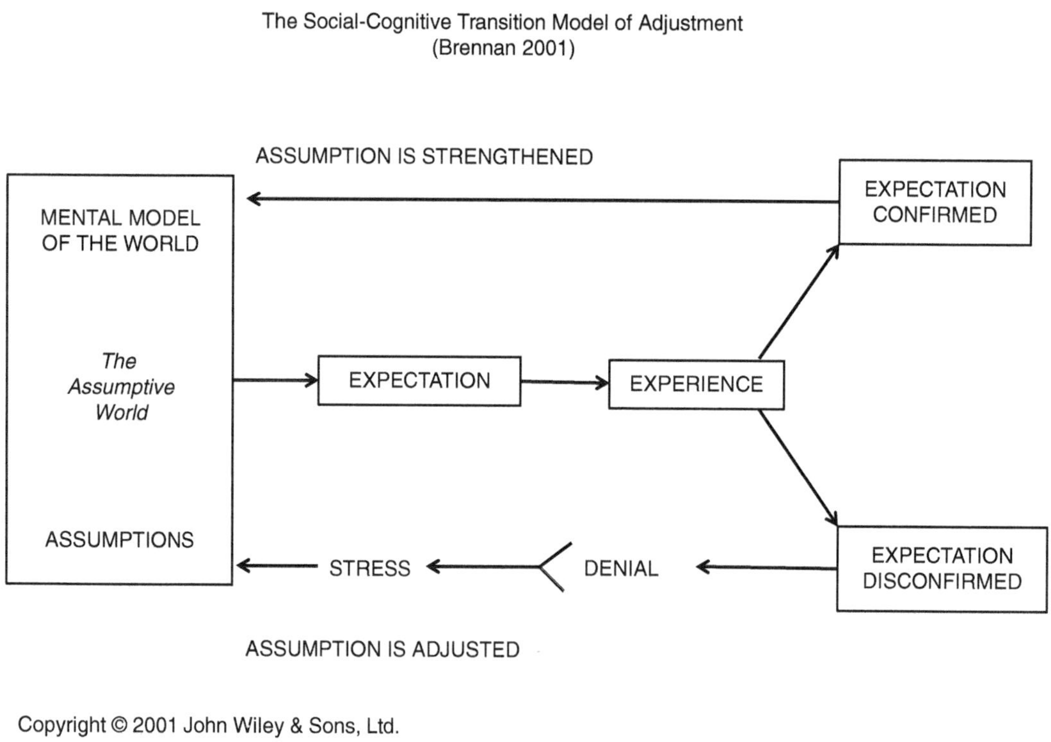

Fig. 27.1 The social-cognitive transition model of adjustment from Brennan J. Adjustment to cancer-coping or personal transition? In Psycho-oncology 2001;10:1–18. p8. By permission of John Wiley & Sons, Ltd

cratic memory of their past life and an image of what their future holds. Idiosyncratic mental maps incorporate beliefs about oneself, other people, the world and the future. As every new experience is interpreted, these mental maps are continually modified in a process known as adjustment or self-regulation. The ability to make sense of the world and to anticipate the future, based on prior learning, gives a sense of safety and control. Many day to day experiences are fairly predictable and can be processed automatically without conscious effort. Experiences that disconfirm expectations lead to some level of stress and require greater modification of the individual's mental maps.

When faced with an unexpected traumatic experience, such as a diagnosis of cancer, a much more fundamental re-organisation of an individual's mental maps is required and may well result in a period of turmoil, uncertainty and distress. Initially many people react with some level of avoidance, ranging from minimising the meaning or emotional impact of diagnosis to denial. Temporary avoidance can be adaptive and understood as a mechanism to slow down the processing of very difficult information. However, the brain also strives to make sense of the new material by assimilating the traumatic experience into the individual's mental maps and ongoing life narrative. Brennan illustrates this as a life story with a break in it where the trauma occurs (Fig. 27.2).

The process of adjustment may take several weeks, months or even years. There may be many periods of adjustment in one cancer journey as a patient is faced with challenges of recurrence, further treatment, or other unwelcome news. "The ultimate task of adjustment is for people to confront and manage the implications of their illness and treatment, to overcome obstacles that are surmountable, and to integrate these events and changes into their mental maps and life narratives, so that they can re-engage productively with the rest of their lives" [49].

The late Paul Kalinithi gives a poignant account of his diagnosis and adjustment to lung cancer, that resonates with the work of both Moorey and Greer, and Brennan. He says of receiving his diagnosis as a 36 year old doctor about to complete specialist training in neurosurgery, "Severe illness wasn't life altering, it was life-shattering .... like someone had just fire-bombed the path forward." In the next stage of his autobiographical account he describes being "determined to restore my life to its prior trajectory." Then sometime later he reveals that "The tricky part of illness is that, as you go through it, your values are constantly changing. You try to figure out what matters to you, and then you keep figuring it out." [50].

Model of Professional Psychological Assessment and Support

NICE recommends a four level model of professional psychological assessment and support. This can be envisaged as a pyramid, with level 1 form-

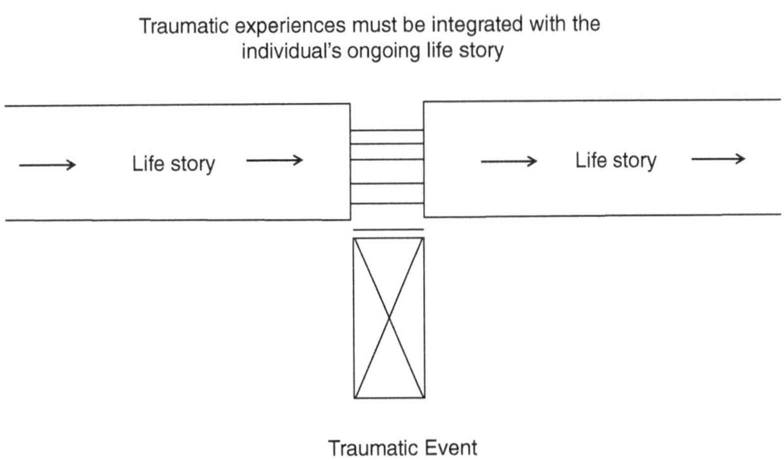

Fig. 27.2 Traumatic experiences must be integrated with the individual's ongoing life story. In Brennan J. Cancer in context: a practical guide to supportive care. 2004. Fig. 1.3 from p. 17. By permission of Oxford University Press

ing the base of the pyramid. Level 1 refers to all clinical staff, all of whom are responsible for "Effective information giving, compassionate communication and general psychological support". Level 2 refers to designated professionals who have received appropriate additional training, to enable them to screen for psychological distress and to utilise simple psychological techniques, within their existing roles. Level 3 refers to trained and accredited practitioners who address mild to moderate psychological distress and cancer-related concerns, through specific psychological interventions, delivered according to an explicit theoretical framework. Level 4, at the apex of the pyramid, refers to mental health specialists (clinical psychologists and liaison psychiatrists) who assess complex psychological problems and deliver specialist interventions for those with moderate to severe levels of distress. A degree of overlap between the levels is likely in practice [19].

The National Peer Review Programme Manual for Cancer Services Head and Neck Measures stipulate that "… at least one clinical core member of the team with direct clinical contact, should have completed the training necessary to enable them to practice at level 2 for the psychological support of cancer patients and carers, and should receive a minimum of 1 hour clinical supervision by a level 3 or level 4 practitioner per month" [51]. As the CNS is ideally placed to provide this level of psychological support it is often expected that they take on this role. In response to a requirement for Cancer Networks to endorse appropriate training for level 2 practitioners, level 3 and 4 practitioners have developed programs to train the identified staff to: recognize psychological distress; assess; and to provide appropriate psychological interventions, such as basic cognitive-behavioural techniques [52].

The Role of the Clinical Nurse Specialist

The management of patient care is to ensure that individuals are provided with appropriate support and representation during their cancer journey, from the point of diagnosis, throughout treatment and into survivorship. Paramount to achieving this objective are the multidisciplinary team and the CNS [8, 53].

The CNS role has become pivotal in many specialities, providing aspects of care such as meeting information needs, holistic nurse led follow up [54, 55], managing care [55, 56] and providing psychological and social interventions, including referral to others, often through the role of keyworker [8, 55].

The experience of care is better from the patient perspective, when access to a CNS is available [57, 58]. In the National Cancer Patient Survey, patients with a CNS reported much more favourably than those without, on a range of items related to information, choice and care [1]. However previous work has shown that patient and family access to a CNS is not consistent [57, 58]. Evidence suggests that there is variation in the proportion of newly diagnosed cancer patients and numbers of specialist nurses across geography and cancer type [56, 59]. Due to the relatively rare occurrence of thyroid cancer, CNS care may be expected to be delivered through other specialities, (e.g. head & neck cancer, breast cancer, endocrinology), where specific care needs differ greatly.

Although practice may vary in different settings, the ultimate goal of the CNS is to ensure that patients receive the highest quality of care, including survivorship care. Key areas addressed in survivorship care are: physical health and activities of daily living; financial difficulties; relationship concerns; emotional problems; and information and communication needs.

Holistic Needs Assessment

An approach that assists with achieving good survivorship care is holistic needs assessment (HNA). HNA "… is a process of gathering and discussing information with the patient and/or carer/supporter in order to develop an understanding of what the person living with and beyond cancer knows, understands and needs. Holistic assessment is focused on the whole person; their entire well-being is discussed—physical, emotional, spiritual, mental, social and environmental" [60]. By identifying these needs, improvements in care can be made in a responsive manner.

Macmillan Cancer Support advises that HNA should be undertaken at diagnosis and re-evaluated at strategic points in every patient's journey. This ensures that concerns are addressed as early as possible, thereby reducing distress [61]. Similarly, the NHS standard contract stipulates that every patient should be offered a HNA at key points in their cancer pathway, leading to the development of a formal care plan. The CNS should ensure that the results of the HNA are taken into account in MDT decision making [1]. Despite being promoted within policy [8, 62, 63], HNAs have not been adopted widely in the UK [64]. This can often be related to time constraints and resources. The need to integrate any new venture into an existing care pathway can cause anxiety for the health care professionals concerned [65].

HNA may be facilitated through use of specifically designed tools e.g. the Distress Thermometer [66, 67] and the Concerns Check List [68]. The Distress Thermometer asks patients to mark their overall level of distress on an illustrated scale from 0- no distress to 10- extreme distress. The National Comprehensive Cancer Network ® (NCCN®) advised that a level of 4 or more is evidence of moderate to severe distress [69]. The Distress Thermometer has been widely used and its psychometric properties have been extensively studied [70].

HNA tools can be viewed as enablers to open up discussion between patients and clinicians [65]. The process of HNA is initiated by the CNS and explained to the patient. Using an HNA tool helps to normalise common concerns. The aim is for the patient to be empowered to talk about their concerns and feelings on their own terms. By acknowledging and discussing problems clinical benefits can be achieved and patient satisfaction increased. Common concerns among patients and survivors of thyroid cancer include:

Social Concerns

The age of patients diagnosed with thyroid cancer varies but will commonly be of working age. Patients may also have dependents in the form of children or ageing parent/s. Many will be concerned regarding their job, finances, social life etc. Discussing these areas can highlight services which may be available to assist e.g. free prescriptions, Macmillan grants and welfare rights services.

Physical/Appearance Concerns

Post-operative changes can be difficult for many patients after thyroid surgery. They include dissatisfaction with scar appearance, neck or shoulder stiffness/restricted movement, increased or ongoing pain and voice changes. Referral back to the original surgeon, ear nose and throat department, speech and language therapy, physiotherapy or pain team, may be necessary.

Other common symptoms after thyroidectomy include: insomnia; fatigue; dyspnoea; bowel changes (constipation/diarrhoea); appetite loss; dry skin; difficulty tolerating cold/heat; hair changes; weight gain/loss; voice changes [71].

It is well known that hypothyroidism causes a broad range of physical as well as psychological symptoms, such as constipation, weight gain, fatigue, depression and slowed cognition, and that the associated distress is high [72, 73].

Emotional Concerns

As discussed previously thyroid cancer is often described as a "good cancer" with a favourable clinical outcome. This can provoke a variety of different responses at the time of diagnosis and throughout the patient cancer journey. Some will gain relief but others will struggle with the term. One author noted that patients felt that their diagnosis of cancer was dismissed as not serious or even a benign cancer [74]. Thyroid patients will often compare their diagnosis to other forms of cancer and may feel a sense of guilt that they have struggled with their diagnosis when they should count themselves "lucky" or "pull themselves together".

With active treatment over, FOR often emerges. Many survivors also find that getting back on with "normal" life is much harder that they or their families imagined it would be. Cancer and its treatment gives rise to many changes, requiring adaptation to a "new normal" [75].

The Role of the Clinical Psychologist

CPs are applied scientists specializing in cognitive, emotional, behavioural and social aspects of human behaviour. They are trained to work with individuals, couples, families and groups and to provide a consultative service to other healthcare professions. Direct clinical work includes detailed psychological assessments, leading to case formulation and when appropriate to the design and provision of evidence-based therapeutic interventions.

Case formulation may be defined as a working hypothesis about the predisposing, precipitating and maintaining factors of an individual's presenting problems. It helps to make sense of and to integrate complex information, drawing on psychological models (and where appropriate, psychiatric diagnoses) and applying these to the unique circumstances of an individual. "As both science and art, a case formulation should embody scientific principles and findings, but also an appreciation of the singularity and humanity of the person in question". It enables anticipation of factors which may interfere with therapy, guides treatment strategies and specific intervention techniques [76]. Case formulations incorporate an individual's strengths and protective factors alongside their difficulties. All or part of a case formulation may be shared with the referrer, multi-disciplinary team and/or the patient, to facilitate understanding, serve as an advocate for the patient and to promote collaborative working.

Indirect roles of the CP include: teaching other healthcare professionals about psychological issues; training non-mental health practitioners in direct clinical skills; providing clinical supervision and support to other healthcare professionals who offer psychological support; providing consultation and advice to clinicians and managers about optimum psychological care; collaboration with multidisciplinary colleagues on research and audit.

The aim of clinical psychology in oncology is to promote psychological wellbeing and to reduce psychological distress associated with diagnosis, treatment and living with disease. These aims are achieved through working directly with patients and carers and indirectly through and with other health care professionals. Promoting the recognition and detection of psychological distress is a high priority. Enabling and supporting other healthcare professionals to provide good psychological care to patients and their families is a key role. Identifying and intervening for people in whom the process of appraisal and adjustment has become stuck or unhelpful is fundamental. Due to the high prevalence of psychological distress and the relative scarcity of clinical psychology resources, individual clinical interventions need to be targeted towards patients and carers with the most complex psychological needs and those most likely to benefit from a specialist psychological intervention.

An Example of Service Delivery

Within the Thyroid MDT based at the Northern Centre for Cancer Care at Newcastle Upon Tyne Hospitals NHS Foundation Trust, the CNS (second author) has initiated a nurse led clinic, to follow up patients initially when they are 2–3 months post radio iodine ablation and thereafter for annual review. An HNA, adapted from the Distress Thermometer, is administered by the CNS at this clinic (Fig. 27.3). Results of the HNA are incorporated into the Nurse led clinic's core letter which (with the patient's consent) is sent to the GP and available to other members of the MDT. Based on the specific concerns indicated by each individual patient, the CNS may offer direct advice, information and support, and/or refer the patient on for further help, e.g.: to another member of the Thyroid MDT; to the GP; for benefits advice; to the CP.

Patients highlighting emotional distress, who may need further input either from the GP (e.g.

NHS
Northern England
Clinical Networks

This screening tool is aimed to encourage professionals and patients to explore current problems and issues that may be affecting patients' physical, psychological, social and spiritual well-being.

The outcome (including patient score) of this assessment is to be documented in the patients ongoing record with an agreed plan of care and referral on for symptom control, rehabilitation, social, spiritual or psychological care where necessary.

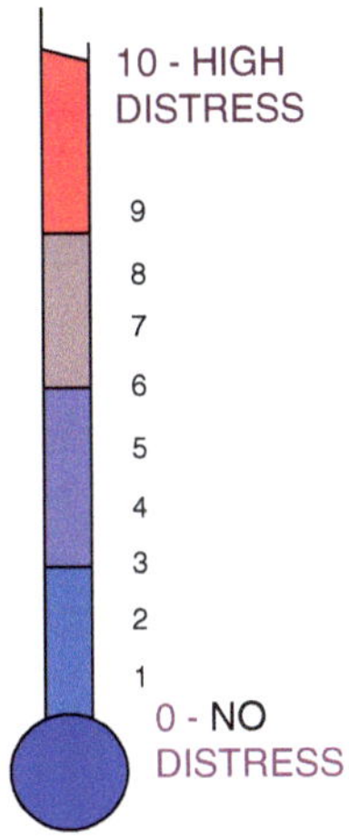

Identify the number (0-10) that best describes how much distress has been experienced over recent weeks, if '0' is no distress and '10' is high levels of distress or anxiety.

Social Concerns
- Coping with dependants
- Work/School
- Hobbies/Leisure activities
- Housing
- Finances
- Travel
- Carer
- Relationships

Emotional Wellbeing
- Sadness
- Fears
- Worries / Anxieties
- Anger
- Alcohol/smoking/other drugs
- Unable to express feelings
- Feeling isolated
- Loss of dignity
- Forgetful/confused
- Stress

Spiritual / Religious Concerns
- Questioning values and beliefs
- Sense of meaning
- Issues relating to dying and death

Rest / Activity
- Sleep
- Fatigue
- Tiredness

My appearance / Body image
- Skin Dry / Itchy / wound healing
- Swollen (limbs/abdomen)
- Weight Changes – loss or gain
- Sexual Problems

Reduced Independence
- Bathing / Dressing
- Getting Around

Toileting Difficulties
- Constipation
- Diarrhoea
- Stoma
- Changes in passing urine

Physical Symptoms
- Difficulties in Communicating
- Breathing
- Pain
- Temperature
- Change in sensation: hands/feet

Eating Difficulties
- Indigestion
- Sores /painful mouth
- Nausea
- Taste changes
- Swallowing difficulties
- Change in appetite

Any other factors

How do you cope at the moment?

What support do you have?

Do you have someone to talk to?

Would you like a copy of this assessment?

Are you happy for us to share this information with the people involved inyour care?

Fig. 27.3 NECN (Northern England Clinical Networks) holistic assessment of concerns. Developed with kind permission of the National Comprehensive Cancer Network (2017) from the NCCN clinical practice guidelines. In Oncology (NCCN Guidelines®) for distress management, version 2.2016

for prescription of anti-depressant medication or referral for psychological support not directly related to thyroid cancer) and/or the CP, will be asked to complete a Hospital Anxiety and Depression scale (HADs) [77]. The HADs was developed as a screening instrument for a non-psychiatric population and performs well in assessing both caseness and symptom severity [78]. In a systematic review of screening instruments used with cancer patients the HADs was identified as a short measure with adequate psychometric properties [70]. In the nurse-led clinic, the HADS can be helpful in demonstrating to a patient why a referral would be indicated, as they may require a higher level of support than can be offered by the CNS alone.

If referral to the CP is indicated, it is suggested and offered to the patient and their consent is sought. Patients who initially decline the referral or need time to consider this option, are made aware that they can request a referral from the CNS at any time. Once in receipt of a referral, the CP aims to offer an appointment within 1–4 weeks, depending on the severity of the difficulties. The patient is offered an initial assessment appointment lasting 90 minutes. Depending on the outcome of assessment, the patient may be offered a series of psychology appointments and an intervention based on the shared case formulation and collaborative discussion of priorities. Consent is sought to share the assessment, formulation and planned intervention in a clinic letter to the CNS which is also copied to the GP and available to other members of the MDT. The patient is also offered a copy of all letters.

Key roles for both the CNS and the CP are to empathise with the difficulties that patients and carers are facing, to help them to make sense of their experiences, and to offer realistic hope.

The authors refer to Brennan's work on psychological adjustment, in order to explain the major cognitive adjustments to mental maps, that take need to take place internally [49]. They refer to Moorey and Greer's work in order to empathise with the many very visible aspects of people's lives that require adjustment e.g. changes to appearance, abilities, work, leisure, and social roles [48]. The authors illustrate the tasks of survivorship with a diagram that acknowledges the enormity of the impact of diagnosis and treatment and that returning to "normal life" exactly as it was before cancer, is often not realistic. The challenge of survivorship is to re-build a "new normal" life. The new normal may well need to incorporate inevitable unwelcome changes, associated with disease and treatment as well as modified assumptions about self, world and future. However there may also be positive re-assessment of personal priorities, benefit finding and post-traumatic growth. This pictorial representation is used to offer some realistic hope, in addition to acknowledging and empathising with the negative impact of diagnosis and treatment (Fig. 27.4).

Level 2 training is provided by the clinical psychology team and clinical supervision is provided by the named CP for the Thyroid MDT (first author) on a monthly basis. This facilitates maintenance and development of the CNS's psychological skills as well as time to discuss new referrals and ongoing reviews.

In addition to direct clinical work, training and supervision, the CNS and CP have run a 6 week Moving on Group for patients with thyroid cancer recently finishing treatment. Cancer survivor groups have been found to be an effective way of facilitating the transition from cancer patient to cancer survivor. They provide continuing contact with familiar healthcare professionals, facilitate psychological processing and enable people to meet others who share similar experiences. However the value of these groups is not always understood by physicians [79]. The Moving on Group run by the authors was fully supported by the rest of the MDT and based on a model developed at a hospice in the region (Cancer Survival and the Moving on Group-returning to psychological & emotional health: The workbook—unpublished). The aim of the Moving on Group was to provide an opportunity to reflect on and reassess personal experiences of diagnosis and treatment and to facilitate a transition to focussing on health and a "new normal" rather than illness. Patients identified by the CNS as having difficulties with adjustment were invited to participate. An in service evaluation was carried out by a psychology assistant, based on verbal feedback collected at each meeting, a written evaluation form at the sixth session and further feedback at a 6 month follow-up meeting. Evaluation identified clear perceived benefits in relation to: emotional processing of a difficult life event; peer support; reduced feelings of isolation; and psychological adjustment to surviving cancer.

The CNS has initiated Survivorship Study Days, also for patients recently completing initial treatment. These comprise a series of informal presentations, based on common themes raised in holistic assessment (e.g.: understanding blood results; symptoms of hypo/hyper thyroid; calcium control; dry mouth; diet & exercise; sleep & relaxation; patient support groups; psychological impact—both professional and service user perspective). These are delivered by healthcare professionals within or allied to the Thyroid MDT, charity representatives and a service user representative. The study days enable patients to dis-

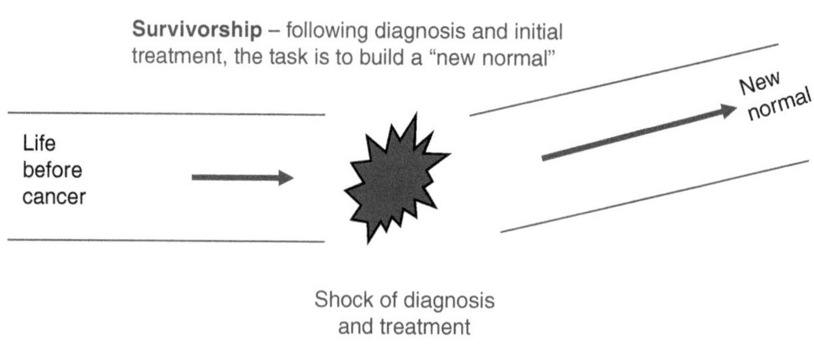

Fig. 27.4 Survivorship-following diagnosis and initial treatment, the task is to re-build a "new normal"

cuss concerns and questions with health care professionals and to meet fellow patients, in a supportive environment. Feedback gathered identified that every person attending these events would recommend them to other patients.

Case Example

The example below is a composite case based on the clinical experience of the authors. It does not represent any individual patient known to the authors.

Keira was a 35 year old woman who was diagnosed with papillary thyroid cancer, 9 months after first presenting to her GP with fatigue and general malaise. She was living with her partner and their three young children. She was employed full time as head of English at a local comprehensive school but had been on sick leave since her diagnosis. Keira underwent total thyroidectomy and radio-iodine ablation and was followed up in the nurse-led clinic 3 months later. During holistic assessment with the CNS, Keira was found to be very anxious about physical symptoms, low in mood and distressed about her thyroidectomy scar and the weight she had gained since her diagnosis. She complained of difficulty sleeping and continuing fatigue. The CNS invited her to complete a HADs which placed her within the severely anxious and moderately depressed range. The CNS also repeated thyroid function tests and other biochemical markers which established that the main cause of Keira's symptoms was unlikely to be physical. Following discussion with the CNS, Keira consented to a referral to the dietician for advice about diet and exercise, to a specialist nursing colleague in plastic surgery regarding camouflage make-up for her scar and to the CP for help with anxiety and low mood. The CNS explained the principles of promoting good sleep and gave Keira some educational material prepared by the Psychology Department.

Psychological assessment revealed that when Keira was 10 years old, her father left the family and did not maintain contact. When Keira was 18 her maternal aunt died aged 35 of breast cancer. Just before Keira's own diagnosis, a colleague, who had previously been treated for a brain tumour, was diagnosed with recurrence and died shortly afterwards, leaving a young son.

Keira also confided that she felt very ambivalent about going back to work. Although her career had always been very important to her and she had been very proud to be made head of department 3 years earlier, she acknowledged that prior to going on sick leave she had been finding managing the increased responsibility at work, alongside family life, very stressful. Due to the delay in diagnosis, Keira found it difficult to fully trust health care professionals and did not feel reassured when she was told that her prognosis was good. Her own belief, based on her vicarious experience of cancer, was that her cancer would recur and that she would die and leave her children motherless. This was an especially poignant fear for Keira in the context of having been "abandoned" as a child by her father. Keira's FOR made her highly sensitive to any physical sensations and she worried that any change or pain was a sign of secondary cancer or a new cancer e.g. if she had a headache she was sure it was a brain tumour and if she had back ache she thought her cancer had spread to her spine. Keira's scar, which she perceived as very ugly, was a daily reminder of her diagnosis. She had an image of herself dying at 35 like her aunt had, i.e. imminently. Keira felt unable to engage fully in activities with her family due to worrying constantly about the possibility of dying and leaving them. As a consequence, she perceived herself as letting her children down and felt guilty and depressed. Often she would wake in the early hours of the morning and dwell on her fears and sense of loss. The "personal meaning of cancer" for Keira was "I am going to die young and leave my children. Therefore I am no longer the good mother I want to be."

In terms of protective factors, Keira's partner was very supportive and she had many friends. She was also able to confide in her mother, who in addition was available for practical support. Keira was motivated to find ways to address her difficulties.

Following assessment, Keira agreed to a course of Cognitive Behavioural Therapy to address her health related anxiety and her FOR. She engaged actively in this treatment and after eight sessions was able to consider alternative non-threatening explanations for bodily symptoms and to think in more rational and helpful ways about her health. She was able to see how her diagnosis differed to those of her aunt and her colleague and to consider that her cancer pathway could take a more positive course, with her living to raise her children. She reported a reduction in her symptoms of anxiety and depression, confirmed by reassessment with the HADs, which by then placed her in the mild range for both anxiety and depression. However, she was still not engaging fully in or enjoying family life.

Therefore Keira was offered and consented to a second phase of psychological therapy, based on Acceptance and Commitment Therapy, to enable her to identify core values that were of importance to her. Being an available and loving mother and also being an excellent teacher were both central to meaning in her life. Once these core values were made explicit, Keira chose to prioritise the first one and was able to make a commitment to spend more quality time with her children, despite not feeling fully well herself. During psychology appointments she planned specific activities with each of them, and for the family as a whole. Implementing these plans at home was challenging initially but gradually her self-esteem as a mother increased and she began to experience pleasure in that role once again. She then began to consider whether returning to work full time was what she really wanted anymore. After some time exploring her thoughts, feelings and potential options, see decided to return to work part-time for 6 months and then to re-consider her position. The CP supported her in planning a phased return to work.

At a psychology review appointment 6 months later, Keira was able to acknowledge that the traumatic experience of diagnosis and treatment had resulted in an unexpected benefit of pushing her to review her life priorities. By then she had made the decision to relinquish her head of department position and to confirm a part-time contract, enabling her to continue to have more time for her children and family life. Work continued to be important to her but she felt that her work-life balance was much more manageable. She and her partner had also made a decision to get married. Due to Keira's reduced income, they had to change their plan to move to a bigger home, but they both felt confident that this decision was right for Keira and the family. Although Keira would never have chosen to undergo a diagnosis and treatment for thyroid cancer, her perception was that she would not have had the courage to change her career path for family life or to make the commitment to marriage without that traumatic experience.

References

1. 2013/14 NHS standard contract for cancer: head and neck (adult). NHS Commissioning Board; 2013.
2. Improving outcomes guidance in head and neck cancer. NICE; 2004.
3. Thyroid cancer statistics. Cancer Research UK; 2017.
4. Mazzaferri EL, Massoll N. Management of papillary and follicular (differentiated) thyroid cancer: new paradigms using recombinant human thyrotropin. Endocr Relat Cancer. 2002;9(4):227–47.
5. Centres of Disease Control and prevention. Cancer survivorship; 2008.
6. Decker C, Haase J, Bell C. Uncertainty in adolescents and young adults with cancer. Oncol Nurs Forum. 2007;34(3):681–8.
7. Hewitt M, Ganz PA. From cancer patient to cancer survivor: lost in transition, an American Society of Clinical Oncology and Institute of Medicine Symposium. Washington, DC: National Academies Press; 2006.
8. Cancer Reform Strategy. Department of Health; 2007.
9. Lee JI, Kim SH, Tan AH, et al. Decreased health-related quality of life in disease-free survivors of differentiated thyroid cancer in Korea. Health Qual Life Outcome. 2010;8:101.
10. Sawka AM, Goldstein DP, Brierley JD. The impact of thyroid cancer and post surgical radioactive iodine treatment on the lives of thyroid cancer survivors: a qualitative study. PLoS One. 2009;4(1):e4191.
11. Gamper EM, Wintner LM, Rodrigues M, Buxbaum S, Nilica B, Singer S, et al. Persistent quality of life impairments in differentiated thyroid cancer patients: results from a monitoring programme. Eur J Nucl Med Mol Imaging. 2015;42:1179–88. https://doi.org/10.1007/s00259-015-3022-9.
12. Singer S, Lincke T, Gamper E, Bhaskaran K, Schreiber S, Hinz A, et al. Quality of life in patients with thyroid cancer compared with the general population. Thyroid. 2012;22:117–24. https://doi.org/10.1089/thy.2011.0139.

13. Applewhite MK, James BC, Kaplan SP, Angelos P, Kaplan EL, Grogan RH, et al. Quality of life in thyroid cancer is similar to that of other cancers with worse survival. World J Surg. 2016;40:551–61. https://doi.org/10.1007/s00268-015-3300-5.
14. James BC, Aschebrook-Kilfoy B, Kaplan S, Kaplan EL, Angelos P, Grogan R. Quality of life in thyroid cancer: physician perceptions. 2016. http://meetinglibrary.asco.org/content/156947-174. Accessed 11 Jan 2017.
15. Banach R, Bartes B, Farnell K, Rimmele H, Shey J, Singer S, et al. Results of the thyroid cancer alliance international patient/survivor survey: psychosocial/informational support needs, treatment side effects and international differences in care. Hormones. 2013;12:428–38.
16. Hoftijzer HC, Heemstra KA, Corssmit EPM, van der Klaauw AA, Romijn JA, Smit JWA. Quality of life in cured patients with differentiated thyroid carcinoma. J Clin Endocrinol Metab. 2008;93:200–3.
17. Ridgway E, Grose J, Charles A, Hewett J, Jarvis M, Benjamin S. Does labelling a rare cancer diagnosis 'good' affect the patient's experience of treatment and recovery? Eur J Cancer Care. 2016;25:348–55. https://doi.org/10.1111/ecc.12258.
18. Roerink SHPP, de Ridder M, Prins J, Huijbers A, de Wilt HJH, Marres H, et al. High levels of distress in long-term survivors of thyroid carcinoma: results of rapid screening using the distress thermometer. Acta Oncol. 2013;52:128–37. https://doi.org/10.3109/0284186X.2012.723822.
19. Improving supportive and palliative care for adults with cancer. The manual. National Institute for Clinical Excellence; March 2004.
20. Walker J, Holm Hansen C, Martin P, Symeonides S, Ramessur R, Murray G, et al. Prevalence, association, and adequacy of treatment of major depression in patients with cancer: a cross-sectional analysis of routinely collected clinical data. Lancet. 2014;1:343–50.
21. Sellick SM, Crooks DL. Depression and cancer: an appraisal of the literature for prevalence, detection, and practice guideline development for psychological interventions. Psycho-Oncology. 1999;8:315–33.
22. Hegel MT, Moore CP, Collins ED, Kearing S, Gillock KL, Riggs RL, et al. Distress, psychiatric syndromes, and impairment of function in women with newly diagnosed breast cancer. Cancer. 2006;107(12):2924–31.
23. Grassi L, Rosti G, Lasalvia A, Marangola M. Psychosocial variables associated with mental adjustment to cancer. Psycho-Oncology. 1993;2:11–20.
24. Grassi L, Sabato S, Rossi E, Biancosino B, Marmai L. Use of the diagnostic criteria for psychosomatic research in oncology. Psychother Psychosom. 2005;74:100–7. https://doi.org/10.1159/000083168.
25. Hubert-Williams NJ. Supporting cancer patients with anxiety. Nurs Pract. 2016;88. Accessed 24 Mar 2017.
26. Simard S, Thewes B, Humphris G, Dixon M, Hayden C, Mireskandari S, et al. Fear of cancer recurrence in adult cancer survivors: a systematic review of quantitative studies. J Cancer Surviv. 2013;7(3):300–22.
27. Stanton AL, Ganz PA, Rowland JH, Meyerowitz BE, Krupnick JL, Sears SR. Promoting adjustment after treatment for cancer. Cancer. 2005;104(11 Suppl):2608–13. https://doi.org/10.1002/cncr.21246.
28. Misono S, Weiss NS, Fann JR, Redman M, Yueh B. Incidence of suicide in persons with cancer. J Clin Oncol. 2008;26:4731–8. https://doi.org/10.1200/JCO.2007.13.8941.
29. London Strategic Clinical Networks. Psychological support for people living with cancer. Commissioning guidance for cancer care in London. June 2015. www.londonscn.nhs.uk. Accessed July 2015.
30. Naylor C, Parsonage M, McDaid D, Knapp M, Fossey M, Galea A. Long-term conditions and mental health. The cost of co-morbidities. London: The King's Fund and Centre for Mental Health; 2012.
31. Tagay S, Herpertz S, Langkafel M, Erim Y, Bockisch A, Senf W, et al. Health-related quality of life, depression and anxiety in thyroid cancer patients. Qual Life Res. 2006;15:695–703. https://doi.org/10.1007/s11136-005-3689-7.
32. Placidi GPA, Boldrini M, Patronelli A, Fiore E, Chiovato L, Prugi G, et al. Prevalence of psychiatric disorders in thyroid diseased patients. Neuropsychobiology. 1998;38:222–5.
33. Ng R. The effect of thyroid cancer on sleep pattern and obstructive sleep apnea. Sleep. 2012;35:A300. 0161-8105 (2012).
34. Yi Y, Zhu Y, Yan Y, Hu F. Analysis of the cause of high doses of 131 iodine treatment induced sleep disorders in patients with differentiated thyroid cancer and nursing experience. Anti-Tumor Pharm. 2014;4(1):71–5. 2095-1264 (February 2014).
35. He Y, Meng Z, Jia Q, Hu F, He X, Tan J, et al. Sleep quality of patients with differentiated thyroid cancer. PLoS One. 2015;10(6):e0130634. 1932-6203 (2015).
36. Uziely B, Ratzon N, Rottenberg Y. Unemployment risk and decreased income 2 and 4 years after thyroid cancer diagnosis: a population based study. J Clin Oncol. 2015;33(15_Suppl):e20618.
37. Rasmussen K, Kilbourn K, Abdel-Maksoud M, Klopper J. Thyroid cancer survivorship: quality of life, mood and fear of recurrence. Endocrine Reviews. 2012. http://press.endocrine.org/doi/abs/10.1210/endo-meetings.2012.THPTA.12.MON-435. Accessed 11 Jan 2017.
38. Bresner L, Banach R, Rodin G, Thabane L, Sawka A. Cancer related worry in the Canadian thyroid cancer survivors. Thyroid. 2012;22:A71–2. 1050-7256 (September 2012).
39. Seok JH, Chang HS, Choi WJ, Oh YJ, Oh JH, Lee YS, et al. Mental adjustment and emotional symptoms of the thyroid cancer patients with psychological distress. Psycho-Oncology. 2011;20:252–3.
40. Seok JH, Choi WJ, Lee YS, Park CS, Oh YJ, Kim JS, et al. Relationship between negative mental adjustment to cancer and distress in thyroid cancer patients. Yonsei Med J. 2013;54(3):658–64.
41. Misra S, Meiyappan S, Heus L, Freeman J, Rotstein L, Brierley JD, et al. Patients' experiences following

local-regional recurrence of thyroid cancer: a qualitative study. J Surg Oncol. 2013;108:47–51. https://doi.org/10.1002/jso.23345.
42. Morley S, Goldfarb M. Support needs and survivorship concerns of thyroid cancer patients. Thyroid. 2015;25:649–56. https://doi.org/10.1089/thy.2015.0032.
43. Harding S, Sanipour F, Moss T. Existence of benefit finding and posttraumatic growth in people treated for head and neck cancer: a systematic review. PeerJ. 2014;2:e256. https://doi.org/10.7717/peerj.256.
44. Galway K, Black A, Cantwell M, Cardwell C, Mills M, Donnelly M. Psychosocial interventions to improve quality of life and emotional wellbeing for recently diagnosed cancer patients. Cochrane Database Syst Rev. 2012;11:CD007064.
45. Dieng M, Cust AE, Kasparian NA, Mann GJ, Morton RL. Economic evaluation of psychosocial interventions in cancer: a systematic review. Psycho-Oncology. 2016;25:1380–92. https://doi.org/10.1002/pon.4075.
46. Jansen F, van Zwieten V, VMH C, Leemans CR, Verdonck-de Leeuw IM. A review on cost-effectiveness and cost-utility of psychosocial care in cancer patients. Asia Pac J Oncol Nurs. 2016;3:125–36. https://doi.org/10.4103/2347-5625.182930.
47. Gordon LG, Beesley VL, Scuffham PA. Evidence on the economic value of psychosocial interventions to alleviate anxiety and depression among cancer survivors: a systematic review. Asia Pac J Clin Oncol. 2011;7:96–105. https://doi.org/10.1111/j.1743-7563.2011.01395.x.
48. Moorey S, Greer S. Cognitive behaviour therapy for people with cancer. Oxford: Oxford University Press; 2002.
49. Brennan J. Cancer in context: a practical guide to supportive care. Oxford: Oxford University Press; 2004.
50. Kalanithi P. When breath becomes air. London: Penguin Random House UK: Vintage; 2017.
51. The national peer review programme manual for cancer services; head and neck measures, version 1.3. National Cancer Action Team; January 2014.
52. Jenkins K, Alberry B, Daniel J, et al. Beyond communication: the development of a training program for hospital and hospice staff in the detection and management of psychological distress – preliminary results. Palliat Support Care. 2010;8:27–33.
53. Tarrant C, Sinfield P, Agarwal S, Baker R. Is seeing a specialist nurse associated with positive experiences of care? The role and value of specialist nurses in prostate cancer care. BMC Health Serv Res. 2008;8:65. https://doi.org/10.1186/1472-6963-8-65.
54. Moore S, Corner J, Haviland J, Wells M, Salmon E, Normand C, et al. Nurse led follow up and conventional medical follow up in management of patients with lung cancer: randomised trial. BMJ. 2002;325:1145.
55. National Cancer Action Team. Excellence in cancer care: the contribution of the clinical nurse specialist. London: NCAT; 2010.
56. Leary A. Lung cancer in England. In: Leary A, editor. Lung cancer: a multidisciplinary approach. Oxford: Wiley-Blackwell; 2011.
57. Department of Health. National Cancer Patient Experience Survey Programme – 2010. National survey report. London: DH, HMSO; 2011.
58. Department of Health. National Cancer Patient Experience Survey Programme – 2012. National Survey Report. London: Department of Health; 2012.
59. National Cancer Action Team. Quality in nursing: clinical nurse specialists in cancer care: provision, proportion and performance. A census of the cancer specialist nurse workforce in England 2011. London: NCAT, Department of Health; 2012.
60. National Cancer Survivorship Initiative. Assessment and care planning definitions; 2013.
61. Macmillan Cancer Support. Holistic needs assessment and care planning – introduction; 2012.
62. The Scottish Government. Better cancer care- an action plan; 2008.
63. All Parliamentary Group on Cancer. Report of all party parliamentary group on cancer's inquiry into inequalities in cancer; 2009.
64. National Cancer Action Team. Holistic needs assessment for people with cancer: a practical guide for healthcare professionals; 2011.
65. Samarasinghe BSW, Wiles L. Meeting patients' needs with risk-stratified colorectal cancer follow up. Gastrointest Nurs. 2012;10:37–43.
66. Roth AJ, Kornblith AB, Batel-Copel L, Peabody E, Scher HI, Holland HC. Rapid screening for psychologic distress in men with prostate carcinoma: a pilot study. Cancer. 1998;82:1904–8.
67. Donovan KA, Grassi I, McGinty IL, Jacobsen PB. Validation of the distress thermometer worldwide: state of the science. Psycho-Oncology. 2014;23:241–50.
68. National Cancer Survivorship Initiative. Living with and beyond cancer – identifying your concerns; 2012.
69. Referenced with permission from the NCCN Clinical Practice Guidelines in Oncology (NCCN Guidelines®) for Distress Management v.1.2017. © National Comprehensive Cancer Network, Inc. 2017. All rights reserved. Accessed June 19 2017. To view the most recent and complete version of the guideline, go online to NCCN.org.
70. Vodermaier A, Linden W, Siu C. Screening for emotional distress in cancer patients: a systemic review of assessment instruments. J Natl Cancer Inst. 2009;101:1464–88. https://doi.org/10.1093/jnci/djp336.
71. Roberts KJ, Lepore SJ, Urken ML. Quality of life after thyroid cancer: an assessment of patients needs and preferences for information and support. J Cancer Educ. 2008;23:186–91.
72. Dagan T, Bedrin L, Horowitz Z, et al. Quality of life of well-differentiated thyroid carcinoma patients. J Laryngol Otol. 2004;118:537–42.
73. Rubic M, Kuna SK, Tesic V, et al. The most common factors influencing on quality of life of thyroid cancer

patients after thyroid hormone withdrawal. Psychiatr Danub. 2014;26(suppl 3):520–7.
74. Husson O, Haak HR, Oranjes WA, Mols F, Reemst PHM, van de Poll-Franse LV. Health-related quality of life among thyroid cancer survivors: a systematic review. Clin Endocrinol. 2011;75:544–54. https://doi.org/10.1111/j.1365-2265.2011.04114.x.
75. Harpham WS. After cancer: a guide to your new life. New York: W. W. Norton and Company; 1994.
76. Eells TD. Psychotherapy case formulation: history and current status. In: Eells TD, editor. Handbook of psychotherapy case formulation. New York: The Guilford Press; 1997. p. 20.
77. Zigmond AS, Snaith RP. The hospital anxiety and depression scale. Acta Psychiatr Scand. 1983;67:361–70.
78. Bjelland I, Dahl AA, Haug TT, Neckelmann D. The validity of the hospital anxiety and depression scale. An updated literature review. J Psychosom Res. 2002;52:69–77.
79. Owen JE, Goldstein MS, Lee JH, Breen N, Rowland JH. Use of health-related and cancer-specific support groups among adult cancer survivors. Cancer. 2007;109:2580–9. https://doi.org/10.1002/cncr.22719.

Index

U. K. Mallick et al. (eds.), *Practical Management of Thyroid Cancer*,
https://doi.org/10.1007/978-3-319-91725-2

D

Q

R

FSC
www.fsc.org
MIX
Papier | Fördert
gute Waldnutzung
FSC® C083411

Kolibri 360 GmbH
Ferdinand-Jühlke-Straße 7
99095 Erfurt, Deutschland
produktsicherheit@kolibri360.de